The Treatment of Anxiety Disorders
Clinician Guides and Patient Manuals

Second Edition

Gavin Andrews
Clinical Research Unit for Anxiety and Depression,
University of New South Wales at St. Vincent's Hospital, Sydney

Mark Creamer
Australian Centre for Posttraumatic Mental Health (ACPMH), Melbourne

Rocco Crino
Anxiety Disorders Clinic, St. Vincent's Hospital, Sydney

Caroline Hunt
School of Psychology, University of Sydney, Sydney

Lisa Lampe
Clinical Research Unit for Anxiety and Depression,
University of New South Wales at St. Vincent's Hospital, Sydney

Andrew Page
School of Psychology, University of Western Australia, Perth

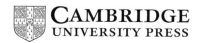
CAMBRIDGE
UNIVERSITY PRESS

PUBLISHED BY THE PRESS SYNDICATE OF THE UNIVERSITY OF CAMBRIDGE
The Pitt Building, Trumpington Street, Cambridge, United Kingdom

CAMBRIDGE UNIVERSITY PRESS
The Edinburgh Building, Cambridge CB2 2RU, UK
40 West 20th Street, New York NY, 10011–4211, USA
477 Williamstown Road, Port Melbourne, VIC 3207, Australia
Ruiz de Alarcón 13, 28014 Madrid, Spain
Dock House, The Waterfront, Cape Town 8001, South Africa

http://www.cambridge.org

First published 1994 (0 521 46521 4)
Reprinted 1995, 1996, 1997, 1998, 1999
Second edition 2003 (0 521 78877 3)
Reprinted 2003, 2004

Printed in the United Kingdom at the University Press, Cambridge

Typeface Minion 10.5/14pt   *System* Poltype® [v N]

A catalogue record for this book is available from the British Library

Library of Congress Cataloguing in Publication data

The treatment of anxiety disorders: clinician guides and patient manuals / Gavin Andrews . . . [et al.]. –
2nd ed.
    p. ; cm.
Includes bibliographical references and index.
ISBN 0 521 78877 3
1. Anxiety – Handbooks, manuals, etc.   2. Anxiety – Treatment – Handbooks, manuals, etc.
I. Andrews, Gavin.
[DNLM: 1. Anxiety Disorders – therapy. WM 172 T7842 2002]
RC531.T68   2002
616.85'223 – dc21   2001052852

ISBN 0 521 78877 3 paperback

The Treatment of Anxiety Disorders
Clinician Guides and Patient Manuals

The Treatment of Anxiety Disorders brought together concise yet thorough theoretical reviews with practical guides to treatment. In this completely revised second edition Gavin Andrews and his co-authors review new developments in the research and treatment of anxiety disorders and provide up-to-date treatment materials. Over half the material in the second edition is new, and there is an entirely new section covering posttraumatic stress disorder. This is a unique and authoritative overview of the recognition and treatment of anxiety disorders, giving Clinician Guides and Patient Treatment Manuals for each. The Clinician Guides describe how to create treatment programs, drawing upon materials and methods that the authors have used success-fully in clinical practice for 15 years. The Patient Treatment Manuals provide session-by-session resources for clinician and patient to work through, enabling each patient to better understand and put into effect the strategies of cognitive behavior therapy.

From reviews of the first edition:

"In my opinion this book deserves a place in any medical library for its clear and comprehensive theoretical overview, and its synthesis of theory and practice for all doctors whose work brings them into contact with anxious patients."
  Journal of the Royal Society of Medicine

"*The Treatment of Anxiety Disorders* is a well-referenced resource book and treatment guide."
  ADAA Reporter

Contents

List of authors

Gavin Andrews is Professor of Psychiatry in the School of Psychiatry at the University of New South Wales, and Director of the Clinical Research Unit for Anxiety and Depression at St. Vincent's Hospital, Sydney.

Mark Creamer is Director of the Australian Centre for Posttraumatic Mental Health and a Professor in the Department of Psychiatry at the University of Melbourne. He is a clinical psychologist with many years of experience in the field of traumatic stress.

Rocco Crino is a clinical psychologist at St. Vincent's Hospital. He is Director of the Anxiety Disorders Clinic and Manager of Psychology at St. Vincent's Hospital, Sydney.

Caroline Hunt is a clinical psychologist and Senior Lecturer in the School of Psychology, University of Sydney. She is a clinician with many years of experience in the treatment of anxiety disorders.

Lisa Lampe is a psychiatrist and Lecturer, School of Psychiatry, University of New South Wales. She is a clinician with the Clinical Research Unit for Anxiety and Depression, Sydney, and Director, Anxiety Disorders Program, Evesham Clinic, Cremorne, New South Wales.

Andrew Page is Associate Professor and Director of Clinical Psychology, School of Psychology, University of Western Australia, Perth.

Preface to the second edition

The first edition of this book was developed from the Patient Treatment Manuals that had been used in the Clinical Research Unit for Anxiety and Depression for the treatment of patients with anxiety disorders. Specialized treatment programs for anxiety disorders were initiated in 1978 modeled on the treatment program for adult stutterers with which Dr. Andrews had long been associated. John Franklin designed and tested the first program for patients with agoraphobia in 1979. Since then programs for panic disorder and agoraphobia, social phobia, specific phobias, generalized anxiety disorder, and obsessive–compulsive disorder have been developed and tested. During these 20 years, many people have contributed to the redevelopment and testing of the Manuals for the various programs. Significant contributions have been made by previous staff members of the unit, in particular John Franklin, Paul Friend, Stephen MacMahon, Richard Mattick, Carmen Moran, Conrad Newman, Susan Tanner, and Morison Tarrant. Robin Harvey was the administrator of the Unit. Advice about the first edition of this book was forthcoming from Alex Blaszczynski, Anette Johansson, Colin MacLeod, Richard Mattick, Hugh Morgan, Michael Nicholas, Cindy Page, Ron Rapee, Mark Ryan, Derrick Silove, Michelle Singh, and Beth Spencer: their help is gratefully acknowledged.

The second edition has been a much easier task. First, knowing that the first edition lacked a credible section on posttraumatic stress disorder, we invited Mark Creamer, the Director of the Australian Centre for Posttraumatic Mental Health, to contribute. Second, having taught from the book to graduate students and to practicing clinicians for some 7 years we had clear ideas about the changes that were necessary. Third, the explosive growth in the literature in the past 7 years meant that revising the chapters was exciting, rather than boring. Fourth, the natural development of the treatment programs in the clinic meant that the treatment manuals are themselves quite altered and we are grateful for advice from Stephanie Rosser and Merran Lindsay on this matter. Last, Dr. Page and Dr. Hunt now work in clinics of other universities so their contributions contain knowledge from those environments. Thus the book now comes from the clinics associated with four leading universities and is no longer the partisan view of CRUfAD. Nevertheless we would recommend that readers supplement this book by recourse to the CRUfAD website (www.crufad.org) for themselves and their patients.

The enthusiasm and guidance of Richard Barling and Pauline Graham of Cambridge University Press is gratefully acknowledged.

Abbreviations

Abbreviations have been kept to a minimum. Some are confined to certain chapters and will be defined there. Those used throughout the book are:

DSM-III   *Diagnostic and Statistical Manual,* 3rd edition (APA, 1980)
DSM-III-R   *Diagnostic and Statistical Manual,* 3rd edition (revised) (APA, 1987)
DSM-IV   *Diagnostic and Statistical Manual,* 4th edition (APA, 1994)
ICD-10   *International Classification of Diseases,* 10th revision, *Classification of Mental and Behavioural Disorders, Diagnostic Criteria for Research* (WHO, 1993)
OCD   Obsessive–compulsive disorder
GAD   Generalized anxiety disorder
PTSD   Posttraumatic stress disorder

Read me

How to use this unusual book

This book is about the treatment of anxiety disorders, about helping people with chronic anxiety disorders to become well and stay well. It contains discussions of the nature and treatment of each syndrome, it describes the problems commonly encountered during treatment, and it outlines some management strategies. Of greatest value, it contains Patient Treatment Manuals for the common anxiety disorders.

Anxiety disorders are not simply about being too anxious, they are about irrational worry and avoidance of situations that are the focus of this worry. Persons with panic disorder worry that their panic will result in physical or mental collapse; those with social phobia worry that their behavior will result in shame; and those with specific phobias fear personal harm. Those with obsessive–compulsive disorder (OCD) worry that their obsessions will come true; those with posttraumatic stress disorder (PTSD) worry that their flashbacks will be real; and those with generalized anxiety disorder (GAD) worry that, despite their worry, disaster will occur. People with chronic anxiety disorders are very sensitive to additional stress, and quickly become anxious and upset. They can develop additional symptoms, including those of other anxiety and depressive disorders. They know this, and commonly think that the seed of their disorder lies within their own nature, personality, or temperament. Perceiving their sensitivity to anxiety and their inability to cope with it, they deny or fail to control the events that generated the anxiety and try to cope by avoiding the situations that worsen their anxiety. They focus instead on the physical symptoms that are part of the anxiety response, or on the situations that provoke their anxiety, rather than trying to understand the meaning of their anxiety. The handicap comes from avoidance: the phobic avoidance, the compulsive rituals, the emotional numbing, the preoccupation with the possibility of physical illness, and from the time spent worrying.

Treatment should aim to reduce the emotional sensitivity to stress, the anticipatory anxiety about outcomes, and the avoidance behaviors related to specific situations. The book is written especially for psychiatrists and clinical psychologists to provide detailed knowledge about the process and pitfalls in conducting a comprehensive cognitive behavioral program for the common anxiety disorders. Clinical psychologists and psychiatrists learn about these techniques during their training, but knowing about something is not equivalent to knowing how to do it. The Patient Treatment Manuals are both the guidebook and the journey. They allow clinicians to make the journey with the patient. In skilled hands these programs comfort, commonly relieve, and quite frequently cure the disorder. These programs can also ameliorate the underlying personality vulnerability to anxiety.

This book contains six detailed Patient Treatment Manuals: for panic disorder and agoraphobia, for social phobia, for specific phobias, for obsessive–compulsive disorder, for generalized anxiety disorder and for posttraumatic stress disorder. The publisher, Cambridge University Press, has agreed that these Manuals may be photocopied by the purchaser of the book for the treatment of individual patients. The Manuals are designed to be used as workbooks, and most patients annotate and therefore personalize their copy with their own insights and with comments from their clinician that are relevant to their particular circumstances. Apart from copies of Manuals made by purchasers for their personal use in the treatment of their patients, the Manuals – or indeed any other part of the book – may not be copied, distributed, or sold. The standard provisions of copyright listed in the front of the book apply.

Some patients with anxiety disorders can benefit from simply being given the Manual to read. However, most have already struggled to recover, and in these persons significant improvement and the prospect of cure come when a clinician gives the appropriate Treatment Manual to a patient and then works through the Manual with him or her, explaining, supervising, and supporting the process of recovery. In this way the clinician's expertise enables each patient to understand and put into effect the substance of the treatment. After treatment has concluded, the Manuals, annotated with notes made during treatment, are commonly used by patients to maintain their improvement and to inhibit relapse. In this sense they do eventually become valid self-help manuals.

This book also contains separate Clinician Guides for the treatment of patients with each of these disorders. These guides contain advice about the structures and settings in which these programs have been shown to work, about patient characteristics and behaviors that will require special skills if the progress of therapy is to continue, and about critical issues in the therapeutic process. The guides are about the art of therapy for patients with these disorders, and the Clinician Guides are for clinicians' eyes only. When the first edition of this book was published the Patient Treatment Manuals and the Clinician Guides were without precedent in the therapy literature. They comprise three-quarters of the book. The remaining quarter is much more conventional: an account of the scientific knowledge needed for clinicians to understand the nature of the disorders affecting their patients and to evaluate the treatment options available.

When a clinician sees a patient with, say, agoraphobia and, after discussion of the other possibilities, it is decided that a cognitive behavior therapy program is to be the treatment of choice:

1. The clinician completes an assessment of symptoms and level of handicap, incorporating appropriate rating scales and questionnaires, and then has the patient identify and rate the extent to which their main problem interferes with their life and activities.

2. The clinician explains the treatment to the patient using words like, "I am going to teach you how to control your panics, enter feared situations, and master your worrying thoughts. Here is a Manual that describes the program. I want you to take the Manual home and look through it. Do remember to bring it to your next session when we will begin to work through it together."

3. The patient is seen often, usually more than once per week, and at each session a segment of the Manual is worked through, the clinician modifying the information to make it appropriate to the patient's disorder and level of understanding. Homework exercises are then set and arrangements for the next session are made.

4. Treatment proceeds quickly with most patients with agoraphobia improving their panic control by session 3, being able to travel by session 6, and mastering worrying thoughts by session 10. Treatment should conclude within 20 sessions with the clinician, the patient having spent an additional 40–60 hours on homework during this time. The homework is focused on practicing the anxiety management strategies, on graded exposure to feared situations, and on identifying and combating dysfunctional cognitions.

5. When treatment concludes, the assessment measures made at the beginning are repeated. Areas in which the patient needs to continue to make gains or to consolidate are identified both from the therapy sessions and from the pattern of scores on these measures. Patients are encouraged to continue their own therapy by using both the Manual, now embellished with the additional information, and techniques provided by the clinician during the therapy sessions, and by periodic follow-up sessions with the clinician.

Clinicians of varying levels of expertise will use the book in different ways. Those new to the field, before treating a patient with, say, agoraphobia, should read Chapters 2 and 3, the general overview and the general advice about treatment, then proceed to Chapters 4 and 5 to review the scientific knowledge about the nature and treatment of agoraphobia. Finally they should read Chapter 6, the

Clinician Guide, about issues that may arise while treating patients with agoraphobia, reading that in conjunction with Chapter 7, the Patient Treatment Manual, for panic disorder and agoraphobia. Thus, when they begin to work with the patient, they will be familiar with both the course of treatment outlined in the Patient Treatment Manual and with the background information an experienced clinician already has. Experienced and busy clinicians may initially skip the review chapters but should still find the general advice about treatment and the Clinician Guide to agoraphobia essential, especially when difficulties arise during treatment. In fact the Clinician Guide will be useful even when the Patient Treatment Manual is not the principal treatment. That is to say, these treatment and clinician guide chapters will also be valuable to many clinicians even when drug treatments are being used, simply because many of the same difficulties will arise. In general, clinicians using drugs as their main treatments will find the chapters reviewing the syndromes and those reviewing treatments to be informative, for patients invariably ask about their disorder and expect their clinician to be conversant with the literature.

This book is for practicing clinicians. It provides most of the information needed for the successful treatment of patients with anxiety disorders.

2

General issues in anxiety disorders

Background information about anxiety disorders

Anxiety disorders are not just a matter of being too anxious. Anxiety is normal. Moderate levels of anxiety are often welcomed to improve performance, and quite severe levels of anxiety can be experienced as normal when they are consistent with the demands of the situation. Persons with anxiety disorders are usually not just complaining of being too anxious too often, for they seek help with specific and recurring fears that they recognize as irrational and somewhat intrusive. To paraphrase the description in Chapter 1: the fears are of physical collapse in panic disorder and agoraphobia, of negative evaluation in social phobia, of harm to self or loved ones in GAD, of self-caused harm to self or loved ones in OCD, of improbable harm to self in the specific phobias, and of the intrusive memory of past threats of harm in PTSD.

It is the specific symptoms and the fear of these symptoms that disables, even though the anxiety that follows is the defining symptom for this group of disorders. It is not surprising therefore that anxiolytic drugs such as the benzodiazepines have not proven to be ideal treatments, for though they reduce both state anxiety and anticipatory anxiety, and hence generally improve composure, they do little to reduce the core fears specific to each disorder. There are general factors that seem to predispose to all anxiety disorders, and treatment should be directed to relieving this general vulnerability, as well as to reducing the fears specific to each disorder. This chapter will present a general model for anxiety that clinicians can teach patients. It is consistent with the cognitive behavioral treatments advocated and allows for the extensive comorbidity that is observed. The chapter will also review diagnosis and assessment, and will consider the epidemiology and health service delivery for these disorders.

A model for anxiety

The Yerkes–Dodson curve

The seriousness of the anxiety disorders is frequently underestimated because anxiety is usually a normal, useful, and protective affect. Depression, on the other hand, is seldom undervalued because it is rarely useful and sometimes dangerous. The notion of the usefulness of anxiety is very important in the management of anxiety disorders. Many patients have learned to fear and avoid situations that produce normal anxiety, and so react to anxiety as though it were abnormal, thus generating fear and compounding their complaint.

In 1908 Yerkes and Dodson described a relationship between anxiety and performance that can help patients understand the facilitating and debilitating effects of normal anxiety. Performance on skilled tasks improves as one becomes aroused and thus anxiety is initially facilitating. This performance increment plateaus once the person is tense and alert. Increases in the anxiety level beyond this optimal level can debilitate, rapidly reducing the capacity for skilled motor movements, complex intellectual tasks, and impairing the perception of new information. "He plays better if he is psyched up" is a colloquial description of facilitating anxiety and "he lost his head" is an apt description of the effects of debilitating anxiety.

Patients with anxiety disorders suffer considerably from the debilitating effects of their excessive anxiety, for it impairs their work and personal relationships, and limits their activities and opportunities. Aware that their excessive anxiety can lead them to make a mess of things, they tend to avoid difficult situations so as not to appear unnecessarily stupid, and defer to others rather than run the risk of asserting themselves and becoming unnecessarily upset. Treatment has to begin slowly because of the debilitating effects of anxiety. In fact, many patients later report that the first sessions of treatment "were all a blur, I was too anxious to concentrate". Some understanding of the effect of anxiety on performance is useful for patients. It is included in many of the treatment manuals.

Components of the model

Clinicians will find a hypothetical model of the relationship among adversity, personality, arousal, coping, and symptoms useful if they are to teach their patients appropriately. The model used by the authors is presented in Figure 2.1. The model will be illustrated by research data – predominantly data from this unit – because to do so makes for a simple and coherent body of information. The reader interested in more detailed models of the nature of anxiety should consult Barlow (2000) and Gray and McNaughton (2000). In most models, threat is regarded as a trigger stimulus for arousal that leads to symptoms. The level of arousal depends on three factors: the extent to which the potentially adverse event is appraised by the individual as being a threat, the extent to which the individual habitually responds to a threat with high arousal, and the individual's sense of being able to control both the arousal and the threat. The arousal is experienced as symptoms consistent with those of the flight or fight response,

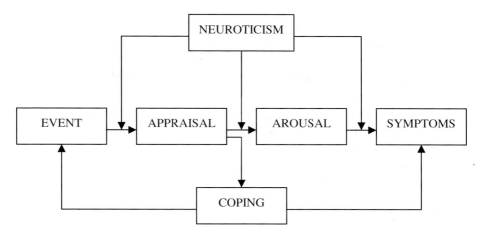

Figure 2.1   A model of the relationship among neuroticism, life events, appraisal, arousal, coping, and symptoms of anxiety.

symptoms that, if chronic, become transmuted into despair or irrational fears.

Most individuals try to cope with arousal by attempting to nullify the threat that provoked the arousal. Any serious threat is unlikely to be solved quickly. In fact, most real threats are partly unresolvable and often lead to loss. So the task is to remain in control, calm and rational, avoiding the deleterious effects of high anxiety, until the best strategy to minimize the problem can be completed. The elements of this model – life events, appraisal, symptoms, trait anxiety or neuroticism, and coping by problem solving – will be discussed in turn.

Untoward life events

Most people become anxious when threatened by loss of love, position, wealth, or safety. Life event research has repeatedly demonstrated the relationship between such threats and state anxiety (Andrews et al., 1978) but has also shown that this relationship is time limited and that most people recover quite quickly, which suggests that the average person is good at coping with normal adversity (Andrews, 1981). Loss of money or position can be accepted within months; loss of parent, child, or spouse within a year or two; but there are some experiences so severe that they continue to produce arousal and increased sensitivity to other threats for a very long time. Adverse life events can be measured by questionnaires (Tennant and Andrews, 1976) or by detailed interviews about the context in which the event occurred (Brown and Harris, 1978). We have used both methods satisfactorily, and while they identify events at quite different thresholds they seem to generate the same associations (Andrews, 1988). Extremely adverse life events are a necessary, and can be a sufficient, cause of PTSD. A surfeit of adverse life events is reported to precede the onset of panic disorder, social phobia, and OCD;

but adverse life events are neither necessary nor sufficient to explain the onset of GAD. Many untoward life events that appear threatening at the time are found to be benign. It is the appraisal of the event that conditionally identifies an event as potentially threatening.

Appraisal

When an untoward and potentially threatening event occurs one asks "Is this a threat to me?", meaning is the threat unpredictable and uncontrollable. The event is appraised in terms of one's prior experience with similar events and in terms of community knowledge about the level of threat associated with such events. Some of this appraisal is deliberate whereas some, conducted at an automatic or unconscious level, seems more driven by irrational thoughts of danger. When the threat is ambiguous and accurate appraisal is difficult, the automatic danger schemas become more influential.

It is not the "things that go bump in the night" that produce anxiety but the meaning given to them. For example, if one is awakened by a creaking door and decides that the cat has caused the door to creak, then it is easy to go back to sleep. If one decides that the noise could be caused by intruders, one instantly becomes alert and anxious, with heart pounding and mouth dry as one rehearses what to do. Once it has been established that the noise was caused by the cat, it is easy to go back to sleep. Thus it is not the event but the thoughts about the event that cause anxiety. Therefore the best way to reduce the anxiety is to evaluate the situation carefully, decide what to do, then just do it. Most events that cause significant anxiety are complex and, as the full import of the event takes time to unfold, appraisal and coping are iterative processes.

Arousal and the symptoms of anxiety

When a situation is identified as being a threat, the automatic response is arousal that leads to action, provided action is possible. When action is not possible then the physiological arousal that would have facilitated the action is experienced as symptoms, symptoms that represent the physiological changes associated with the flight or fight response. These symptoms are: increased circulation (experienced as palpitations) with shift of blood from gut to muscles (experienced as dry mouth, nausea, abdominal distress); increased respiratory drive (experienced as difficulty breathing or feeling of choking, and then – if the person hyperventilates – numbness and tingling, dizziness, light headedness, and chest discomfort); increased muscle tension (experienced as trembling and shaking, muscle tension and pain); and a narrowing of attention (producing difficulty concentrating on other things and, if prolonged, derealization and depersonalization).

Many persons fail to associate these symptoms with the antecedent threat and instead identify the symptoms as evidence that some physiological catastrophe is imminent. They fear they are about to have a heart attack, collapse, faint, go crazy, or die. This perceived threat of physical collapse then functions as an additional uncontrollable threat, thereby increasing the arousal and consequent symptoms even further. All patients with anxiety disorders need to understand the normal physiology of anxiety if they are to manage their own anxiety in a more rational fashion.

Neuroticism or trait anxiety

Some persons, year after year, are noted to be more sensitive, more emotional, and more prone to experience anxiety than are their peers exposed to the same situations. Psychologists, such as Eysenck and Eysenck (1975, neuroticism), Spielberger et al. (1983, trait anxiety), Costa and McCrae (1992, neuroticism) and Tellegen (1982, stress reaction), have developed questionnaires to describe variations in human personality that consistently show the trait of proneness to anxiety to be a major component of personality that determines behavior. Barlow (2000) uses the term "negative affect", based on Clark and Watson's (1991) model. Tellegans's higher-order construct of negative emotionality with which it is often confused is much broader and includes the traits of alienation and aggression as well as stress reaction. We will use the term neuroticism.

The questionnaires used to identify this trait tend to ask questions such as "Are you usually anxious?" and thus appear to be little more than a list of chronic symptoms. As originally conceived, at least by Eysenck in relation to the Neuroticism Scale, this trait was seen as temperament, characteristic of the individual over time, and reflecting structural characteristics of the nervous system. It is stable over time, animal models have been developed, homologs identified in nonhuman species, and the genetics (about half the variance is under genetic control) and likely neurophysiology have been explored (DeFries et al., 1978; Andrews, 1991; Eley and Plomin, 1997; Gosling and John, 1997; Costa et al., 2000).

To understand the influence of this trait, it is helpful to consider the influence of neuroticism on the experience of anxiety symptoms during an eventful but, we hope, hypothetical drive to work that involves a speeding fine and then being hit by a runaway truck. Calm when leaving home, the person with an average neuroticism score becomes aroused, alert, and efficient when stopped by the police for speeding, but becomes so aroused when confronted by the truck that they are debilitated by the anxiety and unable to avoid being sideswiped. Theoretically, the person with low neuroticism will hardly be aroused when stopped by the police and, when faced with the collision with the truck, will use the facilitatory effects of anxiety to skillfully avoid any collision. In contrast, a person with high neuroticism, who was equally calm when leaving home, will become dysfunctional when stopped for speeding, will get fines for noncompliance as well as for speeding, and will remain aroused for a considerable time afterward. When confronted with the truck, they will become so debilitated by anxiety that they will do exactly the wrong thing and be killed.

Precisely because of the influence of trait anxiety or neuroticism on state anxiety, the anxiety disorders used to be considered manifestations of personality vulnerability. Neuroticism is probably the single most powerful risk factor and determinant of symptoms. In our large twin sample (Andrews et al., 1990c), we found neuroticism, measured by the Eysenck Personality Questionnaire Neuroticism Scale (Eysenck and Eysenck, 1975), to be a stable characteristic, with test–retest polychoric correlations of 0.9 at 4-, 8-, and 12-month intervals, even though there is evidence of a gradual reduction over longer time periods. Krueger et al. (2000) reported that the construct "stress reaction" was related (effect size 0.7) to current and future anxiety and depressive disorders. Neuroticism is clearly a surface marker for some underlying trait related to the appearance of anxiety and depressive symptoms.

There is a strong relationship between high neuroticism and anxiety disorders (Brown et al., 1998). Patients with panic and agoraphobia, social phobia, OCD, and GAD who do not have scores more than one standard deviation above the mean are rare (Andrews et al., 1989), and should be investigated further. While significant, the association of neuroticism with PTSD is less absolute. Persons with high neuroticism have been shown to experience an increased level of significant interpersonal life events regardless of whether questionnaire or interview methods are used to determine the occurrence of significant events (Poulton and Andrews, 1992). That both methods have confirmed the relationship suggests that the finding is not simply an artifact of a plaintive set. It is probably evidence of the debilitating effects of neuroticism and anxiety on interpersonal relationships.

High neuroticism scores are associated with the major anxiety disorders. A high score is also associated with a more extensive lifetime history of neurotic illness (Andrews et al., 1990c) and with a higher likelihood of relapse after treatment (Andrews and Moran, 1988).

Coping with adversity

The impact of adverse life events is moderated by neuroticism to produce arousal, which, although experienced negatively as symptoms, does not always lead to appropriate control. Reality-based coping means accurate and considered apprai-sal of the problem, rehearsal and then implementation of possible solutions, and, finally, continual reassessment after any such attempts, much like the steps outlined in the structured problem-solving technique (D'Zurilla, 1986). We use the Locus of Control of Behavior Scale (Craig et al., 1984) to measure the propensity to carry out this type of behavior. Locus of control scores behave as though they were trait measures, being stable over time (test–retest polychoric correlations at 4, 8, and 12 months being 0.7). Patients with anxiety disorders characterize themselves as powerless on measures of locus of control, not only unable to cope with adversity but unable to use external help to enable them to do so (Sandler and Lakey, 1982). The higher the score (higher is used to mean more external in orientation, more powerless), the greater is the history of past anxiety disorder and the higher the probability of relapse after apparently successful treatment (Andrews and Craig, 1988; Andrews and Moran, 1988).

Moderate anxiety can act as a positive force, potentiating effective action. However, anxiety that is too severe debilitates and reduces the individual's ability to perceive, reason, and act appropriately. Hence, integral to any notion of coping with stress is the salience of some automatic defensive mechanism that functions to maintain composure and limit the debilitating effects of high anxiety. Vaillant (1971) has shown the importance of such defense mechanisms in the long-term adaptation of university graduates followed for 30 years. Mature defenses (anticipation, suppression, sublimation, humor) acknowledge the nature and extent of the threat but directly limit the level of arousal and consequent anxiety. We have used the Defense Style Questionnaire (Andrews et al., 1989; Andrews et al., 1993b) to describe such mechanisms. The questionnaire functions as a trait measure (test–retest correlation 0.75 over 1 to 18 months), shows a gradual maturation with age, and discriminates people with anxiety disorders from normal controls. This measure is abnormal in people with panic and agoraphobia, social phobia and OCD, but, like neuroticism and locus of control, does not distinguish between these disorders (Andrews et al., 1993b).

The vulnerability factors

Duncan-Jones (1987) followed a sample population of adults for a year and, using structural equation modeling techniques, estimated that 70% of the fluctuation in anxiety and depression could be best accounted for by stable factors either within the environment or within the personality of the individual. He found that neuroticism alone accounted for 44% of the total variance, leaving 26% to be accounted for by other stable personality or environmental measures. We confirmed Duncan-Jones' (1987) structural equation model using neuroticism and locus of control, and these two measures together explained some 60% of the variation in symptoms over the 16-month period of our study (Andrews, 1991; see Figure 2.2). Figure 2.2 shows the relation between the latent variable of vulnerability to illness, here estimated from Neuroticism and Locus of Control Scores, and the latent variable of illness estimated from the lifetime diagnoses and from

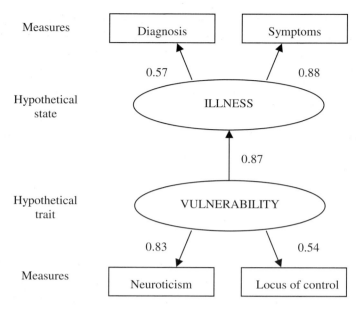

Figure 2.2   The relation between the latent variable of vulnerability to illness as measured from Neuroticism and Locus of Control measures and the latent variable of illness as measured from lifetime prevalence of a neurotic diagnosis and symptoms of anxiety and depression over a 16-month period.

symptom measures taken on four occasions over the 16 months. Because the three vulnerability measures (trait anxiety, locus of control, and defense style) are correlated, there must be overlap in the domains of information tapped by each questionnaire (Andrews et al., 1989). To elucidate this hypothesis we conducted a multivariate genetic analysis of these three vulnerability factors. Results are displayed in Table 2.1 (for the full analysis, see Andrews, 1991). While each of the three measures appears to be influenced by specific genetic and environmental factors, there is a significant loading on common genetic and environmental factors that contributes to each measure. This finding is consistent with the proposition that the three measures are interrelated – perhaps showing that externalized locus of control and immature defense style are the consequence of neuroticism, or perhaps showing that all three of these measures reflect some common underlying pattern of neurological organization.

We have used canonical correlations in a group of adolescents to estimate the relative importance of these three measures in determining anxiety and depressive symptoms and report the following values: neuroticism 0.6, locus 0.2, defense style 0.3 (Andrews et al., 1993a). Their relative roles in determining chronicity once a person is ill with the specific symptoms of an anxiety disorder may, of course, be quite different.

Table 2.1 Parameter estimates for the preferred multivariate model of the unique and common individual environment (E) and additive genetic (H) components of the vulnerability factors: neuroticism, locus of control and defense style

	Unique factors		Common	
Vulnerability factor	E	H	E	H
Neuroticism	0.62	0.44	0.28	0.58
Locus of control	0.61	0.35	0.50	0.53
Defense style	0.60	0.43	0.51	0.44

Comorbidity

The occurrence of other disorders in association with specific anxiety disorders is frequent (Kessler et al., 1994; Andrews, 1996a; Andrews et al., 2001a) and is of therapeutic interest. If the association is because both disorders are due to the same causative factor, then good treatment should target this vulnerability factor. If the comorbid condition is secondary to the anxiety disorder, then treatment of the anxiety disorder should also relieve this secondary illness. Finally, if the anxiety disorder is secondary to the associated condition, then treatment of the primary condition is essential.

Comorbidity due to the effect of the shared vulnerability factors

Support for a general model of anxiety disorders, or of anxiety and depressive disorders, is not convincing when the model depends solely on data from general population samples. There is a strong feeling, perhaps without much evidence, that people who seek treatment for a mental disorder are in some way different, quite apart from severity, from people in the general population who report symptoms consistent with a diagnosis but do not seek treatment. We examined this problem by comparing our sample of 243 twins who reported symptoms that satisfied one or more of the six common DSM-III diagnoses (major depressive episode, dysthymia, panic and agoraphobia, social phobia, OCD, GAD) with a group of 165 patients treated for panic and agoraphobia.

We measured the vulnerability factors of neuroticism and locus of control, and lifetime illness experience in both groups (Andrews et al., 1990b). Ninety-one of the 243 diagnostic twins met criteria for more than one of the six neurotic diagnoses in their lifetime to date. Single diagnoses were much less frequent and multiple diagnoses were much more frequent than is predicted from the prevalences of the individual diagnoses, as though some general factor, such as that

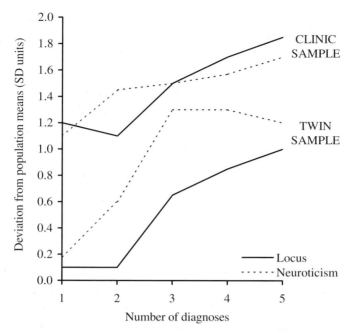

Figure 2.3   The relation between vulnerability factors as measured by Locus of Control and Neuroticism and number of neurotic diagnoses reported in lifetime to date for two samples – one drawn from an anxiety disorders clinic and one from a quasi-population sample of adult twins (redrawn from Andrews, 1991).

hypothesized earlier, was rendering some individuals especially vulnerable to episodes of anxiety and depressive disorders.

All the 165 patients in the clinic sample met criteria for panic and agoraphobia and their experience of other disorders was also extensive. Eighty-six percent had met criteria for other anxiety and depressive diagnoses in their lifetimes to date. The comorbidities in the clinic and twin samples of individuals who had met criteria for panic and agoraphobia were comparable, with both groups reporting an average of 1.8 additional neurotic diagnoses other than their index diagnosis. In the twin sample, co-occurrence occurred whatever diagnosis was taken as the starting point. In fact, after we extracted a common factor of illness co-occurrence, we searched the residual matrix for specific or unique associations between pairs of diagnoses and found none.

In the general model, personality variables such as neuroticism and locus of control were strongly related to the occurrence of symptoms. This relationship also holds for the number of different anxiety and depressive diagnostic criteria met in the lifetimes of the two samples. Such data are presented in Figure 2.3. The association is significant in both twin and clinic groups: the higher the scores on these scales measuring vulnerability to anxiety and depression, the more extensive is the lifetime history of illness. The clinic attenders showed significantly higher vulnerability scores for a given illness history, which may indicate that illness in the setting of a vulnerable personality determines the need to seek specialist treatment, whereas illness alone is not so directly related to treatment-seeking. Good treatment should therefore seek not only to remedy the individual symptoms but also to change the underlying vulnerability. If patients are to be cured, i.e., after treatment have only the population risk of developing the same illness anew, then such vulnerability must be lessened.

In an earlier study that involved a 15-year follow-up of patients initially hospitalized with anxiety or depressive neuroses (Andrews et al., 1990a), we searched for information available at the initial admission that might predict long-term outcome. Personality was found to be the most important of the items measured at intake. In a structural equation model, personality vulnerability, as judged from measures of neuroticism at the initial admission, accounted for 20% of the variance in outcome over 15 years. This effect was not evident in patients with affective psychoses. We see this result as further support for the importance of personality traits as determinants of the genesis and chronicity of anxiety and depression, and another reason to recommend that attention to personality traits be required if a treatment program seeks to do more than remedy the current episode of illness.

The information from this method of examining the meaning behind the comorbidity information is consistent with a two-factor theory of neurosis. The first factor is a general vulnerability to neurosis as evidenced by high trait anxiety and poor coping. The second factor is a vulnerability to a specific disorder that is presumably related (as most of the core disorders have first symptoms in adolescence or in early adult life) to familial, even nongenetic, influences that sensitize one person to fears of bodily dysfunction, another to fears of social disapproval, and a third to fears of harmful thoughts, and so on.

Comorbidity: personality disorder and substance use disorders

In the previous section the high rates of comorbidity between anxiety and depressive disorders were associated with vulnerability as evidenced by elevated Neuroticism, Locus of Control, and Defense Style Scores. In this section, we shall discuss co-occurrence of disorders that may be independent of the association determined by personality trait abnormality. Personality disorders are seen as largely independent and separate conditions that do not influence the symptoms of anxiety disorders even though particular associations with the avoidant, borderline, and obsessive–compulsive personality disorders have been suggested. The reports in the literature differ. Some have reported nonspecific increases in prevalence of all personality disorders in all anxiety disorders. Others report an increase in borderline-type disorders with panic and agoraphobia, an increase in obsessive–compulsive personality disorder with OCD, and an increase of avoidant personality disorder with social phobia (for a review, see Mulder et al., 1991).

There are a number of issues to be discussed. First, it is important to disentangle the effects of the Axis I acute illness symptoms on the behavior of the individual. For example, many clinicians mistake the emotional dyscontrol in patients on the verge of panic as evidence of a cluster B disorder and presume an association between these personality disorders and panic and agoraphobia that is false. In similar vein, many confuse chronic OCD with the related personality disorder. This is not surprising given that OCD – which commonly begins in adolescence – seems to become part of the individual's personality. A similar issue occurs in social phobia and avoidant personality disorder. Simply because of the way avoidant personality disorder is defined, most subjects who are positive for this personality disorder also meet criteria for social phobia. As they usually use the phobia as their presenting symptom when seeking treatment, it is not surprising that a large number of patients in any social phobia program are found to be comorbid for avoidant personality disorder.

The other concern is with the methods used to detect personality disorder. Some questionnaires with good face validity perform very poorly, and only lengthy interviews such as the Personality Disorder Examination appear to be able to identify personality disorder reliably in the setting of concurrent anxiety disorder (Hunt and Andrews, 1992). The results in this clinic show that 35% of patients with social phobia met stringent criteria for avoidant personality disorder. Only 8% of OCD patients met criteria for obsessive–compulsive personality disorder, and only 1% of patients with panic or agoraphobia met criteria for borderline personality disorder. The low rates in this clinic may be because patients with comorbid personality disorder do not seek a behavioral treatment for their anxiety disorders, or the low rates may be because our careful assessment has shown that some of the presumed association is an artifact. Certainly, we encounter patients who, although not meeting criteria for personality disorder, have borderline or narcissistic or paranoid traits sufficient to be of concern. We sometimes find that, as treatment proceeds and they learn to control their anxiety, their need to resort to such behavior becomes less frequent and is no longer of concern.

In summary, the association of personality disorder and anxiety disorder does not appear to be of etiological relevance. Furthermore, given a strong treatment, it is probably of lesser therapeutic relevance than is commonly believed. The specific steps to be taken in respect to individuals who are comorbid for personality disorder are discussed in the Clinician Guide.

Substance abuse disorders are the other conditions that are reported to be more frequent than expected in patients with anxiety disorders. There are three possible mechanisms for such an association. First, a drug such as amphetamine or cocaine could produce the symptoms of anxiety and, conceivably, those of an anxiety disorder. There is a literature that the first panic attack can occur while using drugs (Moran, 1986) and that the first panic can also follow drug or alcohol withdrawal. The second association concerns the observation that many alcoholics and drug users report that their dependence began as a mechanism to reduce their anxiety. Reporting biases do affect such rates, and Mulder et al. (1991) have discussed these effects. In which direction is the association? A review by Kushner et al. (1990) concluded that in agoraphobia and social phobia the alcohol problems are more likely to follow from attempts at self-medication of anxiety symptoms, whereas the association in panic and GAD is more likely to follow pathological alcohol consumption.

In our own clinic we examined the prevalence of substance use disorders among patients being treated for panic, agoraphobia, or social phobia and compared these rates with the risks in the general population. When the effects of sex were controlled, the overuse of alcohol and medication was raised in all diagnoses, with the exception of males with panic disorder. Social phobics exhibited rates of problem alcohol use three to five times greater than those in the control group. In all diagnoses and sexes, rates of sedative or hypnotic abuse were six to 12 times greater than the rates in the population. These high rates were deemed to be secondary to the anxiety disorder.

The specificity of the individual anxiety disorders

Patients who currently meet criteria for panic and agoraphobia, social phobia, or OCD present very differently, even though they all share personality traits that have made them vulnerable to their anxiety disorder. In terms of diagnostic separation, they can be reliably identified by structured diagnostic interviews, although factor analysis of symptom patterns does emphasize the communality between syndromes (Krueger, 1999).

The DSM-IV and ICD-10 classifications

The DSM-IV criteria and the ICD-10 Diagnostic Criteria for Research use similar criteria to define the major anxiety disorders. We have reported on differences in prevalence rates in community surveys that use the Composite International Diagnostic Interview (CIDI) to identify both classifications (Andrews et al., 1999b; Andrews, 2000). Nevertheless we think that in clinical practice the two classifications will be functionally equivalent. "Panic disorder" is described in both classifications as recurrent, abrupt, unexpected or unpredictable attacks of fear or discomfort, peaking in minutes and accompanied by the symptoms and outcome fears listed earlier in this chapter. The criteria for "agoraphobia with panic disorder" do differ in detail. ICD-10 follows the traditional description of excessive or unreasonable fear or avoidance of crowds, public places, traveling alone or when away from home, accompanied by anxiety symptoms when in or thinking about the situation. DSM-IV encapsulates the key features of the disorder better: first, panic attacks themselves must worry or handicap; and, second, the panic attacks lead to avoidance or endurance of situations from which escape might be difficult or help unavailable.

"Specific phobias" are defined as an excessive or unreasonable fear of specific objects or situations, with DSM-IV also requiring that the phobia interfere with one's life and activities. "Social phobia" is defined as excessive and unreasonable fear and avoidance of scrutiny or of being the focus of attention in social situations in case one acts in a way that will result in humiliation or embarrassment. ICD-10 requires that specific symptoms be present, while in DSM-IV a level of handicap is required.

"Obsessive–compulsive disorder" is defined as obsessions (one's own thoughts are intrusive) or compulsions, both being repetitive, unable to be resisted, and excessive and inappropriate, and distress or handicap by occupying time. DSM-IV also requires compulsions to be experienced as repetitive behaviors or mental acts designed to neutralize, while ICD-10 requires a minimum duration of symptoms of two weeks. The two sets of criteria will probably be functionally equivalent. "Generalized anxiety disorder" is defined as more than six months of tension or anxiety and worry over everyday events and problems, accompanied by somatic symptoms of anxiety. ICD-10 requires more anxiety symptoms than DSM-IV, while DSM-IV requires that the worry handicaps and cannot be controlled. Again, despite specific differences (Slade and Andrews, 2001) the two definitions should be comparable in clinical practice. There is considerable difference in the threshold for PTSD, with ICD-10 identifying twice as many cases as DSM-IV. This is due to the absence of the numbing and clinical significance criteria in ICD-10 (Peters et al., 1999).

Diagnostic and assessment instruments

The treatment programs for each anxiety disorder described in subsequent chapters are designed to be used with patients whose disorders are consistent with the above DSM-IV and ICD-10 criteria. Although many of the elements of treatment occur in the different programs, the programs are still diagnosis specific. Accurate diagnosis and assessment of each patient is critical for effective treatment. The detailed issues about diagnosis and behavioral analysis in each disorder will be discussed in the relevant chapters, but some of the general issues will be mentioned here. A clinical diagnosis unsupported by other assessment tools may no longer be good mental health practice. Unsupported diagnoses are no longer good practice in any other branch of clinical medicine.

Forty-eight years ago, Meehl (1954) compared the accuracy of clinical versus statistical prediction on the same data. He concluded that statistical predictions were as least as accurate, and often more accurate, than the judgments of trained clinicians. Clinicians were indignant at Meehl's conclusions, for they considered that their judgments were the "gold standard" against which the tests had been developed and standardized. How could a statistical compilation of the tests be better than their judgments about the tests? The answer lies in reliability. Clinical judgment about the same data may vary from occasion to occasion and between any two sets of clinicians. Statistical compilations do not vary in this manner. Reliability is important because it is a prerequisite for validity. If a clinician cannot reach the same diagnosis on two occasions when reviewing the same clinical data, then the validity of at least one of the decisions is questionable. If two clinicians given the same clinical data cannot agree, then both cannot be correct, and the treatment prescribed by at least one of them will be wrong. Valid judgments depend on reliable judgments.

Structured diagnostic instruments were developed to improve the reliability of the clinical judgment as to how well a patient's complaints satisfied the diagnostic criteria. Such interviews have usually achieved their goal by modeling a clinical interview, the gains in validity coming from standardizing the content of the questions, as well as from the form of the interview and the scoring process. No matter how perfect the structured diagnostic interview, validity will be limited to the validity inherent in the diagnostic criteria on which that interview is based, and by the exactness with which the interview elicits the behaviors, thoughts, and feelings described by those diagnostic criteria. Interviews presently available were reviewed by Page (1991b).

The Anxiety Disorders Interview Schedule for DSM-IV (ADIS-IV) (Brown et al., 1994) is a semi-structured clinician administered diagnostic interview that produces DSM-III-R diagnoses. This schedule is very thorough, covers all the anxiety disorders, but can take two hours to administer. If the interviewer is appropriately trained, the ADIS-IV can provide a detailed and reliable assessment. The principal use is in small-scale clinical research requiring a very detailed assessment.

The CIDI is a fully structured diagnostic interview that can be administered by a trained interviewer. The computerized CIDI-Auto can be completed by an interviewer or directly by the patient, the computer taking care of the logic of this complex interview (Andrews and Peters, 1998). It was developed from the

Diagnostic Interview Schedule under the auspices of the World Health Organization and generates both ICD-10 and DSM-IV diagnoses. The CIDI is in modular form and covers the major categories of mental disorders. The interviewer version takes 30 minutes to cover the anxiety disorders, while the computerized version takes virtually no clinician time. The CIDI is reliable and widely used, being available in 14 languages. The principal uses are in epidemiological surveys, clinical research, and in clinical practice. Validity studies suggest a need for greater specificity, as the CIDI commonly identifies more comorbid diagnoses than do clinicians. However, diagnoses that are not critical can be quickly dismissed by the clinician, while false negative diagnoses, which would be of greater concern, are rare.

The Schedule for Affective Disorders and Schizophrenia (Endicott and Spitzer, 1978) is a semi-structured interview that has acceptable reliability and validity but, being time consuming, is most appropriate for clinical research. The Schedule for Clinical Assessment in Neuropsychiatry is a semi-structured diagnostic interview for experienced clinicians that can generate DSM-IV and ICD-10 diagnoses, although the scoring can be complex. This schedule aims to describe symptoms in a fashion that is independent of the current classifications. Good clinical judgment and considerable training is required before reliability is obtained. The Structured Clinical Interview for DSM-IV (First et al., 1997) is a semi-structured interview. The anxiety subsection is reliable and suitable for clinical research and practice. However, training is required.

There are a large number of questionnaires and rating scales that have been developed for the assessment of patients with anxiety disorders. Most clinicians have areas of special interest and will already be using appropriate scales. Test batteries suitable for clinical practice are described in subsequent chapters.

Epidemiology and health service utilization

Epidemiology is usually thought to have little to do with clinical practice. However, clinicians function in a real world where money and political decisions affect the ease with which they can provide their patients with good treatment. Information about disorder prevalence and health service financing is therefore an essential survival tool for clinicians. The Global Burden of Disease project (Murray and Lopez, 1996) defined the burden of any disease as the sum of the years of life lost plus the years lived with a disability weighted according to the severity of the disability associated with the disease. This sum was expressed as Disability Adjusted Life Years lost. In 1990 they reported that mental disorders accounted for 9% of the global burden of disease. The figure for established market economies like those of the USA, the UK and Australia was 22%, not because the burden of mental disorders was larger in those countries but because the burden of infectious and perinatal diseases was less. Only three anxiety disorders, PTSD, OCD and panic disorder, were included in the 1996 report, but it was of interest that the burden of those three disorders was, in the established market economies, equivalent to the burden of schizophrenia, each accounting for one-tenth of the burden of the mental disorders. The first set of burden calculations to include all the anxiety disorders was that published by Mathers et al. (1999). They reported that the anxiety disorders accounted for 24% of the burden of mental disorders in Australia. Affective disorders accounted for a third of the burden and schizophrenia 5% of the burden. Accompanying their estimates was a table of expenditure that showed that the anxiety disorders accounted for only 8% of the mental health system costs, despite accounting for 24% of the burden.

The anxiety disorders are common, probably the most common of all the mental disorders. The reported lifetime risks for each disorder have varied considerably according to the population being studied and the method being used. The USA national comorbidity survey of adults aged 15 to 54 years reported that 17.2% of adults had met criteria for an anxiety disorder in the past 12 months. These are the highest rates ever reported and this may be due to methodological factors: Kessler et al. (1994) used commitment and stem probes to enhance responses, adjusted for the higher morbidity among nonrespondents, used DSM-III-R criteria that did not have the clinical significance of DSM-IV criteria. Furthermore they asked about simple phobias that are not often a focus of clinical practice, utilized the wider DSM-III-R criteria for social phobia, and of unknown importance, inferred 12-month risk by asking whether respondents, who had met criteria in their lifetime, had had symptoms in the past 12 months, not whether they had met criteria during that time. The matching 12-month data from the Australian survey are presented in Table 2.2 (Andrews et al., 2001a). In this survey it was ascertained that people had met criteria for an anxiety disorder during the 12-month period. In both surveys the anxiety disorders were the most common class of mental disorder.

In the Australian survey of people aged 18 to 99 years (i.e., being representative of the whole adult population), with exclusion criteria operationalized, DSM-IV anxiety disorders had a 12-month prevalence of 5.6% and a one-month prevalence of 3.8%. Those with current symptoms reported being unable to work, or having to cut down on what they did, an average of 10 days out of the past 28 days, and their SF-12 mental competency score was 35.9, significantly below that of the average for all people with a current mental disorder. Anxiety disorders are disabling. Anxiety disorders were more common in females (odds ratio or OR = 1.6), less common in people over 54 (OR 0.4), more common among those separated, widowed or divorced (OR 1.9) or never married (OR 1.4), and less

Table 2.2 Twelve month prevalences of anxiety disorders in Australia (DSM-IV) and the USA (DSM-III-R), exclusion criteria not operationalized

	Australia, $N = 10\,641$ (DSM-IV, aged 18–54 years)		United States, $N = 8098$ (DSM-III-R, aged 15–54 years)	
	%	SE	%	SE
Panic disorder ± agoraphobia	2.3	0.2	2.3	0.3
Agoraphobia without panic	1.7	0.2	2.8	0.3
Social phobia	2.8	0.3	7.9	0.4
Simple phobia	Not assessed		8.8	0.5
Generalized anxiety disorder	4.1	0.4	3.1	0.3
Obsessive–compulsive disorder	0.8	0.1	Not assessed	
Posttraumatic stress disorder	1.7	0.2	Not assessed	
Any anxiety disorder	9.3	0.5	17.2	0.7

SE, standard error.

common among those with tertiary education or in the labor force (0.6). The demographic correlates of depression were virtually identical.

These disorders commonly begin early. The median age of onset for specific phobias is in childhood, for social phobias and OCD is in middle and late teenage, respectively, and for panic, agoraphobia, and GAD it is between 20 and 30 years of age. Many years pass between the onset of most disorders and patients obtaining treatment. Overall females are more commonly affected than males but in treatment programs for social phobia, OCD, and GAD, the sex ratios are close to parity. There is an important association between suicide attempts and anxiety disorders in young people.

In the Australian survey (Andrews et al., 2001b), only 44% of current cases had sought help "for a mental problem" in the previous 12 months. They were equally distributed between people who saw a general practitioner only, who saw a psychiatrist or psychologist as well, or who saw other health professionals. They averaged nine consultations in the year and accounted for 39% of all consultations for a mental problem. Half got a prescription, half got nonspecific counseling, and only one-sixth got cognitive behavioral therapy, the treatment of choice. The probability of seeking help was related to age, sex, disability, and marital status. Only 20% of males aged less than 24 years or over 54 years consulted, whereas 75% of females, aged 25 to 54 years and disabled and no longer married, consulted. The perceived need for treatment among those who did not consult was for information and psychological treatment, not for medication, the treatment most commonly offered. Perhaps that is why they did not consult.

In the past 20 years, there has been an explosive growth in knowledge about the anxiety disorders. Diagnostic criteria are agreed upon, and diagnostic and other assessment instruments have been shown to be reliable and valid. This book will demonstrate that the treatments are efficient and effective. Information as to causes, both specific and general, is emerging. It now behooves clinicians to treat patients with anxiety disorders actively and well.

3

General issues in treatment

Clinician Guide

Effective treatments for the anxiety disorders are reviewed in this book. Some treatments – the cognitive behavioral therapies (CBTs) for the major anxiety disorders – are described in considerable detail. The background to the principal cognitive behavioral techniques will be described in this chapter, together with the clinical issues that are important if clinicians are to convert this group of techniques into an effective treatment.

Cognitive behavioral techniques

In Chapter 2 we presented a model of anxiety in which current adverse life events or mental images of adverse events would cause a person to appraise the events for threat. If the decision was that the event, real or imagined, would be an unpredictable and uncontrollable threat, then the level of neuroticism moderated the extent of the arousal and the symptoms experienced. Once threatened and aroused, the individual had two tasks, to take control to ensure that anxiety was facilitating not debilitating, and to take control over strategies to negate the threat. The problem is that most people with high neuroticism quickly decide that threats, being unpredictable and uncontrollable, are unmanageable. Treatment should make most threats understandable and controllable. Dearousal strategies such as hyperventilation control, and to a lesser extent, meditation and relaxation, are methods to limit arousal. Graded exposure, either to symptoms of the disorder or to phobic situations, is the key to limiting arousal and mastering avoidance. Cognitive therapy is focused on the appraisal process: "Is this event or predicament really a threat?". Structured problem solving is about defining the threat or problem in such a way that solutions to some or all of the threat can be attempted and the problem, no longer uncontrollable, can gradually be mastered. Skilled therapists can help patients to recover by using only one of these techniques, say cognitive therapy or graded exposure, but most of us are pleased to use all four, albeit modified for the particular anxiety disorder. Marks (see Marks and Dar, 2000), once a strong proponent of exposure therapy, has argued that fear reduction is possible by all of the above techniques.

Dearousal strategies

Hyperventilation control

Breathing more deeply than is normal is part of the normal physiological response to threat. Hyperventilation to the point of developing symptoms (lightheadedness, dizziness, shortness of breath, feelings of suffocation, tingling or numbness in limbs, rapid heartbeat, chest pain or pressure, feelings of unreality) has long been observed in patients with anxiety disorders (Lowry, 1967; de Ruiter et al., 1989a; Holt and Andrews, 1989b). Kerr et al. (1937) used voluntary hyperventilation as an educational technique for such patients, presumably to familiarize patients with the cause of their symptoms. The emphasis in recent years has been on the importance of the hyperventilation response as a complication to panic (Garssen et al., 1983), and investigation of the treatment of overbreathing has been almost totally confined to this disorder. Rapee (1985b) presented a single case study in which the importance of hyperventilation in panic attacks was demonstrated to the patient by drawing attention to the similarity between the symptoms of panic and the symptoms produced by voluntary hyperventilation. He then had the patient repeatedly count her respiration rate at rest. Finally, the patient practiced slowing her respiration to an 8-second cycle and was encouraged to use this breathing rate whenever she noticed a panic attack beginning.

Clark et al. (1985) and Salkovskis (1986a) published two series of cases illustrating the effectiveness of voluntary hyperventilation for treating panic. After experiencing the symptoms produced by a period of voluntary hyperventilation (a form of interoceptive exposure), patients were able to control their panics better because they could reattribute the cause of their panic symptoms. These patients were then trained to breathe at a 5-second cycle and instructed to use this rate to control panics whenever they occurred.

The traditional cure for the symptoms of hyperventilation is to breathe into a paper bag to let the carbon dioxide level increase. There is no evidence that this technique is effective, presumably because it is never done as soon as the anxiety begins, or continued for long enough to produce the desired effect. The slow-breathing technique appears to work because the patient can initiate the slow breathing immediately anxiety or panic is anticipated and, because of the overlearning produced by regular practice, the technique can be deployed even when the patient is debilitated by the imminent anxiety or panic. Whether it works because it corrects the hyperventilation, because it distracts from the situation, or because it produces a relaxation response is unknown. There is sensible evidence that total reliance on controlling panic attacks by hyperventilation control may be maladaptive as the person never learns that panic attacks are not dangerous (Schmidt et al., 2000) but when coupled with interoceptive exposure to panic symptoms it remains of value. Hyperventilation control is one control technique that remains valuable when people are acutely anxious for whatever reason.

Meditation

Benson (1976) introduced a simplified yoga technique to the Western world in which subjects were instructed to sit quietly in a comfortable position, close their eyes, and concentrate on breathing and saying the word "one" each time they breathed out. Continuing this for 10 to 20 minutes and concentrating on the task whenever thoughts wandered, they would benefit by a feeling of calmness and a reversion of the flight or fight response. Benson produced data on the short-term changes that would result. It has never been shown to be of benefit in an anxiety disorder but patients, especially those with high neuroticism scores, report benefit. Again this is a control of arousal technique but not one that can be used in any acute situation.

Deep muscle relaxation was introduced to the Western world by Jacobson (1962). This technique involves the alternate tensing and relaxing of all muscle groups, often guided by a tape-recorded script. It, too, produces a lowering of arousal but the results have never been shown to be superior to placebo in people with anxiety disorders. Once people have learnt to use muscle contraction and release to produce a relaxation response they can use the abbreviated form of isometric deep muscle relaxation to produce a relaxation response in stressful situations. The experience of being able to control arousal by using isometric relaxation is beneficial, and regular practice of progressive muscular relaxation is beneficial for the muscle tension that is seen in people with GAD.

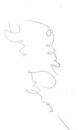

Exposure

Graded exposure is perhaps the most powerful technique assisting patients to overcome feared situations. The roots of these procedures are firmly based in learning theory as habituation or graduated extinction. In short, the procedures involve the gradual re-exposure of the individual to the fear- or anxiety-evoking stimuli. On the basis of information supplied by the patient, the therapist devises a series of exposure tasks arranged hierarchically, so that engagement in those behaviors can be performed without overwhelming anxiety. Progress through the hierarchy is systematic, commencing with behaviors that are minimally anxiety provoking and progressing through mastery of those to tasks that are more anxiety provoking.

Although similarities in form and mechanism may be noted with systematic desensitization (which primarily involves exposure in imagination), the procedures involved in graded exposure differ in two important ways. First, as much as possible of the exposure is conducted in the real world rather than in imagination. Second, no competing response such as relaxation is taught, and no response is designed to replace the anxiety response when the individual is exposed to the fear-evoking stimuli. All persons have to learn for themselves that their anxiety is groundless.

Exposure to fear-evoking cues as a method of alleviating anxiety is by no means a new procedure. Johann Wolfgang von Goethe provided an excellent account of self-directed exposure undertaken in the early 1770s to overcome a fear of heights, noise, darkness, and blood injury. In describing his self-administered treatment, he states, "Such troublesome and painful sensations I repeated until the impressions became quite indifferent to me" (cited by Eysenck, 1990).

Herzberg (1941) used graded exposure techniques to successfully treat a severely agoraphobic woman who was previously unable to leave her house. Grossberg (1965) utilized graded exposure techniques in the treatment of a woman with a circumscribed social phobia (fear of public speaking), allowing her to complete the graduation requirements of the college. Since these early investigations, controlled replication and extension of these applications have been undertaken, with the result that exposure therapy has become an integral part of the behavioral treatment of panic/agoraphobia, social phobia, specific phobias, OCD, and PTSD.

Exposure to the feared stimulus, leading to the conclusion that the fear is groundless, is the key. For many people the feared stimuli are the symptoms themselves, e.g., rapid heart beat in panic, or intrusive thoughts in OCD. Interoceptive exposure refers to the graded exposure to such internal symptoms until the sufferers lose their power to evoke anxiety. In panic disorder, interoceptive exposure is especially important in providing control.

Cognitive therapy

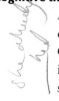

Although cognitive therapy is a relatively recent addition to behavioral procedures, the premise behind these techniques has a long history. The first century Greek philosopher Epictetus asserted that we are not affected by events but by our interpretation of those events. Changing the interpretation of events therefore should exert an influence on the effect those events have over the individual. Cognitive methods such as those espoused by Ellis (1957, 1962) derive directly from the belief that psychological disorders are the result of faulty or irrational patterns of thinking. The therapeutic techniques utilized in Rational Emotive Therapy aim to modify the irrational and faulty thinking and beliefs, replacing them with more rational patterns, and therefore alleviating the disorder. The essential feature is seen in the A-B-C-D-E paradigm.

"A"   refers to the event to which the individual is exposed.

"B"   refers to the chain of thoughts or self-verbalizations that the individual engages in as a response to "A".

"C"   is the emotional and behavioral responses that are a consequence of "B".

"D"   refers to the therapist's attempts at modification of the self-verbalizations and beliefs that occur at "B".

"E"   stands for the modified and beneficial emotional and behavioral consequences.

Another form of cognitive therapy was proposed by Beck (1976). As with Rational Emotive Therapy, the ultimate goal is the development of rational, adaptive thought patterns. Briefly, these patterns are achieved by making patients aware of their thoughts, a process by which they learn to identify inaccurate or distorted thinking. These inaccurate thoughts are replaced with more objective and accurate cognitions through a process of therapist feedback and through behavioral experiments designed to test the illogical thoughts. In the final stages of treatment, attention is given to challenging the underlying assumptions thought to generate the maladaptive cognitions in the first place.

Structured problem solving

Seeking to generate an application suitable for use in behavior modification, D'Zurilla and Goldfried (1971) reviewed the extensive literature on human problem solving. They conceptualized that patients, previously helpless and unable to solve their difficulties, could learn ways of approaching problems that would enable them to become more effective and eventually function "as their own therapists". They suggested that there was a consensus that effective problem solving was characterized by five general stages: a general orientation or set, problem definition and formulation, generation of alternatives, decision making, and verification. D'Zurilla and Goldfried also presented guidelines for clinical application, but the examples given did not seem particularly relevant to clinical practice.

Falloon et al. (1988) adapted the technique to form part of their effective behavioral family therapy package in schizophrenia. The structured problem-solving component encouraged patients and their families to identify the problem, generate a range of alternatives, identify the preferred alternative, and then implement this alternative. Then Falloon trained community mental health nurses to use the technique when working with patients with other mental disorders who were referred by their general practitioners. These patients commonly suffered from anxiety or depressive neuroses and the general practitioners reported (Andrews, 1990c) that the technique was of considerable benefit in converting previously dependent patients into persons who could cope better with, and control, subsequent problems and difficulties.

Structured problem solving with the characteristics identified by D'Zurilla and Goldfried (1971) has been shown to be better than group therapy or wait-list in patients with unipolar depression. Problem-solving effectiveness covaried with reduction in depression in the short and long term, as well as with the internalization of locus of control (Nezu, 1986). Salkovskis et al., (1990) showed that the technique, when compared with treatment as usual, was of benefit in patients at high risk of repeated suicide attempts, by reducing their target problems and depression and suicidal ideation, both at the end of treatment and 1 year later.

There are no controlled trials of the utility of the technique in patients with a specific anxiety disorder. On the basis of Falloon et al.'s (1988) work with patients identified in general practice, we included it as a component of the Patient Treatment Manuals and as a key component of the GAD treatment program. The steps are not different from those originally summarized by D'Zurilla and Goldfried (1971):

1. *Pinpoint the problem*: The first step is to get the patient to specify the key threat or problem and to ensure that it is a threat to them that will not be dealt with by any other person or agency. Overwhelming and complex problems can usually be broken down into a series of component parts, best specified as a list of discrete goals, one of which is identified as the target.

2. *List all possible solutions*: Next, have the patient specify a number of ideas to solve this problem. In this brainstorming approach, it does not matter if some of the solutions are impractical because even bizarre solutions may contain the germ of a good idea.

3. *Evaluate potential consequences*: Discuss the main advantages and disadvantages of each solution.

4. *Agree on the best strategy*: It is usually obvious that a particular solution is to be preferred. Practicality and the ability to carry out the solution now take precedence over better solutions that cannot be implemented promptly.

5. *Plan and implementation*: Patients should plan in considerable detail how to carry out the problem-solving behaviors. These plans must be written down in detail (telephone numbers, names and addresses, key phrases). When people implement the solution they will become anxious and fearful and will all too often forget or confuse the rational steps they had decided to use.

6. *Review results*: The results of the problem-solving attempt should then be reviewed and the clinician should applaud all attempts. Real problems are complicated, and further problem-solving endeavors are usually required. Importantly the problem can usually be redefined in the light of the progress made. Even if the first solution proves to be totally ineffective, something will have been learned that can be used to redefine the goal or the solution when the process is repeated.

Clinical issues

Diagnosis

All persons likely to benefit from treatments described in the manuals in this book suffer from panic disorder, agoraphobia, social phobia, specific phobia, OCD, GAD or PTSD. Failure to respond to previous treatment is not in itself a contraindication. Severity and chronicity are, if anything, positive criteria on which to select patients. Being severely handicapped and outraged at the interference that the disorder has produced in their freedom to live normally provides many patients with the impetus needed to work hard to recover. Recovery from an anxiety disorder is hard work and requires considerable courage.

The clinician is responsible for the accurate diagnostic work-up required to ensure that the symptoms meet the diagnostic criteria of ICD-10 or DSM-IV. A behavioral analysis that makes clear the circumstances that affect the occurrence of the symptoms and the cognitions that co-occur is also required. Curiosity seems to be the greatest attribute for a cautious clinician. "In case what occurred?" is the key question that is commonly used to elucidate the final fear. "In case I had a heart attack", "In case others saw me anxious and thought me weak", "in case harm to my family occurred", "In case everything went wrong", "In case the memories came back" are the thoughts characteristic of the individual anxiety disorders. Once the principal complaint is identified we recommend that the patients rate the extent that the disorder interferes with their life and activities (Figure 3.1). This scale serves two purposes: (1) it identifies the patient's principal goal in coming for treatment right at the beginning; and (2), when used repeatedly, it provides a sensitive and personalized measure to assess the reduction in handicap that follows good treatment.

Comorbidity

If two disorders coexist, and the anxiety disorder is judged to be primary and the comorbid condition secondary, then obviously it is better to treat the anxiety disorder. The single exception is substance abuse. Even persons who originally took alcohol or benzodiazepines for their anxiety disorder must cease their drug use before treatment for their anxiety disorder will be practical. Persons who have taken benzodiazepines for a long time and have become very dependent on them may not be able to be withdrawn and hence will not be able to fully benefit from the cognitive behavioral techniques. Some persons adjust to chronic benzodiazepine intake and it is a foolish clinician who seeks to get each and every such patient to cease this medication. One must consider the gains and costs of such a step. Withdrawal from benzodiazepines is difficult. We recommend that persons transfer to a long-acting benzodiazepine such as diazepam and then reduce their

After having discussed things with the doctor, you have said that your main problem is:

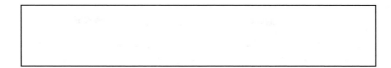

At the present time, how much does this problem interfere with your life and activities?

(please circle the number closest to your response on the rating scale below)

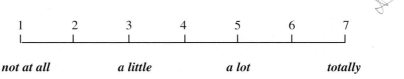

Figure 3.1   Main problem questionnaire.

dose by 10% of the preceding dose every 3 days. Even so it may take 10 weeks to withdraw and the last stages will be the most difficult.

If the anxiety disorder appears in the setting of another disorder, and is secondary to this disorder, then it will do little good to offer treatment for anxiety until the primary condition is resolved. If two conditions coexist but neither is causative, then the clinician should treat either the disorder that is more disabling or that which is easiest to remedy. The contraindication to treatment for anxiety disorders is concurrent substance abuse, because people cannot learn to control their anxiety while affected by, or still craving, drugs or alcohol.

Florid and severe personality disorder is another contraindication, simply because the anxiety is likely to be the least of the patient's difficulties. Often referrals of such patients to cognitive behavioral clinicians are acts of desperation in the hope that, somewhere, something can be done. Patients with psychoses certainly become anxious, and while the essential treatment should be aimed at the psychosis, help with anxiety using cognitive behavioral techniques can be of value. In our experience it is best if the therapist responsible for treating the psychosis carries out the CBT, simply because this therapy has to blend with the other treatments.

Patient motivation

The first question to be asked is "Why did you come for treatment now?". If the answer involves family, medical advisors, or other external factors then clinicians should be cautious before accepting the patient for treatment and inquire further as to whether the patient wants to work at recovering. We do not accept for treatment patients whose disorder is the subject of litigation, simply because motivation for recovery can be severely compromised by the prospect of monetary compensation. Recovery from an anxiety disorder requires courage. Persons have to be motivated if they are going to discipline themselves to manage their anxiety and confront their fears.

Patients need to become their own therapists. Most anxiety disorders are chronic and some patients have learned to be dependent on others or on drugs to solve their bad moments. They must learn to rely on themselves and accept that in the future they will not use medication or the protection of others when things become difficult. The more that the disorder has truly handicapped and produced suffering, the more likely the patients are to accept such responsibility. The more that they have been insulated from the pain of the anxiety by protective relatives or easily available medication, the less they are likely to make the independent steps required for recovery. It seems trite to say it, but patients do have to want to change if they are to benefit from these cognitive behavioral techniques.

After many years of illness and misguided or neglectful attempts at treatment, many patients are quite angry and dismissive about the possibility of successful treatment. It pays to explore this anger. "How do you feel about your previous treatment?" and "Do you believe that recovery is a possibility?" are two opening sentences that can be helpful. Most patients do want to recover. Some evidence that the clinician empathizes with the cost and hurt of prior poor treatment can facilitate an alliance that is essential to the therapeutic process.

The average clinician will be well aware that cognitive behavioral techniques are powerful and effective procedures that can be applied to a variety of other disorders including depression, schizophrenia, eating disorders, sexual and marital dysfunction, and to even less well-defined psychological problems and psychiatric difficulties. There are clinicians who view CBT as a superficial form of treatment that deals only with symptoms, while others abhor the idea that patients should be instructed in how to get better. Neither view is correct, and both views interfere with therapy.

Controlled trials have shown that dealing with symptoms can be an effective and permanent method of treating otherwise chronic and incapacitating disorders. The situation in the anxiety disorders is no different. Similarly, the notion that CBT is merely telling the patient what to do and think is a fallacy. Effective application of the techniques described in this book requires that patient and therapist collaborate. The primary roles of the therapist range from teaching patients how they could manage their disorders, guiding them through difficulties and, when required, supporting them as they reduce their avoidance and minimize other tactics they may implement to delay having to confront their fears and concerns. Achievement of these aims is impossible if the patient is merely told what to do. By the time they present for treatment, they have certainly been told what to do by innumerable concerned friends, relatives, and well-meaning but poorly trained health professionals.

Guiding patients as they become free from pathological fears is different from telling patients what to think. Clinicians must encourage patients to become actively engaged in the treatment process. An understanding, empathic approach is required if the relationship is to be therapeutic. Patients present for treatment when they are distressed, and many are acutely aware of inadvertent comments or behaviors that appear to minimize their condition. If a clinician appears dismissive, it will inhibit progress and undermine commitment to treatment. Similarly, hearing that other patients have similar difficulties may provide reassurance. However, treating complaints as commonplace (and therefore boring) will serve only to alienate the individual who has finally plucked up the courage to attend for treatment. Thus, apart from being understanding and empathic, the treating clinician should have a genuine interest in the welfare and recovery of the patient.

Rabavilas et al. (1979) asked phobic and obsessive–compulsive patients who had been treated with behavioral techniques to rate their therapists on 16 variables related either to the therapist's attitude or to the way in which the therapist conducted treatment. Patients who rated their therapists as respectful, understanding, interested, encouraging, challenging, and explicit, improved the most. Patients who rated their therapist as gratifying their dependency needs, or as permissive and tolerant did less well.

Given the nature of treatment and the primary goal of having patients learn techniques to deal with their symptoms, it is important for the clinician to discourage dependency. An effective teacher of cognitive behavioral techniques will rarely run into difficulties with dependency, primarily because the treatment gains are always attributed to the patients having learned, adopted, and implemented the effective procedures being taught by the therapist. Difficulties with people with dependency needs will arise when the therapist projects the image of an omnipotent expert who fails to educate the patient about the condition and its treatment, and who attributes change to their own therapeutic skill rather than to the work of the patient.

Although CBT procedures are effective and the benefits long lasting, the progress of treatment requires some discussion. Rarely will the application of these procedures run smoothly and be trouble free. The rate of progress fluctuates and problems with patient motivation appear as therapy progresses. Patients come for treatment when their desire to overcome their disorder is stronger than their fear of confronting their feared situations. Progress falters when the tasks being set appear too difficult. Clinicians confronted with an apparent loss of motivation should determine the reasons for the hesitation and encourage the patient to continue. Encouragement may take the form of pointing out the patient's achievements to date, as well as the personal cost of continuing to be affected by the condition. Commonly, patients are more concerned with the tasks they must complete as part of treatment. By focusing only on the task at hand, they tend to lose sight of their achievements, as well as forgetting the distress and discomfort their condition has caused them. Focusing the patient on these wider issues in times of waning motivation often helps to stabilize the situation. Motivational interviewing is discussed in Chapter 14.

In all anxiety disorders, patients have to face their fears if fears are to lose their salience. Refusal by the patient may reflect poor program design or may be a function of anticipatory anxiety. A re-examination of the program with the patient may be required in order to determine whether the expected rate of progress is too rapid or unrealistic. If it is, a more graded program of exposure can be set. If anticipatory anxiety is the key, then reinforcing achievements as well as analyzing the expected difficulties using cognitive restructuring may assist. Finally, and of considerable importance, humor is an essential and invaluable tool for assisting patients to deal with, and face, difficult situations. Humor is, and always has been, one of the best defenses against anxiety.

The role of concurrent medication

Benzodiazepine drugs, as will be discussed in the appropriate chapters, seem to be contraindicated on two grounds. First, they interfere with the generalization of new skills learned during psychotherapy to a drug-free state. Second, even when the pharmacodynamics make benefit impossible, patients misattribute successes to having taken a tablet and attribute failures to their own poor grasp of technique. No one should be asked to do a task where the ownership of success can never be theirs. Antidepressant drugs seem to be different. Although these drugs do not interfere with treatment, it is our practice to withdraw medication from those patients who were given it for their anxiety disorder and to continue medication in those patients who were given it for depression. Serotonergic antidepressants in OCD should be regarded similarly and their continuation discussed with the patient. Most wish to try to control their disorder without drugs, even if they are somewhat apprehensive. Some want to remain on drugs and hope that the CBT will produce additional benefit. Whatever the rationale, no medication should be withdrawn abruptly.

Therapist motivation

It is very easy for clinicians to become demoralized. By definition, all clinicians see the difficult-to-treat and slow-to-recover patients a large number of times. They see the quick-to-recover patients much less frequently. Thus, whenever they look at their appointment books they experience a sense of relative failure; the book is full of the slow-to-improve patients. This is as it should be, for once the quick-to-improve patients have recovered they do not return but continue with their lives independently of continuing medical or psychological help. Colleagues reinforce this whole process by saying they have just seen your patient who is once again having difficulties. One forgets that, by definition, they will never see your other patients who are doing well. We have done a number of follow-up studies and the results have routinely been reassuring; the total cohort of patients does, on average, twice as well as the patients who currently fill the waiting room.

All this angst over therapist effectiveness would be academic if demoralization in the clinician did not lead to a sense of futility, a sense that carrying out specific treatment programs may not be worthwhile, and the nihilistic idea that the "What shall we do today?" type of therapy is permissible. It is not. The key message of this book is that specific and effective treatments exist. Therapists must therefore make an accurate diagnosis and from this develop an appropriate therapy plan. Once this plan is made, there is only one step to take. Just do the therapy to the best of your, and your patient's, abilities.

4

Panic disorder and agoraphobia

Syndrome

Individuals with panic disorder and agoraphobia present for treatment describing "panic attacks" and varying degrees of fear-driven situational avoidance. Correspondingly, treatment aims to modify the symptoms that the person labels as "panic attacks" and to reduce any avoidance. Even though the causal link between panic disorder and fearful avoidance is recognized, the major diagnostic systems draw a qualitative distinction between the panic attacks and agoraphobic avoidance.

Diagnosis

DSM-IV implies a temporal relationship between panic attacks and agoraphobic avoidance. A panic attack is characterized by: fear; feeling dizzy or faint; choking, shortness of breath, or smothering; and fears of dying, going crazy, or losing control. Primacy is given to panic disorder, which describes recurrent unexpected panic attacks or incapacitation caused by panic attacks (characterized by concern about additional attacks or worry about the consequences of future attacks). A diagnosis of panic disorder is typically given as occurring with or without agoraphobia. Agoraphobia is defined as "anxiety about being in places or situations in which escape might be difficult (or embarrassing) or in which help may not be available in the event of having an unexpected or situationally predisposed panic attack". Situations characteristically avoided include being outside the home alone, traveling alone, being in tunnels, on bridges, and in open spaces. Agoraphobia without a history of panic attacks remains in the nosology, probably for historical reasons. In epidemiological studies, the diagnosis appears not infrequently (e.g., Robins and Regier, 1991), but such cases are rarely seen in clinical practice. When individual cases are examined, either they involve anxiety attacks that do not meet the particular cut-off scores for a DSM or ICD diagnosis of a panic attack (Barlow, 1988), or they appear to be better described as a specific phobia (i.e., claustrophobia; Friend and Andrews, 1990). In contrast to DSM-IV,

ICD-10 does not imply a primacy of panic attacks in its nosological structure. Agoraphobia is listed under phobic anxiety disorders and is defined behaviorally by "an interrelated and often overlapping cluster of phobias embracing fears of leaving home: fear of entering shops, crowds, and public places, or of traveling alone in trains, buses, or planes... The lack of an immediately available exit is one of the key features of many of these agoraphobic situations." Although agoraphobia is acknowledged to occur with or without panic disorder, panic disorder (or "episodic paroxysmal anxiety") itself is placed within a category of "other anxiety disorders".

Empirical studies favor the organization found in DSM-IV rather than in ICD-10. In patients who seek treatment, panic disorder typically occurs before agoraphobia (Aronson and Logue, 1987; Franklin, 1987; Garvey et al., 1987). Agoraphobia is characterized less by a fear of certain situations and more by a fear of having a panic in those situations (Franklin, 1987).

In terms of clinical practice, the separation between the two disorders primarily serves a descriptive function indicating the extent to which a person is going to require treatment that targets the agoraphobic avoidance in addition to merely the panic. The greater the avoidance, the greater the amount and proportion of time that will be spent modifying the avoidance. In our experience, it is very rare to see an individual with long-standing panic attacks who has no situational avoidance at all, just as it is very rare to see someone with agoraphobic avoidance who has no attacks of anxiety.

In clinical settings, diagnoses are typically made following an interview with the patient. When greater reliability and validity than the typical interview is desired, structured diagnostic interviews provide an important and valuable clinical and research resource. Selection of a structured diagnostic interview will ultimately depend upon local needs, but arguably the most comprehensive, valid interview is the revised Anxiety Disorders Interview Schedule (ADIS-R; Di Nardo and Barlow, 1988). It achieves in-depth coverage of the anxiety disorders, albeit at the expense of covering a narrow range of disorders (Page, 1991b). If broader coverage is required, the (computerized) Composite International Diagnostic Interview (Peters and Andrews, 1995; Andrews et al., 1999b) is a particularly good candidate.

Clinical description
CASE STUDY

Ms. W., a 33-year-old female, presented to an anxiety clinic after reading a magazine article describing hypochondriasis. For the past 10 years, she has received "far too many" medical investigations because of her belief that she is having a heart attack.

History of presenting complaint

Ten years ago, while attending a postnatal exercise class following the birth of her only child, she noticed a dramatic increase in her heart rate. Afraid she was going to die of a heart attack, she also noted a series of other symptoms. Her breathing became difficult, there was tingling in her hands, her muscles (most noticeably on the left side) became stiff, she was sweating, trembling, and she reported intense stabbing pains in the chest. She left her baby at the class and ran for help. An electrocardiograph was administered but no abnormality was detected. From that time on, a pattern developed in which at least three times a month she notices heart palpitations, becomes frightened that they signal a heart attack, and seeks reassuring medical advice. Since the first "heart attack", Ms. W. has had great difficulty going on her own to places where medical help could not be obtained quickly. She can travel alone, provided she takes her new mobile telephone with her, for she perceives that this will enable her to contact emergency services. Even so, she avoids crowded banks, shopping centers, and movie theaters in case her escape is blocked. Without her telephone she is not prepared to leave home alone.

Previous personal and psychiatric history

Initially she was treated with a variety of beta blockers for an "irritable heart". Her local medical practitioner has prescribed diazepam for the past eight years. The diazepam (present dose is 30 mg per day) appears to make no difference to the frequency of her "heart attacks". An only child, she describes her parents as being "worriers" but they have had no contact with psychiatric services. Born and raised in a large city, she left school to attend secretarial college. After working for 6 years she became pregnant, married, and remained at home thereafter. She presently works part-time for her solicitor husband.

Investigations

A routine physical check-up, full blood count, and thyroid function test detected no pathology. She reports drinking three cups of weak coffee per day and consumes one glass of wine per day after reading that alcohol decreases the risk of heart attacks. She describes herself as always being a "quiet, nervous type" with labile moods. Her responses to the Eysenck Personality Questionnaire indicate high neuroticism and moderate introversion. Her scores on the Agoraphobic Cognitions Questionnaire and the Anxiety Sensitivity Inventory were both very high, while her score on the Beck Depression Inventory indicated very mild depressive symptoms.

The above case study illustrates three common observations about panic disorder with agoraphobia. First, the disorder had a clear onset, which the sufferer dated to her first attack of panic (Uhde et al., 1985; Aronson and Logue, 1987; Franklin, 1987; Garvey et al., 1987). Second, the avoidance of situations developed subsequent to the panic attack, because she feared the consequences of having a panic in certain situations (Goldstein and Chambless, 1978). Third, the panic attack involved a dramatic increase in sympathetic arousal, the true origin of which was unclear to the individual (Franklin, 1990b) and subsequently was misinterpreted as a sign of serious physical pathology (Clark, 1986, 1988).

Differential diagnosis

A diagnosis of panic disorder must rule out physical and other psychological pathology. Typically, individuals have first presented to a medical practitioner who will have conducted a full medical assessment. It is useful to ensure that diseases that mimic panic attacks have been excluded at this time. Such pathologies include hypoglycemia, hyperthyroidism, Cushing syndrome, pheochromocytoma, vestibular disturbances, and mitral valve prolapse syndrome. It is also necessary to evaluate the extent to which substance problems have caused or exacerbated the presenting problem. Although the illicit drugs and alcohol quickly come to mind, it is important to exclude excessive caffeine intake. Differential diagnosis from other psychopathology can be more problematic. Disorders that need to be actively excluded include many of the other anxiety disorders. In OCD, the individual worries less that anxiety will cause a disease (e.g., a heart attack), but that, by an act of omission or commission, some thought or behavior will cause disease or injury. Although individuals with panic disorder exhibit PTSD-like symptoms in response to their panic attacks (Barlow, 1988), the focus in PTSD is the traumatic event that is the cause of the panicky symptoms. Although people with agoraphobic avoidance may fear negative evaluation in social settings, their fear is a consequence of what they believe the panic may cause them to do (e.g., lose bladder control). In contrast, in social phobia, the panic is a consequence of the scrutiny of others (see Page, 1994c). When differential diagnosis between social phobia and agoraphobia is difficult, a potentially useful algorithm involves coding +1 every time a patient endorses (1) feeling dizzy or lightheaded in a panic attack, (2) avoiding traveling on public transportation alone, and a score of −1 every time a patient endorses (3) avoiding speaking to strangers, (4) fearing blushing, shaking, or feeling foolish, and (5) fearing eating with others. Patients with a score of zero or above are more likely to suffer from panic disorder and agoraphobia, whereas patients who score −1 and lower are more likely to suffer from social phobia (Page, 1994c). Separation anxiety disorder also needs to be ruled out when making a diagnosis of agoraphobia. The principal difference will be in terms of the age of onset, with separation anxiety disorder occurring in children. In separation anxiety disorder, the child often (although not always) worries about traumatic consequences happening to others (e.g., a parent) when separated. In agoraphobia, individuals worry about possible traumatic events befalling themselves when separated from supports and sources of help.

The most difficult differential diagnosis is between claustrophobia and agoraphobia. Agoraphobia has been defined (in DSM-IV), in part, as anxiety about being in places or situations from which escape might be difficult or embarrassing. Individuals with claustrophobia will report anxiety in the very same situations.

DSM-IV suggests that if "agoraphobia" is limited to a few specific situations (e.g., enclosed spaces, such as in claustrophobia), then consider a diagnosis of specific phobia. Conceptually and practically, it is difficult to separate claustrophobia from agoraphobia. When the ages of onset of all the different phobias are examined, two patterns emerge. Most of the phobias emerge in childhood and early adolescence, except for agoraphobia and claustrophobia (Ost, 1987a). These two disorders tend to emerge after adolescence, suggesting that other similarities may exist. In fact, Friend and Andrews (1990) followed up people reporting agoraphobia without panic attacks, and found that in most cases the person met diagnostic criteria for a specific phobia, usually claustrophobia. Although sufferers of either disorder may report fear in situations from which escape may be difficult, our clinical rule of thumb is to ask individuals to identify the primary source of their fear. We ask, "Do you fear having a panic attack in an enclosed space because you cannot escape with ease (i.e., agoraphobia), or does being in an enclosed space and unable to get out make you panic (i.e., claustrophobia)?". However, since cognitive behavioral treatment will involve the patient in controlling anxiety as well as in confronting fears, differential diagnosis will not alter treatment dramatically.

Assessment

Having made a diagnosis, it is useful to assess formally the factors relevant to treatment. While a behavioral analysis (Kirk, 1989; Schulte, 1997) will provide a solid foundation for understanding the individual case and tailoring treatment appropriately, standard assessments provide comparison data otherwise unavailable in a clinical interview.

Given that panic disorder and agoraphobia are argued to be manifestations of a General Neurotic Syndrome (Andrews, 1990b), assessment should cover the underlying neurotic vulnerability as well as the neurotic symptoms. The Neuroticism subscale of the Eysenck Personality Questionnaire Revised (EPQ-R; Eysenck and Eysenck, 1975) has proved itself in both research and clinical practice (Andrews, 1996) as a good measure of the underlying vulnerability. The Depression Anxiety Stress Scale (DASS; Lovibond and Lovibond, 1995) is a particularly useful measure of general neurotic symptoms. The DASS is a noncostly measure that distinguishes between anxiety and depression better than do other measures (Lovibond and Lovibond, 1995), it has excellent psychometric properties (Brown et al., 1997) and the factor structure seems more stable than other measures.

In order to assess the more disorder-specific aspects of panic disorder and agoraphobia, see Bouchard et al. (1997) and Page (1998a) for reviews. However, by way of summary, Shear and Maser (1994) recommended that assessment cover

(1) panic frequency, severity, and duration, (2) panic-related phobias, (3) anticipatory anxiety, (4) impairment and general quality of life, and (5) global problem severity. In this context, the Panic and Agoraphobia Scale (P&A; Bandelow, 1995) is a short clinician- or client-rated scale that is particularly good. A global severity score can be obtained, but five subscales are also available (panic severity, frequency, and duration; phobic avoidance anticipatory anxiety disability and health-related worries). A similar measure is a clinician-scored diary called the Panic-Associated Symptoms Scale (PASS; Scupi et al., 1992). The scale measures situational panics, spontaneous panics, limited symptom attacks, anticipatory anxiety, and phobic avoidance. A general severity score is obtainable by summing the subscales. The P&A and PASS are similar, and clinician-rated versions correlate highly; however, they have different strengths. The PASS does not rely on retrospective reports, but the P&A is more time efficient. Thus the P&A represents a rapid, psychometrically sound (albeit retrospective) instrument to assess the major aspects of panic disorder. If an additional assessment of agoraphobic avoidance is required, the Mobility Inventory for Agoraphobia (Chambless et al., 1985) is a 27-item scale designed to measure agoraphobic avoidance behavior both alone and when accompanied. Further, it also provides an estimate of panic frequency in the last week.

In addition to these general measures of the disorder, specific panic symptom measures fall into two categories (Bouchard et al., 1997): assessments of panic-related symptoms and panic-related cognitions. The panic-related symptom instrument with the most psychometric data is the Panic Attacks Symptom Questionnaire (PASQ; Clum et al., 1990). The PASQ has broad symptom coverage, it focuses on the symptoms, and it measures symptom duration. In terms of assessing panic-related cognitions the Agoraphobic Cognitions Questionnaire (ACQ; Chambless et al., 1984) and the Body Sensations Questionnaire (BSQ) stand out. The BSQ (Chambless, 1988) discriminates panic disorder patients from normals and patients with other anxiety disorders. The ACQ further discriminates panic disorder patients from those who also have agoraphobia (Chambless and Gracely, 1989). Furthermore, the BSQ provides an index of fear intensity, whereas the ACQ measures the frequency of catastrophic cognitions (Chambless, 1988). Together the ACQ and BSQ provide a good assessment of cognitions associated with panic disorder.

In summary, following diagnosis, a comprehensive assessment of panic disorder should include measures of common neurotic symptoms, the underlying vulnerability, a treatment-sensitive assessment of panic and its consequences, and indices of panic-related symptoms and cognitions. Each domain has a number of potential candidate measures, of which a suggested list is included in Table 4.1.

Table 4.1. Domains of a comprehensive assessment of panic disorder, suggested prototype instruments for each domain, and recommendations about when to administer (adapted from Page, 1998a)

Domain	Instrument	Pre	During	Post	Follow-up
Diagnosis	ADIS or CIDI	Yes		If possible	
Neurotic vulnerability	EPQ-N	Yes		Yes	Yes
Neurotic symptoms	DASS	Yes		Yes	Yes
Panic and its effects	P&A	Yes	Yes	Yes	Yes
Panic symptoms	PASQ	Yes		Yes	Yes
Panic cognitions	ACQ & BSQ	Yes		Yes	Yes

EPQ-N, Eysenck Personality Questionnaire – Neuroticism Subscale.
For other abbreviations, see the text.

Etiology

Vulnerability

Initially, it was hoped that there was a unique biological predisposition to panic attacks. The four main pieces of evidence giving rise to this hope were differential responses to particular pharmacological treatments, the specificity of responses to biological challenge tests, the spontaneity of panic attacks, and a unique genetic predisposition. However, when subjected to rigorous evaluation, the specificity hypothesis has been usurped by a hypothesis of a general neurotic vulnerability. First consider the specificity of treatment response: on the basis of pharmacological dissection, Klein (1964) argued for a unique substrate to panic. Tricyclic antidepressants reportedly blocked panic but not anticipatory anxiety, while benzodiazepines reduced anticipatory anxiety but not panic. Although inferring etiology solely on the basis of treatment response is questionable (Barlow and Craske, 1988; Mattick et al., 1995), more recent studies have found that, in contrast to Klein's original position, tricyclics can alleviate generalized anxiety (see Kahn et al., 1986; Hunt and Singh, 1991) and high dose/potency benzodiazepines can reduce panic (Dunner et al., 1986). Second, it was hoped that certain challenge tests would function as biological markers for panic attacks and panic disorder (see Dager et al., 1987). Despite numerous attempts using a variety of substances and procedures (e.g., sodium lactate, hyperventilation, carbon dioxide inhalation), the differences between subjects with and without frequent panic attacks have ultimately been attributable to baseline differences in arousal (e.g., Ehlers et al., 1986a,b; Klein and Ross, 1986; Margraf et al., 1986; Ley, 1988; Holt and

Andrews, 1989a,b). That is to say, anxious subjects reach higher levels of arousal/ anxiety in response to the challenge than do controls, by virtue of their higher baseline levels of arousal/ anxiety before the challenge test. Third, it was originally argued that, because panic attacks were spontaneous, they must solely reflect the operation or "firing" of some endogenous dysfunction (Klein, 1981). The main problem for this assertion is that the apparent spontaneity of panic cannot explain the similarity in symptom profiles between situationally cued and "spontaneous" panic attacks (Margraf et al., 1987). Barlow (1988) has suggested that it is more profitable to describe panic attacks as being expected or unexpected and cued or uncued. The term "uncued" is preferable to "spontaneous" because it describes the phenomenon rather than carrying implicit assumptions about presumed etiology. Furthermore, although the initial panic attack is a surprising and puzzling experience (Franklin, 1990a), the majority of panic disorder patients describe their panic attacks as cued and expected (Goldstein and Chambless, 1978; Street, Craske and Barlow cited by Barlow, 1988). The final set of data expected to support the unique etiology of panic attacks was the familial tendency observed in panic disorder (see Crowe, 1985). As discussed in Chapter 2, the genetic studies support the notion that there is a heritable component to panic disorder and agoraphobia (e.g., Pauls et al., 1980; Crowe et al., 1983; Kendler et al., 1993). However, the predisposition is not specific to panic or agoraphobia. Rather the strongest statement the current data can support is that the predisposition is a general trait of anxiety proneness (e.g., neuroticism; see Torgersen, 1983; Roth, 1984; Andrews et al., 1990b). The notion of a general predisposition to neurosis is consistent with the finding that attacks of panic are found across the anxiety disorders; the main distinctions between disorders can be made whether panics are experienced as expected or unexpected, cued or uncued (Barlow, 1988), and the meaning with which the symptoms are imbued. In addition to the general trait of anxiety proneness, a number of risk factors have been associated with the onset of panic disorder and agoraphobia. First, a variety of studies have found that stressful life events precede the onset of the disorder (Faravelli, 1985; Faravelli and Pallanti, 1989; Franklin and Andrews, 1989; Pollard et al., 1989). Interestingly, it appears that it is not an increased frequency of life events per se that precedes the onset of panic attacks, but a negative perception of the importance of the life events by clinically anxious patients relative to normal controls. (Once again, there were no differences between the various anxiety disordered groups, but all differed from normal controls.) The reason why life events are rated more negatively has been attributed to a variety of factors, including personality factors (such as trait anxiety or neuroticism, discussed in Chapter 2), social supports, physical health (Roth and Holmes, 1985; Andrews, 1990a, 1991), and early loss (Faravelli et al., 1985).

By way of summary: panic disorder and agoraphobia share with the other anxiety disorders a general tendency towards anxiety proneness. While the exact nature of the phenotypic expression of the genotype is still debated (see Chapter 2), more recent theoretical accounts have speculated about the effect of a non-specific proneness to anxiety. Barlow (1988) has suggested that the increased vulnerability implies that the flight or fight response (Cannon, 1927) is more easily triggered. The emergency response may be triggered under potentially dangerous circumstances (i.e., it is a "true alarm"). Alternatively, it may be triggered in the absence of potential danger but in response to the negative perception of life stressors (i.e., it is a "false alarm"). While various biological substrates have been suggested (see Barlow, 1988; Gray, 1988; Gorman et al., 1989; Andrews et al., 1990b), the key point is that the action tendencies of the flight or fight response are triggered inappropriately. Consequently, the individual learns to expect that certain situations will trigger the "alarm", so that one of the strongest predictors of agoraphobic avoidance is the expectation that a panic attack (i.e., a false alarm) will occur in a given situation (Telch et al., 1989). Although the anxiety response may be more easily triggered in individuals with anxiety disorders, the failure to clearly identify a unique biological substrate to panic attacks has meant that attention has moved to searching for the etiological factors that channel an individual with high trait anxiety to develop panic disorder and agoraphobia as opposed to another anxiety disorder. One area of interest has been to examine the cognitive processes of panickers; another has been to examine the role of hyperventilation as a cause or exacerbater of panic attacks.

Hyperventilation

Hyperventilation describes increases in the rate or depth of breathing that produces a higher degree of ventilation than what is necessary to meet the body's demands. The end result is that alveolar and arterial carbon dioxide pressures decrease (P_{CO_2}) and blood pH rises. Sustained hyperventilation produces a variety of changes including arterial constriction, increased neural excitability, increased lactic acid production, lowered arterial phosphate levels, and a decreased ability for oxygen to pass from the blood to the body's cells (Missri and Alexander, 1978; Magarian, 1982; Ley, 1988). These physiological changes are believed to produce a characteristic set of physical changes including dizziness, confusion, disorientation, light-headedness, and parasthesias. The particular pattern of symptoms has been labeled the "hyperventilation syndrome". The similarity of the symptoms of the hyperventilation syndrome to a panic attack (Garssen et al., 1992) has led to two hypotheses. The first hypothesis is that hyperventilation causes panic attacks; the second is that hyperventilation is involved in the exacerbation of panic attacks. The first hypothesis is supported by a number of pieces of data including the finding that patients with panic attacks recognize the symptoms produced by voluntary hyperventilation as similar to the symptoms of panic. In addition, during spontaneous panic attacks, P_{CO_2} levels decrease (Salkovskis et al., 1986b; Griez et al., 1988) suggesting that hyperventilation is occurring. However, there are a number of findings not consistent with the hypothesis that panic attacks are caused by hyperventilation alone (Gorman et al., 1984; Griez et al., 1988). These data include findings that, while reported panic attacks produced by lactate infusions were associated with hyperventilation (Gorman et al., 1984), voluntary hyperventilation did not produce a clear panic attack (Gorman et al., 1984; Griez et al., 1988), and although panics are associated with drops in P_{CO_2}, the decrease is not of a sufficient magnitude to indicate acute hyperventilation (van Zijderveld et al., 1999). Further, Hibbert and Pilsbury (1989) found no difference between the symptoms of panic attacks with and without hyperventilation. Moreover only around 50% of patients with panic disorder demonstrate reductions in arterial P_{CO_2} (Garssen et al., 1992). Finally, Roll (1987, cited by Garssen et al., 1992) has demonstrated that a challenging mental task produced as frequent an endorsement of symptoms associated with the hyperventilation syndrome (despite no evidence of changes in end-tidal P_{CO_2}) as did the hyperventilation provocation test (see also Hornsveld et al., 1990). Data from our group suggest that hyperventilation may be one path leading to panic, but it is neither necessary nor sufficient. Holt and Andrews (1989a) used hyperventilation (as well as other panic provocation procedures) and found that the chief difference between individuals with panic disorder and other anxiety disorders was not in terms of the symptoms generated but in the catastrophic interpretations placed on the symptoms. Furthermore, hyperventilation was not found to be unique to panic disorder and agoraphobia. Instead, hyperventilation appeared to occur during periods of high anxiety (presumably thereby increasing the number of symptoms experienced in a natural episode of high anxiety).

In summary, it appears that hyperventilation can produce symptoms that overlap with those symptoms reported during a panic attack. In addition, a large proportion of patients with panic disorder appear to hyperventilate during panic attacks. However, it cannot be concluded that hyperventilation causes panic attacks, because panic attacks can occur without evidence of hyperventilation, hyperventilation does not always cause panic attacks, and the same symptoms can be produced without hyperventilation. Rather, it appears that (some of) the symptoms of a panic attack can be produced by a variety of methods, one of which is hyperventilation. The question then becomes, how do the symptoms produced by hyperventilation (or any other means) relate to the experience of panic? One answer to the question can be found among cognitive models of panic.

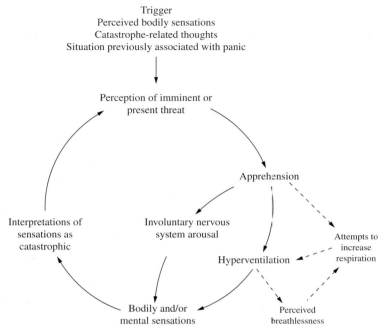

Figure 4.1   A cognitive model of panic attacks. (Modified from Salkovskis, PM (1988) Hyperventilation and anxiety. *Current Opinion in Psychiatry*, **1**, 78.)

Cognitions

Various models of the ways in which cognitive processes contribute to the production of panic attacks (e.g., Clark, 1986, 1988; Beck, 1988, see Figure 4.1) have been proposed. Although there are important differences between the accounts, they share the common premise that patients with panic attacks process information in the external environment, as well as internal somatic stimuli, as though they were threatening. Before considering the models, it is worth examining the data regarding the ways in which individuals with panic attacks process information differently from normal controls and individuals with other anxiety disorders.

The first area in which patients with panic disorder (with and without agoraphobia) have been found to differ from normal individuals is in their expectancies of danger and in their perceptions of control. Individuals with panic attacks report fearing loss of control. Consistent with this is the finding that when patients were informed, during a carbon monoxide challenge test, that they could control the intensity of their bodily sensations using a dial, only 20% reported a panic attack (Sanderson et al., 1989). In contrast, 80% of patients who believed that they had no control over the gas reported panic. Similarly, informing patients of the expected symptoms produced by carbon dioxide inhalation decreased the frequency of catastrophic thoughts and ratings of anxiety (Rapee et al., 1986). One interpretation of these data is that panic attacks occur when people experience sensations over which they feel they have no control.

Related to the supposition that panic attacks are associated with a perception of lack of control is the finding that anxious patients exhibit biases in the interpretation of ambiguous information. For example, McNally and Foa (1987) found that agoraphobics interpret ambiguous scenarios in a more threatening manner than do either normal controls or treated agoraphobics. The interpretation was not specific to internal stimuli, but was found also in response to external stimuli. In addition to the biased interpretations of information, differential encoding of anxiety-related information has been reported. Panic patients allocate attention preferentially towards threat cues in a variety of paradigms (e.g., Burgess et al., 1981; Ehlers et al., 1988; Hope et al., 1990), which is not only a function of familiarity with the stimuli (see McNally, 1990). Furthermore, there is some evidence that individuals with panic disorder have a memory bias for threat-related information. Nunn et al. (1984) reported superior recall of phobic material among agoraphobics as compared with normal controls (see also McNally et al., 1989). However, it should be noted that differential recall may indicate a bias at the input stage (i.e., an attentional bias) or at the output stage (i.e., a retrieval bias). There are some data that imply that the former is more likely (e.g., Mathews et al., 1989; for a discussion, see Williams et al., 1997). For present purposes, it is sufficient to note that there is a body of evidence that individuals with panic disorder – with and without agoraphobia – selectively process threat-related information. The end result is that ambiguous and potentially threatening information is preferentially attended to and recalled by individuals with anxiety disorders.

However, while there is some evidence that particular anxiety disorders exhibit selective processing of material specific to their disorder (Ehlers et al., 1988; Hope et al., 1990; McNally et al., 1990a,b; Foa et al., 1991a), the existence of automatic selective processing favoring threatening information appears to be present across all anxiety disorders (Williams et al., 1997). Putting together these data, a number of statements about cognitive processing in panic disorder and agoraphobia can be made. First, attention will be oriented automatically towards threat-related information; recall for such information will be higher than that for neutral information. Second, ambiguous internal and external stimuli will be interpreted in a threatening manner. These summary statements are consistent with the cognitive models of panic (see Beck, 1988; Clark, 1988). Each argues that certain (otherwise innocuous) cues are interpreted in a threatening manner that triggers anxiety. The elicitation of anxiety (and associated hyperventilation) produces certain bodily sensations that are once again interpreted in a threatening manner and future attacks are anxiously anticipated.

These cognitive models have a rarely noted strength. None of the models is inconsistent with any of the data discussed previously regarding biological predispositions to panic. For cognitive models, however, the sensations produced by any putative pathophysiology are sensations that can be misinterpreted in the same way as any other sensations. Another strength of the cognitive models is that they can account for nocturnal panic attacks. While nocturnal panics have been considered the *sine qua non* of a spontaneous panic (Roy-Byrne et al., 1988), cognitive theorists respond that cognitive processing need not always be conscious (see Mathews and MacLeod, 1986). Rather, since the person has spent their waking hours selectively attuned to certain ("threatening") somatic sensations, when these occur during sleep the person responds to these with panic. That is to say, in just the same way that people will respond to personally relevant material while asleep (see Barlow, 1988), panickers will selectively encode and then respond to panic symptoms.

Cognitive models of panic emphasize the catastrophic misinterpretations placed upon internal bodily cues. Another approach to the same issue has been discussed within the context of anxiety sensitivity. Anxiety sensitivity is a trait construct, which describes individual differences in the tendency to interpret anxiety symptoms in a catastrophic manner. It is acknowledged that somatic symptoms and sensations may be produced by a variety of causes but not all individuals will worry about them to the same extent (e.g., Clark and Hemsley, 1982; Griez and van den Hout, 1982; Starkman et al., 1985). Trait anxiety may predispose individuals to "false alarms", but anxiety sensitivity may encourage an individual to worry about the sensations. Consequently, anxiety sensitivity may be related more strongly to panic disorder and agoraphobia than it will be to other anxiety disorders. The construct of anxiety sensitivity differs from other approaches to cognitive biases in anxiety problems in that it makes particular assumptions about the construct, namely that anxiety sensitivity is a trait conceptually and empirically distinct from trait anxiety (see McNally, 1990).

In summary, cognitive models of anxiety suggest that the critical factor in the development of a panic attack is not the experience of somatic sensations (whatever their origin), but the interpretation placed upon the sensations. In addition to the empirical support for cognitive models of the maintenance of panic attacks, a perhaps unexpected boon has been that cognitive models are becoming increasingly powerful in predicting the degree of agoraphobic avoidance that develops in a person with panic disorder.

Agoraphobic avoidance

The decision to separate individuals with panic disorder into those with and those without agoraphobia is, at one level, a function of a classificatory system with a penchant for categories rather than dimensions. However, people with panic disorder present with varying degrees of agoraphobic avoidance and while border-line cases are hard to dichotomize, there is no denying that individuals with extensive avoidance present very differently from those without avoidance. Agora-phobic avoidance has long been conceptualized in terms of conditioning, so that pairing of situations with aversive events (e.g., panic attacks) leads the contextual stimuli to acquire fear-provoking properties. The treatment consistent with this theory involves exposing the individual to the feared situation until anxiety is substantially reduced. The resulting exposure-based treatments have been repeat-edly demonstrated to be effective in reducing fear-driven avoidance (Emmelkamp, 1979).

Despite the evidence supporting a conditioning model of avoidance (Rachman, 1991), an examination of the predictors of avoidance behavior suggest that cognitive processes are critical in the etiology of agoraphobia. In fact, the cognitive variables appear to predict avoidance better than do those variables implicated by a conditioning model (i.e., the frequency and severity of panics). Clum and Knowles (1991; see also Andrews, 1993b) reviewed the literature pertaining to the reasons for the development of avoidant behavior. They examined eight hypothe-ses and concluded that, while panic attacks almost always precede the develop-ment of agoraphobic avoidance (Uhde et al., 1985; Aronson and Logue, 1987; Franklin, 1987; Garvey et al., 1987), the avoidance was not a function of the severity or frequency of the panic attacks, or age at onset.

The research into the effects of the duration of panic disorder and the location of the first panic attack was less consistent, but the findings could not be taken as providing convincing support for the origin of agoraphobia in the characteristics of the panic. In contrast, Clum and Knowles (1991) argued that the literature supported the hypothesis that agoraphobic avoidance was predicted by three sets of cognitions – situational negative outcome expectancies, catastrophic panic outcomes, and an inability to cope with the panic symptoms. The first cognitive set associated with agoraphobic avoidance involved negative outcome expect-ancies. Extensive avoidance was associated with expectations of situational fears, rather than fears of the panic attack alone (Franklin, 1987; Noyes et al., 1987a; Craske et al., 1988; Fleming and Falk, 1989). In addition, Telch et al. (1989) found that the expectation of negative social (rather than physical) consequences distin-guished avoidant from nonavoidant panickers. The second set of expectations associated with avoidance involved the perception of a link between a given situation and a panic attack. For instance, Rapee and Murrell (1988) found that individuals with panic disorder and marked avoidance were more likely to perceive a link between situations and their panic attacks (see also Craske et al., 1988; Adler et al., 1989; Telch et al., 1989). Finally, Clum and Knowles (1991) suggested that coping strategies and associated self-efficacy predicted the likelihood of avoidance. A perception of being able to tolerate fear predicted less escape and avoidance behavior (Craske et al., 1988). Avoidance behavior was associated with a lack of confidence regarding an ability to cope with future panic attacks (Craske et al., 1988; Mavissakalian, 1988; Telch et al., 1989). Avoiders tended also to use wishful thinking rather than social supports as coping strategies (Vitaliano et al., 1987), and training sufferers in effective coping strategies (e.g., breathing retraining and relaxation) was associated with lower avoidance.

There are a series of important clinical implications that flow from such data. Agoraphobic avoidance is predicted by certain cognitions regarding panic attacks in specific situations. First, people with greater degrees of avoidance tend to perceive an association between certain situations and panic attacks. Therefore, it might be argued that treatment needs to modify these beliefs. One way to achieve this aim is to instruct patients regarding what are currently believed to be the true causes of panic attacks (i.e., personality vulnerability, hyperventilation, catastrophic cognitions), thereby demonstrating that situations cannot in and of themselves cause panic. Another strategy is to teach patients coping strategies so that they are confident that they can stop panic occurring in "panicogenic" situations.

The second cognitive set found to be predictive of avoidance were catastrophic expectations of aversive consequences of panic occurring in particular situations. Treatment will need to modify this belief, especially since patients who cling to these fears will be understandably reluctant to conduct graded exposure exercises to these situations. Cognitive restructuring is one strategy to modify these beliefs, as each catastrophic thought is evaluated and tested. For instance, fears of fainting can be modified by instructing the patient in the origin of the feelings of faintness, discussing why fainting is unlikely to occur (given its etiology), examining the frequency of the feared outcome, and then recording the frequency of fainting in subsequent graded exposure tasks. A perceived inability to cope with panic was identified as the third cognitive set predictive of agoraphobic avoidance. Treatment will need to modify this set of beliefs to fully overcome avoidance. Teaching patients strategies that not only stop panic attacks but that serve to prevent future panics are useful in modifying poor self-efficacy. The perceived ability to cope with panic attacks will be increased once the person has learned effective anxiety-management strategies and found them to be effective while conducting graded exposure exercises.

Course

The modal age for the development of the first panic attack is between 15 and 19 years of age, and the age of onset of panic disorder tends to peak 10 years later in the mid-20s and diminishes by the mid-40s. As with other anxiety disorders, some studies have shown that stressful life events tend to precede the onset of the disorder (e.g., Last et al., 1984; De Loof et al., 1989). However, as discussed earlier, there are additional data suggesting that it is not so much the occurrence of stressful life events that precedes panic, but a negative interpretation of these life events (Rapee et al., 1990).

Epidemiology

Prior to DSM-III, panic disorder was not recognized as a separate diagnostic category and the label agoraphobia did not describe the same disorder as it does today. Therefore, some of the most useful estimates of the prevalence of the disorders currently referred to as panic disorder and agoraphobia come from Robins and Regier (1991). The lifetime frequency of panic disorder alone is just under 2%, while the lifetime prevalence of agoraphobia (usually with panic disorder) is just under 6%. Panic disorder and agoraphobia present differently in terms of their sex distributions. Panic disorder has an annual incidence of 1.43 per 1000, with around a third of cases arising without agoraphobia (Eaton et al., 1998). Panic typically (but not exclusively; Eaton et al., 1998) presents with an equal sex ratio (Myers et al., 1984). This contrasts with agoraphobia, where around three-quarters of sufferers are female (Yonkers et al., 1998). Interestingly, the extent of avoidance appears to be associated with female gender, giving rise to the finding that higher proportions of females with panic disorder also meet criteria for a diagnosis of agoraphobia (see Clum and Knowles, 1991) and are also more likely to experience a recurrence of panic symptoms than men (Yonkers et al., 1998). While many mechanisms may be proposed to explain this, one possibility has been developed following the finding that the tendency to avoid agoraphobic situations is correlated with femininity scores on a sex-role scale (Chambless and Mason, 1986; and see Reich et al., 1987). While being a female is associated with higher femininity scores, males may score relatively highly in terms of femininity and some females may score relatively lowly. Chambless and Mason (1986) found that the more feminine that subjects of both genders rated themselves to be, the greater was the agoraphobic avoidance. Clum and Knowles (1991) have extended this argument by placing this finding against the result that many agoraphobics fear the humiliation that may follow a panic. They suggest that femininity scores are associated with social sensitivity, and that the association between the disorder and gender comes about through the mediation of "femininity". Although one of the more appealing of recent explanations of sex differences, the argument is weakened by the absence of similar differences in the sex ratio of social phobia.

Notwithstanding, females with panic disorder and agoraphobia appear to be more severe than males in terms of avoidance, catastrophic thoughts, number of bodily sensations (Turgeon et al., 1998) and the course of panic disorder may be more severe in women (Yonkers et al., 1998), with women being slightly less than twice as likely to experience a re-emergence of symptoms than men (25% versus 15% at 6 months and 61% versus 41% and 3 years posttreatment). The reasons for these sex differences are not clear, but at present it seems as likely that they reside in psychological (e.g., greater harm avoidance in women, reducing compliance with exposure instructions given in treatment) as in biological (e.g., cyclical hormonal changes that modify the vulnerability to panic) differences (see Bekker, 1996).

Comorbidity

Individuals with panic disorder and agoraphobia tend to suffer additional psychological distress (Katon et al., 1987) and impaired quality of life (Markowitz et al., 1989). Of particular concern is the occurrence of major depression, the preoccupation with death (Overbeek et al., 1998), and elevated suicide rate among individuals with panic disorder (Weissman et al., 1989). A diagnosis of panic disorder is also associated with substance abuse, impaired social and marital function, and financial dependency (Markowitz et al., 1989). Further, if panic disorder is comorbid with another diagnosis, the individual is more likely to seek treatment for the comorbid disorder, than when there is no comorbid panic (Boyd, 1986). In terms of etiology, one comorbidity is that which occurs with specific phobias. Interestingly, Starcevic and Bogojevic (1997) found that death-related phobia was the most proximal specific phobia that preceded the onset of panic disorder and agoraphobia, suggesting that the arousal of these fears may have some etiological significance in the development of panic.

One complication that needs to be borne in mind is the co-occurrence of a personality disorder. Individuals with panic disorder show an increased risk (relative to the population) for personality disorders falling in the "anxious" cluster (i.e., DSM-IV's cluster C, comprising dependent, avoidant, and obsessive–compulsive personality disorders (Klass et al., 1989; Mauri et al., 1992)). As Barlow (1988) noted, this pattern of comorbidity is not surprising, given the postulation of a general neurotic syndrome. The strength of the association appears to be a function of agoraphobic avoidance. That is to say, patients with greater agoraphobic avoidance exhibit a greater number of anxious cluster personality traits because the same vulnerability underlies both disorders.

There is also some evidence for sex differences in comorbidity. Women appear more likely to have comorbid social phobia and PTSD (Turgeon et al., 1998). Both men and women with panic disorder (men 15% and women 9%) and agoraphobia (men 27% and women 9%) show high rates of problem alcohol use; however, the reports of problem use of sedative hypnotics is also disturbingly high among people with panic disorder (men 10% and women 6%) and agoraphobia (men 18% and women 9%; Page and Andrews, 1996).

Summary

Individuals who present to clinics for treatment with agoraphobia almost always have panic disorder. Panic disorder involves extreme attacks of anxiety that perplex the individual, who in turn may misinterpret the anxiety response as a signal of some mental or physical pathology. It appears that those who attribute the causes of panic attacks to certain situations, who feel unable to manage panics in certain situations, or who worry about the aversive consequences of panicking in certain locations will develop agoraphobic avoidances.

5

Panic disorder and agoraphobia

Treatment

In 1988, Barlow examined the evidence from around the world and concluded that "with specifically targeted psychological treatments, panic is eliminated in close to 100% of all cases, and these results are maintained at follow-ups of over 1 year. If these results are confirmed by additional research and replication, it will be one of the most important and exciting developments in the history of psychotherapy" (Barlow, 1988; p. 447). The question facing researchers and clinicians alike is, with the benefit of more than a decade of subsequent research and replication, "Is it possible to concur with Barlow's statement?". The place to begin this evaluation is by addressing the criteria of effective treatment for panic disorder and agoraphobia.

Aims of treatment

Panic disorder and agoraphobia are currently conceptualized as two separate, but frequently related, disorders. Specifically, panic attacks are considered the "motor" that "drives" the agoraphobic avoidance (e.g., Clarke and Jackson, 1983). Therefore, it would be expected that effective long-term treatment for agoraphobia would require effective long-term management of panic attacks. By extension, the first aim of an effective treatment for agoraphobia (with panic disorder) would be to stop panic attacks and their interference in an individual's life. The second aim would be to reduce any concurrent agoraphobic avoidance. Just as with the specific phobias, avoidance will involve anticipatory anxiety and anxiety triggered upon exposure and treatment will be more than simply "turning off" avoidance. However, an ideal treatment would do more than modify the existing symptoms; it would reduce the vulnerability to the disorder. If the vulnerability to panic disorder and agoraphobia (e.g., trait anxiety) could be modified, relapse would presumably be decreased. In summary, effective treatment of panic disorder and agoraphobia will involve (1) the control of panic attacks, (2) the cessation of fear-driven avoidance, and (3) reduction of the vulnerability.

Nondrug treatments

Exposure

In vivo exposure has been one of the strongest and most consistently demonstrated treatments for agoraphobic avoidance. In fact, it has often been demonstrated to be superior to placebo interventions as well as other credible psychological treatments (e.g., Mathews et al., 1981; Mavissakalian and Barlow, 1981;
Emmelkamp, 1982; Teusch and Boehme, 1999) – a none too easy achievement in
psychological research. Furthermore, when anti-exposure instructions are included in comparison therapies, the strength of exposure becomes even more
evident (e.g., Greist et al., 1980; Telch et al., 1985). Barlow's (1988) conclusion
that, following exposure alone, around 75% of agoraphobics (excluding dropouts)
will evidence some clinical benefit is representative of most similar reviews (e.g.,
Mattick et al., 1990). Yet, despite the strength of in vivo exposure in the treatment
of agoraphobia, it is noteworthy that there remains little room for complacency.
Around one-quarter of patients do not experience any clinical improvement
during treatment, not all are completely symptom free at follow-up (e.g.,
McPherson et al., 1980), and not all those who benefit from treatment maintain
their gains (Munby and Johnston, 1980). The research literature provides some
details about the ingredients of a successful exposure package.

First, it appears that the greater the exposure exercises resemble the real
situations avoided by individuals, the better is the outcome. For instance, in vivo
exposure is usually superior to imaginal exposure (e.g., Emmelkamp and Wessels,
1975). Second, the more frequently the person confronts their feared situation and
the greater the duration of exposure sessions, the higher is the proportion of
treatment completers who reach a high end-state functioning (e.g., Vermilyea et
al., 1984). Finally, it is probably the case that exposure that continues until anxiety
has subsided is preferable to shorter exposures (e.g., Stern and Marks, 1973; Foa et
al., 1980). For instance, Rayment and Richards (1998) found that allowing panic
symptoms to develop and pass predicted less avoidance of phobic situations.
However, while among specific phobics (see Marshall, 1985) continuing exposure
until anxiety decreased was superior to "escaping" when anxiety had risen, among
agoraphobics there are some data suggesting that both approaches are equally
effective (de Silva and Rachman, 1984; Rachman et al., 1986; although cf. Rayment
and Richards, 1998).

One additional factor that may enhance exposure programs is an effort to
assure that exposure brings about cognitive changes. Since certain cognitive
variables predict the degree of avoidance (Clum and Knowles, 1991), exposure
should also aim to modify the cognitions predictive of the avoidance. That is
to say, it is important to assure that exposure treatments include instruction

regarding the true causes of panic attacks and be combined with training in anxiety-management strategies. That said, it is apparent that the role that the cognitive variables identified in cognitive theories play in treatment is not completely clear (Oei et al., 1999). For example Soechting et al. (1998) compared the efficacy of a cognitive and a behavioral rationale for exposure treatment among people with panic disorder and agoraphobia, and there was no overall superior efficacy of the cognitive rationale. However, Hoffart (1998) did find that agoraphobics given cognitive therapy showed superior outcomes to those who received guided mastery and that a path analytic strategy implicated the variables identified by cognitive models. In particular, it appears that changes in the situational fear of agoraphobics is particularly mediated by changes in self-efficacy, as opposed to changes in catastrophic beliefs and perceived thought control (Hoffart, 1995).

A further way in which the efficacy of exposure-based programs has been improved is with the involvement of spouses or partners in treatment. While a complete discussion of all the findings regarding marital and family interventions in agoraphobia is beyond the scope of the present book (see Daiuto et al., 1998), a summary statement is in order. Barlow et al. (1984) found that among agoraphobics with apparently well-adjusted relationships, the inclusion of the partner in treatment added little to improvement rates. In contrast, among individuals with poorly adjusted relationships, the inclusion of a partner enhanced treatment outcome, overriding any effects of the poor interactions. Therefore it is useful advice to include partners in exposure-based programs, particularly where there is concern about the negative impact the relationship may have on treatment. Behavioral therapy for couples may be a useful adjunct, but concurrent therapy raises a number of other issues, including the difficulties of combining couple-focused interventions and agoraphobic treatment (Daiuto et al., 1998). Thus our practice is typically to sequence the treatment for agoraphobia and the couples therapy, deciding on a case-by-case basis the order for particular clients.

Finally, one way that in vivo exposure programs have been improved is by the addition of more and different exposure. Fava et al. (1997) reported data that suggested that additional exposure was beneficial for patients who were not initially responding to exposure. More novel treatments, e.g., "interoceptive exposure" have been used to target panic attacks directly. People prone to panic attacks are requested to engage in a series of exercises that produce sensations similar to those that occur during a panic attack (Rapee and Barlow, 1990). For instance, individuals who fear that tachycardia may signal a heart attack are requested to run on the spot. The exercise produces a rapid heartbeat, which can then be included in the person's graded exposure hierarchy. We have demonstrated that among agoraphobics the exercises tend to improve overall treatment outcome (Page, 1994a; see also Ito et al., 1996) and Craske et al. (1997) found that the addition of interoceptive exposure reduced panic frequency posttreatment and at a 6-month follow-up. The Craske et al. study is noteworthy because it also found treatment specificity. That is to say, the interoceptive exposure seemed to exert particular effects upon measures of panic frequency, suggesting that this is a treatment to be stressed with patients who have frequent panic attacks.

In summary, in vivo exposure is the treatment of choice for agoraphobic avoidance. Alone, exposure is a powerful treatment but it is not able to assure a high end-state function in all patients. Therefore, additional treatments need to be considered and combined with exposure. In fact Murphy et al. (1998) found that, while exposure was an important component in treatment, anxiety management added to the overall improvement. Specifically, they argued that once a critical threshold of exposure practice has been achieved, anxiety-management techniques became increasingly important. Therefore, another possible addition to treatment could involve strategies to control the emergence of panic attacks. One such intervention is breathing retraining.

Breathing retraining

Hyperventilation can produce symptoms similar to those experienced during a panic attack and hyperventilation often occurs during a panic attack. Therefore, it is reasonable to suppose that teaching individuals appropriate breathing strategies aimed to control hyperventilation will alleviate panic symptoms and assist long-term symptom management. An analysis of the treatment literature is complicated by the variety of breathing techniques being taught (see Garssen et al., 1992). For present purposes, attention will be limited to studies that compared breathing retraining with exposure-based programs. Although breathing retraining alone can reduce the frequency of panic attacks (Lum, 1983; Rapee, 1985b), given that exposure-based programs have a demonstrated efficacy, the clinically relevant question is "Can breathing retraining enhance the efficacy of standard exposure treatments?". Three studies meet these criteria. One of the studies failed to demonstrate a decrease in panic frequency following breathing retraining and cognitive restructuring (de Ruiter et al., 1989b). This result is surprising, since such a treatment should decrease the frequency of panic attacks (Clark et al., 1985; Salkovskis et al., 1986a). Given the study's failure to demonstrate a treatment effect, it is difficult to interpret the comparisons with exposure treatments. The remaining two studies failed to find any posttreatment differences between exposure-based programs with and without breathing retraining (Bonn et al., 1984; Hibbert and Chan, 1989), leading to the conclusion that, while breathing retraining may reduce panic attacks, it does not improve exposure-based programs in the short term. However, one study (Bonn et al., 1984) examined the patients at a 6-month follow-up point and found that the addition of breathing retraining to exposure enhanced treatment outcome. To summarize, when used alone, breathing retraining can reduce symptoms, but, more importantly, when added to a comprehensive cognitive behavioral exposure-based program, it can improve long-term outcome, perhaps by consolidating the progress made during treatment and enhancing the stability of treatment gains (e.g., Chambless et al., 1986).

Relaxation

Another strategy that has been used in the treatment of panic disorder and agoraphobia is relaxation. When the different forms of relaxation are combined, relaxation alone has been estimated to bring about a clinically significant improvement in around 47% of patients with panic disorder and agoraphobia (Michelson and Marchione, 1991). However, in the context of panic disorder, applied relaxation has been found to be superior to progressive muscle relaxation (Ost, 1987b). Applied relaxation is a rapid form of relaxation that enables individuals to elicit the relaxation response quickly when needed. While effective, Arntz and van den Hout (1996) found that applied relaxation was less effective than cognitive therapy, particularly on measures of panic frequency. There have been some suggestions that progressive muscle relaxation may detract from a cognitive behavioral therapy (CBT) program for agoraphobia (Barlow et al., 1989). However, the design of the study involved the introduction of relaxation as one of the first components into a CBT program. If it is assumed that most individuals with a chronic anxiety disorder will have been taught relaxation skills at some point, the higher dropout rates observed in this condition could have occurred because the patients became disillusioned with receiving a treatment they had already attempted. While further research is needed to address this question, it may be speculated that it may be more helpful to include relaxation later, rather than earlier, in a comprehensive CBT program.

Cognitive restructuring and combined CBT packages

One of the most exciting developments in recent times has been the addition of cognitive techniques to exposure programs. Most often, exposure is targeted at the avoidance behavior, while cognitive interventions are focused at decatastrophizing the interpretations of the panic symptoms. Typically, cognitive approaches are not used alone (although they are somewhat efficacious when used as the sole treatment intervention; Salkovskis et al., 1991; Williams and Falbo, 1996), but are combined with exposure (both to external and internal triggers of panic), relaxation, and breathing retraining. When such combinations are used, the improvement is considerable. While it is not always clear that the addition of cognitive therapy enhances the effects of exposure (Burke et al., 1997), the combined packages are very effective. Barlow et al. (1989), Klosko et al. (1990), and Beck et al. (1992) similarly found that up to 90% of panic-disordered patients were panic free following their combined panic control treatment. Furthermore, it is becoming clear that the effects of these treatment packages have a broader impact on the clients, bringing about an overall improvement in quality of life (Telch et al., 1995).

In addition, it is becoming increasingly clear that these treatment packages are effective not only in clinical research centers. The effects transport well to self-help delivery format (Gould et al., 1993; Gould and Clum, 1995) and can be maintained when face-to-face treatment is reduced in duration but compensated for by a computer program that incorporates the basic principles of cognitive behavioral treatment (Newman et al., 1997). The treatment packages can generalize favorably to adolescent samples (Ollendick, 1995) and to settings that are representative of community treatment, even when the patients are more severe than those typically seen in research trials (e.g., Sanderson et al., 1998). When used in a community mental health center, 87% of panic-disordered patients were panic free after 15 sessions of CBT (Wade et al., 1998); a figure that compares well with that obtained in clinical research settings (e.g., Michelson and Marchione, 1991). The patients also showed reductions in anticipatory anxiety, agoraphobic avoidance, generalized anxiety, and depression; a pattern of data that once again would be expected on the basis of research conducted in clinical research settings (Clum et al., 1993).

Manualized CBT-based treatment packages have also been criticized as being inappropriate for clients with comorbid disorders (see Wilson, 1996). Marchand et al. (1998) examined the rates of change in clients suffering from panic disorder and agoraphobia with and without a comorbid personality disorder and found that both groups responded to the treatment for the anxiety disorder; however, clients with a personality disorder responded more slowly. In addition, Hoffart and Hedley (1997) noted that dependent personality traits appear particularly detrimental to treatment progress, but that CBT for panic disorder and agoraphobia did reduce symptoms of personality disorder (especially avoidant and dependent traits). Thus it seems more reasonable to conclude that clients with comorbid personality disorders may require longer, rather than inherently different, treatment than those without personality disorders.

Drug treatments

Confronted with the increasingly favorable treatment outcomes associated with cognitive behavioral packages, there are three possible reasons why pharmacological interventions might be considered. First, it could be that pharmacological interventions achieve the same outcomes as the CBT packages but at a cheaper cost (financially to the patient or in terms of therapist time), with fewer dropouts, lower relapse rates, and with fewer associated difficulties (such as side-effects). Second, it could be that pharmacological treatments may be useful adjuncts to the CBT packages. Third, it could be that pharmacological interventions are useful treatments to attempt with patients for whom a comprehensive and well-conducted CBT program has failed or to whom such a treatment is unacceptable. Before a therapist can consider each possibility, it is necessary to evaluate the literature regarding pharmacological interventions (Clum, 1989; Michelson and Marchione, 1991; Clum et al., 1993). There are five possible pharmacological interventions, the tricyclic (antidepressants), the benzodiazepines (high and low potencies), the beta blockers, the monoamine oxidase inhibitors, and the selective serotonin re-uptake inhibitors (SSRIs). As with every medication there are pros, cons, and guidelines for use, but at a general level of overall efficacy it appears that the low-dose benzodiazepines and the beta blockers (i.e., propranolol) have limited efficacy.

The tricyclics and the high-potency benzodiazepines have more acceptable success rates. Holland et al. (1999) reported that the tricyclic clomipramine has a slower therapeutic onset than the benzodiazepines alprazolam and adinazolam, but that it reached the same rate of efficacy as alprazolam (both being superior to adinazolam) and had less frequent withdrawal problems. Den Boer (1998) noted that a further advantage of the tricyclics over the benzodiazepines is that the former have greater effects on comorbid depression while being similarly effective in managing anxiety and agoraphobia.

Clum (1989) estimated (when dropouts are included) that behavior therapies in general are successful with 54% of patients, tricyclics with 19%, and the high-potency benzodiazepines with 42%. The unexpectedly low outcomes for the tricyclics (Mattick et al., 1990) probably occur because studies have tended to use people with panic disorder and agoraphobia (who are more difficult to treat), whereas studies with the high-potency benzodiazepines have tended to use subjects with panic disorder alone (Clum, 1989). In a similar comparison, Michelson and Marchione (1991) concluded that CBT packages are generally successful in 74% (including dropouts) of individuals with panic disorder and agoraphobia (86% among panic disorder alone), the tricyclics in 45%, and the high-potency benzodiazepines in 51%. Once again, the treatment outcomes for the low-potency benzodiazepines and beta blockers are relatively low (13% and 8%, respectively). Although the two reviews differ in their final estimates, the pattern of results is similar, suggesting that – of the pharmacological treatments – high-potency benzodiazepines and the tricyclics are the only interventions whose outcomes approach the success obtained with a CBT package. If the choice of pharmacological intervention were limited to these two classes of drug, it would be difficult to choose between them. On the one hand, the dropout rates for the tricyclics are higher than for the high-potency benzodiazepines (although this may reflect different sampling; Clum, 1989); but, on the other hand, the relapse rates for the high-potency benzodiazepines are probably higher (Clum, 1989; Michelson and Marchione, 1991). In terms of unwanted effects, the tricyclics are unpopular because of the anticholinergic side-effects, but the high-potency benzodiazepines are often avoided because of the possibility of dependence and also the negative effects upon memory (Kilic et al., 1999). Indeed, after demonstrating the efficacy of imipramine and (especially) alprazolam in treating panic disorder (Schweizer et al., 1993), Rickels et al. (1993b) identified a "sobering fact [that] over the long term (i.e., after taper), patients originally treated with imipramine or placebo did as well at follow-up as patients treated with alprazolam, without the problems of physical dependence and discontinuation that any long-term alprazolam therapy entails" (ibid., p. 67).

Interestingly, Clum et al. (1993) subsequently identified some methodological weaknesses in Clum's (1989) early analysis. Using more stringent inclusion criteria, the more recent meta-analysis continues to support some of the earlier conclusions. In particular, the antidepressants continued to be identified as a treatment of choice (although dropout rates were high) and psychological interventions were supported once more as a treatment of choice, with exposure or flooding being identified as a successful treatment. However, the support for the high-potency benzodiazepines was much weaker than it had been in the earlier analysis, perhaps because the earlier analysis had included some clinical trials, with no control groups, that included only data from people who completed the trials.

In summary, it appears that the efficacy of the CBT therapies is equaling, and sometimes surpassing, that of the pharmacotherapies (Clum, 1989; Michelson and Marchione, 1991). Furthermore, given the difficulties associated with medications, such as side-effects and the possibility of dependence, psychological interventions should be the treatment of choice for panic disorder and agoraphobia. Pharmacotherapies may be preferred because of their initial low cost; however, the cost of continuing medication and the hidden cost of the higher rates of relapse have yet to be factored into the equation. However, with the relatively recent emergence of the SSRIs it is premature to draw strong conclusions about these drugs. Nevertheless, the data to date are promising (e.g., Pollack et al., 1998; see Boerner and Moeller, 1997). Finally, although rarely discussed in the literature, just as there are some patients who find the prospect of medication unacceptable, there are some who will not participate in a CBT program. Given that the success of a CBT program relies upon active participation, for these individuals pharmacotherapies may be preferred.

Combining drug and nondrug treatments

Examining the effects of combining treatments is not simple. Any grouping runs the risk of combining dissimilar categories (e.g., different drugs within one class, different dosages, different durations of administration, different forms of exposure, different cognitive interventions, etc.; see Oei et al., 1997). The interested reader is referred to recent reviews by Spiegel and Bruce (1997) and Schmidt (1999) for more detailed discussions. For present purposes, the two main classes of drug that have been combined with behavioral treatments are the high-potency benzodiazepines and the tricyclic antidepressants. Van Balkom et al. (1997) conducted a meta-analysis on the combination of pharmacological and cognitive behavioral treatments of panic disorder with and without agoraphobia. Focusing on their indices of panic and agoraphobia, they concluded that among these studies high potency benzodiazepines, antidepressants, and cognitive behavioral treatments were all equally superior to a control and the gains were maintained following the termination of treatment (Bakker et al., 1998). Interestingly, while in vivo exposure was no more effective than the control condition in alleviating panic symptoms, it was markedly effective in alleviating agoraphobic symptoms. Further, the effects of in vivo exposure were dramatically increased (effect size (Cohen's d) = 2.47) by the addition of tricyclic antidepressants. This effect clearly warrants further investigation (especially because Fava et al. (1997) found that supplementing exposure with imipramine reduced the efficacy of in vivo exposure), but some light may be shed on it by the work of Murphy et al. (1998). They found that patients with panic disorder and agoraphobia who were also depressed exhibited a reduction in the benefit derived from in vivo exposure sessions. Thus, given the potential mediating role of depression, antidepressants may enhance the efficacy of in vivo exposure by removing the otherwise inhibiting effects of depression. Continuing this speculation, similar increases in outcome may also be achieved by using the skills the client has acquired in CBT to focus on the symptoms of depression when these are comorbid with the anxiety disorder.

Considering the combination of psychological treatment with benzodiazepines, the picture seems less favorable. For instance, Schmidt (1999) concluded that the combination of CBT and benzodiazepines appears to produce poorer end-state functioning than CBT alone. Wade et al. (1998) found that the only predictor of posttreatment panic was pretreatment anxiolytic medication use, which they noted was primarily benzodiazepines. Further, if nonhuman data are considered, Bouton et al. (1990) found a dose-dependent interference with fear extinction in rats from two benzodiazepines. Thus these animal data suggested that relapse rates may be elevated when behavior therapies are combined with increasingly more potent benzodiazepines. Although the appropriate human studies have not been conducted, it is apparent that there is presently strong support neither for nor against combining benzodiazepines with CBT (see Spiegel and Bruce, 1997). Thus a reasonable position would seem to be that combining benzodiazepines with CBTs should await research support before being recommended as routine clinical practice.

Summary

The treatment of panic disorder with agoraphobia is consistent with the etiology models discussed. A comprehensive nondrug treatment package involves panic control (e.g., education about anxiety, breathing retraining, panic provocation exercises) as well as modification of the agoraphobic avoidance and catastrophic misinterpretations (in vivo exposure and cognitive restructuring). Drug treatments, using high-potency benzodiazepines or the tricyclics, have been found to yield similar rates of treatment success probably because they also decrease anxiety (Barlow, 1988) and thereby facilitate exposure. However, while drug and nondrug treatments are both effective, there is one added bonus that is often not mentioned. There is evidence that CBT modifies the vulnerability factors that give rise to the disorder. For instance, Andrews and Moran (1988) found that an earlier version of the Clinician Guide and Patient Manual substantially reduced neuroticism scores and that the size of the decrease was predictive of subsequent relapse. Given the long-term advantages of reducing vulnerability, a cognitive behavioral intervention should probably be the treatment of choice (see also Nathan and Gorman, 1998).

Yet, despite the success of CBTs for panic disorder and agoraphobia, there are two words of caution. First, surveys of clients serve as a salutary reminder of state of clinical practice. In a survey of 100 patients with panic disorder and agoraphobia, Bandelow et al. (1995) found that unproven treatments (e.g., herbal preparations) were overutilized and treatments with demonstrated efficacy (e.g., CBT and tricyclic antidepressants) were underutilized. Further, Wade et al. (1998) noted that clinicians are often ambivalent about using a structured, short-term treatment that requires adherence to a protocol, preferring to revert to more familiar approaches of selecting treatments that they believe will be effective for this particular patient. Therefore, it is not only important that the outcomes of research be disseminated, it is important that clinicians routinely use (and be encouraged by their management structures to continue to use) established and efficacious treatments.

A closing word of caution can be taken from more recent work of Barlow (1997). The present chapter opened with Barlow's enthusiasm for this form of treatment, and he quite reasonably persists with this enthusiasm, commenting that "cognitive-behavioral treatments yielded the highest mean effect sizes [comparing] favorably with pharmacologic as well as combination drug and CBT treatments" (Barlow, 1997: p. 34). However, his enthusiasm is now tempered by data indicating that not insignificant numbers of patients continue to suffer from panic continuously or continually following treatment. For instance, Barlow described data from his group indicating that "while 74% of our patients remained panic free at a 24-month follow-up when followed cross-sectionally and 57% had reached a state of 'high end-state functioning' that would represent a state close to 'cured,' these numbers dropped notably when patients were followed longitudinally... Thus, it seems that at least some of these patients do reasonably well over the long term but continue to suffer from periods of exacerbation of their Panic Disorder and Agoraphobia" (Barlow, 1997: p. 35). Therefore, attention needs to continue to be allocated to those people who are less successful during therapy and identify how treatment can be delivered or targeted more effectively.

6

Panic disorder and agoraphobia

Clinician Guide

After formal diagnosis and assessment, two issues must be addressed before treatment is planned. First, the clinician, by conducting a thorough behavioral analysis, must identify the factors that trigger and maintain the panic attacks and the avoidance behavior. Second, the clinician must consider the effects of comorbid disorders on treatment.

Behavioral analysis

The general principles and practice of behavioral analysis have been outlined elsewhere (Kirk, 1989; Schulte, 1997). However, in panic disorder and agoraphobia there are unique details to be considered. In terms of the antecedents of panic attacks, it is necessary to evaluate the physical and psychological triggers. These typically include situations previously associated with panic, certain physical sensations, and particular worrying thoughts (e.g., "Oh no! What if I had a panic attack right now?"). In addition, panic attacks will be more likely to occur when the person has been made more physically aroused as a result of being anxious, stressed, hot, smoking, drinking alcohol, taking stimulant drugs (e.g., coffee), and so on. In addition, panic attacks appear more likely when the individual is "run down", perhaps because of illness (e.g., flu), physical and psychological stress (e.g., childbirth), or sleep deprivation. Once a listing of antecedents has been made, the consequences of panic attacks need to be identified. The consequences can be divided into three categories. First, individuals may respond to panic attacks with avoidance behavior. Commonly avoided agoraphobic situations have been described earlier, but for present purposes it is worth noting that identifying the cognitive link between panic attacks and avoidance will facilitate cognitive behavioral treatment (e.g., "I avoid crowded trains because the air may run out when everyone is breathing it"). Second, the subtle avoidance strategies (e.g., the use of safety signals) need to be identified. Finally, the social consequences of avoidance need to be evaluated. For instance, individuals with dependent traits may welcome the increased support given as a consequence of panic attacks and become more dependent. Such behavioral patterns need to be identified to ensure they do not inhibit progress in treatment.

Management of comorbid disorders

The most frequently comorbid axis I disorders are the other anxiety disorders, especially social phobia (Sanderson et al., 1990). One advantage of cognitive behavioral interventions is their applicability to all the anxiety disorders, in that each disorder responds to various combinations of anxiety-management and exposure strategies. Therefore, we tend to treat the primary anxiety disorder first, and then encourage individuals to apply their new skills to manage any associated anxiety disorders. The personality disorders will be the next set of comorbid disorders considered (Klass et al., 1989; Mauri et al., 1992). Cluster C (i.e., anxious) personality disorders can pose a problem because they make achieving treatment goals more difficult. Individuals with avoidant personality disorder tend to require greater encouragement to engage in exposure tasks. Individuals with dependent personality disorders rely excessively on therapists, friends, or partners during exposure tasks and therefore need to learn to function without this support. In contrast, obsessive–compulsive personality disorder can sometimes be an apparent asset when such patients stick rigidly to the guidelines laid down in the treatment program. The lack of flexibility will, however, produce difficulties when cognitive restructuring is begun. Thus a cluster C personality disorder, while requiring additional attention, may not be a contradiction to treatment. The cluster A (eccentric) and cluster B (erratic) personality disorders are more difficult to treat. Persons with cluster B personality disorders can produce disturbances in a group that can interfere with the progress of the other members to a degree that is counterproductive. Individual treatment is, therefore, recommended if the personality disorder is severe. If the person's primary problem is the personality disorder, then treating the anxiety problem may not, in fact, be the best strategy. Some patients who, at the initial interview, appear to have a personality disorder will not meet criteria when structured diagnostic interviews such as the Personality Disorder Examination are administered. Most often the patient will endorse various criteria, but will claim that such behavior was not typical of them before the anxiety disorder began. Furthermore, these apparent "personality disorders" disappear rapidly as the anxiety disorder is treated. The primary anxiety disorder may have led the patient to behave in a way typical of a personality-disordered individual. For example, fear of panic may increase their dependency needs, needs that will remit when the panics are controlled. We have become cautious in diagnosing a personality disorder on the basis of disturbed behavior in the clinical interview.

Format of treatment

Therapeutic outcome is a function of at least two sources of variance. One source of variance is attributable to the treatment package. The second source of variance in treatment outcome corresponds to the therapist's ability to (1) enhance motivation for treatment (discussed in more detail in Chapter 7), (2) enhance treatment comprehension and compliance, and (3) successfully handle problems that arise during treatment. The present chapter aims to make explicit the ways in which a therapist can overcome some of these difficulties and maximize treatment success. The first issue is the structure of a treatment program. We will describe our group program; but, for an individual patient, this would be modified by assigning reading and exposure exercises for homework, reserving treatment sessions for the discussion of progress, and for planning the next stages of the intervention.

Group program structure

The program at the Clinical Research Unit for Anxiety Disorders (CRUfAD) is structured around a 3-week intensive program. At the University of Western Australia, the program is structured in a less intensive 9-week program. Each structure will be described in turn.

Three-week intensive group program structure

Patients attend the clinic from 9 a.m. to 5 p.m. Monday through Friday for 2 weeks, separated by 1 week. During their time at the clinic, patients are given their own copy of the Patient Treatment Manual, have it explained to them, discuss it, and engage in assignments. During the middle week, when they are away from the clinic, patients engage in self-directed exposure assignments planned at the end of the first week of the program. An outline and timetable for this program is provided to acquaint the reader with the rate of progress to be expected. Considerable emphasis is placed on mastering the anxiety-management techniques of monitoring respiration rate, and practicing slow-breathing and relaxation techniques. However, even more time is spent planning and carrying out the graded exposure assignments, and in debriefing patients when those assignments have been completed.

Day one

On the first day most patients are highly anxious and it is most important to establish rapport. After the usual introductions are completed, the therapist should acknowledge the anxiety and make a list of everyone's anxiety symptoms, in part to confirm the nature of panic and, in part, to allow group members to realize that others have the same symptoms. Other things to be done at this stage include the following. Outline the program and distribute the manual.

Explain that the manual is the key to the program, and that patients should personalize their copy by underlining especially relevant sections, and by adding examples which are personally relevant.

Check that each patient has organized transport to and from the clinic.

Indicate that patients will be expected to use public transport or drive alone to and from the clinic towards the end of the program.

If there are still individuals who are taking medication, check on the quantity and type of medication that each person is taking.

To achieve the maximum benefit from this program, encourage patients who are taking benzodiazepines to cease these before beginning treatment. It is important that benzodiazepines are discontinued because they appear to block extinction learning (Bouton et al., 1990). In addition, as they provide a predictable relief of symptoms 30 to 60 minutes after ingestion, patients do not learn that their anxiety symptoms can be controlled by their new anxiety management skills.

The therapist provides specific instructions for the directed exposure program but does not accompany the patients on outings (apart from two brief group trips to familiarize the patients with the local area). Although the itineraries for the group trips and the individual assignments are predetermined, patients are encouraged to modify these assignments, after consulting the therapist, so that they have more relevance for them. As there is some evidence that patients do better if they perceive control over their assignments, it is important to be flexible and take into account each patient's needs. The group trips familiarize patients with the areas to which they will be traveling subsequently on their own. It is important to explain that the program is designed to ensure that they learn to cope with their own anxiety, take responsibility for doing the assignments, and successfully enter previously avoided situations. At all times the therapist aims to use language readily understood by patients (e.g., Page, 1993). The therapist helps patients with their assignments by rehearsing the steps necessary for each of the tasks before the task is attempted. On the first day therapists aim to cover the following material and assignments:

- Material in Patient Treatment Manual: Section 1: The Nature of Anxiety, Panic and Agoraphobia; and Section 2: Control of Hyperventilation.
- Accompanied group walk around the local area (duration 20 minutes).
- Individual assignment 1: Walk to closest bus stop and return to clinic. It is important to emphasize that the assignments should be done in the order shown, from least to most difficult. When individual assignments are completed they are ticked off on a notice board, in part to reinforce the individual's success

and in part to encourage recalcitrant group members. All group trips and individual assignments are reviewed by the therapist. Any specific difficulties, especially the panic-related cognitions, are identified and strategies to overcome these difficulties outlined.

- Homework for day one: Monitor respiration rates and practice the slow-breathing technique.

Day two

At the beginning of day two it is useful to ask about each patient's attitude to the program, to inquire about sleep the previous night, and to ask about each person's current level of anxiety. Patients are reminded that they will be expected to attempt an individual assignment later in the day. Therapists should cover the following material and assignments during day two:

- Review homework: respiratory monitoring, practice of the slow-breathing technique.
- Material in Patient Treatment Manual: Section 3: Relaxation Training; and Section 4: Graded Exposure.
- Group practice of progressive muscle relaxation.
- Unaccompanied group walk around the block, walking further than the bus stop in the previous day's assignment. Individual assignment 2: same as group walk but now completed alone.
- Homework for day two: respiratory rate monitoring, practice of slow-breathing and relaxation techniques.

Day three

Therapists should cover the following material and assignments:

- Review homework: respiratory monitoring, practice of slow-breathing and relaxation techniques.
- Group practice of progressive muscle relaxation.
- Unaccompanied group trip: travel by bus for two stops.
- Material in Patient Treatment Manual, Section 5: Thinking Straight.
- Homework for day three: respiratory monitoring, practice of slow-breathing and relaxation techniques.

Day four

We remind patients about the group trip and the individual assignment scheduled for later in the day. The section on Thinking Straight must be completed. All free time is spent preparing and reviewing group and individual assignments, with an emphasis on cognitive strategies. Therapists should cover the following assignments:

- Review homework: respiratory monitoring, practice of slow-breathing and relaxation techniques.
- Group practice of progressive muscle relaxation.
- Unaccompanied group bus trip of about 10 stops to a small shopping center. Patients should remain there for 30 minutes and are encouraged to enter shops, go to the bank, and walk about the shopping center alone.
- Individual assignment 3: Repeat the 10-stop bus journey and the visit to the shopping center alone.
- Debriefing after assignments: Review how the anxiety-management and cognitive restructuring techniques were applied.
- Homework for day four: respiratory monitoring, practice of slow-breathing and relaxation techniques.

Day five

Therapists should cover the following material and assignments:
- Review homework: respiratory monitoring, slow-breathing and relaxation techniques.
- Group practice of progressive muscle relaxation.
- Material in Patient Treatment Manual, Section 6: Producing the Panic Sensations.
- Unaccompanied group bus trip (15 stops) to major shopping center or mall, remaining there for coffee. The purpose of this trip is to extend the patients' range of travel away from the clinic and to expose them to a more crowded shopping center with multilevel shops.
- Individual assignment 4: Repeat this day's group assignment alone.
- Debriefing after assignments: Review how the anxiety-management and cognitive restructuring techniques were applied.
- Planning for week two: Before the end of the first week all patients should have a detailed plan for week two written in a diary format. Each patient should aim to complete one Graded Exposure exercise and one Producing Panic Sensations exercise every day. The therapist should help each patient to design their individual assignments, using the goals and Graded Exposure hierarchies from Section 3 and the Panic Sensations hierarchy from Section 5 of the Patient Treatment Manual. The assignments should be relevant to the patient and compatible with their usual activities. If any individual has not completed the first week's individual assignments, they should complete those assignments before continuing with the tasks for week two.

Day fifteen

Therapists should cover the following material and assignments:
- Review week two homework: respiratory monitoring, slow-breathing and relax-

ation techniques. Carefully review the individual assignments and determine which were completed and how each patient feels about their achievements. Patients frequently overestimate their ability to enter previously avoided situations when planning their assignments. If this has happened, they can become demoralized. The therapist should analyze these situations carefully, determining whether there were any mitigating factors and – using a problem-solving approach within the group – identify new approaches or strategies that might be used when the patient attempts to re-enter the situation. By adopting this approach the therapist demonstrates to the patients how to think rationally about, and plan for, difficult anxiety-provoking situations.

- Group practice of progressive muscle relaxation.
- Accompanied group walk to closest railway station and return to clinic.
- Material in Patient Treatment Manual, Section 7: Producing Panic Sensations in Your Daily Life.
- Individual assignment 5: Travel 20 bus stops and remain at the destination for 20 minutes.
- Debriefing after assignments: Review how the anxiety-management and cognitive restructuring techniques were applied.
- Homework for day fifteen: respiratory monitoring, practice of slow-breathing and relaxation techniques.

Day sixteen

Therapists should cover the following material and assignments:
- Review: respiratory monitoring, practice of slow-breathing and relaxation techniques.
- Group practice of progressive muscle relaxation.
- Unaccompanied group trip around the city. The purpose of this trip is to demonstrate to the patients that they can cope with a 6-hour outing. A possible trip can include lengthy bus trips, very short train trips, as well as the use of elevators and escalators.
- Debriefing after assignment: It is important to emphasize that this last exercise has been long and tiring, and that tiredness should not be misidentified as anxiety. Review how the anxiety-management and cognitive restructuring techniques were applied.
- Homework for day sixteen: respiratory monitoring, practice of slow-breathing and relaxation techniques.

Day seventeen

Therapists should cover the following material and assignments:
- Review: respiratory monitoring, practice of slow-breathing and relaxation techniques.

- Material in Patient Treatment Manual, Section 8: More About Thinking Straight.
- Group practice of progressive muscle relaxation.
- Individual assignment 6: Repeat yesterday's assignment, this time alone.
- Debriefing after assignment: Review how the anxiety-management and cognitive restructuring techniques were applied.
- Homework for day seventeen: respiratory monitoring, practice of slow-breathing and relaxation techniques.

Day eighteen

Therapists should cover the following material and assignments:

- Review: respiratory monitoring, practice of slow-breathing and relaxation techniques.
- Group practice of progressive muscle relaxation.
- Individual assignment 7: Travel by train for six stops, changing trains at one station, using both surface and subway trains, if available.
- Debriefing after assignments: Review how the anxiety-management and cognitive restructuring techniques were applied.
- Homework for day eighteen: respiratory monitoring, practice of slow-breathing and relaxation techniques.

Day nineteen

Therapists should cover the following material and assignments:

- Review: respiratory monitoring, practice of slow-breathing and relaxation techniques.
- Group practice of progressive muscle relaxation.
- Material in Patient Treatment Manual, Section 9: Keeping Your Progress Going.
- Individual assignment 8: Travel 30–40 stops by train, walking and catching buses between stations and the clinic (this exercise should take 3–4 hours).
- Review of course: In this session the therapist reviews all the techniques that have been taught during the course and restates how and when each technique may be used. The essential instructions, printed on a card that may be carried in a pocket or purse, are given to patients.

When you panic

1. Recognize that this is a panic attack and that the physical symptoms are due to the panic.
2. Use the slow-breathing technique until the panic subsides.
3. When ready, continue what you were doing.

When you are anxious

    1. Recognize that this is anxiety and that the physical symptoms and thoughts are due to this.

    2. Remember the techniques you have learned and choose an appropriate one. Do you need to use the slow-breathing technique, isometric exercises, or the progressive muscle relaxation tape? Do you need to counter irrational thinking?

    3. When your anxiety falls, plan your next move positively.

    4. When ready, continue appropriately.

- Final instructions: Practice each day and do not make excuses for avoiding anxiety-provoking situations or activities. Improvement will continue provided you are prepared to keep entering anxiety-provoking situations and using the anxiety-management techniques.

Nine-week less intensive group program structure

Broadly speaking, the same material is covered that has been discussed above; however, it is done so in the context of nine, 2-hour weekly group sessions comprising up to 10 clients. Each session follows a structure that involves setting an agenda (and review of homework assignments when appropriate), discussion of the relevant section in the Patient Treatment Manual and training and practice of the particular skills, the setting of homework assignments (which involve reading the relevant section in the Manual and exposure exercises that follow a hierarchical pattern similar to those in the 3-week structure). Each of the nine weekly sessions focuses on one of the nine main sections in the Patient Treatment Manual. The chief differences in format are that exposure exercises are conducted between, rather than within, treatment sessions and they are conducted in the person's typical environment, rather than in the area surrounding the clinic.

The treatment process

The therapist's task is not only to teach the cognitive behavioral techniques, but also to ensure that obstacles to progress are managed effectively. Hindrances to treatment comprehension and compliance can be grouped according to problems in (1) education, (2) slow breathing, (3) relaxation, (4) graded exposure, and (5) cognitive restructuring.

Problems with education

Franklin (1990b) found that sufferers of generalized anxiety disorder were able to explain their initial panic attacks in terms of a stress reaction, while 90% of sufferers of agoraphobia were perplexed about the origin and real meaning of their symptoms. The goal of the educational component of the Patient Treatment Manual is to rectify this problem by providing a complete understanding of the origin of every physical sensation and symptom. Doing so not only decreases anxiety, but also lays the groundwork for cognitive restructuring. The first two sections in the Treatment Manual serve to bring the patient to the understanding that panic attacks represent a misfiring of the flight or fight response exacerbated by hyperventilation and maladaptive cognitions. The flight or fight response has misfired because its threshold for activation is too low. The increased sensitivity of the flight or fight response has been caused by a nervous temperament, stress, and a tendency to over breathe (see Chapter 4). The first step in providing a new conceptualization of panic is to agree upon a common domain of conversation. The Manual achieves this by defining agoraphobic avoidance and the symptoms of a panic attack. When conducting group treatment, it is useful to construct a table that all can see (on a blackboard or a sheet of paper) of each patient and their symptoms. Doing so allows patients to see the similarities and differences between themselves and other group members and defines the range of symptoms experienced during panic attacks publicly. It is then possible to demonstrate that many of the symptoms are similar to those found in the naturally occurring flight or fight response. Worry about each symptom of panic can then be decreased by drawing attention to the purpose of each physical change as a preparation for danger. As a result, the person's perception of panic changes from being just a loose conglomeration of worrying symptoms to an ordered emergency response, brilliantly designed to keep the individual safe. In a panic, it is not that the symptoms are inherently dangerous it is just that the response is being triggered at the wrong time and in the wrong place. Once a link has been made between the flight or fight response and a panic attack, it is necessary to consolidate this learning by explaining the origin of panic by discussing the putative etiology of a decreased threshold of the flight or fight response. It identifies stress, a nervous temperament, and hyperventilation as three key causes of initial panic attacks. The Patient Treatment Manual uses the metaphor of a car alarm to convey the message that the flight or fight response can be triggered inappropriately if the firing mechanism is too sensitive. The metaphor helps patients to grasp the otherwise abstract concept of a differential temperamental sensitivity to react to stressors with anxiety. The Treatment Manual describes the mechanism of breathing and the effects of over breathing in detail. Consequently, it is necessary to take patients slowly through the details to ensure understanding. Laying the groundwork at this point makes it easier to respond to the complaint that slow breathing is simplistic by referring the patient back to the explanation that panic attacks are the misfiring of the flight or fight response exacerbated by hyperventilation. It is not simplistic, because it is able to modify a complex set of mechanisms responsible for the escalation of anxiety into panic. Nevertheless, the slow-breathing technique, in practice, is elegantly simple. Once the putative processes responsible for a panic are understood, reversing the changes with slow breathing is straightforward. Once the details of the slow-breathing technique are outlined, the therapist is in a position to begin to help to modify the inaccurate and irrational beliefs regarding panic attacks and agoraphobic situations. The Treatment Manual moves on to explicitly address the worrying thoughts that trigger and exacerbate panic attacks. To modify maladaptive beliefs, the therapist will switch between a number of strategies. These involve (1) replacing inaccurate with accurate information, (2) explaining the origin (and therefore the benign nature) of the symptoms of panic, and (3) reiterating the purpose of the flight or fight response. Later in therapy it becomes increasingly important to avoid giving reassurance; therefore, in the early stages, it is necessary to provide a foundation for the person to reconceptualize their panic attacks in terms of normal physiology. It is important to consolidate the new conceptualization of the experience of panic. If the flight or fight response is an emergency response designed to protect the person from danger, it is possible to evaluate each disturbing symptom in this light. For example, a patient who worries that a panic attack is going to cause them to run around in circles yelling obscenities may benefit from considering whether there is any adaptive advantage to such behavior, if it were to be triggered in the presence of a physical danger. When the absurdity of the situation has been seen, the patient can be asked why such behavior should be triggered when the flight or fight response is triggered as a false alarm (i.e., during a panic). After many years of interpreting symptoms in a particular way, it takes time for the new conceptualization of panic to modify the person's thinking more generally. Therefore expect each person to continue to offer previously unexplained symptoms to the therapist for explanation through-out therapy. Once again, respond to these inquiries in an empathic manner, not seeking to reassure, but seeking to educate and explain each symptom in terms of the model of anxiety and panic presented earlier.

Problems with slow breathing

After patients have been taught the principles behind a technique it is important to ensure correct practice. Slow breathing, while simple, is often not practiced correctly. To ensure correct practice, model one slow breathing cycle, count patients through at least one cycle, and then observe them engaging in slow breathing. Checking that patients have initially learned the technique correctly avoids the problems of the patient having to unlearn bad habits later in therapy. Two common mistakes with slow breathing are: (1) beginning to use the technique too late, and (2) finishing it too early. Slow breathing is to be used at the first sign of anxiety to stop the spiral of anxiety into panic. Done at this time, the person will be able to reverse quite quickly any changes caused by hyperventilation. It will take longer to reverse the changes if they wait until hyperventilation has affected blood carbon dioxide levels. Even when slow breathing is used successfully to control the beginning of a panic attack, it is useful to continue the slow breathing for a couple more cycles. Otherwise, the person may continue with their activity and notice the re-emergence of physical sensations that may initiate the processes responsible for a panic. Another difficulty with the implementation of the slow-breathing technique is when people take very large breaths. Consequently, their breathing rate is reduced to a reasonable level, but the quantity of carbon dioxide being expelled remains high. If this problem is suspected, the typical signs that the therapist may observe include significant rising and falling of the shoulders and overextension of the chest area. A related difficulty is that the person may breathe from the chest rather than from the diaphragm. Diaphragmatic breathing is usually recommended as the "correct" form of breathing at rest and for patients with a tendency to overbreathe it is probably sensible, although there is no empirical basis for this assertion (Weiss, 1989). Logically, it would be expected that a person breathing from the chest would tend to take short shallow breaths, which increase the amount of carbon dioxide expelled. Since expansion of the chest is constrained by the rib cage it is also probable that a slow breathing rate will be difficult to sustain comfortably unless breathing is diaphragmatic. For these reasons, we discourage chest breathing in patients prone to panic attacks (for a discussion of teaching diaphragmatic breathing, see Weiss, 1989). A common difficulty with slow breathing is neglecting to hold the breath at the start of each slow-breathing cycle. This error, as well as decreasing the technique's effectiveness, draws the attention of the therapist to a possible misunderstanding of the principles underlying slow breathing. Holding the breath aims to increase blood levels of carbon dioxide (by decreasing the rate with which the gas is expelled). Breathing in and out on a 6-second cycle aims to ensure a respiration rate that is slow and balanced (thereby preventing any new imbalance). Since the two components aim to bring about different effects, it is equally important for patients not only to slow their breathing frequency but also to regularly hold their breath to further increase blood carbon dioxide levels. Therefore if the patient neglects one part of the technique it is probable that the rationale has not been completely understood.

Problems with relaxation

As a complement to slow breathing, the Patient Treatment Manual (Chapter 7) presents relaxation as an anxiety-management technique. We include relaxation in the treatment program as a prophylactic anxiety-management strategy. Patients are encouraged to use progressive muscle relaxation before confronting feared objects and situations. Isometric relaxation is used to combat anxiety in vivo, in a manner similar to Ost's (1987b) applied relaxation. One frequently cited difficulty with isometric relaxation as a panic control skill is the speed with which panic attacks occur. Patients argue that almost before they know it, the panic is rising rapidly, and they do not have the time to engage their relaxation techniques. Because of the ubiquitousness of this difficulty we have taken to encouraging patients to engage in progressive muscle relaxation before entering anxiety-provoking situations, as a prophylactic measure. Isometric relaxation can be used to manage tension during a panic, but in our program emphasis is placed upon the need to first bring hyperventilation under control. Patients are taught to hold their breath at the first sign of panic, to stop the spiral of anxiety into panic. Once the slow breathing starts to work, the person is in a better position to tackle associated problems such as muscle tension. They can then use cognitive restructuring techniques to control worrying thoughts and they can use isometric relaxation to reduce any tension. This choice of emphasis (i.e., stopping the escalation of hyperventilation-induced symptoms versus stopping the escalation of physical tension) is governed principally by reports from patients. They say that during a panic their principal concern is the uncontrollable and rapid rise of the symptoms. Therefore, we emphasize the need to use hyperventilation control to tackle this part of the problem first – only then moving on to modify other parts of the vicious cycle of panic.

Problems with graded exposure

As soon as patients have learned some anxiety-management strategies, it is essential that they be encouraged to face their fears. Without confronting feared somatic sensations, patients may accept the theory of the treatment program but remain skeptical about the ability of the techniques to help them to overcome panics. It is only when an individual is successfully able to control panic in a phobic situation that the treatment is perceived to be credible. For this reason, the Patient Treatment Manual introduces two forms of exposure: in vivo exposure to feared situations and interoceptive exposure to the bodily sensations associated with panic attacks. While the former is aimed primarily towards decreasing fearful avoidance of certain locations, the latter is aimed specifically towards decreasing panic frequency by reducing the fear of bodily sensations. Mattick et al. (1990) demonstrated that in vivo exposure has an antipanic effect in addition to its antiphobic effect, and Page (1994) has suggested that interoceptive exposure has additional antipanic effects. Nevertheless, beginning to confront feared situations is often a source of considerable anxiety to patients because setbacks in progress are immediately obvious, the associated anxiety is intensely aversive, and the feelings of demoralization can be profound. For these reasons graded exposure needs to be planned carefully and conducted consistently. Many of the general issues regarding graded exposure will be discussed in Chapter 14, and therefore the present section will consider only issues unique to agoraphobia. One common difficulty in constructing a hierarchy is the patient who wants to dispense with steps along the way, facing immediately the most feared situation. This desire comes from two sources. First, the patient may be impatient and therefore unwilling to "waste time" breaking the goal down (see Chapter 14). The second reason why patients opt for flooding is because panics are no longer frightening. If they now consider that they have avoided situations for fear of panic and they can now control panic attacks, all situations become equally safe. With such individuals we have found it easiest to let them attempt to face the (previously) most fear-provoking situation first, simply because they invariably do it anyway. Nevertheless, it is useful to get the patients to agree to view the attempt as an experiment and, if it fails, to commit themselves to trying a graded hierarchy (Miller and Page, 1991). Although patients may be timid about confronting their feared situations, a related fear is therapist timidity. Timidity and maladaptive cognitions appear to strike the novice therapist most commonly when conducting panic provocation exercises, even though these exercises are intrinsically safe. The therapist must communicate, in a calm manner, that to overcome fears those fears must be faced. If the fear is of the internal bodily sensations, then these too must be confronted. Only by facing the feared situation will anxiety be truly overcome. When the rationale is clearly presented to patients who have had some success in controlling panic attacks, we have found no difficulties with compliance. The panic provocation exercises function as a useful method for bringing about cognitive change as well as rapidly decreasing the frequency of panic symptoms (Page, 1994). When encouraging exposure to feared situations therapists must avoid a common trap. Because individuals with panic disorder and agoraphobia are often afraid that some catastrophe is imminent, they seek reassurance or safety in some person or object (Rachman, 1984). Since these people and objects then become anxiety-reducing mechanisms, they can attenuate the power of exposure-based programs. Patients also have a tendency to attribute success to the presence of the safety signal, thereby negating the hard-won gains of exposure therapy. There is a degree of consistency across patients with panic and agoraphobia regarding the subtle avoidance strategies used; the most common talismans that are carried in case they may be needed to abort panic include anxiety medication, food, or drink (Barlow, 1988). Therapists should identify such safety signals and persuade patients to relinquish them. Another common strategy used by patients to minimize anxiety during exposure is distraction (see Clarke and Jackson, 1983). While distraction may have helped sufferers of panic to cope with anxiety in the past, it does not allow anxiety to extinguish or habituate. In addition, patients often spend so much time distracting themselves that they fail to implement the new anxiety-management techniques. While it is difficult to encourage patients to give up one of the few techniques that they have found useful, it is profitable to do so. Once the person can actively control panic attacks, the fear of panic decreases. Since panic disorder is fundamentally a fear of future panics, it is only when the patient is given a sense of true mastery over the panic that fear decreases (de Silva and Rachman, 1984; Rachman et al., 1986). In addition to difficulties with grading exposure tasks, there are some situations that are ungradable. Usually, difficulty in grading a specified task can be overcome by imaginative and lateral thinking. However, the feared outcome may be truly ungradable. For instance, one patient with long-standing agoraphobia identified a primary fear to be "What if I panic, and it lasts forever?". Every effort to grade exposure tasks failed to modify this fearful belief, because the patient was able to respond, "But I knew that the task would be over in a set time and then the panic would end". It was only when ungraded and essentially "open-ended" situations (e.g., long-distance train travel) were attempted that anxiety began to decrease and the irrational cognition was successfully challenged.

Problems with cognitive restructuring

One of the advantages of exposure, whether to external situations or to internal somatic sensations, is that it permits patients to challenge catastrophic panic-related cognitions. For this reason, it is probable that exposure alone would serve as a cognitive restructuring technique. However, many patients misattribute treatment gains to external factors (e.g., "I was having a good day") and they misattribute treatment setbacks to internal factors (e.g., "I'm such a weak person, I can't even get on a bus"). They can also draw false conclusions from exposure exercises (e.g., "I didn't panic because my partner was nearby"). Given the propensity for exposure alone to fail to modify maladaptive cognitions in the best possible way, it is important that patients be given a method for challenging cognitions. The Patient Treatment Manual uses Ellis' model (Ellis and Harper, 1975), which asserts that emotions are the consequence of beliefs about certain activating events. The reason for this choice is primarily because patients find the model intuitively appealing, the corresponding treatments have good empirical support (see Chapter 4), and it is consistent with Clark's (1986, 1988) model of panic presented in Section 1.13 of the Treatment Manual. Therapists have moved to draw upon other cognitive techniques (e.g., testing inaccurate beliefs; Beck et al., 1985) but even these remain within the framework provided in Ellis' model. Even though the model of cognitive restructuring is not presented until a reasonable portion of the program has been conducted, it should not be new to patients. Educating about anxiety, the cognitive model of panic, and the purpose of graded exposure to test maladaptive beliefs have all set the stage for cognitive restructuring. Most often patients see the sections on cognitive restructuring as making explicit the cognitive therapy that has, until now, been only modeled by the therapist. This perception is fostered as patients are encouraged to increasingly take responsibility for their own cognitive therapy. Patient independence in cognitive therapy is developed by moving through three stages during treatment. In the first few days of therapy, the therapist models cognitive therapy by reconceptualizing panic and agoraphobic avoidances as well as explicitly and forcibly challenging any inaccurate and maladaptive beliefs. In the second stage, Ellis' model of cognitions is made explicit and panic attacks and agoraphobic avoidance are conceptualized in cognitive terms. Patients are taught to challenge and dispute irrational and maladaptive cognitions in the therapeutic context. Therapist and patient work together, refining the challenges so that they are accurate, believable, and acceptable to the patient. Following this, the patient is encouraged at every opportunity to identify and challenge any maladaptive cognitions that occur, especially during panic attacks and graded exposure tasks. In the final stage, the therapist moves from a collaborative to provocative role. Once the patient has begun to understand and successfully apply the cognitive skills, the therapist begins to raise the stakes by deliberately finding weaknesses in the person's challenges. Patients do not find this a novel situation, because whenever they have previously tried to challenge maladaptive thoughts before, an internal provocateur has attempted to pick holes in their new thoughts. However, for this to be therapeutic, it is important to bring patients to a point where they begin to flounder, but then, using a careful Socratic approach, encourage development of greater cognitive restructuring abilities. If the therapist provides a clear and simple resolution when patients begin to flounder, they will not acquire any greater skills at challenging maladaptive cognitions. If the therapist leads them to develop a new understanding, they acquire not only the adaptive cognition but also the means to develop such thoughts in the future.

Problem solving

As the therapist works through the treatment program, challenges and questions arise. Responding openly to any query encourages patients to express their doubts and misgivings about the details of the program. Otherwise, the therapist runs the risk of blithely progressing under the false impression that the patients have not only understood but also accepted everything. In this context, it is useful to bear in mind that, because anxiety-disordered patients are usually anxious, they may have poor concentration. It is therefore important to speak slowly, using illustrations where necessary. Complaints, difficulties, and questions commonly occur, despite the best teaching. The following section provides some suggested answers and resolutions. One problem often encountered among patients with severe agoraphobic avoidance is "secondary gain". It appears that the person or a significant other serves to gain more from the continuation of the disorder than from its amelioration. Although this behavior is by no means universal and almost certainly does not cause agoraphobia, when present it makes therapeutic progress more difficult. Although such behavior can be construed as passive-aggressive, it is perhaps more profitable to conceptualize the actions as a problem requiring great therapeutic skill to resolve. At the risk of trivializing the complexity of resolving therapeutic resistance of this kind, it is useful to outline some principles. First, if "secondary gain" is considered a form of resistance, then motivational interviewing can be used to guide the therapist's approach (see Chapter 14). The primary aim will be to develop a discrepancy, so that the gains of recovery outweigh the gains of remaining incapacitated. Second, it is probably helpful to view the behavior as a sensible response to particular environmental contingencies (which can be modified), rather than a defect in the person's personality. Third, when the partner (rather than the patient) is the primary hindrance, it is useful either to discuss with the patient strategies whereby they may alter their partner's behavior or to involve the partner in treatment and perhaps offer additional behavioral relationship counseling (e.g., Barlow et al., 1984). One other problem encountered during treatment is the effect of intrusive or obsessional thoughts. It has been documented that intrusive and obsessional thoughts are common in the general population (Rachman, 1981). Similarly, individuals with panic disorder and agoraphobia can worry about having unpleasant intrusive thoughts. Although the problem may not warrant a diagnosis of OCD, patients will often reluctantly confess, late in treatment, bizarre intrusive thoughts. They have secretly endured these thoughts, convinced that they are true evidence of insanity. In group treatment, when such "confessions" can be elicited, they are often greeted with relief from other group members who too can "confess" to similar ideation. Once brought into the open, the problem (if severe) can be tackled in the manner described in Chapter 17.

Typical complaints

"I have had this problem for years, I've had numerous treatments, I can't get better in three weeks!" Our group program for panic disorder with agoraphobia is run intensively over 10 days spread over 3 weeks and concludes with patients making a solo trip by bus, by train, and on foot that takes them many kilometers from the clinic, a journey that takes the greater part of a day. For people who at the start of treatment have great difficulty even coming to the clinic and who may have been effectively housebound for years, this rate of progress is hard to believe. This is even more difficult for patients who have had numerous failed treatment attempts. Indeed, we too are constantly amazed at the degree and speed of recovery that occurs. We have found the best way to handle this comment, if it arises at the initial treatment session, is to draw attention to the number of hours the person will spend in the program. If the treatment program were spread over individual 1-hour weekly sessions, the person would be in treatment for 2 years. Patients can conceive that they may be brought to this point within 2 years. The therapist can then suggest that the group program compresses this treatment and allows patients to rapidly build on their successes. If the comment arises later in therapy, it is more useful to direct attention to the task at hand. That is to say, rather than thinking (and usually worrying) about goals that are perceived to be unattainable, the patient can be encouraged to successfully work to master the present task, which is one step towards the seemingly impossible goal. "I can't get to your clinic, will you come to me?" Having made numerous failed attempts to take treatment to housebound agoraphobics, we now insist that patients come to the clinic. Although this may sound harsh, we have found that doing otherwise fosters dependency. Patients do find ways to attend the clinic – even individuals who have been housebound. We have developed this practice from our experience and it is for the same reason, the fostering of dependency, that we refuse to conduct an inpatient program. If you elect to offer a home-based program for those confined to their homes and find it successful, please publish how you did it. A related issue is accompanying patients upon their graded exposure assignments. We accompany patients only on their very first graded exposure assignment. After the first group walk, patients conduct the therapist-directed exposure tasks first as a group and then alone. Most patients are able to master fearful situations much more easily when accompanied by the therapist. Although not accompanying patients initially slows the rate of progress, in the long-term this strategy appears preferable because the therapist does not become a safety signal (Rachman, 1984). In addition, the patient learns from the beginning of therapy that self-control of panics is possible and it is the way to overcome phobic disorders and ensure independence. The one exception is the first assignment after patients have returned for the second half of their program. Many patients are demoralized at this time, believing wrongly that they have made little progress. The therapist is able to analyze what has been achieved, provide support and, more importantly, observe each patient's performance in vivo so that accurate feedback can be provided. "Panics are unbearable, I can't live like this any more!" Individuals with panic disorder and agoraphobia have higher suicide rates than the general population. Furthermore, given the comorbidity of the disorders with depression (Andrews et al., 1990c) and alcohol problems (Page and Andrews, 1996), expressions of hopelessness need to be taken seriously. Most often patients are using the strongest language available to them, to communicate the incapacitation caused by panics and the terror that haunts them. Therefore, the therapist must disentangle whether the patient is communicating a suicidal intent or the enormity of the disorder. If it is the former, the therapist must pursue standard practice for intervening with suicidal patients. If it is the latter, begin the program that has been outlined.

General summary

Conducting treatment for panic disorder and agoraphobia requires a thorough understanding of the science behind the disorder and its treatment. However, there is an art to presenting empirically validated techniques. This may explain why clinicians unfamiliar with a cognitive behavioral formulation may have slightly less impressive treatment outcomes when compared with those who are more familiar with cognitive behavioral theories and interventions (e.g., compare Welkowitz et al. (1991) and Gournay (1991) with Klosko et al. (1990)). The present chapter has outlined the art of delivering an empirically validated treatment technique, suggesting that maximum success attends those who can enhance motivation for treatment, enhance treatment comprehension and compliance, and successfully handle patients' criticisms and difficulties.

Panic disorder and agoraphobia

Patient Treatment Manual*

This Manual is both a guide to treatment and a workbook for persons who suffer from panic disorder and agoraphobia. During treatment, it is a workbook in which individuals can record their own experience of their disorder, together with the additional advice for their particular case given by their clinician. After treatment has concluded, this Manual will serve as a self-help resource enabling those who have recovered, but who encounter further stressors or difficulties, to read the appropriate section and, by putting the content into action, stay well.

Contents

*Gavin Andrews, Mark Creamer, Rocco Crino, Caroline Hunt, Lisa Lampe and Andrew Page *The Treatment of Anxiety Disorders* second edition © 2002 Cambridge University Press. All rights reserved.

SECTION 1

1 The nature of anxiety, panic, and agoraphobia

Since the time of the ancient Greeks there have been consistent reports of a disorder causing the most irrational fears in otherwise sane persons. It was not until the latter part of the nineteenth century that this came to be known as agoraphobia, which literally translated means "fear of the market place". More recently, it has come to be known more generally as a fear of public places or open spaces.

While fear of public places or open spaces does characterize the majority of sufferers of agoraphobia, recent evidence suggests that these situational fears are not the primary fears in agoraphobia. It is the *fear of panic or anxiety attacks*, regardless of where they occur, that is the primary fear in panic disorder and agoraphobia.

Many people have attacks of panic. However, only a few people continue to have frequent or distressing attacks of panic that begin to interfere with their day-to-day functioning. When panic attacks are very frequent or when a person spends a considerable amount of time fearfully anticipating the next attack of panic, that individual may be said to suffer from panic disorder.

Some people with panic continue their daily lives despite the attacks of anxiety that strike them out of the blue. For other people with panic, the attacks of anxiety lead them to avoid situations for fear of panic. Typically, people who panic do so for one of three reasons. First, they may avoid situations because they see a link between the various situations and their panics. For example, panic attacks may occur regularly in shopping centers, so the person comes to avoid these places. Second, people with panic can avoid situations where a panic may occur because of the physical or social effects of panicking in that place. For instance, someone who fears urinating during a panic may avoid places where people easily may observe the consequences of such a loss of control. Finally, individuals may avoid situations where they perceive that they do not have the resources to manage a panic. For instance, a person may avoid driving if they fear that a panic may rob them of the capacity to drive safely.

The avoidance of situations for fear of panic typically includes crowded areas, open spaces, buses, trains, closed-in places, and being a long way from home or help. Remember, these fearful avoidances are secondary to the basic fear: the fear of panic. It is, therefore, more appropriate to describe agoraphobia as a fear of panic attacks that may lead a person to avoid any situation or activities that they think will provoke these attacks or prevent escape or hinder help arriving.

The distinction between primary and secondary fears is important. For individuals with panic disorder it will be necessary to learn to control the primary fear, the panic attacks. For individuals with panic disorder and agoraphobic avoidances, the fact that the fear of situations is secondary to the fear of anxiety means that to overcome the problems of agoraphobia it is necessary to learn to control the anxiety and panic attacks. Once this primary fear is controlled, an individual with agoraphobia can learn to overcome the situational fears. As individuals learn that they can control their anxiety and their panics, they can confront those situations that they have previously avoided, secured by the knowledge that they can prevent panic attacks.

This primary fear in agoraphobia is often described as a fear of fainting or collapsing, having a heart attack, going crazy, losing control of bowel or bladder, or in any other way losing personal control. The secondary or situational fears are many and varied. These fears include any situation that an individual believes will provoke or is associated with high anxiety. The important point here is that one does not actually have to experience an anxiety attack in all of these situations, but need only believe that the situation might provoke an attack. In this sense it is not only the attacks of anxiety but the way in which an individual thinks about the attacks that determines which situational fears develop. In our experience, almost all people with a long-standing panic disorder come to avoid some situations for fear of panic. The extent of your avoidance will determine the amount of time and energy you will need to allocate to overcoming this problem.

Some disorders occasionally mistaken for agoraphobia include depression, schizophrenia, social phobia, and obsessive–compulsive disorder. However, a reasonable understanding of the nature of agoraphobia as previously described generally allows for easy classification of these disorders as not constituting agoraphobia.

1.1 How do panic disorder and agoraphobia develop?

1.1.1 Stress

For many people, the first panic attack occurs during a period of increased stress. Stress can be psychological or physical.

Psychological stress: such as arguments with parents or partner, death or illness in the family, problems with others outside the home, financial problems, or work pressure.

Physical stress: resulting from personal illness, exhaustion from overworking, excessive use of alcohol or drugs, lack of sleep, low blood sugar as a result of dieting.

1.1.2 Anxiety

Both physical and psychological stress can produce an anxiety reaction. Becoming anxious is not the inevitable consequence of stress, but it is a common result. Often these stresses and the associated anxiety can be quite subtle, but it is in these situations that a person is more vulnerable to a panic attack.

At some time or another everyone experiences stress and reacts by becoming anxious. However, not everyone who experiences anxiety develops panic attacks. The question arises why some people develop panics while others don't. Unfortunately, there is no single answer to this question as yet. There are, however, various possible explanations. First, there is some evidence that people who develop panic disorder and agoraphobia have been subjected to greater than normal amounts of stress just prior to their first attack, thus making them more vulnerable than others. Second, it may be the case that people who develop panic attacks are more vulnerable than others to stress and to worry about panic attacks.

1.1.3 Hyperventilation or overbreathing

To hyperventilate means to overbreathe, either by breathing too quickly or too deeply. The actual abnormal breathing often goes unnoticed by the sufferer; however, the effects of hyperventilation do not. The symptoms include dizziness, light-headedness, tingling sensations in hands or feet, weakness in the legs, palpitations, tightness and pains in the chest, and rising panic. These symptoms are the result of reduced carbon dioxide in the blood as a result of overbreathing. Control of these symptoms will be discussed in Section 2.

1.1.4 Personality characteristics

Another possible reason why panic disorder and agoraphobia afflicts some and not others is that people have different natures. Most sufferers of panic disorder and agoraphobia have a tendency to worry. They are often overly concerned with many aspects of their lives, especially their health. When things go wrong, or do not turn out as expected, some of us consider that it is a more drastic or serious problem than is actually the case. Control of these worrying and self-defeating thoughts, which often contribute to anxiety, will be discussed in detail later in the Manual.

For the present, we shall turn our attention to the attack of panic.

1.2 The nature of panic

A panic attack is a sudden spell or attack when you feel frightened, anxious or terrified in a situation when most people would not feel afraid. During one of these attacks you may have noticed some of the following sensations:

- Shortness of breath
- Pounding heart
- Dizzy or light headed
- Tingling fingers or feet
- Tightness or pain in the chest
- A choking or smothering feeling
- Feeling faint
- Sweating
- Trembling or shaking
- Hot or cold flushes
- Things around you feel unreal
- Dry mouth
- Nausea or butterflies

- "Jelly legs"
- Blurred vision
- Muscle tension
- Feeling you can't get your thoughts together or speak
- Fear you might die, lose control or act in a crazy way

When the panic becomes severe, most people try to get out of the particular situation in the hope that the panic will stop, or else they get help so that should they collapse, have a heart attack, or go crazy, there will be somebody with them who will look after them. Occasionally, some people want to go somewhere alone so that they do not embarrass themselves in some way.

The first few times that someone experiences a panic attack are usually very frightening because this is a new experience that is strange and abnormal. However, after many such experiences most people know deep down that they're unlikely to lose control, collapse, die, or go crazy. At least, they haven't up till now. However, many fear that the next time may be different, that the next panic may be the worst. Some people manage to resign themselves to the experience of panic, even though they never like the experience.

Panics rarely come truly out of the blue. Even the first attack usually occurs at a time when the individual is under emotional pressure, or unwell (e.g., recovering from the flu), or when they are tired and exhausted and beginning to feel at the end of their tether. A person's first panic attack is very uncommon when someone is truly safe, genuinely relaxed, and free from stress.

1.3 The development of situational fears

Most people rapidly learn to predict the situations in which the panic is likely to occur. It is not that the situation is so dangerous; it is just that they can identify it as an awkward place to have a panic. Planes, trains, buses, elevators, or escalators are often seen as awkward places to panic, since you have to wait until they stop in order to get off. Having to wait in a line in a bank or a shop is often difficult for the same reason. Being truly alone, as in being at home with no neighbors to call, or driving on a lonely road, or being in a lonely place like a beach or a field can have the same effect: who would come to your aid if you panicked? Driving on your own and being caught in a traffic jam has all these problems: being alone, help can't get to you, but you can't really leave the car should you panic. Of course, for some, the fear of making a fool of yourself outweighs the need for help, and so you'd do anything to be alone.

When an event occurs in our lives, we seek an explanation for that event. Also, when a panic attack is experienced, an individual will seek an explanation for it. At the time of the attack, 90% of people with agoraphobia will have no true explanation of why the attack occurred. Stress, anxiety, and hyperventilation, which have in fact caused the attack, are not seen as the reasons by the sufferer. This is because stress, anxiety, and overbreathing develop gradually, and the individual is often unaware of their presence.

The individual with agoraphobia mistakenly explains the panic attack in terms of the situation in which the panic was experienced. One way that this association is made is by the process of conditioning. Because the experience of the panic and the place in which it happened both occurred at the same time, the conditioning process leads to an association between the two events being made in memory. Your memory of the attack is associated with your memory of the situation in which it occurred. It is this association that leads to the belief that the situation caused the attack. This belief leads to the development of the situational fears and the avoidance of certain situations.

As was mentioned previously, not all situations avoided by people with agoraphobia have necessarily been the site of previous panic attacks. These individuals need only think that a certain situation may provoke an attack to avoid it. This explains the often widespread fears and avoidances held by people with agoraphobia. It also explains the speed with which these fears can develop. In fact, in 30% of people with agoraphobia, widespread avoidance develops within one week of the first panic attack. The process by which these avoidance behaviors or fears spread is known as generalization.

It is important that you understand the concepts of conditioning and generalization because the successful treatment involves the breaking down of the associations between the panic attacks and the avoided situations that have been built up by these two processes.

Another reason why people with panic attacks develop avoidance of feared situations is because they see themselves as being unable to control a panic in that situation. Because the panic is out of control, the person begins to worry about the possible consequences of having a panic, the embarrassment or possible injury. For example, you may worry that people will think less of you if you collapse in public, or you may worry that if you were to lose control of your actions you may injure yourself or loved ones. Whatever the reason, it appears sensible to avoid situations in which the consequences of having a panic (such as driving a car) are frightening.

Remember, the primary fear in agoraphobia is the fear of panic or anxiety attacks, not the fear of certain places or situations. The situational fears are secondary. Successful treatment involves, first, learning to manage and control the anxiety and panic attacks and then, second, with that knowledge, learning to overcome the situational fears.

1.4 Subtle avoidances

We have already talked about avoidance of actual situations, but there are also other types of avoidance which, although more subtle, are nevertheless connected to panic attacks.

- Do you avoid medication of any kind even if your doctor prescribes it?
- Alternatively, do you avoid going out without medication?
- Do you avoid exercise?
- Do you avoid becoming very angry?
- Do you avoid sexual relations?
- Do you avoid very emotional movies such as horror movies or even very sad movies?
- Do you avoid being outside in very hot or very cold conditions?
- Do you hate being startled or frightened?
- Do you avoid being away from medical help?
- Do you keep an eye out for exit routes?
- Do you avoid standing and walking without structural support?

If so, these forms of avoidance may well be connected to panic attacks and will need to be overcome.

Distraction can act as another form of avoidance. Many people attempt to "get through" situations in which they are afraid of having panic attacks by distracting themselves. For example, if you feel yourself becoming anxious or panicky do you:

- Carry around something to read and then read it as intensely as you can?
- Open windows?
- Play loud music?
- Try to imagine yourself somewhere else?
- Tell somebody who is with you to talk to you about something – anything?
- Seek reassurance
- Play counting games?

If you have tried many of these tricks (or are still using them), then the chances are that they have helped you to get through a panic attack in the past and may well help you in the future. However, these tricks often become strong habits in themselves to the extent that many people come to depend on them. In the long run, these strategies, while not harmful, are not helpful, since they do not change the core element of panic attacks or your anxiety over the future occurrence of panic attacks.

In addition, if you are too busy distracting yourself, you will be unable to employ the techniques we will be teaching you to control worrying thoughts. During a panic attack, the thoughts and statements that one tells oneself involve the sense of impending doom, that something terrible is about to happen, and involve a great deal of worrying about the present and future. There is an anticipation of the worst and apprehension about what may be going to happen. In addition, there are feelings that events could proceed uncontrollably or that one may not have control over one's own reactions. We will be looking at how such thoughts can trigger, intensify, and prolong our anxiety reactions.

1.5 Rationale of the program

This program will teach you to alter your responses by learning to change the way you think and the way you react to certain events. In essence, you will be learning new methods of control. The program covers three basic strategies:

Techniques designed to modify what you say to yourself,

Techniques designed to control physical sensations, and

Techniques to help you to face more comfortably the things you currently fear and avoid.

We will begin by teaching you techniques to directly control many of your physical sensations. This will be done through control of your breathing and muscle tension. Many people breathe too much when they have a panic attack, even though it sometimes feels like the opposite. Overbreathing is a major reason for the worsening of the panic sensations that you experience and learning to control your breathing will help to reduce many of the panic symptoms. In addition, muscle relaxation exercises will lower your general level of stress and tension as well as relieving muscle tension when you get uptight.

Some people quickly begin to avoid the situations that might trigger the panics, particularly those situations from which there is no easy escape or in which help is not available should a panic occur. This avoidance seems to limit the panics in the short term, but in the long term most people need to avoid more and more situations and they may even become housebound or unable to be left on their own.

Avoiding situations in which panic has occurred at first seems to be a sensible thing to do because it initially reduces the number of panic attacks. One of the problems with avoiding situations in which panic has occurred is that each time a situation is avoided, the need to avoid it the next time is heightened or increased. In this way, the panics are no longer the only problem because the individual often structures his or her life around the panics, and spends considerable effort and anxiety planning what to do in case a panic should occur or how to avoid being in a situation where a panic is possible. In this way, agoraphobia can take on a life of its own.

The next part of treatment entails exposure or practice in the situations that you have been avoiding, which in the past have become associated with panic and anxiety. Another important component of treatment involves looking at the things you say to yourself before, during, or after a panic attack and looking at the specific kinds of misinterpretations and assumptions that contribute to your anxiety. You will be shown how to question and challenge these assumptions and misinterpretations by examining the evidence.

In addition, treatment will involve examining the physical sensations that have become part of your panic response and helping you to repeatedly experience those sensations so that they become less fear provoking.

It is important to realize that achieving control of your anxiety and panic is a skill that has to be learned. To be effective, these skills must be practiced regularly. The more you put in, the more you will get out of the program. It is not the severity of your panic or avoidance, how long you have been panicking, or how old you are that predicts the success of this program, but, rather, it is your motivation to change your reactions.

1.6 Hindrances to recovery

Another factor to consider is the maintenance of agoraphobia. In some cases, there are various hindrances to recovery that maintain the phobia. One particularly difficult situation is when the person with agoraphobia or some important person in his or her life actually gains something from the person remaining agoraphobic. For example, a person might be able to accept his or her partner's agoraphobia quite readily because the person then feels confident that their partner will remain faithful since they are so dependent on them. A person with agoraphobia might prefer to remain disabled in order to avoid making decisions about what to do for the rest of his or her life. Such dependencies do not appear to cause the initial panic attacks, but they can make recovery difficult. In this program, you will be taught how to deal with panic attacks. It may also be necessary to consider whether there are any hindrances involved in remaining agoraphobic and how to deal with them. We will return to this factor later in the program.

1.7 The nature of anxiety: a true alarm

People who have suffered panic attacks soon become afraid of even small amounts of anxiety for they know that a rise in anxiety occurs at the beginning of a panic. But anxiety is useful.

Consider the following: just as you are about to cross the road, a bus hurtles straight through the intersection, just 2 meters away from you. You are startled and you run back onto the footpath. Yet even before you begin to run, your brain becomes aware of danger. Immediately, adrenaline is released to activate the involuntary nervous system. Activation of the involuntary nervous system instantly causes a set of bodily changes. Every one of the changes enables you to act quickly, avoid injury, and escape danger. By examining each of the changes in turn, the advantages of this alarm response can be made clear.

- Breathing speeds up and the nostrils and lungs open wider. This increases the amount of oxygen available for the muscles.
- Heart rate and blood pressure increase so that the oxygen and nutrients required by the muscles can be transported quickly to where they are needed.
- Blood is diverted to muscles, particularly the large muscles in the legs. Less blood is allocated to areas that do not immediately require nutrition. Blood moves away from the face and you may "pale with fear".
- Muscles tense, preparing you to respond quickly.
- Blood-clotting ability increases so that, were physical injury to occur, blood loss would be minimized.
- Sweating increases to cool the body, stopping it from overheating when strenuous physical activity begins. Blood vessels expand and move towards the skin to cool the blood.
- The mind becomes focused. It becomes so preoccupied with the thought, "What is the danger and how can I get to safety?" that other things pass unnoticed.
- Digestion is put on hold. The stomach stops digesting food. The mouth dries as less saliva is produced. Food sits heavily in the stomach and nausea or "butterflies" may occur. Instead, glucose is released to provide energy.
- The immune system slows down. In the short term, the body puts all of its efforts into escaping.
- Sphincter muscles around the bowel and bladder constrict so that no trail is left by which a predator could track you down.

It is the automatic activation of this flight or fight response that allows you to run and escape. The flight or fight response is an automatic reaction that will first lead you to flee from danger. Only when escape is impossible will you turn and fight for your life. In contrast to this life-saving alarm, it is clear that not all anxiety is of the same intensity. The prospect of examinations or a job interview may increase anxiety but not usually to the same degree as if one were faced with a vicious dog. However, whatever the degree of anxiety experienced, it is controlled by the involuntary nervous system. Whether panic or vague worries, it is the flight or fight response being triggered. The alarm is triggered, but to a lesser degree.

Also consider that anxiety helps you perform any skilled activity. If you are totally relaxed when you take an exam, play a game, solve a quarrel between your children or discuss a problem with your in-laws you will not do your best. To do anything really well you need to be alert, anxious to do well, or "focused". Anxiety in moderation can work well to make you more efficient. People with anxiety disorders often fear all anxiety, even anxiety that can help them to perform well. They often worry that it may spiral out of control, and they may panic, and hence try to avoid any anxiety.

When people do get too anxious, the anxiety can interfere with performance, as they are focused on the symptoms of anxiety and want to escape. High levels of anxiety may lead to mistakes. The more difficult the task, the more important it is to manage anxiety carefully; ideally one should remain alert, tense and in control for maximum efficiency. The relationship between anxiety and skill is shown in the diagram. On this course we will teach a number of techniques for remaining calm when the situation is appropriate, and alert, tense, and in control in difficult situations.

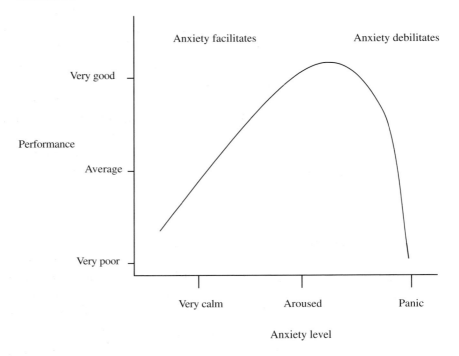

1.8 Anxiety: a false alarm

Anxiety problems originate when the flight or fight response is too sensitive. Like an overly sensitive car alarm that goes off at the wrong time, if the body's alarm is too sensitive, the flight or fight response will be triggered at the wrong time. If your anxiety alarm goes off too easily, you will be more likely to become anxious in situations where other people would not feel anxious. For example, someone with panic disorder and agoraphobia may become worried in the supermarket. Standing in a shopping line you may feel dizzy, light-headed, and slightly unreal. Having an easily triggered alarm reaction, you may then think, "What if I go crazy and I run amok in the local shops, shouting, swearing, and hitting people?". As a result, you may find yourself retreating to the safety of your home.

If you have become anxious in situations in which other individuals would not be so anxious, it suggests that your anxiety "alarm" (the flight or fight response) is too sensitive. The alarm reaction, designed to protect you from dangerous buses, charging bulls and other physical dangers, has been triggered at the wrong time.

The flight or fight response is useful in the short term, especially if the danger can be avoided by physical exertion. But it is of no use in the long term and certainly of little use in most stressful situations in the modern world. It doesn't help to run when the traffic cop pulls you over and it doesn't help to fight physically when the boss threatens you. However, because the flight or fight response was useful to our ancestors, it is still a part of our bodily make-up. It is no wonder, then, that when we are threatened, we can't get enough air, our hearts pound, we feel nauseated, and the muscles in our arms and legs tingle and shake, for all these responses would be useful if we could flee or fight.

The symptoms of a panic attack are, of course, very similar. This is because a panic attack is the flight or fight response being triggered at the wrong time. But as we know, there is no outside danger: the train is most probably not going to crash, the supermarket will not catch fire, we won't suffocate waiting in the bank queue. We know our anxiety is unreasonable. So people with panic attacks come to fear themselves, fear that the panic will lead them to have a heart attack, lose control, or die.

1.9 Why do I have false alarms?

If panic attacks are false alarms, because your flight or fight response is too sensitive, why has this happened? What has made you more likely to react with the flight or fight response than other people? Psychological research has revealed three causes of a sensitive anxiety alarm. The first is stress, and we have already talked about how stress increases anxiety. The second is overbreathing (or hyper-ventilation), and we will discuss this soon. The third reason why false alarms may be more likely to occur is due to your nature or your personality.

1.10 The effect of personality

Personality refers to the usual way we react, feel, and behave year in and year out. Most people who seek treatment have come to regard themselves as nervous people in general. They consider themselves to be people who are usually sensitive, emotional, and worry easily. This has advantages including being sensitive to other people. But the emotionality and the proneness to worry can make you more vulnerable to developing panic disorder. People with a high degree of or general nervousness tend to respond to stressful events with more physical arousal. They may then tend to become overly aware of slight changes in body sensations and wrongly treat these as signs of panic. The thinking techniques and relaxation strategies that we will teach you will aid you to control this aspect of your personality.

1.11 Summary

When people find themselves in stressful or threatening situations, an automatic physiological response is triggered. This response has been part of our physiological make-up for perhaps thousands of years. It is a primitive response that prepares people to protect themselves or escape from the source of stress. It produces changes that prepare the body for vigorous physical action.

All of these changes are quickly reversed once vigorous physical activity has been carried out. This explains why many people report the desire to run or in some other way expend physical energy when placed in stressful situations. Today, however, it is often the case that we are unable to immediately engage in such physical activity and, therefore, are less able to reverse these changes.

This problem of reversing the flight or fight response is especially the case when the response is activated by stressful or disturbing thoughts rather than physically threatening situations. In this situation, the physical changes persist for longer than they would in other situations. For people who are prone to worry excessively, these changes can be quite disturbing and a source of considerable anxiety. This, of course, leads to further activation of the flight or fight response and the whole cycle is continued. Treatment must therefore aim to break this vicious cycle. One way is by controlling hyperventilation.

1.12 Hyperventilation

For the present, we shall turn our attention to one particular aspect of the flight or fight response that is of most concern in panic disorder and agoraphobia, namely the increase in rate of respiration, or overbreathing.

As we discussed in the context of the fight or flight response, the anxiety alarm involves an increase in breathing. This overbreathing can make many of the symptoms that occur in panic disorders and agoraphobia much worse than they otherwise would be. These symptoms are important because people fear the occurrence of the anxiety reaction even more than they fear danger in a feared situation. Overbreathing has the power to make anxiety symptoms worse. Let us see how this can happen. The diagram shows how the major components of breathing link together.

Whenever we breathe in, oxygen goes into the lungs. The oxygen travels to the blood where it is picked up by an "oxygen-sticky" chemical. This oxygen-sticky chemical, called hemoglobin, carries the oxygen around the body. Oxygen is then released by the hemoglobin for use by the body's cells. The cells use the oxygen and

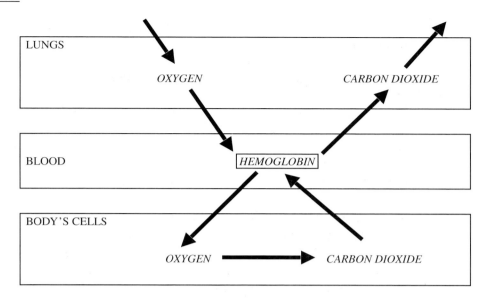

generate a waste product – carbon dioxide. The carbon dioxide is released back to the blood, taken to the lungs, and breathed out.

The puzzle is, if hemoglobin is "oxygen-sticky", then how did the oxygen become unstuck? What is the key that unlocks the oxygen? The key is carbon dioxide. Whenever the hemoglobin meets some carbon dioxide, the oxygen is unlocked so that it can go into the body's cells. Therefore, while it is important to breathe in oxygen, it is just as important that there is carbon dioxide in the blood to release the oxygen. Overbreathing makes anxiety worse not because you breathe in too much oxygen but because you breathe out too much carbon dioxide.

Breathing "too much" has the effect of decreasing the levels of carbon dioxide, while breathing "too little" has the effect of increasing levels of carbon dioxide. The body works best when there is a balance between oxygen and carbon dioxide. When you overbreathe, you end up with more oxygen than carbon dioxide in your blood. When this imbalance happens a number of changes in the body occur.

One of the most important changes is a narrowing of certain blood vessels. In particular, blood going to the brain is somewhat decreased. Coupled together with this tightening of blood vessels is the fact that the hemoglobin increases its "stickiness" for oxygen. Thus less blood reaches certain areas of the body. Furthermore, the oxygen carried by this blood is less likely to be released to the cells. Paradoxically, then, while overbreathing means we are taking in more oxygen, we are actually getting less oxygen to certain areas of our brain and body. This results in two broad categories of sensations.

Some sensations are produced by the slight reduction in oxygen to certain parts of the brain. These symptoms include:

- Breathlessness
- Light-headedness
- Dizziness
- Body feels different or unreal
- Things around you seem unreal
- Confusion
- Increased heart rate
- Tingling, "pins and needles" or numbness in hands, feet or face
- Muscle stiffness
- Sweating hands
- Dry mouth or throat

It is important to remember that the reductions in oxygen are slight and totally harmless.

One of the most distressing sensations caused by hyperventilation is a feeling that you cannot get enough air. This can trick you into breathing even harder or faster, which will just make the symptoms worse. If overbreathing continues, further symptoms can appear such as:

- Vertigo
- Nausea
- A feeling of restricted breathing
- Chest pain, constriction or tenderness
- Muscle paralysis
- Increasing apprehension or fear
- Rising terror that something terrible is about to happen, for example, a heart attack, brain hemorrhage, or even death

When individuals hyperventilate, they use more energy than they need to. This may cause other symptoms:

- Feeling hot or flushed
- Sweating
- Feeling tired
- Muscle fatigue, especially chest muscles

Looking at the lists of physical sensations produced by hyperventilation, there is some overlap with symptoms commonly reported in panic attacks. It is also easy to see how individuals might mistake the sensations produced by hyperventilation as signs of some serious physical illness. When individuals do this, their anxiety increases, they hyperventilate more, and thus worsen or prolong their symptoms.

It is important to remember that hyperventilation produces physical sensations that are unpleasant (and, for some, frightening) but they are not dangerous. The physical sensations produced may be experienced as physically unpleasant, but will not harm you. When you stop hyperventilating (or when your body's protective mechanisms step in), the sensations will go away.

Another requirement for survival is that the levels of oxygen and carbon dioxide in the body are balanced. The body has a number of protective mechanisms that prevent this relationship from becoming too unbalanced. When hyperventilation occurs for a while, the body takes steps to correct it. There are many examples of protective mechanisms in the body that maintain the body's function. For example, there is a protective mechanism that maintains blood pressure at a stable level, thus preventing people from fainting every time they stand up. Other protective mechanisms exist to regulate eating, sleep, and temperature. These mechanisms are in-built, long lasting, and generally automatic.

Breathing has automatic and voluntary control. That is to say, when you are not thinking about it, your body maintains your breathing rate. When you want to, you can change your breathing rate, e.g., holding your breath under water. In Section 1.13, you will learn that you can take advantage of this voluntary aspect of breathing control to reduce the panic symptoms produced by hyperventilation.

Although people vary greatly in their response to overbreathing, the symptoms listed are those most commonly reported. It is these symptoms of hyperventilation that can make the symptoms of panic attacks much worse than they otherwise would have been. Mild hyperventilation can also cause an individual to remain in a state of perpetual apprehension.

At the risk of repetition, the most important point to be made about hyperventilation is that it is not dangerous. Even though it can feel uncomfortable and sometimes very unpleasant, severe anxiety alone does not harm you physically. Increased breathing is part of the flight or fight response and so is part of a natural biological response aimed at protecting the body from harm. Thus it is an automatic reaction for the brain to immediately expect danger and for the individual to feel the urge to escape.

Hyperventilation is often not obvious to the observer, or even to the persons, themselves. It can be very subtle. This is especially true if the individual has been slightly overbreathing over a long period of time. In this case, there can be a marked drop in carbon dioxide but, because the body is able to compensate for this drop, symptoms may not be produced. However, because carbon dioxide levels are kept low, the body is less able to cope with further decreases and even a slight change of breathing (e.g., a sigh, yawn, or gasp) can be enough to trigger symptoms.

1.13 Types of overbreathing

There are at least four types of overbreathing that you should learn to recognize. The first three tend to be episodic and are probably more common among people with specific phobias. That is to say, they occur only during episodes of high

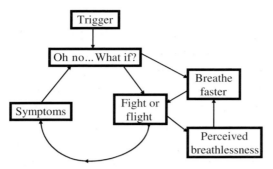

(Modified from Salkovskis, PM (1988) Hyperventilation and anxiety. *Current Opinion in Psychiatry*, **1**, 78.)

anxiety, such as when you are exposed to what you fear. The other is habitual: it occurs most of the time and is essentially a bad breathing habit or style.

- *Panting or rapid breathing:* Such breathing tends to occur during periods of acute anxiety or fear. This type of breathing will reduce carbon dioxide levels very quickly and produce a rapid increase in anxiety.
- *Sighing and yawning:* Sighing and yawning tend to occur during periods of disappointment or depression and both involve excessively deep breathing.
- *Gasping:* Gasping occurs when people think of frightening things such as doing something that they have avoided for a long time.
- *Chronic or habitual overbreathing:* This type of breathing involves slight increases in depth or speed of breathing sustained over a long period. Generally, this happens during periods of worry. It is not enough to bring on a sense of panic, but leaves the person feeling apprehensive, dizzy, and unable to think clearly. If such people are placed in the presence of what they fear and increase their breathing even by a little, this may trigger panic.

The relationship between phobic triggers and hyperventilation is summarized in the above diagram.

1.14 Common myths about anxiety symptoms

When fear is intense, people often worry about the possible consequences of extreme levels of anxiety. They may worry that anxiety will escalate out of control or that some serious physical or mental problem may result. As a result, the sensations themselves become threatening and can trigger the whole anxiety response again. It is therefore important to review the common misinterpretations about anxiety that some people have.

1.14.1 Going crazy

Many people fear they are going crazy when they experience the physical sensations of a panic attack. They may think they have the severe mental disorder called schizophrenia. However, schizophrenia and panic attacks are quite different. Panic attacks begin suddenly and tend to occur again and again. Schizophrenia begins gradually and once the symptoms are present, they do not come and go like panic attacks. The experience of panic is also quite different from schizophrenia. People with schizophrenia experience disjointed thoughts and speech, delusions or strange beliefs, and hallucinations. This is not the same as having your mind go blank or worrying about things that other people do not worry about. The strange beliefs might include the receiving of bizarre messages from outer space. Examples of hallucinations may be the hearing of voices that are not really there. Additionally, because schizophrenia runs strongly in families and has a genetic base, only a certain number of people can become schizophrenic and in other people no amount of stress will cause the disorder. Finally, people who develop schizophrenia usually show some mild symptoms for most of their adult lives. Thus, if this has not been noticed in you then it is unlikely that you would develop schizophrenia. This is especially true if you are over 25 years of age, as schizophrenia usually first appears in the late teens to early 20s.

1.14.2 Losing control

Some people believe that they will "lose control" when they panic. Sometimes they mean that they will become totally paralyzed and not be able to move. Other times they mean that they will not know what they are doing and will run around wild, hurting people or swearing and embarrassing themselves. It is clear where this feeling may come from when you remember our discussion of the fight or flight response. Your body is ready for action when the anxiety response is triggered and there is often an overpowering desire to get away from any danger. The problem is that when you do not use the anxiety response to flee or fight, you may feel confused, unreal and distracted. Nevertheless, you are still able to think and function normally. You are still able to decide what action to take in response to panic; that is, whether to stay or leave.

1.14.3 Heart attacks

At first glance it seems quite reasonable to worry that you might be dying of a heart attack when you notice that you have chest pains, tingling in your hands, shortness of breath, and so on. Fortunately, most people have never experienced a heart attack and therefore never know how this differs from a panic attack. Although the symptoms of a heart attack include breathlessness and chest pain, they tend to be related to effort and will go away once you rest. In contrast, the symptoms of a panic attack can happen at any time. While panic symptoms can occur during exercise and feel worse with exercise, they appear out of the blue and can even occur during sleep. Lastly, if a doctor has checked your heart with an electrocardiogram (a device which measures electrical changes in the heart) and has given you the all clear, then heart disease is unlikely to be causing the attacks. Heart disease produces obvious changes in the electrical activity of the heart; panic attacks just cause an increase in heart rate.

SECTION 2

2 Control of hyperventilation

2.1 Recognizing hyperventilation

The first step in preventing and controlling hyperventilation is to recognize how and when you overbreathe.

Try monitoring your breathing rate now. Count one breath in and out as 1, the next breath in and out as 2, and so on. It may be difficult at first, but don't try to change your breathing rate voluntarily. Write the answer here ____. As part of treatment you will be required to monitor your breathing rate for 1 minute during various times of the day. The form in Section 2.3 should be used for this purpose. Now consider the following:

- *Do you breathe too quickly?* The average person only needs to take 10 to 12 normal breaths per minute at rest. If your rate of breathing is greater than this then you must reduce it.
- *Do you breathe too deeply?* Does your chest sometimes feel overexpanded? You should breathe from the abdomen and through the nose, consciously attempting to breathe in a smooth and light way. Breathing through the mouth is a bad habit in most cases, and can be controlled by practice.
- *Do you sigh or yawn more than others?* Excessive sighing or yawning may be a sign of hyperventilation.
- *Do you gasp or take in a deep breath when for example, someone suggests an outing or you hear the telephone ring?* Taking one deep breath can trigger the hyperventilation cycle in many people.

Apart from recognizing the way in which you overbreathe, it is also important that you recognize the sorts of activities or events that may trigger overbreathing.

- *Are you smoking too much or drinking too much tea or coffee?* Tobacco, tea and coffee are all stimulants that will accelerate the fight or flight response. Try to reduce your smoking to a minimum and do not smoke just before anxiety-provoking situations. Switch to decaffeinated coffee or tea during the program, and later keep the number of cups you have to one or two per day. A significant percentage of people have their panic attacks triggered by caffeine, and if you find you are one of these it will be better to avoid all caffeine.

- *Are you drinking too much alcohol?* Initially alcohol acts as a depressant; however, a few hours after drinking it acts as a stimulant. At this time and at times when you experience "hangover" symptoms you are more susceptible to hyperventilation attacks.

- *Are you suffering from premenstrual tension or period pain?* Some women experience an increase in bodily sensations in the week before their periods. For this reason you may experience a worsening of panic-like sensations prior to menstruation. Become aware of these changes and use the opportunity to deal with a predictable period of increased bodily sensations and panic.

- *Are you always rushing?* Are you over conscientious – working too hard or too fast? Slow down and give yourself adequate time to do things. Organize events so that you are not always rushing from place to place. Physical activity will increase your body's need for oxygen, and, as a result, breathing rate and depth of breathing will increase. You will achieve more by staying calm and working at a reasonable pace.

2.2 Slow-breathing technique

This technique is to be used at first signs of anxiety or panic.

You must learn to recognize the first signs of overbreathing and immediately do the following:

- Stop what you are doing and sit down or lean against something.
- Hold your breath and count to 10 (don't take a deep breath).
- When you get to 10, breathe out and mentally say the word "relax" to yourself in a calm, soothing manner.
- Breathe in and out slowly in a 6-second cycle. Breathe in for 3 seconds and out for 3 seconds. This will produce a breathing rate of 10 breaths per minute. Mentally say the word "relax" to yourself every time you breathe out.
- At the end of each minute (after 10 breaths), hold your breath again for 10 seconds, and then continue breathing in the 6-second cycle.
- Continue breathing in this way until all the symptoms of overbreathing have gone.

If you do these things as soon as you notice the first signs of overbreathing, the symptoms should subside within a minute or two and you will not experience any panic attacks. The more you practice, the better you will become at using it to bring your phobic fear under control. Remember that your goal should always be to stay calm and prevent the anxiety and fear from developing into panic. You need to identify the very first symptoms of hyperventilation, and the moment you experience any of these, use the above slow-breathing techniques immediately.

2.2.1 Troubleshooting

You may find the slow-breathing technique "unnatural" or uncomfortable. Breathing at a rate of 10 breaths per minute is not unnatural, though for people who have been overbreathing for a long time it may not be habitual. Regular practice in a variety of settings will make the slow-breathing technique comfortable and habitual.

If you feel your symptoms are getting worse using this technique, ensure you are keeping time with a watch. Simply counting to yourself may lead to accelerated breathing.

Don't expect too much too soon. Regular practice in ideal circumstances will make it easier for you to use the technique in more tricky situations.

Focusing on breathing may seem "strange" for some people. Persevering with the technique will reduce this feeling.

2.3 Daily record of breathing rate

Instructions

Your breathing rate should be monitored at the times shown opposite unless you are performing some activity that will inflate your rate, such as walking upstairs. In this case wait for about 10 minutes. Try to be sitting or standing quietly when you count your breathing. Each breath in and out counts as 1: so, on the first breath in and out, count 1; on the next breath in and out count 2, and so on. Count your breathing rate in this way for 1 minute, then do the slow-breathing exercise for 5 minutes. After this, count your breathing rate again for 1 minute. Your therapist will be able to check whether your breathing rate remains low following the exercise.

Date	8:00 a.m.		12:00 noon		6:00 p.m.		10:00 p.m.	
	Before	After	Before	After	Before	After	Before	After

SECTION 3

3 Relaxation training

3.1 The importance of relaxation training

Human beings have a built-in response to threat or stress known as the flight or fight response. Part of this flight or fight response involves the activation of muscle tension, which helps us to perform many tasks in a more alert and efficient manner. In normal circumstances, the muscles do not remain at a high level of tension all the time but become tensed and relaxed according to a person's needs. Thus a person may show fluctuating patterns of tension and relaxation over a single day according to the demands of the day, but this person would not be considered to be suffering from tension.

If you remain tense after demanding or stressful periods have passed, you remain more alert than is necessary and this sense of alertness ends up turning into apprehension and anxiety. Constant tension makes people oversensitive and they respond to smaller and smaller events as though they were threatening. By learning to relax, you can gain control over these feelings of anxiety. In this program, you will be taught how to recognize tension, how to achieve deep relaxation, and how to relax in everyday situations. You will need to be an active participant, committed to daily practice for 2 months or longer.

Since some tension may be good for you, it is important to discriminate when tension is useful and when it is unnecessary. Actually, much everyday tension is unnecessary. Only a few muscles are involved in maintaining normal posture, e.g., sitting, standing, or walking. Most people use more tension than is necessary to perform these activities. Occasionally, an increase in tension is extremely beneficial. For example, it is usually helpful to tense up when you are about to receive a serve in a tennis game. Tension is unnecessary when (1) it performs no useful alerting function, (2) when it is too high for the activity involved, or (3) when it remains high after the activating situation has passed.

In order to be more in control of your anxiety, emotions, and general physical well being, it is important to learn to relax. To do this you need to learn to recognize tension; learn to relax your body in a general, total sense; and learn to let tension go in specific muscles.

3.2 Recognizing tension

When people have been tense and anxious for a long period, they are frequently not aware of how tense they are, even while at home. Being tense has become normal to them and may even feel relaxed compared with the times they feel extremely anxious or panicky. However, a high level of background tension is undesirable, because other symptoms, such as hyperventilation and panic, can be easily triggered by small increases in arousal brought on by even trivial events.

Where do you feel tension? For the next 12 days we want you to monitor the tension in your body. Use the following form to indicate the location of your tension and the degree of tension. Always choose approximately the same time each day to monitor your tension. Before your evening meal is usually a good time for this.

In each box of the Muscle tension rating form, place the number corresponding to your level of tension:

```
0          1          2          3
└──────────┴──────────┴──────────┘
Nil        Low      Medium      High
```

Muscle tension rating

Location of tension	D1	D2	D3	D4	D5	D6	D7	D8	D9	D10	D11	D12
Around eyes												
Jaw												
Side of neck												
Top of scalp												
Back of neck												
Shoulders												
Top of back												
Lower back												
Chest												
Abdomen												
Groin												
Buttocks												
Thighs												
Knees												
Calves												
Feet												
Upper arms												
Lower arms												
Hands												

3.3 Relaxation training

3.3.1 Progressive muscle relaxation

Progressive relaxation means that the muscles are relaxed in a progressive manner. This section will outline how to use both progressive relaxation and "isometric" relaxation. You should master both forms of relaxation, because the progressive muscle relaxation exercises are useful for becoming relaxed (before you confront your fears) and the isometric relaxation is useful for remaining relaxed (while you confront your fears).

Relaxation exercises should be done at least once a day to begin with, preferably before any activity that might prove difficult. Select a comfortable chair with good support for your head and shoulders. If a chair does not provide good support, use cushions placed against a wall. Some people prefer to do the exercises lying down, but do not use this position if you are likely to fall asleep. These relaxation exercises are not meant to put you to sleep, since you cannot learn to relax while asleep. Sleep is not the same as relaxation. Consider those times when you have awakened tense. When possible, it is advisable that you use a relaxation tape as a preparation before you expose yourself to what you fear.

You will need to commit yourself to daily practice in order to achieve really long-lasting effects. Some people continue daily relaxation many years after leaving treatment. If you can do this, we strongly advise it. However, not all people continue relaxation in this way. People who benefit most from relaxation either practice regularly, or practice immediately after they notice any increase in tension or anxiety.

3.3.2 Isometric relaxation

Isometric relaxation exercises can be done when you experience fear. Most of the exercises do not involve any obvious change in posture or movement. This is because "isometric" refers to exercises in which the length of the muscle remains the same. Because it stays the same length, there is no obvious movement.

The most common mistake that people make with isometric exercises is putting the tension in too quickly or putting in too much tension. These are meant to be gentle and slow exercises. The aim of the exercise is to relax you, not get you even more tense. If circumstances do not allow you to hold the tension for 7 seconds, you can still benefit from putting in the tension slowly over some period of time and releasing it in the same manner.

When sitting in a public place:

- Take a small breath and hold it for up to 7 seconds.
- At the same time, slowly tense leg muscles by crossing your feet at the ankles and press down with the upper leg while trying to lift the lower leg.

  Or

- Pull the legs sideways in opposite directions while keeping them locked together at the ankles.

    Or
- After 7 seconds, breathe out and slowly say the word "relax" to yourself.
- Let all the tension go from your muscles.
- Close your eyes.
- For the next minute, each time you breathe out, say the word "relax" to yourself and let all the tension flow out of your muscles.

    Choose other parts of the body to relax, e.g., the hands and arms:
- Take a small breath and hold it for up to 7 seconds.
- At the same time, tense hand and arm muscles by placing hands comfortably in your lap, palm against palm, and pressing down with the top hand while trying to lift the lower hand.

    Or
- Place hands under the sides of chair and pull into the chair.

    Or
- Grasp hands behind chair and try to pull them apart while simultaneously pushing them in against the back of the chair.

    Or
- Place hands behind the head, interlocking the fingers, and while pushing the head backward into hands try to pull hands apart.
- After 7 seconds, breathe out and slowly say the word "relax" to yourself.
- Let all the tension go from your muscles.
- Close your eyes.
- For the next minute, each time you breathe out, say the word "relax" to yourself and let all the tension flow from your muscles.

    If circumstances permit, continue with various muscle groups.

    When standing in a public place:
- Take a small breath and hold it for up to 7 seconds.
- At the same time, straighten legs to tense all muscles, bending the knees back almost as far as they will go.
- After 7 seconds, breathe out and slowly say the word "relax" to yourself.
- Let all the tension go from your muscles.
- Close your eyes.
- For the next minute, each time you breathe out, say the word "relax" to yourself and let all the tension flow from your muscles.

    Other exercises for hand and arm muscles:
- Take a small breath and hold it for up to 7 seconds.
- At the same time, cup hands together in front and try to pull them apart.

    Or

- Cup hands together behind and try to pull them apart.
  Or
- Tightly grip an immovable rail or bar and let the tension flow up the arms.
- After 7 seconds, breathe out and slowly say the word "relax" to yourself.
- Let all the tension go from your muscles.
- Close your eyes.
- For the next minute, each time you breathe out, say the word "relax" to yourself and let all the tension flow from your muscles.

3.3.3 Further isometric exercises

Various muscles that can be tensed and relaxed in order to make up additional isometric exercises. You need first to decide which of your muscles tense up most readily. (If you have difficulty deciding, consider what people say to you: "Your forehead is tense"; "You're tapping your feet again"; "You're clenching your jaw".) Once you have decided on a muscle or muscle group, decide how you can voluntarily tense these muscles, and finally how you can relax them. In this way, you can design your own tailor-made set of isometric exercises.

Instructions

Some example exercises are given below. Complete the remainder by starting with those muscles that you rated as highly tense on the muscle tension rating form earlier in this section. Write down some suggestions for putting tension in the muscle area and then suggestions for relaxing that muscle. Give the suggestions a try, but remember to tense gently and slowly.

Site of tension	Manner of tensing	Manner of relaxing
Shoulders and neck	Hunching shoulders up towards the head	Letting shoulders drop and let arms hang loose
Hand tension	Make a fist	Let all fingers go loose. Place hands palm facing upward on lap

---

Important points about learning to relax quickly

1. Relaxing is a skill – it improves with frequent and regular practice.
2. Do the exercises immediately whenever you notice yourself becoming tense.
3. Develop the habit of reacting to tension by relaxing.
4. With practice the tensing of your hand and leg muscles can be done without any movement that would attract attention. It helps to slowly tense and relax the muscles.
5. When circumstances prevent you holding the tension for 7 seconds, shorter periods will still help but you may have to repeat it a few more times.
6. Do not tense your muscles to the point of discomfort or hold the tension for longer than 7 seconds.
7. Each of these exercises can be adapted to help in problem settings such as working at a desk or waiting in a queue. Use them whenever you need to relax.
8. Using these exercises you should in a few weeks be able to reduce your tension, prevent yourself from becoming overly tense, and increase your self-control and confidence.

3.3.4 Difficulties with relaxation

Some people report they can't relax, or they can't bring themselves to practice relaxation. Since all human beings share the same biological make-up there is no purely physical reason why relaxation should work for some and not others. The reason relaxation may not work for some people is usually due to some psychological factor or insufficient practice. These problems can be overcome. If you are experiencing difficulty in relaxing you should discuss this with your therapist. Some examples of difficulties are given below.

1. *"I am too tense to relax."* In this case the individual uses the very symptom that needs treating as an excuse for not relaxing. Relaxation may take longer than expected, but there is no reason why someone should have to remain tense. It might be useful to consider whether there is some other factor getting in the way of relaxation.

2. *"I don't like the feelings of relaxation."* About 1 in 10 people report that when they relax they come into contact with feelings they don't like or that frighten them. These feelings indicate that you are coming into contact with your body again and noticing sensations that may have been kept under check for many years. You do not have to worry about losing control during relaxation sessions. You can always let a little tension back in until you get used to the sensations. As you keep practicing these sensations will pass.

3. *"I feel guilty wasting so much time."* You need to see relaxation as an important part of your recovery. Relaxation exercises take time, just like many other therapies.

4. *"I can't find the place or time."* Be adaptive. If you can't find 20 minutes, find 10 minutes somewhere in the day to relax. If you do not have a private room at

work, go to a park. You may need to consider whether other factors are pre-venting you from relaxing if you keep making the excuse that there's no time.

5. *"I'm not getting anything out of this."* Unfortunately, many people expect too much too soon from relaxation training. People often exaggerate the speed of recovery. You cannot expect to undo years of habitual tensing in a few relaxation sessions. Impatience is one of the symptoms of anxiety and often indicates a need to continue with relaxation training. Give the training time to take effect.

6. *"I haven't got the self-control."* You need to realize that quick, easy cures for panic disorder calling for no effort from you do not exist. The longest-lasting treatment effects occur when an individual takes responsibility for his or her recovery. Responsibility means self-control, but self-control is difficult if you are not motivated.

SECTION 4

4 Graded exposure

When a panic attack occurs for the first time in a certain situation, most people believe that, should they find themselves in that same situation again, they would be more than likely to panic. The occurrence of severe panics is very frightening and so, as any sensible person would, sufferers soon learn to try to anticipate situations likely to trigger their panics. For most people with panic disorder and agoraphobia, these situations involve public transport, crowded, lonely, or closed-in places – all situations from which it is impossible to escape easily or in which help couldn't easily arrive. The person usually feels that help is what is needed in a severe panic. Occasionally, some people prefer to panic on their own, to save themselves from possible embarrassment should they lose control.

Each time an individual with panic disorder and agoraphobia approaches some feared situation worry and anxiety may begin to rise. If the person then avoids it, in whole or in part, the fear increases because the drop in anxiety (which follows the "escape") tells the person that the avoidance was a sensible strategy. Thus the avoidance behavior is strengthened: after all if you can avoid panics by avoiding situations, why not do so? Unfortunately, the panics really don't stop; you just find more and more situations that could be "dangerous" and avoid them, too.

4.1 More about avoidance

Situational fears are fears of places or situations in which the panic sufferer thinks a panic attack could occur. The individual may have experienced such attacks in the same or similar situations in the past. But, due to the process of generalization, a person need not actually have experienced a panic attack in a certain situation in order to develop a fear of that situation.

Once situational fears are established, the individual with panic disorder and agoraphobia develops an avoidance of the situation. The avoidance can be of sufficient strength that the person never again enters the situation and therefore never knows whether or not it would, in fact, trigger a panic attack. This is similar to someone who, having once been frightened by a dog in a particular area, thereafter avoids going down that street and thus never learns that the dog is no longer there or is now tied up.

It is the goal of treatment to have you overcome avoidances and to break down the association between panic attacks and specific situations, such as traveling by bus or train, going far from home, or staying in small or closed-in places. The process is gradual, as fears can often be made worse if the person suddenly forces himself or herself without sufficient preparation and training in anxiety-management skills to confront something he or she may have avoided for years. In this situation, the anxiety produced by such a sudden exposure can actually strengthen the association between the situation and the fear.

What then is the cure? If the fear is reinforced by leaving the situation, what would happen if you stayed put? Actually, if you stayed in the situation for an hour or so, the fear would eventually go, and the fear the next time you entered that situation would be less. But few people with situational fears can actually stay in the situation for the 1 or 2 hours required for a really big panic to wear off. So they keep avoiding those situations.

Instead, if the associations are to be weakened, exposure to the feared situations must be gradual. First, you must learn to master situations associated with mild anxiety and then progressively master situations associated with greater levels of anxiety. It should be remembered that anxiety is different from panic, and moderate anxiety in new or previously feared situations is a perfectly normal and reasonable response. Thus we do not expect you to wait until you are anxiety free before you enter a situation. This program requires that you identify specific goals that you wish to achieve and then break them down into small steps. Each step is practiced and mastered before you move onto the next step. The skills you have learned for the control of anxiety and hyperventilation are to be used when practicing each step.

4.2 Planning your program

1. Draw up a list of goals that you would like to be able to achieve. These should be specific goals that vary from being mildly to extremely difficult. You may have many goals but the ones that are relevant are those involving anxiety in

specific situations. Examples of general goals that do not lend themselves to graded exposure could include:

- "I want to get better."
- "I want to know what sort of person I am."
- "I want to have purpose and meaning in life."

Although they are appropriate goals to have, they do not allow you to work out practical steps by which such problems can be solved. Your goals should be precise and clear situations that you can approach in a series of graded steps. The following examples are based on fears that some individuals with agoraphobia have:

- To travel to the city by underground train in rush hour.
- To shop alone in the local supermarket and do the weekly shopping.
- To go to the movies in company to a crowded performance and sit in the center of a row.

2. Break each of these goals down into easier, smaller steps that enable you to work up to the goal a little at a time. Note that the first goal comes from an individual with a fear of traveling by train. In order to be able to work towards eliminating this fear, you would need to start with (1) small trips by train, starting with traveling one station above ground, and (2) uncrowded trains. Then, gradually, you would increase the number of stations, the number of people likely to be on the train, and eventually go underground. The first goal mentioned above could be broken down into the following steps, organized like a stepladder:

- Traveling one stop on an above-ground train, quiet time of day.
- Traveling two stops in an above-ground train, quiet time of day.
- Traveling two stops in an above-ground train, rush hour.
- Traveling one stop on an underground train, quiet time of day.
- Traveling two stops in an underground train, rush hour.
- Traveling five stops in an underground train, quiet time of day.
- Traveling five stops in an underground train, rush hour.

The number of steps involved depends upon the level of difficulty of the task. To make the above steps a little easier, you might wish to do them in the company of a friend or partner to begin with, and then do them alone. For other people, these steps might be too easy. In that case you would eliminate those that are too easy. All of your goals can be broken down into smaller steps within your capabilities. Use this method to more easily achieve your goals.

3. You may also need to consider the practical aspects of how you are going to organize your exposure tasks.

4. You should always be working on those activities that you can perform, knowing you have a reasonably good chance of managing your anxiety. Some people use the 75% rule: undertaking activities that you are 75% confident you will be able to perform while managing your anxiety. If you use this rule you can determine whether you are going from one step to another with too big a jump, i.e., attempting a level that you are not ready for. If you feel less than 75% certain of controlling your panic, modify that step so as to increase your confidence. Note: Do not use the 75% rule as a reason for avoiding activities – you can always modify the activity in some way. All of your goals can be broken down into smaller steps. Use this method to more easily achieve your goals.

We would now like you to practice making out a set of steps for each of the following goals:

1. *Goal:*   Traveling up the tallest available building in an elevator.

   Steps: _____

             _____

             _____

             _____

             _____

             _____

             _____

2. *Goal:*   Doing the weekly shopping alone at a busy shopping center.

   Steps: _____

             _____

             _____

             _____

             _____

             _____

             _____

4.3 Implementing your program

1. Make sure that you perform some activity related to your phobia every day. Avoidance makes fears worse. If you are having a bad day, you should always do something, but you need only go over the steps that you have already mastered.

2. Confront a situation frequently and regularly until you overcome the fear. Many fears need to be confronted frequently (i.e., three to four times a week) at first, otherwise your fear will rise again by the time you do it next. Once you have largely overcome the fear, you need do it less frequently.

   The general rule is: *The more you fear it, the more frequently you need to confront it.*

3. Try to be working on at least three goals at any one time. When you have finished one, move on to another more difficult goal.

4. Carefully monitor and record your progress. Keep a diary of your goals, steps, and achievements, together with comments about how you felt and how you dealt with particular situations. This will help you to structure your progress and also to give you feedback on how you are doing.

4.4 Practicing the steps

1. Use the progressive relaxation exercises before you perform the activity.

2. Mentally rehearse successful performance of your activity. A good time is at the end of the relaxation session.

3. Perform all activities in a slow and relaxed manner. This means giving yourself plenty of time.

4. Monitor your breathing rate at regular intervals during the activity. This may be once every 5 or 10 minutes for an extended activity or more frequently if it is shorter.

5. When the circumstances allow it, stop your activity at the point at which you become anxious. Stop and implement the strategies you have learned in order to overcome your fear, and then wait for it to pass.

6. Do not leave a situation until you feel your fear decline substantially. This means you need to agree with yourself (and anyone who accompanies you) exactly how long or exactly how much your anxiety must decrease before you leave the situation. Never leave the situation out of fear: face it, accept it, let it fade away, and then either move on or return. If you do not do this, you may see it as a failure and lose confidence.

7. Try to remain in the situation as long as possible.

8. Congratulate yourself for successful achievements.

4.5 Facing fears in imagination

In a few instances, it may be difficult to approach your goal in a series of "real-life" steps. In such cases, some steps can be practiced in imagination. This is slower than real-life exposure, but it does provide a useful way of adding in-between steps in some "all-or-none" types of activity. In order to use exposure in imagination, you will need to specify the characteristics of the type of step you would ideally like to perform, write this on a card or series of cards, and then practice the activity specified on the card in your imagination after your next relaxation session. You will need to use cards so that you can read predetermined details about the situation that you are "rehearsing". We do not want you to let your imagination run riot. Simply imagine yourself performing the activity in a calm, collected manner. If you imagine yourself getting overly anxious or panicking, continue the session, using one of the various techniques outlined in previous sections to control anxiety.

Remember, you imagine yourself in these scenes operating in a competent manner. Even if you do not think you would, you *imagine* that you are. In this way, you can rehearse competent behavior at the same time as facing your fears. Only imagine one scene at a time. You do not have to imagine all scenes in a single session.

Other situations that can be practiced in imagination are plane travel, train travel, weddings, and being with people with whom you let yourself feel awkward.

Note that imaginal exposure should be used only where you are unable to perform a step in real life. It should also be used in combination with real-life exposure to feared situations. Imaginal practice alone will not cure agoraphobia.

4.6 Achieving your own personal goals

As we have mentioned, an essential skill in overcoming situational fears is the ability to establish clear, realistic goals for yourself and to break these down into a number of smaller, easier steps through which you can progress. Nothing will encourage you like previous success and you should learn to judge the size of the steps so that you are at least confident of controlling your panics when doing the next step.

An essential skill in overcoming situational fears is the ability to establish clear, helpful goals for yourself and to break these down into a number of smaller, easier steps through which you can progress. Nothing will encourage you like previous success.

A goal can always be broken down into a series of smaller, easier steps by varying the following:

• Whether you do the activity in company or with a companion.
• How far you are from help.

- How long you stay in the feared situation.
- How many things you do while you are there.
- How close you go to what you fear.

Using various combinations of these, you can easily build up a set of steps that enable you to more easily achieve your goals.

In the space below, we would like you to work out 10 goals of your own choosing. These goals should vary in difficulty from those things that you hope to achieve in the next few weeks, to those that may take 6 months to attain. Remember that your goals should be clear and precise situations in which you become anxious.

Before working out your own goals, read the examples of well-defined and less well-defined goals.

Less well-defined goal	Well-defined goal
I want to get out and about by myself	I want to spend two hours a week shopping alone in the nearest shops
I want to travel on buses	I want to be able to travel from my home to the city by bus alone

Now write out up to 10 goals of your own choosing.

1. _____

2. _____

3. _____

4. _____

5. _____

6. _____

7. _____

8. _____

9. _____

10. _____

Now select three (at the most) of the above goals that you would like to work on first, and write these below. Set out beneath each goal the steps you intend to take in order to achieve it.

1. *Goal:* _____

   Steps: _____

   _____

   _____

   _____

   _____

   _____

   _____

   _____

2. *Goal:* _____

   Steps: _____

   _____

   _____

   _____

   _____

   _____

   _____

3. *Goal:* _____

   Steps: _____

   _____

   _____

   _____

   _____

   _____

   _____

SECTION 5

5 Thinking straight

This part of the program will help you to control the thoughts that accompany and promote anxiety. This will be done by learning to label situations more appropriately and reduce the frequency, intensity and duration of upsetting emotional reactions. The techniques in this chapter should be used along with other parts of the treatment program.

All people have various thoughts, feelings, and behaviors in response to experiences throughout their days. These thoughts, feelings, and behaviors influence each other. Sometimes, however, people are unaware of these influences, especially the influence of thoughts on feelings. It is easy to assume that events lead directly to emotional responses (see the following diagram). This is very important, because it may lead people to believe they have no influence over the way they think, feel, or behave. The consequences are caused by the activating events. However, in the same way that the roman alphabet does not run from A to C without going through B, **A**ctivating events do not cause emotional **C**onsequences without going through our **B**eliefs. Let us consider for a moment what this means. It means that the situations that appear to **A**ctivate the **C**onsequence of a **P**anic **A**ttack, do so because of what we **B**elieve about them.

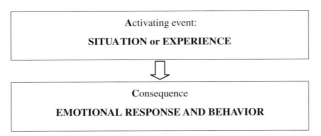

Rather than **A**ctivating events causing emotional **C**onsequences, **B**eliefs intervene.

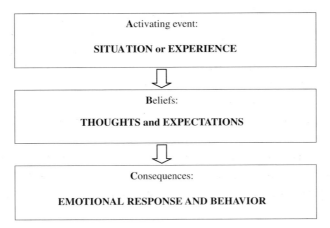

To make this more concrete, consider the following comparison between people with and without panic disorder.

Individual *with* Panic Disorder	Individual *without* Panic Disorder
Activating event: Crowded cinema	**Activating event:** Crowded cinema
Beliefs: What if I panic and can t get out? What if others can see I m anxious?	**Beliefs:** There are a lot of people here. I m glad I got a good seat in the middle.
Consequences: Anxious and tense Sits on aisle, near exit	**Consequences:** Relaxed Settles down to watch movie

As you can see, the situation or **Activating** event is the same for both people. What are different are the **Beliefs** that they have. Therefore the emotional and behavioral **Consequences** are quite different too. Thus many individuals with panic disorder and agoraphobia recognize that their emotional responses to various situations (e.g., a cinema or a boat ride) differ from those of others around them. This occurs because the individual with panic labels such situations as threatening or dangerous, and therefore feels anxious. It is important to realize it is appropriate to feel anxious in response to objectively threatening or dangerous situations. The problem in panic disorder is that the label is clearly unhelpful and in many cases it is incorrect, because it is based on an exaggerated threat.

The individual with panic disorder and agoraphobia is responding appropriately to their thoughts; it's just that the thoughts are not appropriate to the situation. They have labeled the situation as being more threatening than they need to. By changing the way you label or interpret events, you can gain more control over your feelings, in a more helpful and adaptive way.

Some individuals with panic disorder and agoraphobia have been labeling or interpreting places, events or interactions in unhelpful and fear-producing ways for months to years. After many repetitions, such patterns of thinking may occur extremely quickly, and almost seem automatic. Some people even seem to become experts at such unhelpful thinking patterns, and are able to make themselves anxious in many different situations, by applying unhelpful thinking patterns.

Avoiding situations only reinforces unhelpful and fear-producing thinking habits, as it prevents individuals from getting new, helpful information. This means they cannot prove their unhelpful beliefs to be wrong.

It is important to recognize that unhelpful thinking patterns are habits, and that habits can be changed with effort and practice. Identifying unhelpful thoughts associated with anxiety is the first step in changing your thinking.

Step 1:	*Identify* anxiety-provoking thoughts.
Step 2:	*Challenge* unhelpful anxiety-provoking thoughts.
Step 3:	*Generate* more helpful alternatives.

5.1 Step 1: Identifying anxiety-provoking thoughts

It may be difficult to detect anxiety-provoking thoughts at first, especially if they have been around for a long time. In situations where you feel anxious or uncomfortable, ask yourself:
1. What do I think about myself?
2. What do I fear will happen?
3. What do I think about the situation?
4. How do I think I will cope?
5. What will I do?

5.1.1 Anxiety-provoking thoughts in panic disorder

Common errors in thinking that produce anxiety in individuals with panic disorder include:
1. *Overestimating the chance they will panic:* Individuals with panic disorder often believe they are more likely to have a panic attack than they really are.
2. *Exaggerating the feared consequences of panic:* Individuals with panic often believe the medical, psychological, or social consequences of panic are more obvious, longer lasting or serious than they are.
3. *Underestimating their own ability to cope:* Individuals with panic often judge themselves as being unable to cope. In most cases, they are able to perform their activities on some level; it's just that they feel very anxious while doing so.
4. *Misinterpreting normal and anxiety-related physical sensations:* Individuals with panic often mistake day-to-day physical sensations as dangerous. They also misinterpret the physical sensations of panic as dangerous, rather than unpleasant.

5.1.2 Misinterpreting physical sensations

Many individuals with panic disorder and agoraphobia misinterpret the symptoms of a panic attack as being the sign of some immediate medical illness. This is understandable, given the intense physical symptoms that occur, especially the first few times panic occurs. Some people also start to misinterpret normal physical sensations, such as those that occur during exercise. Some common misinterpretations are listed below.

Physical sensation	Common misinterpretation
Pounding heart	I'm having a heart attack
	I'm going to drop dead
Feeling short of breath	I'm going to stop breathing
	I'm choking
Feeling lightheaded	I'm going to pass out or collapse
	I'm having a stroke

Look through the list of physical sensations commonly associated with panic attacks. Write down those physical sensations that occur during your panic attacks and the beliefs you have about those sensations. When you have done this, we will later find alternative, less threatening, thoughts to challenge your original beliefs.

5.1.3 Situational fears and unhelpful thinking

As mentioned earlier, unhelpful thinking patterns may explain why some people generally feel uncomfortable in specific situations, such as a lift or train. These situational fears may be explained by two basic groups of unhelpful thoughts:

- If I have a panic attack, I won't be able to get out.
- If I have a panic attack, help won't be able to get to me.

Of course, some situations involve both types of thought. For example, a crowded underground train may be anxiety producing because it is difficult to get out, because the train only stops at stations, and because it is difficult for help to get to it.

Individuals can also apply anxiety-provoking thoughts about one situation to other situations, and then start to become more anxious in those situations. This process is known as generalization. For example, an individual who is worried about panicking on a train may start to worry about being on buses and planes. This is understandable, because all three of the situations share some features: other people, limited opportunities to leave, and limited control over their direction.

This technique should be used with the technique of graded exposure, to help you re-enter situations that you currently avoid because of anxiety.

The following examples come from individuals with panic disorder and agoraphobia.

Example 1

Description of situation	Anxiety-provoking thoughts and first anxiety rating	Helpful thoughts and second anxiety rating
Catching an express train, where I couldn't get off if I wanted to	I'll panic – being on a train makes be lose control and panic	I probably won't lose control, I'll just feel anxious
	I'll go crazy if I can't get out	Even if I do feel anxious and uncomfortable, that doesn't mean the situation is dangerous
	What'll people think of me?	I've never done something out of control on a train, and probably won't do something this time either
	If I can't get out I'll do something stupid or out of control. Everyone is watching me	I can use my techniques to manage my anxiety. People won't notice me, and even if they do, they'll just think I'm a little tense
	No one else feels this way	I know other people have panic attacks too
	I must be loopy to feel this way	I'm not loopy, just anxious, and I'm doing something about that
	Anxiety: 100%	**Anxiety: 40%**

Example 2

Description of situation	Anxiety-provoking thoughts and first anxiety rating	Helpful thoughts and second anxiety rating
Walking into a train station, noticing a pounding heart, and getting suddenly anxious	I'm going to have a heart attack and die immediately	I'm not having a heart attack. I'm experiencing an anxiety reaction
	There is something physically wrong with me	The unpleasant physical sensations are due to anxiety, which I have learned to control
		Breathing too hard will make the symptoms worse, which proves it is not a heart attack
		I've never had a heart attack, collapsed or died as a result of a panic attack
	I'd better sit down before I collapse **Anxiety: 90%**	I don't need to sit down, I can do my breathing exercise **Anxiety: 35%**

5.1.4 Wishful thinking

Helpful thinking is not simply positive thinking; it does not reject all negative thoughts. It is looking at things in a way that is most helpful given the facts. It is therefore important to distinguish helpful thinking from "positive", or wishful, thinking.

Some examples of the difference between unhelpful, helpful, and wishful thinking are

Unhelpful	I didn't get the job, which proves that I'm a failure. I'll never get a job or have things go right for me.
Wishful	Who cares! I didn't want the job anyway.
Helpful	I'm disappointed I didn't get the job, but I'll get over it and cope in the meantime.

Unhelpful	I feel really worthless now that I know what John's been saying about me.
Wishful	He can say what he likes – it doesn't worry me a bit.
Helpful	I'm sorry to hear John said that about me, but I'm not going to let myself get too upset by it.

Unhelpful	What if I can't cope with this? I just know I'll do something wrong.
Wishful	I wish I didn't have this problem.
Helpful	I'm going to give this a try. I'll do my best, and see how it goes.

5.1.5 More tips on detecting unhelpful thoughts

If you have an unpleasant experience or event, go through the questions listed earlier in this chapter. At the same time, check whether your response is reasonable. If so, face your disappointment, but don't make a catastrophe of it either! It is sometimes difficult to tell the difference between unhelpful, wishful, and helpful thinking. Here are some clues to help to clarify these.

Unhelpful thinking
- I must...
- I've got to...
- What if... [something happened] ... that would be terrible.
- I couldn't stand it if...

Wishful thinking
- It'll work out.
- I don't care...
- It wouldn't have done any good anyway.
- I won't be anxious at all.

Helpful thinking
- I'd like to...
- I'd prefer not to...
- It's unlikely that... [something] ... will actually happen.
- If things don't go the way I want, I might be disappointed, but I'll probably cope.

5.2 Step 2: Challenging anxiety-provoking thoughts

It may be difficult to challenge anxiety-provoking thoughts, especially when they have been present for a long time. Some thoughts may even appear to be automatic. One of the best ways to challenge unhelpful thinking is to write them down on paper, and replace the unhelpful beliefs with more helpful or rational alternatives.

Some important questions to help you to challenge unhelpful thoughts are:

1. What is the evidence for what I fear?
2. How likely is what I fear to happen?
3. What is the worst possible thing that will realistically happen?
4. What alternatives are there?
5. How helpful is the way I'm thinking?

5.3 Step 3: Generating alternative thoughts

Through the process of challenging unhelpful thoughts, you may have started to generate more helpful thoughts. We will begin by starting with common examples of unhelpful thoughts that individuals with panic disorder report. After this, we will look at specific examples from your own experience.

Generating alternative, more helpful, thoughts is not easy to do at first. It will take time and practice, but your skill at this will improve if you apply the technique consistently. Start with the following examples of thoughts reported by individuals with panic disorder.

Anxiety-provoking thought	Helpful thoughts
I could faint the next time I panic – that'd be awful. People would think I was strange	
If I feel dizzy the next time I drive I could have an accident and kill someone	
If I'm left alone and panic, I'll really lose it and go crazy	
What if I get trapped in the elevator for an hour and panic the whole time? I couldn't cope	
What if all the doctors have been wrong and I've really got something seriously wrong with me? I could have only weeks to live	
I can't stand the way I'm feeling. Maybe I'll be like this for the rest of my life	

Now think of a recent situation where you felt anxious or had a panic attack. Write down a description of the situation, and any anxiety-provoking thoughts you may have had. Then write down some more helpful thoughts that could be applied to that situation, in order to reduce your anxiety. There is also space for an additional individual example.

Description of situation	Anxiety-provoking thoughts and first anxiety rating	Helpful thoughts and second anxiety rating

5.4 Troubleshooting

1. *"I don't know what I'm thinking – I'm too scared."* Ask yourself, "What am I scared of? What am I scared might happen?". It is difficult to identify unhelpful fears, especially to begin with. It may help to wait until the anxiety has dropped, then think about the situation and associated fears. Re-entering a situation may make the fears clearer.

2. *"I can't think of alternatives."* After many months to years of having anxiety-provoking thoughts, it may be difficult to think up less threatening alternatives. Look at all available evidence, especially evidence that contradicts your thoughts. Ask yourself why others around you do not fear the situation, and try to consider what they might be thinking about the situation.

3. *"I'm doing it and it's not working."* Use all available techniques, including relaxation and slow breathing, to reduce your anxiety. Do not expect to be perfect at cognitive restructuring or expect the technique to work immediately.

Changing well-established patterns takes time and effort.

4. *"I still feel anxious."* Cognitive restructuring is designed to provide more helpful and appropriate responses to given situations, events or interactions. If the reality is that a particular situation is associated with some anxiety for most people, do not expect to use the technique to reduce all anxiety.

5. *"I don't believe my new thoughts."* This may occur if you have not addressed all of your anxiety-provoking thoughts. Go back and look at the original thought, and try to think whether there are any related thoughts that still cause anxiety. Also, you don't have to believe your new thoughts immediately, as part of the exercise is to disprove your old, unhelpful thoughts. Try to act as if your new thoughts are true, and see what happens.

5.5 Summary

Let us take a moment to see where we are up to and to summarize what we have learned by putting it into a series of steps.

When you are anxious:
- Breathe slowly using the breathing exercise and say "relax" as you breathe out.
- Sit down, stop, or rest.
- Use quick isometric relaxation.
- Challenge and replace any unhelpful thinking.
- Plan your next move positively.
- Slowly move on when ready.

These summary instructions, or your own version of them, can be written on a small card that you can carry with you and use to remind yourself of what to do when you are in the early stages of learning the strategies.

Remember: The anxiety will always begin to fall within a few minutes and, if you act promptly in controlling your breathing, you can prevent panic attacks.

SECTION 6

6 Producing the panic sensations

One of the elements central to panic is the fearful reaction to bodily sensations, such as a pounding heart, dizziness, etc. We deal with this subject towards the end of the first part of the program because the techniques involved are not easy for all people to do and we want to be sure that you have some anxiety-management techniques. In this chapter we will deal with your reactivity to different panic sensations.

As we noted in the first section of the Manual, different sensations frighten some people more than they frighten others. Just as you have been learning to reduce your fear of particular sensations through regular graded exposure, you can now begin to learn to reduce your fear of the frightening bodily sensations by regular graded exposure. If you are not sure which symptoms are most relevant to your fear we can use a series of exercises that bring on sensations similar to the sensations experienced during anxiety and panic. In other words, you will expose yourself to internal bodily feelings in the same way that you expose yourself to feared situations through graded exposure. Fear reduction can be accomplished only by repeatedly confronting the things that frighten you, in this case the bodily feelings associated with panic.

Although you may not like the idea of deliberately bringing on the feelings that are similar to those you experience when you panic, dealing with these fears is very important. Many everyday experiences will cause you to feel sensations that are similar to panic sensations. For example, any individual who engages in a hard game of squash or goes for a jog may experience breathlessness, sweating and light-headedness. These are normal reactions to the stress of exercise and should not lead to fears of panic. In this part of the program we wish to dampen down, or even extinguish, the anxiety produced by these harmless sensations.

In addition, performance of the exercises will provide you with a chance to practice more purposefully the strategies you have acquired up to this point, especially the rational thinking exercises. Their application during these repeated practices will enhance their effectiveness and their preparedness. The more you rehearse a particular strategy, the more powerful and natural it becomes.

6.1 Panic sensations exercises

First we will begin by working through some specific exercises. Your task is to identify any sensations that the exercise causes you to feel. After performing the exercises set out below, write down all the physical sensations you experienced during or after the exercise, as well as any anxiety-provoking thoughts. After you have done this, rate three different aspects of the sensations:

1. The physical unpleasantness of the sensations (rated on a 0 to 8 scale where 0 = not at all and 8 = extreme).
2. The maximum level of anxiety you experience in response to those physical sensations (rated on a 0 to 8 scale where 0 = not at all and 8 = extreme).
3. How similar the physical sensations are to the physical sensations you experience in a panic attack (rated on a 0 to 8 scale were 0 = no similarity at all and 8 = identical).

Panic sensations exercises

1. Hyperventilate for 1 minute. Breathe deeply and quickly, using a lot of force.
2. Shake head from side to side for 30 seconds.
3. Place your head between your legs for 30 seconds, then stand upright quickly.
4. Step up on a step or box, then step down again, quickly, for 1 minute.
5. Hold your breath for 30 seconds, holding your nose shut at the same time.
6. Maintain complete body tension for 1 minute. Hold a push-up position for 1 minute, or, alternatively, tense every muscle in your body for 1 minute.
7. Spin for 30 seconds while standing. Don't hold onto things or sit down immediately afterwards.
8. Breathe through a straw for 1 minute. Hold your nose whilst you do this.
9. Breathe with chest fully expanded for 1 minute. Fill your lungs with air until your chest feels fully expanded. Take quick, shallow breaths, and breathe from your chest.

	Physical unpleasantness (0 to 8)	Anxiety or fear (0 to 8)	Physical similarity (0 to 8)
1. Hyperventilation			
2. Shaking head			
3. Head between legs			
4. Step-ups			
5. Holding breath			
6. Body tension			
7. Spinning			
8. Breathe through straw			
9. Chest breathing			

If none of these exercises triggers some or other of your sensations, then you can try to come up with some exercises of your own. For instance, if you are most distressed by a dry mouth, you may wish to get some dental rolls and put them in your mouth to soak up the saliva. Staring at a light for a few seconds and then looking at a blank wall can create visual distortions that other people find distressing. Talk to your therapist about ways of creating the particular symptoms that trouble you most.

6.2 Constructing a stepladder of panic sensation exercises

1. Asterisk (*) or circle the exercises that produced a score of 3 or more on the physical similarity scale.
2. Rank the list of asterisked exercises from the least anxiety provoking (i.e., the lowest score) to the most anxiety provoking.

6.3 Practicing the panic sensation exercises

1. Start with the two asterisked exercises that produced the least anxiety.
2. Perform the exercises as described earlier in the manual. You will need to organize a clock or watch.
3. If you feel like stopping before the time for the exercise is up, try to persevere with the exercise for as long as you can. If necessary, reduce the intensity of the exercise a little, but try to keep on going.
4. Once the exercise is over, allow the physical sensations to gradually diminish. When the physical sensations are finished, write down:
   - All the physical sensations experienced.
   - Any anxiety-provoking thoughts about the exercise (before, during or after).
   - Physical unpleasantness, anxiety and physical similarity scores.

Do

- Bring on the sensations as strongly as you can during the exercises.
- Try to experience the sensations fully.
- Use the exercises as a chance to identify and challenge anxiety-provoking thoughts.

Don't

- Use anxiety-management techniques before doing the exercises.
- Use distraction techniques during the exercises.
- Try to stop the sensations as soon as the time is up.

6.4 Scheduling the panic sensation exercises during the program

1. Practice two exercises each day. Plan in advance which two exercises you intend to do, and write them down in the diary forms provided.
2. If you have an anxiety rating of more than 2 after any exercise, you should repeat it (either once later that day, or on another day), until the anxiety rating is 2 or less.
3. You may wish to repeat these exercises once again later in the day. More than this is not necessary.

4. Once you have managed to bring anxiety associated with these exercises to a minimal level (or even have no anxiety whilst doing them), you can extend them by doing the following:
   • Increasing the length of time by another 30 to 60 seconds.
   • Standing up whilst doing the exercises.
   • Doing the exercises in a park or other place away from help.

6.5 Troubleshooting

1. *"I don't need to do these exercises – I already know what my panic feels like."* These exercises allow controlled exposure to physical sensations associated with panic attacks. Repeated exposure *will* reduce the amount of anxiety that these normal, everyday physical sensations produce.

2. *"These exercises don't work, because I know that I'm safe."* Try doing these exercises in a variety of settings: in the clinic, at home, or in a park. If you have anxiety in any of these situations, try to examine the thoughts that are behind this anxiety. For example, you may be more anxious at home than in the clinic, because of a belief that you are somehow more at risk alone. Spend some time challenging these unhelpful thoughts.

3. *"I don't feel anxious, because I'm in control of these physical sensations."* The physical sensations produced are normal, everyday physical sensations. They are the same as the physical sensations produced by daily activities, which may trigger panic attacks in some people. Later in the program, we will be instructing people in how to incorporate these kinds of exercises in their day-to-day lives.

4. *"I can't stand these sensations."* Try to identify the underlying thoughts that are producing these fears, and challenge them. It is important to persevere with these exercises, and gradually reduce your fear of them. This may take several repetitions for some people. Some sensations may be unpleasant, but they need not produce anxiety.

5. *"I'm not having a good day today."* Most day-to-day illnesses can't be predicted, and sometimes it isn't possible to avoid commitments because of them. It is better to prepare for the colds and viral illnesses that affect most people each year, increasing your chances at better coping when they happen.

6. *"These exercises will trigger a panic attack."* These exercises may increase anxiety, because the physical sensations they cause generate anxiety-producing thoughts. Try to identify these thoughts and challenge them with more adaptive and helpful thoughts. If necessary, use other techniques you have learned to reduce your anxiety. Avoidance of physical sensations, like avoidance of situations, does reduce anxiety in the long-term.

6.6 Plan for break

During your time away from the clinic, you will need to keep a record of your daily activities. This will help you to remember what you did, the steps forward, and the difficulties. When you return, we will then be able to discuss the ways in which you best managed your panics. To help in planning, below is a schedule you can complete.

On the first page, you can plan what you are going to do. Remember that your aim should be to attempt a graded exposure exercise, a producing panic sensations exercise, and a relaxation session every day.

Following the plan is room for you to write any comments that you may have about the activities.

On the next pages are tables for you to write in the irrational thoughts and level of fear that occur during your graded exposure and producing panic sensations exercises. You can then write down rational thoughts so that you will be better able to manage your panic attacks.

DIARY

Day: _____

Graded exposure exercise: _____
Panic sensations exercise: _____

Time
7–8
8–9   Breathing exercise
9–10
10–11
11–12
12–1   Breathing exercise
1–2
2–3
3–4
4–5
5–6
6–7   Breathing exercise
7–8
8–9
9–10   Breathing exercise

Comments and notes

_____

_____

_____

_____

_____

_____

_____

_____

_____

_____

_____

_____

_____

Graded exposure exercise

Situation	Unhelpful thoughts and first anxiety rating	Helpful thoughts and second anxiety rating

Panic sensations exercise

Panic sensations exercise	Unhelpful thoughts and first anxiety rating	Helpful thoughts and second anxiety rating

SECTION 7

7 Producing panic sensations in your daily life

Once panic attacks become regular, individuals with panic disorder and agora-phobia can begin to misinterpret the physical sensations caused by everyday activities as signals of panic. You may even have found that you avoid certain activities because you are frightened by the sensations they produce. You might avoid aerobic exercise because it makes your heart beat faster. You might not lift heavy objects because it causes unpleasant physical sensations as a result of the increased blood pressure. If the activities cause the sensations, you can then misinterpret the sensations as signals of danger and a panic attack might occur. The aim of this part of the program is to reduce any anxiety associated with physical sensations produced by everyday activities.

As you begin these activities, it is important to note a difference between the panic sensation exercises done previously and the activities outlined in this chapter. When you did the exercises to produce the panic sensations, you would have noticed that the sensations started and stopped roughly when the exercises started and stopped. In contrast, when panic-like sensations are generated by daily activities, their onset and offset will be less clear. Do not worry about this. The more natural the activity is, the less likely it is that the sensations will start when the activity begins and stop when the activity stops. Take, for example, going out on a hot day. It takes some time to become hot and sweaty when you go outside and it will take some time to cool down once you come inside again. This is just what happens with natural everyday activities. However, if you worry about the fact that the sensations are no longer as predictable as before and do not stop the instant you stop the activity, you are just going to make the symptoms worse and make it more likely that you will have a panic attack.

Following is a list of activities or places that may produce panic-like sensations. Consider these activities and decide whether you avoid, or find uncomfortable, any of these activities *for fear of having a panic attack*. There may be other activities of your own that you wish to add to the list.

- Heated vehicles or public transport
- Hot stuffy shops or shopping centers
- Watching medical programs
- Watching suspenseful TV programs or movies
- Watching sporting events on TV or in person
- Eating rich or heavy meals
- Arguments
- Amusement park rides
- Riding on boats or ferries
- Sexual activity
- Bushwalking
- Jogging or exercising of any kind
- Going to the gym or lifting weights
- Sports
- Dancing
- Surfing or swimming
- Getting up quickly from lying down
- Running up hills or stairs
- Walking in hot or humid conditions
- Heavily air-conditioned places
- Having showers with doors and windows closed
- Hot or steamy rooms

If you avoid any of these activities or places *for fear of panic* you should apply your anxiety-management techniques, specifically graded exposure and straight thinking. Begin with exposure to the least anxiety-provoking activity. The goal is to repeat the activity a number of times until only mild anxiety is experienced. Then move on to the next most anxiety-provoking activity. Below list up to five activities you are aware of avoiding for fear of panic:

Goals: _____

_____

_____

_____

_____

Now choose one goal you would like to start working on in the near future. Write down the goal in the space provided, then break it down into steps. Also, write down any anxiety-provoking thoughts you may have about doing this activity, and then challenge and replace those thoughts.

Goal: _____

Steps: _____

_____

_____

_____

_____

Anxiety-provoking thoughts

_____

_____

_____

Helpful thoughts

_____

_____

_____

As with the graded exposure tasks you have been carrying out the important points to remember are:

---

1. Clearly specify the task you are to attempt in advance.
2. Continue the activity until a decrease in anxiety is experienced.
3. Use your anxiety-management skills such as breathing control, relaxation and thinking straight (of course you will not be able to slow your breathing if you are engaging in an activity that requires increased oxygen, e.g., walking quickly).
4. Make sure that you practice some activity every day.

SECTION 8

8 More about thinking straight

Having discussed previously how unhelpful thoughts can be identified, challenged, and disputed we shall consider another method. Rather than engaging in a mental exercise of weighing up the evidence a person can actively go out and seek evidence for and against the belief.

Examples of unhelpful thoughts include:

- I will never be able to go out without my tablets.
- If my heart starts pounding and I exert myself, I could have a heart attack.
- If I sit in a tiny room, the air could run out and I might suffocate.

If you had these thoughts you could argue with yourself about their truth. However, a better test would be to try to go out without the tablets, to see whether the anxiety decreased if you went near what you feared and stayed there, or to see whether the air ran out and you suffocated in a tiny room. Obviously to achieve this result the graded exposure exercises you planned are very relevant. Not only will they help to elicit the thoughts (what better time to identify thoughts than when you're afraid) but you will be able to test them at the same time.

We now know that unhelpful thoughts (e.g., "I will panic and collapse") can make your fears much worse than they otherwise would have been. Sometimes it is possible to think yourself into a fearful state without even being near what you fear. Disputing the unhelpful thought will decrease the power they have over your feelings. As you begin to replace the unhelpful thoughts with helpful ones, your feelings will become more appropriate to the situation you face.

You have all been identifying, challenging and disputing your unhelpful thoughts, but it is not always that easy. To give you some extra help there are four types of question you can ask yourself that may make the unhelpful aspects of the thoughts more clear.

1. *"What is the evidence for what I thought?"* Ask yourself whether other people would accept the thought as correct. From your or other people's experience, what is the evidence that what you believe is true? Ask yourself whether you are jumping to conclusions by basing what you think on poor evidence. How do you know what you think is right?

    e.g., If I panic I will definitely lose control.

2. *"What alternatives are there to what I thought?"* Is the thought the only one you could have? Perhaps there are alternative explanations of an event or ways of thinking about something. Determine whether any of these have better evidence for them or would be more helpful in overcoming your feelings.

    e.g., My heart is beating fast – I must be having a heart attack.

3. *"What is the effect of thinking the way I do?"* Establish in your own mind what your goals are and then ask whether the way you are thinking is helping you to achieve those goals or is it taking you further away.

    e.g., I failed in my exposure task, I'll never improve, I might as well give up.

4. *"What thinking errors am I making?"* Some examples of common thinking errors include:

    (i)   Thinking in *all-or-nothing* terms. This is black-and-white thinking in which things are seen as all good or all bad, safe or dangerous – there is no middle ground.

        e.g., I know panic attacks are very dangerous.

    (ii) *Using ultimatums.* Beware of words like always, never, everyone, no-one, everything, or nothing. Ask yourself whether the situation really is as clear-cut as you are thinking.

        e.g., No-one else has a fear like mine, everyone else in the group is improving so much faster than me.

    (iii) *Condemning yourself* on the basis of a single event. Because there is one thing that you cannot or have not done you then label yourself a failure or worthless.

        e.g., I avoided doing my exposure task today, I am a complete failure.

    (iv) *Concentrating on weaknesses and forgetting strengths.* Try to think of other times you have attempted or even been successful at something and think about the resources that you really do have.

        e.g., I haven't made any progress and that's just typical of me.

    (v)   *Overestimating the chances of disaster.* Things will certainly go wrong and there is danger in the world, but are you overestimating these? How likely is it that what you expect will really happen?

        e.g., I could never hyperventilate alone because I might go crazy or die.

(vi) *Exaggerating the importance* of events. Often we think that some event will be much more important than it turns out to be. Ask yourself, "What difference will it make in a week or 10 years? Will I still feel this way?"

   e.g., My breathing rate is not decreasing as fast as everyone else in the group.

(vii) *Fretting about the way things ought to be.* Telling yourself that things *should* be different or that you *must* act in a certain way indicates that you may be worrying about how things "ought" to be rather than dealing with them as they are. Challenge the "should's" and "must's". Why should it be that way? Why must you act that way?

   e.g., I ought to be better by now.

(viii) *Pessimism* about a lack of ability to change a situation leads to feelings of depression and lowered self-esteem. There may be no solution but you will not know until you try. Ask yourself whether you are really trying to find answers and solutions.

   e.g., I'll never completely get over my panics.

(ix) *Predicting the future.* Just because you acted a certain way in the past does not mean that you have to act that way forever more. Predicting what you will do on the basis of past behavior means that you will cut yourself off from the possibility of change.

   e.g., I'm a nervous person, I'll always be afraid.

8.1 Coping statements

There are times when you may need some short cuts to coping with feelings. Here are a few.

1. Have a cue that makes you turn a potentially bad feeling into a coping one. For example, if you feel butterflies in the stomach, instead of saying "Oh no, I'm really getting anxious and upset" say "I know what these feelings mean. They mean I'm getting anxious. That means: slow down, regulate my breathing and do some isometric exercises."

2. Develop some personal self-statements, such as "Take this step by step", "Don't jump to conclusions" or "This fear can't hurt me – I can tolerate it". Make these statements up yourself so that they are relevant to your life.

3. Don't always put yourself down. Don't say, "A baby should be able to do this", "I'm hopeless" or "I'll never get the hang of this". As long as you say these sorts of things to yourself you make them come true (but only for as long as you say them, fortunately).

4. Praise yourself. Say things like "That was good" or "I felt I was having a bad day this morning, but I still managed to get on the crowded train". Remember the

most important source of praise is from inside you, because you know yourself best and what your actions mean to you.

8.2 Summary

When you are aware of upset feelings, do the following:

- Discover what your feelings really mean (e.g., are you hurt or really angry, or perhaps even tired?).
- Identify what assumptions you are making in what you are saying to yourself.
- Question the assumption. Accept what is true and accurate.
- Change those thoughts and assumptions that are unhelpful and inaccurate by substituting more accurate, helpful thoughts.

SECTION 9

9 Keeping your progress going

9.1 Coping with setbacks or difficulties in making progress

Setbacks or difficulties in making progress are generally the consequence of either poor management or poor planning of goals and steps. If you should experience such difficulties, you must carefully analyze the way in which you carry out these two exercises.

9.1.1 Managing anxiety and hyperventilation

- Are you regularly monitoring your breathing while performing activities?
- Are you using the isometric relaxation exercises and the slow-breathing technique when you experience the first signs of anxiety?
- Are you regularly practicing the progressive muscle relaxation exercises, especially prior to entering a situation?
- Are you too obsessed about having anti-anxiety medication with you?
- Are there mounting background stresses in your life that need to be defused? For example, marital, family, or financial problems.
- Are you suffering from any form of physical stress? For example, illness, premenstrual tension, poor diet, lack of sleep, overwork.

9.1.2 Planning of goals and steps

- Are you trying to progress too quickly or too slowly?
- Is the difference between levels of difficulty at each step too great?
- Do you need to develop in-between steps of gradually increasing difficulty that

lie between the last step you completed successfully and the step with which you are now having difficulty?

- Do you need to practice new steps more frequently and for longer periods before moving on to more difficult ones?
- Is your level of certainty of success too high or too low?
- If your objectives are too easy or too difficult you will not make progress. Are you sure that you are not expecting too much of yourself?
- Make sure that you give yourself sufficient praise for your achievements. Remember that the key to success is gradual but regular progress.

9.2 Emotional problems during setbacks

Setbacks do occur occasionally, even in persons who are making excellent progress. When this happens, some people become alarmed and despondent, fearing they have gone back to their very worst. Remember, no matter how badly you feel during a setback, it is very rare for you to go all the way back to your worst level of incapacitation. For most people, the apparent setback is only a passing phase, due to factors such as outside stressors, the 'flu, or school holidays. In such cases, the setback is often viewed as devastating because it has a lot of emotional meaning for the person who has put considerable effort into recovering. This effort is not wasted, and after the stressors pass you will find it easier to get yourself out and about again. This pattern has been demonstrated again and again. Therefore, if you have a setback, don't add to the problem with all the old catastrophic, emotional, and self-destructive ideas. Keep practicing all the techniques you have been taught and you will be able to make progress.

If you feel that you have genuinely lost the skills necessary to control anxiety and panic, then you may want to consider retreatment. Most people do not lose the skills but need some fine-tuning of their skills.

"Booster" sessions or follow-up meetings are the best way to receive this form of assistance.

9.3 Expect lapse occasionally

Here, a lapse means that you stop listening to your relaxation tape, start to worry about having a panic attack, or stopping slow breathing. Most people will have some sort of lapse when they are trying to change their behavior.

The trick is not to turn a lapse into a relapse and exaggerate the lapse into being bigger than it really is. If you have noticed that you have stopped using your panic control skills, don't say things to yourself like "I'm really hopeless, I'm right back where I started from, I'll never be able to change". Instead, you should view your lapse in the following light: "I'm disappointed that I have let things slip, but I can cope with that and I'm not going to turn it into an excuse for giving up altogether. Now I'll get out my Manual and start again." Of course, some people do stop things like relaxation training or slow breathing when they have been feeling okay for some time.

This is fine, so long as you keep aware of any stress or anxiety that may be creeping back into your life, and restart the training as soon as you become aware of any increase. Also, it will be important to reinstate such techniques if you have recently experienced any stressful life event.

9.4 Conclusion

You now have three skills that you have been taught and now need to practice. You need to use the various exposure tasks, working up the graded "stepladders" of anxiety, to reduce your fear of your panic. *Relaxation exercises* will help to reduce your general level of tension before the exposure task and the isometric exercises will regulate tension during exposure. *Slow breathing* will help to keep control of any anxiety you may experience. By *thinking straight* you will be able to stop anxiety from spiraling into panic.

SECTION 10

10 Recommended resources

The following books are available from most good bookstores, some news-stands, and over the internet. If in doubt, ask whether the book can be ordered. We also suggest that you use your local library to gain access to many of these books. When you read these or any similar books on the management of anxiety or depression, remember that they are best regarded as guidelines only. Be critical in both a positive and negative sense when reading these books, so that you get what is best for you out of them. Most of these books are inexpensive.

10.1 Books

Barlow D and Rapee R. (1997) *Mastering Stress: A Lifestyle Approach*. Killara, NSW: Lifestyle Press.

Burns DD. (1999) *The Feeling Good Handbook*, revised edition. New York: Penguin.

Copeland ME. (1992) *The Depression Workbook: A Guide for Living with Depression and Manic Depression*. New York: New Harbinger.

Davis M, Eshelman ER and McKay M. (1995) *The Relaxation and Stress Reduction Workbook*, fourth edition. Oakland, CA: New Harbinger.

Ellis A and Harper R. (1979) *A New Guide to Rational Living*. Hollywood, CA: Wilshire Book

Company.

Emery G. (2000) *Overcoming Depression: A Cognitive-Behavior Protocol for the Treatment of Depression.* Oakland, CA: New Harbinger.

Greenberger D and Padesky C. (1995) *Mind Over Mood.* New York: Guilford.

Marks IM. (2001) *Living with Fear.* New York: McGraw-Hill.

McKay M and Fanning P. (1987) *Self-Esteem: A Proven Program of Cognitive Techniques for Assessing, Improving and Maintaining Your Self-Esteem.* Oakland, CA: New Harbinger.

McKay M, Davis M, and Fanning P. (1995) *Messages: The Communication Skills Book.* Oakland, CA: New Harbinger.

McKay M, Davis M, and Fanning P. (1997) *Thoughts and Feelings: Taking Control of Your Moods and Your Life.* Oakland, CA: New Harbinger.

Meichenbaum D. (1983) *Coping With Stress.* London: Century Publishing.

Page A. (1993) *Don't Panic! Overcoming Anxiety, Phobias and Tension.* Sydney: Gore Osment.

Walker CE. (1975) *Learn to Relax: 13 Ways to Reduce Tension.* Englewood Cliffs, NJ: Prentice Hall.

Weekes C. (1966) *Self-Help For Your Nerves.* Sydney: Angus and Robertson.

Weekes C. (1972) *Peace From Nervous Suffering.* Sydney: Angus and Robertson.

10.2 Video

Rapee R, Lampe L. (1998). *Fight or flight? Overcoming Panic and Agoraphobia.* Available from Monkey See Productions. P.O. Box 167, Waverley, NSW 2024 Australia.

10.3 Internet resources

Anxiety And Panic Internet Resource: http://www.algy.com/anxiety/

Clinical Research Unit for Anxiety and Depression: http://www.crufad.unsw.edu.au/

Internet Mental Health: http://www.mentalhealth.com/

Mental Health Net: http://mentalhelp.net/

Robin Winkler Clinic (Printable handouts on psychological problems): http://www.psy.uwa.edu.au/rwclinic/

8

Social phobia

Syndrome

Clinical description

Social phobia is characterized by phobic anxiety and avoidance of social or performance situations. There is fear of scrutiny, of doing or saying something that would be embarrassing, and of being seen to be anxious. Central to the disorder is an underlying fear of negative evaluation (Beck et al., 1985; Liebowitz et al., 1985; Lucock and Salkovskis, 1988; Mattick and Peters, 1988; Mattick et al., 1989). Both the probability and anticipated detrimental consequences (cost) of negative evaluation are exaggerated. Social phobia for many patients is a chronic and disabling condition, with a significant morbidity in terms of personal distress, failure to achieve full social, occupational and personal potential, and significant psychiatric comorbidity. Cognitive, behavioral, and physiological aspects of the disorder have been recognized.

Individuals with social phobia experience many of the same anxiety symptoms as people with other anxiety disorders. However, the symptoms that are most troubling are those which are most visible to others: 77% reported blushing, sweating or trembling as an accompanying symptom in one study (Mersch et al., 1995). Individuals with social phobia worry that these symptoms indicate to others that they are anxious. They worry that if they are viewed as being inappropriately anxious they will be evaluated negatively.

Avoidance is the most prominent behavioral symptom of social phobia. Many patients will avoid the feared situations when possible, but will endure with intense anxiety when the negative consequences of avoidance are perceived to outweigh the negative consequences of attending. Social situations that cause anxiety may have primarily an interactional focus (e.g., initiating and maintaining conversations, meeting or "getting to know" others) or a performance focus (e.g., public speaking, presentations in meetings and tutorials, writing or signing one's name in front of others). Situations that involve actual or possible scrutiny may also trigger anxiety (e.g., standing in line, using public transport, using public toilets, using the telephone when others are around, eating or drinking in public, crowded situations including shops and cinemas). Most patients with social phobia fear more than one situation (Turner and Beidel, 1989; Manuzza et al., 1995).

Classification, subtypes and relationship to avoidant personality disorder

Social phobia has relatively recently been recognized as a diagnostic entity. ✗ Problems of social anxiety had often been thought of as an aspect of personality (Turner and Beidel, 1989). However, in the 1960s, more detailed syndromic descriptions emerged with arguments supporting the classification of social anxiety as a phobia (Taylor, 1966; Marks, 1969, 1970). Following the work of Marks (1969) in distinguishing social phobia, specific phobia, and agoraphobia, DSM-III in 1980 introduced the disorder to the psychiatric taxonomy. Subsequent revisions have attempted to increase the sensitivity and specificity of the diagnostic criteria, particularly with respect to other anxiety disorders and to avoidant personality disorder (APD). DSM-IV also aimed to enhance parity with ICD-10. ICD-10 differs from DSM-IV principally in the requirement that certain physiological symptoms of anxiety be present and in the greater emphasis on excluding psychotic disorders in the differential diagnosis.

DSM-III-R introduced generalized and discrete subtypes of social phobia. DSM-IV has retained the generalized specifier but as yet the definition has not been operationalized. Generalized social phobia is defined simply as including "most social situations". In clinical samples it is more common than discrete social phobia, but comprises only one-third or less of epidemiological samples (Wittchen et al., 1999; Furmark et al., 2000). Allowing for variation in the strategies different teams of investigators have used to assign generalized versus nongeneralized subtype status, there do appear to be significant differences between these groups. Public-speaking fears are the most common fears in both subtypes but interactional fears are more common in the generalized compared to discrete subtype (Manuzza et al., 1995; Kessler et al., 1998). Recently, a three-cluster solution of "pervasive social anxiety" (public speaking + social interaction anxiety + scrutiny fears + fears of eating and drinking in public), "moderate social anxiety" (fear of public speaking + moderate social interaction anxiety) and "dominant public-speaking anxiety" has been suggested (Eng et al., 2000) based on Liebowitz Social Anxiety Scale (LSAS) data from a large clinical sample. Social Phobia Scale (SPS) and Social Interaction Anxiety Scale (SIAS) scores from an epidemiological population also yielded a three-cluster solution in broad agreement with that above (Furmark et al., 2000). Significant differences exist between pure public-speaking (social) phobia and generalized social phobia (Kessler et al., 1998, 1999b). Social phobia limited to one or a few social situations is generally less disabling, associated with less comorbidity and better prognosis (Manuzza et al., 1995; Kessler et al., 1999b). Comorbid depression and alcohol abuse become increasingly more common along the spectrum from discrete to generalized social phobia to social phobia comorbid with APD (Turner et al., 1986; Holt et al., 1992; Lepine and Pelissolo, 1998; Stein and Chavira, 1998). Greater autonomic arousal is evident in social phobia limited to a fear of public speaking (Stein, 1998).

Currently there is most support for the view that social phobia and APD represent different points on a spectrum whereby the comorbid condition is associated with greater severity and pervasiveness of anxiety and distress, more comorbidity, and greater functional impairment (Holt et al., 1992; Turner et al., 1992b; Rapee, 1995; Boone et al., 1999). Estimated rates of comorbid APD in social phobia vary from 18% to 84% (Alnaes and Torgersen, 1988b; Schneier et al., 1991; Turner et al., 1991; Holt et al., 1992; Mersch et al., 1995; Baillie and Lampe, 1998; Turk et al., 1998). In studies utilizing DSM-III-R criteria there is little to distinguish between those with generalized social phobia alone and those in whom the condition is comorbid with APD on feared situations, general cognitive focus, subjective situational anxiety and perceived impairment of performance (Holt et al., 1992; Turner et al., 1992b) but the latter exhibit greater avoidance and overall distress (Turner et al., 1986). First-degree relatives of probands with generalized social phobia show markedly elevated rates of APD as compared with relatives of controls without social phobia (Stein et al., 1998). DSM-IV made significant revisions to the criteria for APD, for which there is some empirical support (Baillie and Lampe, 1998). The greater emphasis on fears of rejection and humiliation, and the sense of personal inadequacy and inferiority required to make the diagnosis may enable the identification of a group of individuals who differ in significant ways from the currently recognized subtypes of social phobia and who may have needs currently unmet by existing treatment programs.

CASE EXAMPLES

Case 1

Patient identification

Mrs. B is a 45-year-old woman who is married with two children. She works part-time with her husband in their own business.

History of presenting complaint

Mrs. B complains of anxiety when entertaining clients of the business in their home. She enjoys entertaining their mutual friends, but becomes anxious as soon as she knows she will be entertaining business associates. In the days leading up to the event her anxiety becomes increasingly severe. She fears she will say something foolish or inappropriate, have nothing to say at all, or will simply look so anxious and uncomfortable that others will think it odd. She worries about blushing and fears her hands may shake as she is serving guests or eating, and others will think her odd or weak. Her anxiety is worst when she feels she is the center of attention. Recently Mrs. B felt so anxious before the event she convinced her husband to make an excuse and take their guests to a restaurant without her. When asked about other difficult situations Mrs. B says that she is comfortable with friends she knows well, but that she does become very anxious about meeting new people socially and would prefer to avoid it. She is uncomfortable signing anything with someone watching and will avoid doing so whenever possible. She is highly anxious about public speaking and her husband takes responsibility for any meetings or presentations that are necessary to advance the business. She also never joined parent or community groups, despite having some interest in doing so.

Family history
Mrs. B described her father as a quiet, gentle man who socialized little outside the family, but her mother was sociable and outgoing. She has one brother who is much like her in personality.

Premorbid personality
She describes herself as always having been "shy", meaning that she has always felt anxious meeting new people, feeling self-conscious and fearful of saying something foolish or appearing socially inadequate. She was always a little anxious at the start of each school year, but quickly settled in, enjoyed school, and always had a small group of close friends. She is confident with people she knows well, in knowing her job and in her intimate relationships.

Mental state at presentation
Mrs. B was a neatly groomed woman who appeared a little ill at ease but who was able to make normal eye contact with the interviewer and relate her history fluently and spontaneously.

Diagnosis
Social phobia, generalized subtype.
   Mrs. B is typical of patients at the milder end of the social phobia spectrum, who are able to enjoy some satisfying social relationships and who are minimally impaired. This case illustrates the problems of making the generalized versus discrete distinction: Mrs. B's fears involve only two types of situation, meeting new people and public speaking. However, she encounters, or avoids because of her anxiety, many situations of these types. She also admits to a fear of scrutiny, and it may emerge during treatment that she has problems with a wider range of situations than she currently realizes, because she has adapted her activities around her fears over the years.

Case 2

Patient identification
Mr. P is a 35-year-old single clerk.

History of presenting complaint
Mr. P complains of feeling "stressed". He has worked for the same local government

department since he left school, and in the same position for the past 10 years. However, his employer is "restructuring" and he has learned that he is to be moved to a different position where he will be expected to learn new skills and be part of a team. This has made Mr. P extremely anxious and he does not think he will be able to cope. Getting to know new people terrifies him: "I never know what to say. I make people uncomfortable and they don't want me around." However, he can cope better if he knows he will only have to see someone once or twice – when he has to establish any type of relationship with another person he becomes convinced that they will soon learn that he is inadequate, even worthless, and will reject him. He is fearful of meeting the new demands that will be placed on him: "If I can't do it they'll be angry [and reject me]." Mr. P also worries about others seeing his anxiety, especially the fact that he tends to sweat profusely when anxious, but says that this does not tend to be much of a problem in practice because for years he has avoided any situation that will trigger his anxiety. Mr. P lives with his parents, and they take care of all outside chores such as shopping and even buying his clothes. Mr. P's only outings are to work. He utilizes his employer's flexible hours arrangement to avoid traveling on the bus at peak hours, because he is acutely uncomfortable in crowds. In his current work situation he shares a large office with two others who are often out on field work. He has one friend from school who visits him occasionally, and on very rare occasions he has gone out with this friend to a bar, where the alcohol has enabled him to tolerate the situation. He has never had an intimate relationship and never accepts social invitations.

Previous history
Mr. P was treated for depression in his early 20s. There have been other periods of his life where he has felt depressed but has not sought treatment. Mr. P has used alcohol to excess intermittently but has never missed work because of his drinking.

Family history
Mr. P is an only child. His parents are both quiet and have never socialized outside the home. Mrs. P had postnatal depression after Mr. P's birth. He describes her as "nervy".

Personal history and premorbid personality
Mr. P said that from his earliest years at school he felt "different" and as though he did not "fit in". Later, he saw himself as somehow inferior to others. He only ever tended to have one friend, and never initiated contact with others. From his first schooldays onwards he never spoke up in class, even to answer questions, because he was too anxious of being humiliated if he gave a wrong answer, and teachers often thought him of low intelligence. Mr. P left school as soon as it was legal for him to do so. He spent the next 2 years at home until his father managed to find him a job at the local government department where he himself had worked for 20 years. He was offered promotions but refused them because of his anxiety, fearing that he would be unable to meet new demands or that he would be placed in a situation that may require more interpersonal interaction with colleagues. He dated a woman at work on one occasion after she asked him out, but did not return any of her calls, "She'd only reject me when she realized what I was really like".

Mental state examination
Mr. P was neatly attired. He appeared extremely ill at ease, fidgeted in his seat and avoided

almost all eye contact, although this improved somewhat as the interview progressed. His history was halting and his speech was quiet and colorless. His affect was anxious and dysphoric. There was no evidence of thought disorder, delusions, or hallucinations.

Diagnosis
  Social phobia, generalized subtype.
  Avoidant personality disorder.
  This example illustrates the typically earlier onset of symptoms when social phobia is comorbid with APD, the typically very negative self-beliefs and the generalized anxiety and avoidance that is driven primarily by fear of rejection. Mr. P expects rejection because he believes himself inferior and unable to meet the social expectations of others. The avoidance in APD is so extensive that anxiety may not be a prominent presenting complaint, in contrast to social phobia. An earlier age at onset of symptoms has been associated with greater disability in social phobia. This may explain at least some of the greater disability and impairment seen in APD. Although duration of illness is not linked to outcome, age at onset was found to be a powerful predictor of recovery in a Canadian epidemiological study (DeWit et al., 1999). Those aged 7 years or less at onset of the disorder were least likely to recover.

Relationship of social phobia to "shyness" and social anxiety

Shyness has not been adequately defined. It encompasses elements of "self-consciousness" and may be equated with mild social anxiety that involves some fear of negative evaluation but does not lead to significant distress or avoidance. The prevalence rate of self-reported shyness has been found to be as high as 40% (Turner and Beidel, 1989). It is thus more common, but less disabling, than social phobia. Even for those who have not been shy, some social anxiety commonly develops in adolescence. It may arise out of normal intellectual development whereby adolescents become aware of themselves as social objects. The National Comorbidity Survey asked respondents whether there had ever been a time in their lives when one or more of six social situations had made them so afraid that they tried to avoid the situation or felt very uncomfortable in it. At least one social fear was endorsed by 38.6% of the sample. The single most common fear was of public speaking, reported by 30.2% to have been present at some time in their life (Kessler et al., 1998). There is some evidence that social anxiety that results in avoidance may cause measurable impairment even when limited to one situation and not perceived by the individual to cause functional impairment (Davidson et al., 1994).

Epidemiology

Epidemiological and clinical surveys in the past decade have put the lifetime prevalence of social phobia at between 9.5% and 16% in Western nations, depending on whether DSM-III-R, DSM-IV or ICD-10 criteria have been used and the number and range of situations probed for in the surveys (Magee et al., 1996; Weiller et al., 1996; Ballenger et al., 1998; Fones et al., 1998; Turk et al., 1998; Furmark et al., 1999). Social phobia has been reported across cultures (Chaleby and Raslan, 1990; Tseng et al., 1992; Walker and Stein, 1995, pp. 54, 57–58), but varies widely in incidence and presentation. Lifetime prevalence rates show a five-fold variation across countries (Kasper, 1998) and lesser but still significant variation between different racial groups within the same country (Eaton et al., 1991). Cross-cultural differences in social and gender role expectations may influence the decision as to whether a given case of social anxiety fulfils the disability and distress requirements of DSM-IV and ICD-10.

In contrast to panic disorder, the gender ratio approaches equality in social phobia. The female excess in epidemiological samples varies from 1.1 to 2.3 (Bourdon et al., 1988; Schneier et al., 1992; Andrews et al., 1999a). In clinical samples the ratio may be even closer to 1.0. Across studies that used DSM-III criteria to diagnose social phobia in clinic attenders or media respondents, 145 (49.7%) of a total of 292 patients were female (Butler et al., 1984; Emmelkamp et al., 1985b; Heimberg et al., 1985; Solyom et al., 1986; Mattick and Peters, 1988; Mattick et al., 1989). Of reviewed studies employing DSM-III-R criteria, 50.3% (238) of the total 473 patients were female (Manuzza et al., 1995; Mersch et al., 1995; Feske et al., 1996; Turner et al., 1996; Chambless et al., 1997; Van Velzen et al., 1997; Cox et al., 1998; Morgan and Raffle, 1999). The higher proportion of men in clinical as compared with epidemiological samples is thought likely to be due to differences in treatment-seeking behavior: data from an Australian epidemiological survey indicate that slightly more men (65.2% of those meeting criteria for DSM-IV social phobia in the past month) than women (57.9%) had used outpatient mental health services in the past 12 months (L. Lampe, T. Slade, C. Issakidis and G. Andrews, unpublished data). Weiller et al. (1996) found that men with social phobia consulted more frequently than women, for psychological reasons.

Course and disability

Patients who present for treatment typically report an early onset and chronic course of the disorder. Social phobia typically becomes a problem later in life than specific phobias and earlier than panic disorder and generalized anxiety disorder. Most estimates put the age at onset in the mid teens, but it is clear that a significant minority of individuals experience distressing and disabling social anxiety from early childhood. The mean duration of "social fears" was reported by Heimberg et al. (1990b) to be 6 or more years in 80% of the sample, 15 or more years in 28%, and "as long as I can remember" in 9%. In an epidemiological sample

(Epidemiological Catchment Area (ECA) data; Schneier et al., 1992) of DSM-III social phobia, 15 of 97 subjects (15%) reported that social phobia had been present their whole lives; age at onset occurred in a bimodal distribution with a mean reported age at onset of 15.5 (standard deviation (SD) 13.3) years and peaks at the interval 0 to 5 years and at age 13 years. This study did not find differences in age at onset between uncomplicated and comorbid social phobia. Manuzza et al. (1995) in a large clinical sample found that the age at onset was significantly earlier for generalized as compared with circumscribed social phobia. In contrast to the early age at onset, the average age at presentation is much higher: typically between 30 and 41 years (Marks, 1970; Mattick et al., 1989; Mersch et al., 1989; Heimberg et al., 1990b; Turner et al., 1991; Manuzza et al., 1995; Feske et al., 1996; Van Velzen et al., 1997). A recent study has allowed some estimate to be made of the risk of developing social phobia later in life. The Baltimore ECA follow-up study, in which a substantial proportion of the original Baltimore ECA cohort were reinterviewed, estimated the weighted 13-year incidence of DSM-IV social phobia to be 0.4% to 0.5% per year (Neufeld et al., 1999), although these individuals reported the onset of *social fears* to have been in childhood. Social phobia was more likely to develop in individuals who had met criteria for depression, dysthymia, panic disorder or phobias at the time of the original ECA study. There is no evidence from recent studies to suggest that the average age or duration of symptoms at presentation is reducing, implying that, despite greater awareness of social phobia amongst health care workers, individuals are still suffering with this condition for many years before finding treatment. Van Velzen et al. (1997) reported that 29% of their sample had never been treated before, and none of 35 individuals meeting criteria for lifetime social phobia in an epidemiological sample had ever been treated (Neufeld et al., 1999). A French study of primary care attenders found that psychological problems were given as the reason for contact by only 5.6% of individuals with social phobia not comorbid with depression; patients with social phobia, both with and without depression, were significantly more likely to consider their health as poor compared with that of controls (Weiller et al., 1996). However, recent Australian epidemiological data may be more encouraging: approximately 61% of individuals who would have met criteria for social phobia in the past 12 months sought help from outpatient services for mental health in the 12 months prior to the survey (Issakidis and Andrews, 2002). Other data from this survey indicate that persons over the age of 24 years were most likely to seek help, and, of those who sought help, almost half visited their general practitioner.

There is a considerable associated disability in social phobia that has been under-recognized. There is impairment of role functioning across several domains and significant comorbidity. Individuals with social phobia fail to achieve their full educational and occupational potential and are less likely to marry than the general population: 37% with nongeneralized social phobia and 64% with generalized social phobia in a clinical sample had never married (Manuzza et al., 1995). A small study of media respondents found that those meeting criteria for social phobia were significantly more likely than a group meeting criteria for panic disorder to be single, living alone and unemployed, despite a higher level of education (Norton et al., 1996). The degree of impairment, disability and comorbidity increases along the spectrum from discrete to generalized social phobia to social phobia comorbid with APD.

Differential diagnosis

Axis I disorders

Social phobia may be confused with agoraphobia, since many of the same types of situation will be avoided. However, the underlying fearful cognitions, the *reasons* for avoiding, will differ. The person with social phobia may dislike shopping centers, crowded trains, and queues because of the risk of scrutiny and the difficulty of escaping in case they embarrass themselves. The person with agoraphobia may dislike these same situations because of the difficulty of escaping in case of physical harm. Embarrassment will not be the main focus of the fear. A useful distinguishing exercise can be to ask a patient whether they would be anxious if they could be completely alone in the feared situations: the person with agoraphobia will find this a frightening proposition, whereas an individual with social phobia will report that if there were no one else around they would not have the problem. Social phobia may also be confused with simple phobia when there appears to be only one feared situation. If the fear is of scrutiny or embarrassment, a diagnosis of social phobia takes precedence, but may be subtyped as non-generalized. In clinical practice, a careful history will usually reveal that more than one situation is avoided. A loss of confidence and social withdrawal are common features of major depression. There may even be associated social anxiety. However, the history of premorbidly normal social functioning excludes social phobia. Social anxiety and avoidance is frequently reported in body dysmorphic disorder and to exclude this condition it can be helpful to ask patients whether there is some particular aspect of their appearance or behavior that they fear will attract a negative reaction from others. Whilst individuals with social phobia may have a range of concerns regarding their presentation to others, individuals with body dysmorphic disorder typically manifest a marked preoccupation with a quite specific perceived defect while appearing normal in reality. Social phobia may be comorbid with body dysmorphic disorder in 11% to 12% of cases (Wilhelm et al., 1997).

Axis II: Personality disorder

A diagnosis of APD should be considered in every case, and may be given concurrently with social phobia. Occasionally, clinicians may encounter patients who report anxiety in social situations in which the underlying fear is that others will not perceive the individual's true greatness or superiority. In this case, a diagnosis of narcissistic personality disorder should be considered. For most patients with social phobia, just being like everyone else would bring great happiness. The fear of negative evaluation and rejection for some patients may be part of an underlying paranoid personality style in which there is the expectation of harm from others. Social phobia may be comorbid, but careful inquiry is needed to establish whether criteria for the Axis I disorder are met. Anxiety in social situations without the desire for social attachments may be indicative of schizotypal personality disorder.

Assessment

There are now a large number of measures specifically designed for use in social phobia. The choice of assessment instrument will be affected by whether the clinician wishes to measure symptoms, discriminate between individuals with social phobia and nonanxious individuals or those meeting criteria for other anxiety disorders, measure treatment outcome, or conduct research. The Fear of Negative Evaluation Scale (FNE; Watson and Friend, 1969) is a 30-item true–false self-report questionnaire that provides a measure of apprehension about others' evaluations, distress over negative evaluations, and the expectation of negative evaluation. Means of around 24 have been described in social phobic populations (Heimberg et al., 1988). The FNE is useful in confirming the presence, and perhaps extent, of social evaluative anxiety. However, available evidence suggests that it does not reliably discriminate social phobia from other anxiety disorders (apart from specific phobias), and it is not recommended for use as a diagnostic tool (Turner et al., 1987; Oei et al., 1991). Several newer measures have been developed, including the Social Phobia Scale (SPS; Mattick and Clarke, 1998), the Social Interaction Anxiety Scale (SIAS; Mattick and Clarke, 1998), the Social Phobia and Anxiety Inventory (SPAI; Turner et al., 1989, 1996), and the Liebowitz Social Anxiety Scale (LSAS; Liebowitz, 1987). The psychometric properties of these scales are gradually being established. The SPS has been shown to be most closely associated with scrutiny fears, and the SIAS with fears of social interaction (Cox et al., 1998; Ries et al., 1998). The SPAI asks individuals about somatic symptoms of social anxiety. The SPAI and LSAS also aim to measure avoidance behaviors in social phobia, although the fear/anxiety and avoidance subscales of the LSAS have been shown to be highly correlated (Cox et al., 1998; Safren et al.,

1999). Overall, there has been consistent failure to demonstrate any reliable association between verbal report measures and observable behavior. The SPAI and SIAS may be particularly sensitive measures in their ability to distinguish between specific and generalized subtypes of social phobia (Ries et al., 1998), and the SPAI also has a high degree of specificity in distinguishing social phobia from other anxiety disorders (Cox et al., 1998; Peters, 2000). All the newer measures appear sensitive to treatment change (Ries et al., 1998).

Etiology

Etiological theories of social phobia have been proposed, encompassing genetic/ biological, environmental and cognitive behavioral domains. Research to date has suggested heritable factors that include a general vulnerability to anxiety disorders (Andrews et al., 1990a; Kendler et al., 1992a; Manuzza et al., 1995; Beidel, 1998). The general vulnerability probably corresponds to an elevated trait anxiety, common to all anxiety disorders and also found in some depressive disorders (Andrews et al., 1990a; Parker et al., 1999).

Several family studies have now shown an increased incidence of social phobia in first-degree relatives of probands with social phobia. A recent study using twin data across two measurement occasions (allowing better control over sources of measurement error, including diagnostic unreliability) has found substantial increases in the heritability estimates for all phobias. It is now estimated that genetic factors account for approximately 50% of the variance in liability to develop social phobia (Kendler et al., 1999). Generalized social phobia appears to show the strongest association with genetic/biological factors. More relatives of probands with social phobia than control probands met criteria for social phobia in the study of Manuzza et al. (1995), although there did not appear to be a greater rate of generalized than nongeneralized social phobia in these relatives. In a later study utilizing a similar design, Stein et al. (1998a) found a greatly increased incidence of generalized social phobia (26.4%) but not the nongeneralized form in the relatives of clinic attenders with generalized social phobia as compared with relatives of controls (2.7%).

In their seminal work, Kagan et al. (1988) identified a temperamental construct, which they referred to as behavioral inhibition to the unfamiliar (BI), and suggested that it represents a putative biological basis for shy behavior. They found in a longitudinal study that extreme shyness (defined as inhibition in social situations) at age 2 years was predictive of inhibition at age 7 years. Similarly, extreme disinhibition remained relatively stable over time. Further research has sought to establish the relationship of BI to the later emergence of anxiety disorders and the utility of early intervention strategies. Behavioral inhibition has since been linked both to panic disorder/agoraphobia and to social phobia, but not to specific phobia, OCD, GAD or affective disorder (Beidel, 1998; Mick and Telch, 1998; Cooper and Eke, 1999). The children in the longitudinal cohort described by Kagan had significantly higher rates of phobic disorder of childhood than the uninhibited children. Inhibited children also seem more likely to have parents with social phobia, especially if the child has BI in association with multiple anxiety disorders (Knowles et al., 1995). Definitions of the BI construct encompassed both social and nonsocial novelty. Preliminary evidence suggests that BI in response to social novelty may be more linked to later social phobia, but the same study failed to find a close relationship between panic/agoraphobia and nonsocial novelty (Van Ameringen et al., 1998). A stronger association with generalized than with nongeneralized social phobia has been reported (Wittchen et al., 1999). It remains unclear at present whether BI is a general vulnerability factor related to the development of social phobia and agoraphobia but not that of specific phobias or whether there is a particular relationship with social anxiety.

The neurobiology of social phobia remains poorly understood. Biological correlates of social dominance, social affiliation and attachment have been identified in animals (e.g., Stein, 1998) that have potential for the development and study of human models. There is preliminary evidence for both serotonergic and, alone of the anxiety disorders, dopaminergic dysfunction in social phobia (Nutt et al., 1998; Stein, 1998).

Several psychological models of social phobia have been proposed (for a review, see Mattick et al., 1995). Many studies have sought to assess the association of social phobia with childhood environmental factors but rely on recall of distant events, and hence are subject to unreliable accuracy of both recall and causal attribution. Aversive conditioning models have been proposed but the data suffer from the limitations of retrospective studies. There may be some role for aversive social events, perhaps making some contribution to the initiation or maintenance of social phobia: typically 60% of subjects report such events (Mattick et al., 1995). Preparedness conditioning theories of social phobia suggest that certain types of social interaction may have a particular salience such that individuals may more readily learn particular associations. Öhman's (1986) work strongly suggests that humans readily learn to fear critical, angry or rejecting faces but does not explain fear of scrutiny (Mattick et al., 1995). The social learning model (e.g., Bandura, 1977) may have some relevance to the acquisition of phobias (there is some experimental evidence for this in primates), but has not yet been studied with respect to social phobia. However, Kendler et al. (1992a, 1999) concluded that familial environmental influences on social phobia are small or insignificant. Individual-specific environmental influences may account for 40% to 60% of the etiology of social phobia. A model of social skills deficits as a causal influence in social phobia has also been suggested. It is now realized that an apparent lack of skill may represent either a true skills deficit or an inhibition of skill expression. There is an association between severity of social phobia and poor social skills, but a causal relationship has not been established.

Cognitive theories of the initiation and maintenance of emotional disorder have been applied to social phobia, and now represent the strongest area of research interest among psychological theories (e.g., Clark and Wells, 1995; Rapee and Heimberg, 1997). In social phobia, the underlying cognitive set, or "schema", is seen to include beliefs that negative evaluation is a catastrophic outcome with a high probability of occurring as a result of any one of several contingencies specific to the individual (e.g., Clark and Wells, 1995; Leary and Kowalski, 1995: Rapee and Heimberg, 1997). Evidence is available, from our laboratory and others (Lucock and Salkovskis, 1988; Rapee and Lim, 1992), that individuals with social phobia underestimate their social performance, overestimate the probability of negative social outcome, and overestimate how bad it would be if the feared outcome occurred. Individuals with social phobia have more negative thoughts in social situations than other anxious and nonanxious controls and show a preponderance of negative thoughts prior to treatment (Bruch et al., 1991). Data are available that support a cognitive vulnerability factor of discrepancy between individuals' views of themselves as they are and their view of how others see them (Mattick et al., 1995). These patients also tend to attribute more responsibility for negative outcomes to themselves rather than to external factors, in a pattern opposite to those who are not particularly socially anxious (Hope et al., 1989).

Recently, there has been considerable research interest from an information-processing perspective, seeking to understand how individuals with social phobia process information about themselves and their environment in social situations. Several cognitive "biases" have been identified that result in hypervigilance for social cues and influence the individual to interpret the cues in a manner consistent with the underlying cognitive schemas of social phobia, even though the interpretations may not be particularly realistic or helpful to that individual. An interpretive bias ensures that scrutiny, criticism, and negative evaluation are detected even when realistically not apparent, and an attentional bias towards threat cues (physiological symptoms of anxiety, presence of others who may potentially scrutinize) maintains overestimates of probability and cost of negative social outcomes (Hope et al., 1989; Mattick et al., 1995). Interpretation bias may also lead an individual to misinterpret interoceptive information as disastrous and to interpret an ambiguous social situation as negative. Individuals with social phobia consistently tended towards a negative interpretation of self-relevant situations, even when presented with positive alternatives in one study (Amir et al., 1998a). It is suggested that this may be a relative negative bias as compared with the generally more positive interpretations that nonsocially anxious individuals make (Constans et al., 1999). Individuals with prominent social-evaluative concerns have been shown to focus their attention on themselves in social situations, attempting to create an image of how they would appear to others, often referred to as "the observer perspective" (Wells and Papageorgiou, 1999). This contrasts with the cognitive experience of individuals with normal levels of social anxiety whose attention is focused mostly on aspects of the social interaction or situation. Self-focused attention is postulated to prevent the individual from gaining more accurate information about the situation and others' responses that might disconfirm negative expectations. The benefits of exposure were enhanced in a single small case series when individuals with social phobia were encouraged to focus attention on actual social cues rather than becoming preoccupied with their own thoughts and feelings (Wells and Papageorgiou, 1998) and reduced self-focused attention was linked to better outcome in a study of group cognitive behavioral therapy (Woody et al., 1997).

Memory and judgment biases have also been reported in socially anxious individuals, although there have also been negative findings for memory bias (Hope et al., 1989; Mattick et al., 1995; Amir et al., 1998b; Constans et al., 1999).

Comorbidity

ECA (Schneier et al., 1992), National Comorbidity Survey (NCS; Magee et al., 1996) and National Survey of Mental Health and Wellbeing in Australia (NSMHWB, Lampe et al., unpublished data) data indicate a high rate of comorbidity between social phobia and other Axis I conditions, particularly other anxiety disorders and major depression (Table 8.1). In the NCS, 81% of persons with social phobia reported at least one other lifetime DSM-III-R disorder. In contrast to other anxiety disorders (excluding specific phobia) and to depression, social phobia most often preceded the comorbid disorder (typically in about 70% to 80% of cases in both the ECA and NCS studies; Schneier et al., 1992; Kessler et al., 1999b).

Depression, suicidal ideation and suicide attempts occur in social phobia at greater than population rates. However, an elevated frequency of suicide attempts in social phobia appears to be mostly, though not completely, related to the presence of comorbid conditions. According to ECA data, the rate was approximately 14 times the population frequency. In the NSMHWB survey, the presence of a comorbid Axis I disorder resulted in a tripling of the rate of suicidal ideation, but without a corresponding increase in suicide attempts. When social phobia was comorbid with anxious personality disorder (closely related to APD) both suicidal ideation and attempts were reported at significantly higher rates – suicide

Table 8.1. Comorbidity in social phobia compared across three epidemiological surveys

Axis I disorder comorbid with social phobia (lifetime or 12 month)	% comorbid for disorder, lifetime or 12 month (odds ratios)[a]		
	ECA (Schneier et al., 1992; DSM-III)	NCS (Magee et al., 1996; DSM-III-R)	NSMHWB (Andrews et al., 1999a; DSM-IV)
Major depression	16.6 (4.4)	37.2 (3.6)	52.8 (4.7)
Agoraphobia	44.9 (11.8)	23.3 (7.1)	24.3 (4.8)
Panic disorder	4.7 (3.2)	10.9 (4.8)	25.7 (4.4)
GAD		13.3 (3.8)	48.2 (5.4)
OCD	11.1 (4.3)		10.2 (3.3)
Simple phobia	59.0 (11.8)	37.6 (7.7)	
Any anxiety		56.9 (5.8)	68.8 (4.7)
Alcohol abuse	18.8 (2.2)	10.9 (1.2)	16.7 (3.7)
Alcohol dependence		23.9 (2.1)	
Somatization disorder	1.9 (8.02)		
Dysthymia	12.5 (4.3)	14.6 (3.1)	16.6 (4.1)
PTSD			17.9 (3.1)

[a] For abbreviations, see the text.

attempts were reported at almost four times the frequency of that in uncomplicated social phobia. An early study (Amies et al., 1983) found that parasuicidal acts were more common in a socially phobic sample than in a comparison group meeting criteria for agoraphobia, but more recent epidemiological and clinical studies have failed to confirm this finding (Cox et al., 1994; Norton et al., 1996; Montgomery, 1998). The risk of depression does not appear to increase with duration of social phobia, but may be reduced if social phobia remits (Kessler et al., 1999a). Clinical samples have also shown elevated rates of depression, suicidal ideation and suicide attempts in social phobia comorbid with other Axis I or with Axis II conditions (Amies et al., 1983; Turner et al., 1991; Weiller et al., 1996). The presence of depression is likely to obscure the diagnosis of social phobia in primary care (Weiller et al., 1996). Alcohol abuse is another important area of comorbidity. Excessive use of alcohol has been reported in 16% to 36% in clinical samples with social phobia (Amies et al., 1983; Liebowitz et al., 1985; Schneier et al., 1989). Significantly, in the Schneier et al. (1989) study, the rate of alcoholism as defined by research diagnostic criteria was twice the population rate for men, but three to four times the population rate for women, suggesting that women with social phobia may be particularly at risk of developing alcohol abuse. Epidemiological studies generally find the rate of alcohol abuse or dependence in social phobia to be one to two times the population prevalence but have not reported gender differences. Alcohol abuse is more likely in the generalized subtype of social phobia and has been strongly associated with comorbid APD (Stravynski et al., 1986; Morgenstern et al., 1997). The risk of alcohol abuse also appears to increase with an earlier age at onset of social phobia (Lecrubier, 1998; Regier et al., 1998). Studies of populations described as "alcoholic" have shown high rates of social phobia, estimated at between 16% and 25%, concurrent with the period of alcohol abuse (Mullaney and Trippett, 1979; Smail et al., 1984; Thomas et al., 1999). ECA data (Schneier et al., 1992) indicate that social phobia was temporally primary in 85% of subjects with comorbid alcohol abuse, and 76.7% of those with comorbid drug abuse. The prevalence of comorbid depression and alcohol abuse is higher in those with an early onset (prior to age 15 years) of social phobia and is more likely to result in service utilization and overtly psychological presentations (Lecrubier and Weiller, 1997). In a large clinical study, alcoholics with social phobia were more likely to have a lifetime history of depression and show greater severity of alcohol dependence than those without social phobia (Thomas et al., 1999).

Personality disorders have been reported as comorbid with social phobia in a significant proportion of patients. Estimated rates of comorbid ICD-10 personality disorders in the NSMHWB were anxious (avoidant) 35.8%, anankastic 24.3%, schizoid 27.2%, dependent 20.7% and paranoid, impulsive and borderline about 12%. Individuals with a comorbid personality disorder are likely to show higher symptom levels and disability, but appear no less likely to improve with treatment. APD is invariably the personality disorder most frequently reported as comorbid. Other cluster C personality disorders are also frequently reported as comorbid in clinic samples, including dependent personality disorder (Alnaes and Torgersen, 1988b), and obsessive–compulsive personality disorder (Turner et al., 1991).

Summary

Social phobia is a fear of negative evaluation that results in significant avoidance of social situations. Affected individuals overestimate the probability and adverse consequences of negative evaluation and process social information in ways that maintain such estimates. The disorder affects men and women almost equally, begins most commonly in the second decade of life, and has a chronic course. It is associated with significant personal distress and secondary morbidity, and commonly results in failure to achieve full social and occupational potential.

Social phobia

Treatment

Aims of treatment

The aims of treatment are symptom reduction and improved function. Elimination of all anxiety is unlikely (and unnecessary), and the therapist has a role in helping the patient to set realistic goals for therapy. Psychological and pharmacological treatments are available for social phobia. The treatments for which there is most evidence of efficacy are cognitive and exposure-based treatments, social skills training packages, antidepressant medication and benzodiazepine anxiolytics. In general, outcome is related to severity of symptoms at pretreatment.

Psychological treatments for social phobia

Social skills training

The role of social skills training in the treatment of social phobia continues to be debated. Prior to the publication of DSM-III, social skills training had demonstrated clinical utility in heterogeneous populations of psychiatric outpatients with social skills difficulties or anxieties (Stravynski et al., 1982; Wlazlo et al., 1990). Hence it was proposed that these techniques be applied to the treatment of social phobia. Reviewers agree that few of the early studies that examined social skills treatments were methodologically sound (Marks, 1985; Heimberg, 1989; Stravynski and Greenberg, 1989; Mattick et al., 1995); in particular, only rarely was a control condition in evidence. Diagnostic groups were often heterogeneous or poorly defined. No differentiation was made between those with and those without avoidant personality disorder (APD). In addition, strategies referred to as social skills training often included explicit instructions more consistent with exposure therapies, e.g., to regularly confront their fears and to persist in the situation until anxiety diminished (Wlazlo et al., 1990).

Part of the argument over the role of social skills training centers on whether apparently poor social skills are the result of actual skills deficits, or really due to inhibition of skills expression due to anxiety. Turner et al. (1986) examined the social skills of patients with social phobia, comparing those with and without avoidant personality disorder. They found that patients with social phobia alone felt anxious, and perceived that others found them anxious and inadequate, but in fact had appropriate social skills. Those with APD were found to be markedly lacking in social skills. However, the authors were unable to exclude profound inhibition in social situations as the underlying cause giving rise to the appearance of skills deficits: in APD, severe anxiety related to a core schema that social error will lead to rejection can result in profound social inhibition and avoidance.

Whatever the relation of social skills to social phobia may be, social skills training packages demonstrate an effectiveness equal to exposure therapy. This appears to be the case where participants' existing social skills have not been assessed (Van Dam-Baggen and Kraaimaat, 2000) and is not improved by attempting to direct those with skills deficits towards social skills training (Wlazlo et al., 1990). Maintenance of therapeutic effects to 2 years has been demonstrated. For patients who are "socially dysfunctional" and who have social phobia, social skills training has been reported to be superior to bibliotherapy, group discussion, and psychoanalytical group psychotherapy. For these patients, who would probably meet criteria for APD, it does not seem that the effect of social skills training is enhanced by the addition of propranolol, anxiety-management techniques such as relaxation, or by cognitive strategies. On the other hand, those with APD improve to an equivalent degree when they are treated with cognitive behavioral therapy (CBT). Emmelkamp et al. (1985a), comparing exposure and cognitive therapy, noted that improvement in social anxiety can occur in the presence of persisting poor social skills and that, conversely, treatment failure is not predicted by poor social skills. Social skills training is a complex package with components of exposure and desensitization, behavioral rehearsal, and modeling of appropriate behavior (Emmelkamp et al., 1985a; Marks, 1985) – it remains unclear which aspect(s) of the package may be effective. The most active ingredient appears to be the exposure component, since patients do equally well whether they have formal social skills training or are given homework requiring social interaction (Stravynski and Greenberg, 1989; Stravynski et al., 2000). In patients with APD, social skills training may have the benefit of improving social performance and increasing prosocial behaviors.

Behavioral treatments

Recognition of the success of exposure and desensitization techniques in treating other phobic disorders led to trials of these techniques in the management of social phobia. Studies using imaginal desensitization techniques were largely completed prior to the publication of DSM-III, and used subjects variously diagnosed as socially phobic, socially dysfunctional, and socially anxious. In a review of these techniques, Marks (1985) found that in general they were not very effective in treating the problems under study, although there are some reports of effectiveness equal to social skills training (Shaw, 1979; Stravynski and Greenberg, 1989). Graded exposure to feared social situations, within a group treatment setting and in vivo, is the most common behavioral technique currently in use. It has been shown to reduce the physiological symptoms of anxiety in feared situations, and reduce avoidance of targeted situations (Emmelkamp et al., 1985b; Wlazlo et al., 1990). Exposure alone results in significant improvement in social phobia. However, given the evidence for the importance of cognitive factors in social phobia, it is of significant interest to compare the results of exposure therapy to cognitive therapy and of exposure alone to the combination of cognitive and exposure therapies.

Cognitive-behavioral treatment of social phobia

Concurrently with the trials of social skills training in social phobia, and spurred by the publication of DSM-III, research was directed at elucidating the core features of the disorder. It was proposed that cognitive factors were particularly important in the genesis and maintenance of social phobia (Emmelkamp et al., 1985a) and, hence, that cognitive therapeutic strategies would be necessary components of treatment (Butler, 1989a; Mattick et al., 1989). A consensus was reached that excessive fear of negative evaluation was a central feature of social phobia. Mattick and Peters (1988) and Mattick et al. (1989) demonstrated that a reduction in the degree of concern over the opinions of others (fear of negative evaluation) was the most important mediating attitudinal variable effecting improvement in their trials of exposure, cognitive therapy, and CBT. Most early studies based the cognitive therapeutic component on the work of Ellis (1962), Beck (1976), or Meichenbaum (1977). Heimberg and associates (1995) have since described a group therapy program that is widely used as a model for CBT programs. The efficacy of cognitive behavioral treatments was suggested initially by a number of uncontrolled studies. These findings have been confirmed by a large number of studies employing a variety of control conditions including wait-list (Butler et al., 1984; Mattick et al., 1989) and conditions controlling for attention and support, including "nonspecific therapy" (Butler et al., 1984), education and supportive psychotherapy (Heimberg et al., 1990a, 1998), and "associative therapy", where subjects were asked to free-associate to thoughts and memories of social encounters (Taylor et al., 1997).

Having established that both cognitive and exposure-based therapies are effective in treating social phobia, debate has arisen over whether the combination is superior to either treatment alone. Both negative and positive findings have been reported. Case reports and treatment studies of nongeneralized social phobia

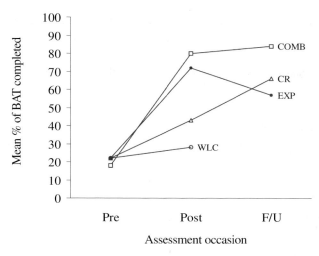

Figure 9.1   Behavioral approach test (BAT) mean scores (percentage) before (Pre) and after (Post) treatment, and at 3-month follow-up (F/U). CR, cognitive restructuring without exposure; EXP, guided exposure; COMB, guided exposure with cognitive restructuring; WLC, wait-list control. (Redrawn with permission from Peters (1985), unpublished honors thesis, University of New South Wales.)

suggest that the addition of cognitive therapy may provide no advantage over exposure alone (Biran et al., 1981; Stravynski et al., 1983; Van Velzen et al., 1997). Taylor (1996), in a recent meta-analysis, located 25 studies using DSM criteria and comparing two active treatments or using a placebo or wait-list control. Most studies included a majority of participants with generalized social phobia. In this analysis, exposure therapy, cognitive therapy, social skills training and combined cognitive therapy and exposure were all effective relative to wait-list control, but only combined cognitive therapy and exposure yielded a significantly greater effect size than a placebo. There was a trend for the combined treatment to show larger effect sizes. In this analysis the effect sizes for both pill- and attention-control placebo were similar at 0.4 to 0.5, while effect sizes of the active treatments ranged from 0.6 (for social skills training and for cognitive therapy alone) to 1.0 (for combined cognitive and exposure therapy). All active treatment conditions showed *increased* effect sizes at 3 months posttreatment, at which time there was little difference between them due largely to the significant gains that occurred in the cognitive therapy and social skills training groups. At 3 months all effect sizes were close to 1.0.

A similar finding has been reported by Mattick et al. (1989; see Figure 9.1) and Salaberria and Echeburua (1998). In these studies, the exposure-only group actually showed some deterioration at follow-up. Gould et al. (1997a) required a no-treatment or wait-list control or psychological placebo for studies selected for meta-analysis. Sixteen studies were identified, of which six were also included in the Taylor (1996) meta-analysis. Most of the differences are explained by the inclusion of more early studies (including pre-DSM-III) and exclusion of studies comparing only active treatments in the Gould et al. (1997) meta-analysis. Despite these, and other minor methodological differences, the findings were similar, with average effect sizes of 0.8 for combined exposure plus cognitive restructuring, and 0.6 for cognitive therapy alone and for social skills training. However, a slight advantage was reported for exposure alone, with an average effect size of 0.89. Most studies did not report follow-up data for the control condition (understandably, since most such research is conducted in clinical settings where patients who meet criteria for social phobia are seeking treatment and those randomized to wait-list or placebo already suffer considerable delay). Therefore, effect sizes were calculated comparing posttreatment and 3-month follow-up data for the active treatment conditions only. Mean effect sizes for different treatments, based on seven studies were: exposure alone (four studies; two negative effect sizes) 0.16; cognitive therapy alone (one study) 0.62; social skills training (one study) 0; combined exposure plus cognitive therapy (six studies; one negative effect size) 0.23.

On reviewing individual studies that compare exposure with cognitive interventions and anxiety management strategies, it seems that slightly different symptoms (behavioral, cognitive, and physiological) may be targeted by each treatment, but that these differences largely disappear at follow-up (Butler et al., 1984; Heimberg et al., 1985; Jerremalm et al., 1986; Mattick et al., 1989; Hope et al., 1995). It has also been suggested by some authors that certain symptom profiles may respond best to particular aspects of a cognitive behavioral package and that not all components may be necessary for all patients. The limited evidence from studies of circumscribed social phobia would support this view. Ost et al. (1981) found some evidence for this view in an early study, but were unable to replicate their findings later (Jerremalm et al., 1986). Negative findings were also reported by Wlazlo et al. (1990).

In summary, we recommend a combined cognitive behavioral treatment package for social phobia because it is not yet possible to match symptom profiles with specific treatment strategies, and because there is some evidence to suggest that gains from exposure-only treatments may not be as well maintained in the long term as the gains that result from combined cognitive behavioral treatments.

Treatment effect sizes and dropout rates

The effect sizes of both pill placebo and attention placebo have been estimated at 0.4 to 0.5 in social phobia (Taylor, 1996). Dropout rates average 10% to 15% for CBT (Taylor, 1996; Turner et al., 1996; Gould et al., 1997) but rates around 25% are also commonly reported (e.g., Salaberria and Echeburua, 1998; Otto et al.,

2000). A dropout rate of 34% was reported by Van Velzen et al. (1997) from their exposure-based individual treatment, which they argued may have been more frightening for participants without the assistance of cognitive strategies or the support of a group (although clinical observation would suggest that the *prospect* of group treatment can be frightening: perhaps once enrolled in group treatment, the support provided may enhance continuation). Dropout rates for social skills training show more variation, having been estimated as ranging between 4% and 25% (Taylor, 1996; Gould et al., 1997a; Stravynski and Greenberg, 1998).

Long-term outcome

All the studies reviewed demonstrated maintenance of gains at follow-up periods of 3 to 6 months. It is important to determine whether results can be maintained in the longer term. There is now preliminary evidence of sustained improvement over 5 years (Heimberg et al., 1993). Patients who had earlier received treatment in either cognitive behavioral group therapy or a control condition comprising education and supportive psychotherapy (reported by Heimberg et al., 1990a) were re-evaluated after a period of 4.5 to 6.25 years after treatment. Those who had received the CBT remained more improved on a variety of behavioral and self-report measures than those treated in the alternative condition. More importantly, global measures suggested that they continued to function well. It was noted that patients who participated in the long-term follow-up were less impaired pre- and posttreatment than those who were not re-evaluated at the long-term follow-up (Heimberg et al., 1993). However, there were no differences in pretreatment severity between long-term follow-up participants who received education support or CBT.

Predictors of outcome

Symptom severity at baseline is the strongest and most consistent predictor of outcome, for both drug and psychological treatments (Otto et al., 2000). Symptom severity in turn is related to the subtype of social phobia (generalized versus nongeneralized) and the presence of comorbid conditions, the most studied being depression and APD. Consistent findings are that the rate of improvement, or degree of change, in social phobia is very similar no matter what the comorbidity or pretreatment symptom burden, but severity of symptoms and degree of impairment posttreatment are most closely related to pretreatment levels. In other words, CBT is likely to be of benefit no matter how severe symptoms are, but functional outcome will be poorer for the more severely impaired individual. Predictive factors that have been identified generally account for only a small part of the variance, and seem to become of even less predictive value as follow-up periods lengthen.

Depression

Individuals with generalized social phobia and avoidant personality disorder but no depression improve to the same degree as those with generalized social phobia alone, but show more impairment before and after treatment (Heimberg et al., 1990b; Hope et al., 1995; Feske et al., 1996; Turner et al., 1996). At least some of the difference in symptom severity has been attributed to the presence of comorbid depression, depression and APD showing some independence of effects in one study (Feske et al., 1996). In this study, the presence of comorbid APD was related to a poorer functional outcome, while comorbid depression reduced the degree of improvement/rate of change. The presence of depressive symptoms accounted for 5% of the variance in outcome at 6-month follow-up, as did treatment expectancy, in the study of Chambless et al. (1997). At follow-up, depression was a more important predictor of outcome than APD. Scholing and Emmelkamp (1999) found that depression was a weak predictor of outcome at posttreatment but not at 18-month follow-up.

Avoidant personality disorder

As noted above, individuals who meet criteria for comorbid APD appear more impaired both before and after treatment, with a poorer functional outcome, despite showing a similar degree of response to treatment. A few studies have examined comorbidity for other personality traits or disorder. A worse outcome was related to histrionic traits in the specific subtype of social phobia and avoidant traits in generalized social phobia at posttreatment, but at 18-month follow-up only dependent traits were modestly (positively) correlated with outcome for the total group, in a study using the Millon Clinical Multiaxial Inventory for personality diagnosis (Scholing and Emmelkamp, 1999). APD as the only comorbid axis II diagnosis did not adversely affect outcome, with the exception of measures of avoidance at 3-month follow-up, in a study employing the Structured Clinical Interview for DSM-III-R (Van Velzen et al., 1997). Depression was more closely linked to the presence of multiple personality disorder diagnoses, both pre- and posttreatment, and this was the group that tended to do worse overall. No other study as yet has controlled for the presence of personality disorders other than APD, and it may prove that total symptom burden is more closely related to both comorbid depressive symptoms and functional outcome than to avoidant personality disorder per se.

Frequency of negative cognitions

Reduction in frequency of negative cognitions appears to be related to improvement posttreatment and in the short term (Mattick et al., 1989; Chambless et al., 1997; Coles and Heimberg, 2000), but there is no evidence that it is either causal or necessary to recovery and it may have less relevance to longer-term outcome (Scholing and Emmelkamp, 1999). A reduction in negative self-focused thoughts was also linked to improvement in an exposure-based treatment without an explicit component of cognitive therapy (Hofmann, 2000).

Treatment format

Most reported studies conducted group cognitive behavioral treatment of social phobia. Wlazlo et al. (1990) compared individual with group social skills training and found an advantage for the group condition. There are few trials comparing group with individual cognitive behavioral treatment, but neither Scholing and Emmelkamp (1993) nor a recent meta-analysis (Gould et al., 1997a) found significant differences between reported outcomes of group and individual treatment programs. Butler (1989a), in an excellent review, has commented on the difficulties of creating adequate exposure conditions for social phobia as a function of the often brief and unexpected nature of many types of social interaction. For this reason, group treatment might be expected to have an advantage because of the prolonged exposure intrinsic to this treatment format. A prolonged group exposure situation provides the opportunity to habituate to the anxiety provoked by exposure to strangers. As the group becomes acquainted, there is also the opportunity for exposure to fears of interacting with a group of people who are better known, and whose opinions may therefore matter more to the individual.

Research limitations

Existing CBT treatment literature suffers from several methodological limitations. Early studies using DSM-III may have excluded more severe cases of social phobia, since hierarchical rules prevented those diagnosed with APD from also being given a diagnosis of social phobia. Studies that employ clinical samples often also have a significant proportion of participants on psychotropic medication, including benzodiazepines and antidepressants, who are free to seek additional treatment between posttreatment and follow-up: such factors cannot always be controlled for given small sample sizes. The specific requirements of an adequate and appropriate control condition for trials of psychological treatments were recognized years ago (Heimberg et al., 1990a; Kendall and Lipman, 1991), yet there are still relatively few reported trials employing the type of placebo condition that provides a more robust test of psychological treatments. However, the number of trials using at least a wait-list control is large enough to establish the efficacy of the psychological treatments reviewed above in relieving at least some of the burden of social phobia. Comparison between studies and treatments is rendered difficult by the wide range of outcome measures used across studies, and the adoption of a small number of well-validated measures of symptom burden and social functioning (e.g., see Bobes, 1998; Cox et al., 1998; Lampe, 2000) would assist the interpretation of results.

Pharmacological treatments

Several classes of drug have been the subject of research. These are beta blockers, anxiolytics of the benzodiazepine class, and antidepressants.

Beta blockers

Beta blockers – such as propranolol or atenolol – may be of value in reducing peripheral symptoms resulting from hyperactivity of the beta-adrenergic nervous system, such as tremor, sweating, blushing, dry mouth, and palpitations (Marshall, 1992; Roy-Byrne and Wingerson, 1992). In this context, beta blockers are frequently used in the management of performance anxiety. Twenty-seven percent of performing artists reported using them in one study (Marshall, 1992). Individuals with performance anxiety will in many cases meet criteria for social phobia, DSM-III-R circumscribed type (Clark and Agras, 1991). There is some rationale for the use of beta blockers in that physiological symptoms of anxiety are often interpreted catastrophically, a factor that has been proposed as important in the maintenance of social phobia (Clark and Wells, 1995; Wells and Papageorgiou, 2000). Therefore, minimizing or eliminating these symptoms may result in fewer anxiety-provoking irrational cognitions and less anxiety. However, evidence for the efficacy of beta blockers in generalized social phobia is lacking. Atenolol was no better than placebo in the studies by Liebowitz et al. (1988) and Turner et al. (1994). Side-effects may include depression, sleep disturbance, and broncho-constriction in susceptible patients, especially with noncardioselective beta blockers. Beta blockers may also cause bradycardia and hypotension and possibly dose-related cognitive and psychomotor impairment. In those whose social anxiety is not limited to public speaking or other discrete performance situations, a beta blocker is likely to be of little value.

Benzodiazepines

Uncontrolled trials have suggested that benzodiazepines can be of value in the treatment of social phobia (Ontiveros and Fontaine, 1990). Munjack et al. (1990) compared clonazepam to no treatment for patients meeting DSM-III-R criteria for social phobia, generalized subtype. Patients receiving the drug (average dose 2.75 mg per day) improved on cognitive measures of social phobia, but at post-treatment were not engaging in any more exposure than the nontreatment group, and there was no real difference between the groups in level of disability secondary to social phobia. No follow-up was reported. Clonazepam (up to 4 mg per day) and encouragement to engage in new social situations was as effective as CBT in a study with no placebo control (Otto et al., 2000). Two placebo-controlled studies also reported positive findings for clonazepam or alprazolam (Gelernter et al., 1991; Davidson et al., 1993) but overall there remains a scarcity of such studies. Risks include dependence, tolerance and relapse when the medication is ceased, and changes in cognition and psychomotor performance that may have deleterious effects on functioning. In addition, the associated high lifetime risk of alcohol abuse warrants cautious prescribing and may suggest a higher risk of becoming benzodiazepine dependent for patients with social phobia. Benzodiazepines are also ineffective for depression, which so often complicates social phobia. A recent review of evidence-based treatments has recommended that they be reserved for patients who are nonresponsive or intolerant to other treatments (Roy-Byrne and Cowley, 1998).

Monoamine oxidase inhibitors (MAOIs)

A number of randomized, placebo-controlled studies have demonstrated the effectiveness of irreversible inhibitors of monoamine oxidase. Phenelzine was superior to atenolol and placebo in a study by Liebowitz et al. (1988, 1992). Atenolol did not differ significantly from placebo. Patients with circumscribed social phobia appeared to have a better response to atenolol than those with generalized social phobia, but the sample size (N=18, five to seven in each group) was said to be too small for statistical analysis. Moclobemide, a reversible inhibitor of monoamine oxidase, performed well in an early randomized controlled trial against both placebo and phenelzine (Versiani et al., 1992), with 91% of the phenelzine group, 82% of the moclobemide group, and 43% of the placebo group meeting criteria said to equate to an almost symptom-free condition after completing 16 weeks of treatment. These investigators noted that patients who met criteria for APD also showed significant improvement on the active drugs, with the majority no longer meeting criteria for APD by week 8 (24/27, as opposed to 2/16 in the placebo group). However, more recent trials of moclobemide in doses of up to 800–900 mg per day have consistently shown a much weaker effect, with generally low response rates (International Multicenter Clinical Trial Group on Moclobemide in Social Phobia, 1997; Noyes et al., 1997; Schneier et al., 1998).

Selective serotonin reuptake inhibitors (SSRIs)

All available SSRIs have now been the subject of case studies (Liebowitz et al., 1991), open studies (Van Ameringen et al., 1994; Bouwer and Stein, 1998) or randomized, placebo-controlled trials (Stein et al., 1998b; Allgulander, 1999; Baldwin et al., 1999; Stein et al., 1999). Their efficacy is well established, to the point that they are now regarded as first-line pharmacological treatment in social phobia. It is consistently reported that about twice as many subjects on an SSRI as on placebo are classified as much or very much improved. Favorable outcomes on the Sheehan Disability Scale have also been reported in all studies that used this measure (mainly recent studies). In flexible dosing studies, the average dose required by participants has often been of the order of 1.5 to 2 times the usual starting dose, e.g., approximately 35 mg for paroxetine, the most widely studied drug (Stein et al., 1998; Baldwin et al., 1999), 150 mg for sertraline (Van Ameringen et al., 1994) and 200 mg for fluvoxamine (Stein et al., 1999).

Most studies have reported significant numbers of participants meeting criteria for generalized social phobia, and a few have also identified comorbid APD: no differences in response have been reported from those with nongeneralized social phobia or social phobia without APD, indicating that SSRIs are also effective for more severe forms of social phobia. In fact, some studies reported a tendency for a greater response in more severe levels of illness (Montgomery, 1998; Schneier et al., 1998).

Treatment effect sizes and dropout rates

Dropout rates in antidepressant therapy appear comparable to or perhaps slightly higher than CBT at approximately 25% of participants (Schneier et al., 1998; Baldwin et al., 1999). Effect sizes are generally not reported in the pharmacological literature, but it would greatly assist comparisons with psychological treatments were this to become more usual (Lampe, 2000).

Comparison trials: pharmacological versus psychological treatment for social phobia

There remain few controlled trials comparing psychological and pharmacological therapies in the treatment of social phobia. All patients showed significant improvements in self-report measures of fear, avoidance and disability in a study where the active treatments of phenelzine, alprazolam or cognitive behavioral group therapy (CBGT) were no more effective than a placebo given with instructions for self-exposure (Gelernter et al., 1991; drug treatment groups were also given self-exposure instructions). Subjects who completed CBGT, with or without buspirone, had a greater reduction in subjective anxiety during musical performance and a greater improvement in quality of performance than those treated with buspirone or placebo alone in a study of musicians with performance anxiety (92 of 99 subjects met criteria for DSM-III-R social phobia, discrete subtype; Clark and Agras, 1991). A comparison of CBGT versus clonazepam (up to 4 mg per day) with encouragement to engage in new social interactions revealed no significant posttreatment differences between treatment groups for any clinician- or patient-rated variable using the last observation carried forward method (Otto et al., 2000). Dropout rates of 25% for CBGT and 40% for clonazepam were reported as not significantly different. Both conditions showed improvement with effect sizes of 0.92 for CBGT and 0.99 for clonazepam (calculated from data provided in Otto et al., 2000, Table 1, p. 352). CBGT and phenelzine were superior to placebo and an Education + Support control condition, with the phenelzine group showing an earlier improvement and superiority to CBGT on some measures (Heimberg et al., 1998). Effect sizes for phenelzine over placebo were of the order of 0.6 to 0.7 and for CBGT were more variable, ranging from 0.1 to 0.44.

Limited evidence suggests that individuals treated with both medication and CBT do no better than those treated with a single therapeutic modality, or may even do somewhat worse (e.g., Clark and Agras, 1991).

Long-term outcome

To date, studies of discontinuation of pharmacotherapy have resulted in high relapse rates, even, in one case, after active treatment had been administered for up to 2 years (Versiani et al., 1996). The depression literature has shown that CBT results in a reduction in the frequency and severity of relapse. Future research in social phobia must be directed towards establishing whether treatment gains are maintained and whether maintenance of gains requires continued administration of the drug or could be improved with the addition of CBT.

Summary

The core elements of social phobia are now well defined. Successful treatments have been identified and include CBT, MAOIs and SSRIs. Functional outcome of CBT is related to pretreatment symptom severity. There is reasonable evidence that gains from CBT can be maintained in the medium term, with a need for more long-term studies. There is as yet no evidence that gains from drug treatment can be maintained once medication is withdrawn. The specific active ingredients of CBT programs remain largely unknown, and there remains a need for more dismantling studies. In view of the long-term outcome, CBT is the treatment of choice for social phobia. When social phobia is complicated by conditions for which there are established and indicated drug treatments, these drugs should be used as appropriate. There is good evidence for reduction of reported levels of social anxiety and self-reported avoidance of nominated social situations after treatment with either antidepressant therapy or CBT. It has not been demonstrated that a reduction in measures of social anxiety equates with more functional social interaction in the real world. The challenge for social phobia outcome research in the twenty-first century is to find and implement measures of functional outcome: how well do our treatments assist individuals to achieve their goals of social function in work, family and community social domains? There is also a need for more studies to assess the long-term outcome of treatment, and to maximize therapeutic effectiveness for the individual.

10

Social phobia

Clinician Guide

Chapter 11 (Social phobia: Patient Treatment Manual) contains the information given to patients in our cognitive behavioral treatment program for social phobia. This chapter discusses the issues of relevance to treatment for the therapist: assessing patients for treatment, the treatment process, and solving problems and difficulties that may be encountered.

Working with individuals with social phobia is challenging but rewarding. The treatment program makes significant demands on the patient. Confronting feared situations will generate high levels of anxiety, and doing so consistently is exhausting. To support the person with social phobia in this task requires genuineness, respect, and empathic firmness. Appropriate empathy is assisted by a thorough familiarity with the physiological, cognitive, and behavioral experience of social phobia. Reading case examples can be helpful, but the best learning experience is talking to individuals with a personal experience of social phobia.

Assessment

Diagnosis

This aspect has been covered in detail in Chapter 9. Correct diagnosis is essential. The core cognitions of social phobia differ from those of the other anxiety disorders: the cognitive component of treatment must be directed at the core cognitive distortions of social phobia to be maximally effective.

The presence or absence of comorbid conditions will influence treatment priorities, choice of treatment format and response to treatment.

Comorbid anxiety disorders

Many patients presenting for treatment will meet criteria for more than one anxiety disorder, since such comorbidity is common in the community (Turner et al., 1991; Schneier et al., 1992; Magee et al., 1996; Offord et al., 1996). Simple phobia appears to be the anxiety disorder consistently reported as having the highest rate of comorbidity, with panic disorder, agoraphobia and GAD also frequently reported. Conversely, social anxiety and concerns about negative evaluation occur in other anxiety disorders (Rapee et al., 1988). When more than one anxiety disorder is present, the underlying concerns that maintain the anxiety may cover several different cognitive themes. In individual treatment, a comprehensive approach may be planned to cover all areas of concern. Group cognitive behavior therapy (CBT) may be available offering either general anxiety-management strategies or targeting a specific anxiety disorder. In the first case it is important that participants realize that the techniques being taught may be successfully applied to any phobic disorder and may also be useful in a wide range of emotional problems. Ideally, some guidance should be given as to how to apply these techniques. In general, if group treatment with a specific anxiety disorder focus is the available format, the patient should be directed to the group treatment program aimed towards the principal or most disabling concern. The patient can later be assisted to apply learned strategies to other problem areas.

Other Axis I disorders

CBT is best deferred for patients with acute Axis I conditions that interfere with attention, concentration, ability to think rationally or generate alternative points of view. Appropriate treatment for the acute condition is the priority. Patients may be reassessed once the aspects of the more acute disorder that preclude CBT have resolved. For example, patients with a major depressive episode may demonstrate psychomotor slowing, impaired attention and concentration and an intense negativity of outlook that they are unable to challenge.

Comorbid personality disorder

Personality disorder is comorbid with social phobia in a substantial number of cases. There are very few contraindications to individual treatment if a therapeutic alliance can be established. However, for group treatment a careful assessment is required, as many personality disorders when comorbid will preclude or complicate this format of treatment. In particular, group treatment is often unsuitable for patients with cluster A and cluster B disorders (schizoid, schizotypal, paranoid, borderline, histrionic, narcissistic, and antisocial personality disorders). Patients who will become excessively demanding of support and attention when faced with difficult and stressful situations, patients who are excessively preoccupied with themselves and their need for attention, and patients who view the world with suspicion and the expectation of harm cannot focus all their attention on their social phobic concerns. In the group situation, most patients will not share these dysfunctional worldviews, nor will there be enough time to invest in challenging these individual schemas unrelated to social phobia. The extra time that may be required to deal with such issues adversely impacts on the treatment experience of other group members. Cluster C disorders, on the other hand, especially avoidant personality disorder, are commonly comorbid with social phobia and rarely preclude group treatment.

Symptomatic assessment

A detailed history should be taken of the patient's physiological, behavioral, and cognitive symptoms of anxiety. How symptoms are related across these domains is also important. In the behavioral assessment, patients should be asked about situations that are avoided and in which anxiety is experienced. Note that patients may say that they have no trouble with a particular situation because they are avoiding it completely. Individuals may also be using *safety behaviors*, designed to reduce the likelihood of the feared symptom, or to reduce the likelihood of others noticing or thinking negatively of it should it occur (e.g., wearing a high collar to hide any flushing of the neck). Many patients structure their lives around their social phobia, incorporating avoidance into every aspect of their daily routines. Hence, it is important to ask patients what they *would like to be able to do*. This will help to formulate the goals of treatment. Physiological symptoms of anxiety are prominent (Amies et al., 1983) and distressing. It is important to determine which symptoms are experienced as particularly troubling, the frequency with which they occur, and the personal meaning of such symptoms. Some symptoms will be feared but rarely happen; others will in reality occur frequently – different treatment approaches are required. Knowing why such symptoms are feared will assist with effective cognitive challenging and graded exposure. It is important to ask about "embarrassing" types of symptom that patients will not volunteer because they fear your negative evaluation: fear of vomiting, urination, defecation, incontinence, burping, flatus.

Assessment instruments

A number of diagnostic instruments of established reliability and validity are available for use with DSM-IV and ICD-10 (including the Structured Clinical Interview for DSM-IV Axis I Disorders (SCID), Anxiety Disorders Interview Schedule for DSM-IV (ADIS-IV), and the Composite International Diagnostic Interview (CIDI)), although not usually available outside of research settings. Symptom measures have been discussed in Chapter 9. Many patients are interested to know their scores on such measures and those which are sensitive to change, such as the Social Phobia Scale (SPS), Social Interaction Anxiety Scale (SIAS), Social Phobia and Anxiety Inventory (SPAI) and the Liebowitz Social Anxiety Scale (LSAS), are useful aids in assessing treatment effectiveness. The Personality Disorder Examination (Loranger, 1988), the International Personality Disorder Examination (Loranger et al., 1997) and the Structured Clinical Interview for

DSM-IV are semi-structured instruments designed for administration by a clinician. They can assist in confirming the presence of personality disorder or traits.

Treatment format

Social phobia may be treated individually or in a group setting in massed sessions or in sessions distributed over time. Feske et al. (1996) found no difference in outcome between 32 hours of massed group treatment and 42 hours of more spaced group treatment. In many treatment settings, group programs may not be available. Where such programs are available, the following considerations may also assist in deciding on the treatment format to recommend.

1. Individual therapy
   - Will take 10 to 20 hours of therapist time, with social phobia uncomplicated by significant other Axis I disorders or personality disorder.
   - Useful where feared events or situations are unusual or particularly embarrassing to discuss.
   - Preferable when comorbid conditions make a group format unsuitable for the patient, or where the patient is likely to behave in a way that will impair the access of other group members to effective treatment.
   - May represent more efficient use of patient time in circumscribed social phobias: but note that a minority of those who present for treatment of social phobia have truly circumscribed fears (Mattick et al., 1989; Holt et al., 1992; Schneier et al., 1992; Eng et al., 2000).
   - Can provide more flexibility in terms of scheduling and content.

2. Group therapy
   - Generally involves around 24 to 50 hours of treatment over a number of sessions, typically held at weekly intervals.
   - Efficient use of therapist time.
   - Benefit of peer support and modeling.
   - Opportunity not present in the individual therapy setting for exposure experiences such as public speaking, social interaction, scrutiny and performance under observation within a therapeutic setting.

It is our belief that some exposure to group treatment confers a clinical advantage to the majority of sufferers with generalized social phobia. It provides lengthy periods of exposure to others, which permits habituation to anxiety. Given the brief nature of many social interactions, and the often great degree of avoidance, this may be a first opportunity to learn that, with persistence in the anxiety-provoking situation, the level of anxiety will eventually diminish. It may also be the first opportunity that many participants have to meet others with the disorder and to find that they are not alone. Furthermore, in the group setting there is the important advantage of positive peer influence. The reports of peers that practice the recommended techniques resulting in improvement tend to carry more weight than didactic statements by the therapist. The group permits some types of exposure exercise that are not possible in individual therapy, in a supportive setting.

It is entirely understandable that, given the nature of the disorder, many individuals react with anxiety to the suggestion of participating in a group treatment program. In most cases, the individual readily appreciates the potential value of such a program once the rationale for group treatment is described. However, a minority, particularly those who also meet criteria for avoidant personality disorder, may require some individual therapy before they can consider the prospect of group treatment without extreme anxiety.

Special considerations applying to group treatment
Establishing a group

A group of six to eight persons seems to present the optimum number for group treatment: enough to allow useful group interactions and the realistic sense of an audience, but small enough to permit adequate therapist attention to individual concerns. Ideally, at least half the group would have relatively uncomplicated social phobia. We have successfully mixed ages and backgrounds, although more cohesive groups result when patients have similar demographics. It is important to have both men and women in the group, because individuals with social phobia are often most uncomfortable with persons of the gender to which they are sexually oriented. Some treatment programs advocate a male and a female therapist, but this is expensive of therapist time.

Comprehensive individual assessment of patients prior to entering the group will ensure that the therapist is aware of significant comorbid conditions and personality factors and hence can deal with these effectively to prevent any adverse influences should they arise in the group. This is a matter of experience. Awareness of this information can also ensure that individual concerns of participants are addressed.

Treatment schedule

The program is run as a closed group, and patients are expected to attend all sessions. Most cognitive behavioral group programs are scheduled as weekly sessions of 2 to $2\frac{1}{2}$ hours over 10 to 12 weeks. We have also used formats of 3 full days followed by a number of shorter weekly sessions, and a series of 3–5 full days separated by intervals of 1 or 2 weeks. All formats have shown equivalent effectiveness, and hence it appears that groups may be scheduled in a manner that suits the participants and the institution.

We believe that the breaks between treatment sessions are an important part of the therapy; however, since they allow time for participants to practice their new skills, and achieve some success, but also encounter problems and difficulties that can provide the opportunity for discussion in the group and hence further learning and skills enhancement. Recent work on relapse prevention has highlighted the need for patients to learn to cope with failure and difficulties adaptively (Whisman, 1990; Wilson, 1992).

The first few group sessions

It is important to appreciate that to have turned up at all to the first group session represents a feat of great courage for the person with social phobia. Group members will be feeling acutely anxious and uncomfortable, perhaps even to the point of panic, since the small group is one of the most difficult situations for those with generalized social phobia. In dealing with the high level of anxiety of the participants at this first session, the principles of graded exposure are applied. For example, patients need not be expected to start talking about themselves immediately. Instead, at the commencement of the group, the therapist can do the talking. Welcome the participants, tell them about any housekeeping rules, about rules related to groups, such as confidentiality, and give a brief outline of how the sessions will run. Stick-on nametags can be handed around to avoid the need for introductions but begin the process of getting to know each other. Acknowledge participants' anxiety and their courage in overcoming it to attend. It can be helpful to illustrate that everyone is feeling anxious: the therapist can ask for an indication that this is so (a nod will do). Many participants will be thinking "I'm the worst here, I look really anxious, but they don't. They're thinking I'm really bad." As the day goes by, and anxiety lessens, participants can be asked to make brief introductions. Additionally, at appropriate parts of the Patient Treatment Manual, group members can be asked to contribute their own experience. Before concluding for the day, it is important to direct some intervention towards ensuring that all group members return for the next session. This is necessary because, although at the end of the first session participants may have the intention of returning, it is a common experience that anxiety is again severe just prior to the next session, with the strong temptation to avoid. The likelihood of a patient staying in treatment may be enhanced by the following:

- The empathy a therapist is able to demonstrate for the anxiety participants are experiencing.
- The therapist's ability to demonstrate their understanding of the experiences of sufferers.
- Advice that participants are unlikely to experience worse anxiety than those first few hours.

- Early assistance with some strategies to manage this anxiety. For example, participants may find it helpful to remind themselves of their motivation for attending, and to remember that they survived the first day, perhaps even with a gradual reduction in the level of anxiety experienced.

Problem solving

It is not uncommon to have a person fail to turn up at the first session despite confirming their intention to attend perhaps only a short time before the group starts. For some patients, the anxiety on the day seems too great and they deal with it by avoiding the situation. Such individuals will usually be followed up to determine the reasons for nonattendance and the best course of action, but it is not recommended that they attend the current group unless able to come in and start immediately, i.e., in the current session. If the patient returns much later, they will have missed important educational aspects of the program and will not have been part of the developing rapport between group members. These factors may impede the individual's progress and reinforce their anxiety, further diminishing their chances of persisting with the program.

Occasionally, patients will fail to return for the second treatment session. A follow-up phone call as soon as practicable is valuable: it reinforces the supportive aspect of the therapeutic alliance and allows an opportunity to reassess the most appropriate format of treatment. In general, when the individual has unrealistic anxieties about the group that are amenable to cognitive challenge, and when his or her anxiety responds to the empathy and support of the therapist, a successful return to the same group is often possible – preferably that same day, or at the very next session. Otherwise, the same considerations as noted above will apply.

At times during the group, participants may experience extreme distress or anxiety, and may cry or leave the room upset. Common reasons for leaving are severe anxiety, usually related to some particular cognition, especially regarding perceived negative evaluation from other group members. Serious decompensation (e.g., frank paranoia) is occasionally seen and warrants psychiatric assessment. It is appropriate to acknowledge distress but in a way that does not demean or embarrass the patient, or detract from the development of mastery and responsibility. Empathic inquiry into the individual's emotional state, if necessary gentle reminders to use anxiety-management strategies, and permission to do what they feel is necessary to cope, is often sufficient. At a convenient break, the therapist should talk to the patient privately to ascertain what the problem may have been, and devise a management plan if the issue has not resolved. The calm and accepting way in which the disturbance is handled demonstrates that expression of strong emotions does not necessarily attract negative evaluation, that anxiety and distress within the group is not unusual, and that the therapist has faith in the patient's ability to cope. These episodes can be valuable learning experiences for both the patient and the group.

The person with social phobia is likely to be highly anxious and acutely sensitive to criticism. The degree of anxiety, coupled with an underlying cognitive bias to interpret situations negatively, may impair attention and realistic appraisal of the situation. When social phobia is complicated by avoidant personality disorder there are in addition distorted ideas about rejection (e.g., that if someone disagrees with the individual this equals rejection as a person). The person with social phobia also fears negative evaluation from the therapist. In a group situation, the therapist may need to disagree somewhat with a participant's opinion (e.g., that social phobia is caused by one's parents) but must be sensitive about the ways in which such disagreement is expressed. Rather than assert that an expressed opinion is incorrect, it may be more helpful to suggest alternative interpretations. Similarly, when giving feedback about a participant's performance or manner of relating. In general, the fear of negative evaluation also means that individuals with social phobia are very compliant with requests, tasks, and homework. However, they are reluctant to express disagreement or ask questions, so that the therapist should initiate discussion at certain points and be alert for signs of incomprehension or dissension.

Time management

In general the program is worked through in the order in which chapters are set out in the Manual. The first priorities of treatment are to educate about anxiety and panic, and teach methods of anxiety management. Initially participants are taught a technique of hyperventilation control, since most individuals find this a useful anxiety management strategy, which can be quickly mastered. The principles of CBT are outlined, and patients are introduced to a model of social phobia. Some discussion of the individual's experience of social phobia in relation to this model is often useful at this point. This may also be a convenient time to introduce discussion of "embarrassing" symptoms or else fear of negative evaluation may mean that these are never disclosed. Next, work begins to identify and challenge the specific underlying cognitions that drive the individual's social phobia. This work will continue throughout the course of treatment, the eventual goal being the identification and challenge of underlying schemas. Exposure exercises should begin early. At this stage the behavioral analysis may be completed in more detail than may have been possible initially, since many patients have avoidance strategies of which they are unaware prior to treatment. Once this core material has been covered, sessions can usefully be divided into sections comprising review of homework tasks, discussion of any here-and-now issues or problems, the topic for that session (in the early stages), and planning of between-session goals and exercises, including cognitive and exposure-based tasks. Home-work may include reading material (e.g., the appropriate section of the Patient Treatment Manual), exposure tasks, behavioral experiments, and cognitive challenging exercises.

In the group setting, some exposure exercises are usually carried out during the session. These may include various types of interaction or performance, including public-speaking or role-play exercises tailored to individual areas of difficulty.

The sections of the Patient Treatment Manual will be discussed in more detail below.

Education: what is social phobia (Sections 1.1–1.5) and the nature of anxiety (Section 2)

Treatment begins with education about the nature of anxiety and social phobia. At this point, many patients often raise their own theories about why they have social phobia. In some cases, they unequivocally blame some other person, often a parent. This is a good time to discuss the multiple influences (biological, psychological, and environmental) on the development of social phobia, and to stress that, whatever the cause or causes, something can be done to improve the situation. The individual's experience of anxiety should be discussed. In the group situation, the similarities and differences in participants' experience of anxiety can be explored. The exercise, "Make a List of Situations in Which You Would Feel Very Anxious" can be another useful group exercise. Once patients have completed their own list, a group list can be generated for the whiteboard. This may be saved so that the therapist and group members can check that exposure tasks over the coming sessions target these situations. Once again, patients will see how much they have in common. In individual treatment, the list of difficult situations will form the basis of the graded exposure hierarchy. At this stage, patients are often unable to appreciate how so many seemingly different situational fears can have anything in common and may ask about this. They may also point out that "sometimes this is a problem, and sometimes it isn't. It's totally unpredictable". In fact, the list will be logically understandable in terms of the individual's specific underlying fears. Until they have learned about the influence of cognitions on the experience of anxiety it may be difficult to be persuaded of this. It is probably best to say that this issue will be discussed at a later stage, and that it will probably turn out that their fears are more predictable than it currently seems.

It is helpful to discuss the Yerkes–Dodson curve (Yerkes and Dodson, 1908) in detail. We often begin by asking patients to predict what they think might be the relationship between anxiety and performance. The actual shape of the curve usually comes as a surprise. Many patients who attend for treatment believe that any anxiety is abnormal and hope that treatment will eliminate all anxiety. This concept should be discussed with reference to the implications from the Yerkes–Dodson curve (and reinforced by real life experience) that not only is it not necessary to eliminate all anxiety, but some anxiety can even be helpful. Suggest that the aim should be to keep to the left side of the curve, entering situations with as low an initial anxiety level as is reasonable and possible, but remembering that some anxiety can improve performance (Section 2.3).

Anxiety-management strategies (Section 3)

Many patients find hyperventilation control especially helpful. It may assist the individual to feel more in control of their anxiety level, and less likely to make catastrophic interpretations when they experience physiological symptoms of anxiety. The correct procedure should be demonstrated by the therapist, and the patient's technique observed. It is helpful to practice the technique frequently outside of the therapy setting; this can be set as homework – four practice sessions per day. In a massed sessions group, one practice can be done in group time, which gives the therapist an opportunity to check on participants' techniques. Patients may keep a record of their breathing rates before and after each practice. This may be done for a week or two until the technique is well rehearsed. An introduction to relaxation training is included in our program, and many patients report that they find it very helpful. However, there is no research evidence to suggest that it is an essential component of treatment.

Cognitive therapy for social phobia (Section 4)

This section introduces discussion about the underlying fears of social phobia. The Fear of Negative Evaluation scale (Watson and Friend, 1969) may be used as a tool to give individuals some idea of how their level of concern about negative evaluation compares to that of others in the community. This gives support to the model of social phobia introduced in Section 1, which proposed that a key element of social phobia is an excessive concern about being negatively evaluated by others.

Cognitive challenging is then introduced as a technique to help to reduce fear of negative evaluation and modify thinking so that it is more reasonable and self-enhancing. To introduce the concept of hypothesis testing through behavioral experiments, and to illustrate the unreasonable nature of many underlying beliefs and cognitions in social phobia, patients may be asked to carry out an experiment of walking down the street. Specific instructions about the task should be given: how to look at people (only to glance at people, not maintain gaze which could be interpreted as an aggressive challenge, or as an advance of some type), how long to stay out, or how many people to look at, where to go, whether it may be done in company. The likely response is that most people will quickly look away and not pay the individual any particular attention. Hence, the hypothesis in the Patient Treatment Manual (i.e., that no-one is really very interested in the individual with social phobia) is given some support. The technique of guided discovery may be used to help individuals to reach this conclusion and realize that their initial predictions overestimated the probability of a negative outcome. The Patient Treatment Manual details the most common types of cognitive distortions or "errors" in social phobia. This may assist mastery of the skill of cognitive challenging. Individuals usually take a significant amount of time to master the technique and to begin to see results. Once the basic skills have been introduced, a significant proportion of session time is spent in reviewing and fine-tuning an individual's application of the techniques in every day life. In general, patients will need to identify and challenge underlying unhelpful cognitions repeatedly with therapist guidance. As their skill level increases, patients can be gradually encouraged to take more responsibility for identifying and challenging their own beliefs. The "downward arrow" or "flow of thought" techniques are introduced early to help to uncover core schemas. In time, most patients will be able to identify a number of underlying core schemas operating in most social situations. Specific behavioral experiments may be devised to help to challenge these. Cognitive restructuring is most effective in social phobia when it is linked to exposure to feared situations. It is introduced before graded exposure, as we have found that patients find it easier to engage in exposure tasks if they can reduce their level of anxiety beforehand using cognitive challenging.

Problems with cognitive restructuring

Some individuals find it difficult to identify their underlying beliefs and interpretations. They may require more time in therapy to master the skill, and may benefit from more guided discovery. Some strategies that may help an individual to increase awareness of his or her thoughts are given in Section 4.5 of the Manual.

Some patients will resist identifying their anxious thoughts about tasks. Frequent complaints include:

"I am worse since I started the program. Now I worry about things that never used to cause any problems."

"Thinking about my worries only makes it harder to do the tasks. I'd rather not think about it, just go out and do it."

A phase of increased anxiety is common. An essential step in restructuring to a set of more adaptable cognitions is becoming aware of distorted cognitions. As many unrealistic beliefs and underlying maladaptive schemas as possible must be identified and challenged for success. As patients face their fears, they will naturally experience some anxiety. In many ways, it is a sign of progress. With consistent challenging, the distorted views will change and cease to be so anxiety provoking. Techniques of anxiety management are taught concurrently to help to cope with the anxiety. The trouble with the "don't think about it" approach is that it does not develop any real control. It may work or it may not. Things do not improve over time, to which the patient attests by having asked for treatment. These patients are often the ones with the apparently "unpredictable" anxiety pattern.

Those with avoidant personality disorder will often be slowest to accept the potential benefit of exposure and cognitive challenging. Exposure is particularly challenging because of beliefs about the cost and likelihood of rejection. A group therapy setting can be helpful in this regard, where the testimonials of other participants that they find the method working for them are valuable and motivating.

Graded exposure

This concept is one of the more difficult aspects of the program for individuals in therapy to grasp. To be most effective, exposure should be targeted at specific underlying concerns. For example, consider the goal of having a meal at a restaurant with friends. The graded exposure program will be different for the person whose main fear is that their hands will shake as compared with the person whose main fear is that they will not be able to make conversation. The former needs practice with eating, drinking, and writing under scrutiny, but the latter needs practice making social conversation. Patients find it hard to generate steps of variable difficulty. When the goal cannot be easily divided into steps, individuals find it particularly hard to generate steps involving situations that are different from the goal, yet similar enough to provoke the same underlying fear and therefore engage anxiety related to the goal. Versions of a performance target will result in desensitization, generalizing to the principal target when the intermediate step engages the specific underlying fear and is successfully achieved. Considerable practice is usually required. There are several practice examples in the Patient Treatment Manual that are usefully worked through. In a group treatment program, each patient can be asked to volunteer their suggestions in turn. Participants will learn from their peers, and the therapist will have the opportunity to illustrate that there is no single "right" answer, but that there are several useful approaches, and that the specific program will vary according to the specific underlying fears. The "who, what, when, where, how long" format is an attempt to make the process a little easier by using a "formula". Each category can be altered for most tasks. Within these categories much can be modified to alter the degree of difficulty. The following list provides a format for modifying such tasks to form a graded hierarchy.

Who: Vary who will be present and what their relationship is to the patient, e.g., authority figure, family, close friend, acquaintance, colleague, stranger. Vary how many people will be present.

What: Vary exactly what is to be done: should focus on behavior rather than style, e.g., to give a 5-minute talk, but not "to be free from anxiety" or "to give an outstanding oration".

When: Vary the time of day, for this may influence the individual's energy level and motivation and how many other people may be around. The degree of advance warning influences anticipatory anxiety.

Where: Vary the setting. Consider such factors of potential importance as relative ease of escape, how much the setting results in a feeling of being under scrutiny (e.g., open-plan restaurant versus booths), who else is likely to be there. Locations include work, home, public places, friends' homes, family homes.

How long: Vary how long the activity will last. Could the patient leave earlier; how long will the patient expect to perform that activity in that situation; should they remain after the activity has been completed?

Setting exposure tasks

Tasks are chosen over the course of treatment that expose the person with social phobia to a range of situations so that all aspects of their fears will be engaged over time. For most individuals this will include exposure to both performance- or scrutiny-based situations and social interaction. This is always done by negotiation and discussion. In our program, we also routinely ask participants to perform some tasks that are realistically a little out of the ordinary, and might be expected to attract attention. Each is designed to provide some exposure to scrutiny, as well as to the potential for attracting negative evaluation. We believe that if an individual learns that he or she can cope when the "worst" happens (i.e., they *do* behave in an unusual way and come under scrutiny), the fear of negative evaluation is more quickly, and perhaps more effectively, reduced. Such tasks also help individuals to make more accurate appraisals of the likelihood of attracting negative evaluation through doing something unusual or embarrassing, and to be more realistic about how unusual a given behavior or situation really is. Examples include: asking a patient to sit down next to someone on a bus, and then to ask that person to exchange seats without offering any reasons or excuses; the group walking down the street in single file; paying a compliment to a stranger; standing and proposing toasts in turn at a café. It is most helpful if the therapist has a good idea of what is likely to happen when set tasks designed to test particular core beliefs are used: do it yourself, and get some colleagues to do it and report back. Ideally, patients should perform the task without giving reasons and excuses for their behavior, since this represents a greater perceived risk for negative evalu-ation. Posttask discussion may center around how much attention was really paid by others, how unusual various behaviors really are, and how much negative evaluation assertive or unusual behavior really attracts. Participants may be asked to predict the outcome before they set out and compare the actual outcome on their return. Other tasks are negotiated with reference to the hierarchy of feared situations already established for the individual. Throughout the practice of graded exposure it is stressed that the goal is to develop effective anxiety-managment strategies and reduce fear, rather than achieve a "perfect" performance in the practice situation.

In a group program, graded exposure is undertaken within the group, outside the group during therapy time, and by the individual between meetings. Some tasks are set by the therapist to be carried out either as a group, in pairs, or individually: these are usually the tasks that serve as behavioral experiments that will challenge common underlying beliefs in social phobia. Role-play exposure to challenging situations may also be undertaken in the group setting. Types of situation that are challenging for the majority of participants are chosen. Typically these include meeting new people (especially potential dates) and making conver-sation, and various types of situation requiring the exercise of assertiveness skills such as resolving conflicts, making requests, and handling criticism. We have found a public-speaking exercise to be particularly valuable in a group setting. This task is chosen because it will provoke anxiety in the majority of participants. It can be structured to provide a demonstration of the application and effective-ness of graded exposure and of cognitive challenging in reducing the anxiety provoked by exposure situations. Individuals give talks of gradually increasing duration to their fellow participants. We alternate between prepared and im-promptu talks to provide exposure to both anticipatory anxiety as well as give practice at coping with the unexpected. It also provides the opportunity for an extremely useful exercise, which challenges beliefs about how anxious an individ-ual believes they look. In this exercise, participants are videotaped giving their talk in front of the group. Before watching the videos each participant is asked to give a Subjective Units of Distress (SUDs) rating to how anxious they felt while giving their talk. This is recorded against the appropriate individual's name on a white-board. Next, each video is watched in turn. After each video, the individual on the tape is asked to rate how anxious they feel they *looked* on the video. Finally, the group is asked to provide an honest appraisal of how anxious they feel the person looked ((S)UDs scores are roughly averaged to give a group measure). This process is repeated after each video is viewed. Typically, each individual rates himself or herself as highly anxious, then is surprised to see that he or she definitely does not look as anxious as they felt, although he or she still tends to give unrealistically high self-ratings of the appearance of being anxious. Typically, the group rating is lower again (because they do not interpret various mannerisms and gestures as indicative of anxiety, contrary to the individual who feels that these signs make his or her anxiety glaringly obvious to others). This exercise may be repeated a few times to allow participants more time to test this hypothesis and hence trust the repeatedly positive outcome as reliable. Participants consistently report finding this a very valuable exercise. We provide them with a tape of themselves to take home as a reminder. Occasionally, some individuals find it too painful to watch themselves on video (even when others are not present). In our experience there is often an underlying body dysmorphic disorder in such cases. We would not press too hard for them to watch the video, but they can complete the other elements of the task.

Having generated an exposure hierarchy, individuals are shown how to link cognitive challenging with exposure therapy. They are encouraged to identify anxieties about a task *before* entering the situation, and to find effective challenges for these concerns. Challenges are effective when they reduce the level of anxiety an individual experiences. If anxiety does not diminish it is most often because the major underlying concern (usually linked to the core schemas) has not been identified or challenged. Many individuals also like to identify some coping strategies that will help them to manage anxiety in the situation (e.g., "get there in plenty of time", "remember to do my breathing", "focus on the task at hand"). They are encouraged to use the "A–B–C–D" format introduced under Cognitive therapy in Section 4.4 of the Manual and to actually write all their fears and challenges down. We have found in practice that this process results in greater mastery of the techniques. The long-term goal is, of course, for the individual to be able to complete this process *in* the situation in a quick and effective manner, but this level of skill seems to result only from repeated, quality practice, and a quality practice is one that thoroughly examines for both superficial and deeper concerns and challenges these from a range of perspectives (i.e., how likely is it? how much would it really matter? etc.) After completing the exposure task, individuals are encouraged to compare the predicted with actual SUDs in the situation, and to formulate some conclusions about what was learned from it, including implications for previously identified unrealistic beliefs and predictions about outcome. The exposure diary in the Manual illustrates this.

It is also important to extend the principles of cognitive challenging to an individual's interpretation of the outcome of exposure tasks. The attentional and interpretive biases that are common in social phobia often mean that an individual returns from carrying out an exposure task with memories of the experience consisting largely of all the social errors they believe they committed and the negative evaluation they believe they attracted. This is especially likely in severe generalized social phobia and the avoidant personality style. Hence, it is also very important to review an individual's report of the experience in detail, as the alert therapist will usually detect points in the story where alternative interpretations may be more realistic and helpful. For example, a young woman completed a task of asking the person standing in line ahead of her for the correct time. She reported that the task had gone badly. When asked to describe what had happened in detail, she reported that there had been a man standing in front of her, and when she asked him for the time he had looked at her (this appeared to be the point at which she perceived negative evaluation) and *then he smiled* and gave her the time. The experience of scrutiny was so uncomfortable for her that she had not attended to the other part of the man's response, i.e., his smile to her, which was surely more likely to be indicative that he was positively disposed towards her.

A careful history of an individual's exposure task experience will also help to elicit subtle forms of avoidance and safety behaviors. Cognitive challenging can then be used to determine the reasons why the individual is employing these strategies. We believe that a better outcome is likely if the individual can be encouraged to gradually give up these avoidant coping strategies. For example, the therapist sets a task: "To get on a bus, sit down, and after a few stops ask someone sitting near you to change seats with you. Remain on the bus for at least a few more stops." On return of the group, the therapist inquires of a participant "Did you change seats with someone?" and that individual replies "Yes". However, more careful questioning might reveal that what the individual actually did was to ask someone standing if they would like to sit, which was not the intention of the task (i.e., to create a situation where an individual might be exposed to some scrutiny and evaluation) and which would result in a lost opportunity for learning that it may not be as difficult or unpleasant to face the possibility of negative evaluation, and to face the uncertainty of not knowing for sure. Or the therapist may find that the individual completed the task, but in a special way that incorporated avoidance: e.g., waiting for a bus that looked less crowded, catching several buses until they found someone who looked "approachable". Exploring underlying cognitions that resulted in subtle avoidance behavior is usually enlightening for the individual. Similarly, if an individual has become so anxious that they have used escape from, or complete avoidance of, the task, the experience should be discussed and underlying cognitions elicited and challenged. The whole process needs to facilitate learning in a supportive and nonjudgmental setting.

Participants in treatment are asked to bring their diaries, containing their written A–B–C–D exercises linked to exposure practice, and their records of the experience and outcome of this practice, with them to therapy sessions. This diary is used to determine with patients what types of difficulty they are experiencing and what situations need further attention. It also gives an indication of compliance and general grasp of the principles of treatment. It should be stressed that the therapist is not expecting the person to go away and have no problems. In fact, this is a helpful time to experience difficulties, since they still have ready access to the therapist (and the group in this setting), and problems can be more easily solved in these circumstances. It is an opportunity for fine-tuning and problem solving. When a record indicates that little cognitive challenging or exposure practice has been undertaken, this forms the focus of further problem solving.

Problems with graded exposure

The most common problem with set tasks is avoidance in various forms. Often, avoidance may not initially be recognized as such by the patient. Dealing with avoidance has been discussed.

In a group it is not always easy to set common exposure tasks at the right level of difficulty for each participant: one must aim for best fit. A balance needs to be struck between giving the timid and very anxious (usually those with comorbid avoidant personality disorder) some strong encouragement, but not pressing people to do things for which they are really not ready (since we emphasize that they tailor their own program and design exposure steps of manageable difficulty level). The therapist can ask whether anyone has any particular concerns about the task that has been set. Does anyone feel unable to do it? We use the "75% rule". That is to say, that an individual should feel about 75% confident of being able to engage in a given exposure task. This achieves about the right level of difficulty: challenging but not overwhelming. If in doubt, the individual should rate the task as *more* rather than less challenging, as it is preferable to have an experience of success. The usual concerns relate to unrealistic fears about how others will react. If no concerns are volunteered in a group situation, it is unlikely that there are none! It is most likely that fear of negative evaluation from other group members or the therapist is keeping participants from expressing their anxiety. Encourage the process by asking questions that will engage anxiety: "What if the person says no?", "What if everyone looks at you?", "What if you get really anxious?". This usually results in some discussion. If after cognitive challenging the person still feels the task is too hard, the therapist can ask them to set a slightly easier form of the task. Have this easier form of the task "on standby". Often the individual will be able to complete the task in its original form after all. However, if he or she had not been taken through the exercise of modifying the difficulty level, and once in the situation had found that he or she were too anxious, the individual would have been likely to avoid the whole task. This, too, could have been turned into a learning situation ("How could you manage better next time?"), but it involves the risk of further loss of self-esteem and fails to reinforce the principle of facing anxiety and dealing with it effectively.

In a group it seems important that no-one is allowed to fall significantly behind the others in terms of equivalent achievement, because they may lose self-esteem and experience a reduced sense of self-efficacy that would impair further improvement in the group. At the same time, it is essential to stress that it is not what is done; rather, the goal is to successfully manage the anxiety in that situation. In other words, if simply catching the bus causes as much anxiety for one person as asking someone to change seats does for another, then these tasks represent equivalent levels of achievement and this should receive equal recognition in the group, and from the individual.

Individuals commonly confuse what might be called "preparation" or "coping techniques" with exposure steps. Using an example from the Patient Treatment Manual, the goal "to give a five minute speech at a friend's anniversary party", many patients will suggest a graded exposure program along the lines of:

Decide what you want to say.

Practice the speech so you know it really well.

Don't have too much to drink at the party.

Remember to do your breathing.

Do the speech.

These are essentially coping strategies, and many individuals find it useful to prepare such a list, but they also need to be able to devise an individually appropriate exposure hierarchy and may require further assistance in developing this skill.

Many social situations are of such a nature that it is difficult to devise graded exposure programs for them. Examples of such situations include interactions that are brief or unexpected. Situations of brief duration may be practiced frequently and repetitively. Practice for situations that often occur unexpectedly, e.g., running into an acquaintance in the street, may include role-play, particularly in group situations, and imaginal desensitization. Practicing related situations in vivo is also helpful.

A commonly encountered problem is that patients devalue what they achieve. For example, on completing a task and discovering that it was not as difficult as anticipated, an individual may say, "It doesn't really count because it was quite easy". Patients may be reminded that before doing the task they were quite anxious about it, and not completely certain that they could do it. If they subsequently discovered that their anticipatory anxiety was excessive, that is a good learning experience but does not detract from the achievement of performing a task despite being anxious about it. Patients may have difficulty accepting that they are making progress: "Okay, I talked to someone at the party for 5 minutes, but that's hopeless. I should be able to talk to lots of people." Individuals can be reminded that graded exposure involves step-by-step progress, but the steps will eventually reach their target behaviors. People take lessons for things all the time. They could not simply get in a car the first time and drive it away, they could not learn a trade in one lesson, and so forth. Many things take practice and are achieved with stepwise improvement. Note also the use of "should". Where is the rule about what "should" happen at parties?

Assertiveness

This is an important component, since most persons with social phobia are underassertive for fear of rejection or negative evaluation. This section generates a great deal of discussion. One of the most common concerns after fear of negative evaluation is fear that an assertive act by the person with social phobia will damage the other person in some way. This cognitive distortion also arises in response to tasks that require a "false" or "pointless" interaction with another person. For example, asking someone to change seats on the bus when the person asking does not really want the seat but is just doing it as a task, paying someone a compliment that the person doing the task does not really mean ("they'll know I'm not sincere and they will be upset"). In reality, no patient has ever reported a reaction that indicated the other person "knew" they were not sincere. On the contrary, patients are often amazed that many people react to even "insincere" compliments with apparent pleasure. The idea that they can "make" someone else feel or behave in some particular fashion requires vigorous challenge. It is also important to remind participants that the other person in the interaction has the right to choose how to respond, e.g., by refusing their request to change seats.

General progress to be expected

In our 3-week intensive group treatment program the average improvement in symptoms for patients with social phobia without avoidant personality disorder is of the order of one standard deviation. There is improvement in self-report measures of anxiety and depression and in attitudinal variables, and patients report increased engagement in desired social activities. Further significant improvement over time occurs for those who continue to put into practice the principles of treatment. The need, and benefit, of continuing to work on difficulties should be stressed. In our clinic we offer a follow-up meeting where any problems or difficulties may be discussed with the therapist. In individual treatment, the interval and number of follow-up visits may be tailored to the individual. Clinically, improvement occurs rapidly once individuals start to engage actively in exposure, particularly as they recognize themselves starting to tackle tasks perceived as difficult. Patients with comorbid avoidant personality disorder improve to the same degree, but are more impaired prior to treatment and remain so posttreatment. They are likely to need a longer period of treatment.

Problem solving: failure to progress

Few patients fail to improve when the principles of treatment are actively practiced. A patient who is failing to improve after learning the basic principles requires careful assessment:

- Is the diagnosis correct?
- Are they effectively and actively practicing all components of treatment?
- Have they developed a comorbid condition that is preventing full participation in treatment, or has such a diagnosis been missed at assessment? Consider especially depression and substance abuse.
- Are concurrent psychosocial stressors causing disruption?
- Are personality factors interfering with treatment? Consider especially self-defeating and passive–aggressive personality styles.

Clinically, these appear to be the most common factors that prevent expected progress and require assessment and formulation of an appropriate course of action.

Social phobia

Patient Treatment Manual*

This Manual is both a guide to treatment and a workbook for people who suffer from social phobia. During treatment, it is a workbook in which individuals can record their own experience of social phobia, together with the additional advice for their particular case given by their clinician. After treatment has concluded, this Manual can serve as a self-help resource when challenges or difficulties are faced.

Contents

*Gavin Andrews, Mark Creamer, Rocco Crino, Caroline Hunt, Lisa Lampe and Andrew Page *The Treatment of Anxiety Disorders* second edition © 2002 Cambridge University Press. All rights reserved.

SECTION 1

Social phobia is a treatable condition. This Manual takes you step by step through a cognitive behavioral program. By working through it you will learn about the nature of social phobia, anxiety, and panic. Not only will you learn skills that will enable you to develop more control over your anxiety, you will also learn to worry less about appearing anxious and about being evaluated.

To learn these skills will require time and effort. To be effective, they will need to be practiced regularly. The more you put in, the more you will get out of the program. However, you are unlikely to be completely cured by the time you reach the last page, or even the last session of your treatment program. To get lasting improvement you need to be prepared to go on working. Research around the world has demonstrated the possibility of long-term achievements, as well as continued improvement.

1 What is social phobia?

Social phobia is a fear of being scrutinized, evaluated, or the center of attention. However, the real underlying fear is of being evaluated *negatively*. People with social phobia commonly fear that others will find fault with them or think that they are incompetent or strange. They may worry that this will occur during social interaction with one or more other people, when they are doing something under observation or even in situations where there is just the chance that they may attract attention. Sometimes, this may involve simply being with others.

The person with social phobia believes that being judged negatively may result from being seen to be anxious (e.g., blushing, sweating, trembling, or shaking), from saying or doing something they think is embarrassing, appearing awkward or making a mistake. Some also believe that there is some aspect of their appearance or behavior that may attract criticism.

Feared situations include public speaking (including tutorials and presentations), parties, writing or signing one's name under scrutiny, standing in a line, using the phone with others around, eating or drinking in public, using public toilets, and public transportation. Some individuals fear that embarrassing bodily functions will occur inappropriately, e.g., losing control of bowel or bladder, passing flatus, vomiting, stomach noises.

The main fears in social phobia may relate more to *performance* situations or more to *social interaction*. There may be great anxiety about looking anxious or even having a panic attack in these situations. The individual may believe that this anxiety will be obvious and will lead others to evaluate them negatively. When social interaction is the main fear, the individual often worries about having nothing to say, being boring, saying something inappropriate or being judged as inadequate in some way. In any case, social situations are either endured with intense anxiety and discomfort (during which panic attacks may occur), or are avoided. Anxiety and avoidance may be linked to only one situation (circumscribed or nongeneralized social phobia), but commonly occur in many situations (generalized social phobia).

The fears in social phobia are excessive and unreasonable. While in the situation, feeling acutely anxious and convinced that things are going badly, it may not seem that the fear is unreasonable. However, most individuals with social phobia realize that their anxiety in social situations is much greater than for those who do not suffer from the disorder. Thinking about things more calmly once out of the situation it is usually possible to accept that the anxiety triggered by the actual circumstances was excessive. More about this later.

1.1 How does social phobia differ from shyness and normal social anxiety?

Many people describe themselves as shy, although there is no clear definition of what this means! Shyness with others, or increased self-consciousness, occurs in phases through childhood. It is common in the teenage years as an individual starts to think about how others might see them. For most people, this type of social anxiety decreases with age.

Some social situations continue to cause a degree of anxiety for most people. Good examples are public speaking, or arriving alone at a social gathering of unfamiliar people. Normal social anxiety is not disabling, it settles quickly during or after the event, and it does not begin weeks before the event. There is less expectation of negative evaluation. Things are different for the person with social phobia. They tend to start worrying a long way in advance, the discomfort may well get worse as they stay in the situation, and next time they may be even more worried. Afterwards they may go over and over aspects of their performance with which they were unhappy. The reasons for this will be discussed in detail in later sections (Sections 4.4 and 5.4). Severe shyness that causes significant avoidance of social interaction or distressing anxiety in social situations is probably social phobia.

1.2 What is avoidant personality disorder?

Individuals with avoidant personality disorder are anxious in almost all types of social interaction. They fear, and expect, not only negative evaluation, but also rejection or humiliation. There is often a sense of inferiority to others, low self-esteem, and considerable avoidance of social interaction. Interestingly, looking anxious is often not the greatest concern of those with the avoidant personality style. These individuals may be far more anxious about how they are relating to others, and fearful that in some way they will be found inadequate or worthless and be rejected. The problem has usually been present since early childhood, and involves deeply ingrained patterns of thinking. Estimates vary greatly as to how common this problem is, but at least a quarter of those with social phobia will also have the avoidant personality style. Avoidant personality styles can be helped by the social phobia program because there is so much overlap between the two disorders.

If you have an avoidant personality, you must be prepared for the fact that it will probably take some time to overcome your problems to a satisfactory degree because they have been present for so long, and to such an extent. In many cases, you will find it helpful to seek ongoing help with your problems after this program finishes. You can discuss this matter further with your therapist.

1.3 How common is social phobia?

Social phobia has been documented across a range of cultures. It is estimated that between 1.5% and 4.5% of the population have social phobia at any time. Slightly more women are affected than men. However, probably more men are affected by avoidant personality disorder. Social phobia usually starts in the teenage years and tends to be a chronic disorder that does not go away spontaneously. Studies consistently indicate that most people have suffered with social phobia for many years before they seek or find appropriate treatment.

1.4 What causes social phobia?

We still don't know for sure what causes social phobia. It seems that the most important factor related to the development of social phobia is a genetic vulnerability to anxiety in general. This is probably largely due to greater sensitivity and reactivity of the nervous system. Some people tend to react more, often with anxiety or nervousness, when faced with any type of external event. These people seem to be more vulnerable to developing anxiety problems. There is also an increased risk of developing social phobia if a close relative has the disorder. It is unusual for social phobia to develop from a specific incident, although this may happen more often in "circumscribed" social phobia (where only one or a few situations cause anxiety). The nature of the family environment of itself does not appear to be an important causative factor in many cases. However, it is possible that aspects of the family environment might influence an underlying sensitivity or shyness in either a helpful way, to enhance confidence and make it easier to socialize, or by reinforcing these concerns.

1.4.1 The effect of personality

Personality refers to habitual ways of thinking about ourselves, our relationships with others and our environment, and the coping strategies we use in these situations. Individuals with social phobia tend to describe themselves as sensitive, emotional, and prone to worry. As we have seen, this does tend to run in families. People who are very sensitive to criticism, or overly concerned about creating a good impression may be more susceptible to social phobia. Some of these attitudes are learned in childhood, but genetic and temperamental factors also influence personality development in ways we do not fully understand.

Hypersensitivity, emotionality, and proneness to worry can be a handicap. You can't radically alter your personality – but nor should you want to! There are advantages to being sensitive: sensitive individuals care about others and can empathize readily, which are valuable characteristics. We can teach people to be less sensitive but it is very hard to teach someone to be more sensitive! Those with social phobia are "people people". What you *can* change about your personality is the *degree* to which you show various traits. This course aims to help you to learn to be less sensitive and less worried about what others think.

1.5 Treatment of social phobia

Cognitive behavior therapy has been shown to result in long-term improvement. It is based on the principle that how we feel about a situation is determined by how we think about it, and the work of Aaron Beck and Albert Ellis. These principles will be discussed in detail later in the Manual. The components of a cognitive behavioral program for social phobia include:

- Knowledge about anxiety and social phobia.
- Control of anxiety and panic.
- Changing unhelpful thinking patterns.
- Involvement in social interaction.

Drug treatments are also available in social phobia but many people will not need medication. When medication is necessary, it is still important to learn cognitive behavioral techniques for managing social phobia, since this appears to give the best long-term result. Your doctor can give you more information.

1.5.1 The aims of this program

What you can expect by the end of this program is for your symptoms to have shown a noticeable degree of improvement. You should have a good understanding of what is required to treat social phobia and be confident that you can continue to apply the principles you have learned with a good expectation of further success. Your therapist can discuss this with you in more detail.

Summary

Social phobia is an excessive, distressing, and often disabling fear of social situations in which a person fears they may say or do something which may lead to embarrassment, humiliation or rejection. Many types of social situations may be feared or avoided. Social phobia is common among both men and women. Cognitive behavior therapy is an effective treatment for social phobia.

SECTION 2

2 The nature of anxiety

Anxiety is part of an automatic response to threat that all animals share. It is known as the flight or fight response. A series of physiological changes is triggered that is designed to give the animal extra strength and speed in order to successfully escape from the threat, or, if trapped, to fight it.

Changes triggered by the flight or fight response
- Increase in alertness.
- Increase in heart rate and blood pressure, to pump extra blood to the muscles.
- Extra blood goes to the skin and sweating increases to help to cool the body.
- Muscles tense ready for action.
- Blood is diverted away from the gastrointestinal system and digestion of recent meals slows down. Any waste products already in the bowel are hurried along.
- Saliva production decreases, causing a dry mouth.
- Breathing rate speeds up. Nostrils and air passages in lungs open wider to get in air more quickly.
- Liver releases sugar to provide quick energy.
- Sphincter muscles contract to close the openings of the bowel and bladder.

This response is produced by the release of various stress hormones, most notably epinephrine (adrenaline), which occurs instantaneously once a threat is perceived. It is designed as an immediate and *brief* response. Once out of danger the hormones that were released are rapidly metabolized (destroyed) by the body and the flight or fight response ceases. Think about the last time you narrowly avoided a collision on the road ... what happened once you knew you were safe? You probably felt pretty shaky for 10 minutes or so, but then almost back to normal.

In animals the flight or fight response is largely instinctual. Humans may also have instinctive fears, e.g., of snakes, heights, or storms. However, animals and humans also *learn* to fear situations. When an individual feels threatened they will become anxious. This anxiety often becomes linked in the individual's mind with the situation in which it occurred.

The flight or fight response is designed to help us to escape from physically threatening situations. The key point, though, is that it is triggered by *perceived threat*. Whilst this threat may be physical (e.g., a near-miss traffic accident or being followed down a dark alley), it can also be more abstract in nature. We may become anxious when we feel the threat of a loss of some type. In social phobia, the threat is the loss of the approval or acceptance of others, or of the individual's social standing. The *actual* likelihood of being disapproved of or rejected may be small. It is the individual's perception of being under threat of negative evaluation that is the key. To some extent the strength of the anxiety response will relate to the perceived likelihood of the consequences that are felt to threaten the individual, and how catastrophic the individual believes these consequences would be.

An anxiety disorder arises when the flight or fight response is being repeatedly triggered at too low a threshold, or by situations that do not actually represent a threat to survival. The flight or fight response occurs as an automatic reaction to perceived threat. It cannot be eliminated. What needs to change is the individual's tendency to interpret situations as threatening.

2.1 What is a panic attack?

Panic means a sudden spell or attack of feeling frightened, anxious or very uneasy. Typically symptoms come on suddenly and escalate in severity over the next 5 to 10 minutes. A panic attack is essentially a severe flight or fight reaction.

During a panic attack the following symptoms may occur:

- Feeling short of breath
- Pounding heart
- Sweating
- Trembling or shaking
- Blushing
- Trembling or croaking voice
- Nausea or a fear of vomiting
- Dizziness or light-headedness
- Tingling fingers or feet

- Tightness or pain in the chest
- A choking or smothering feeling
- Hot or cold flushes
- Feelings of unreality
- A feeling that you cannot get your thoughts together or speak
- An urge to flee
- A fear that you might die
- A fear that you might act in a crazy way

Any or all of these symptoms may occur. Not everyone with social phobia gets panic attacks. Individuals tend to have their own pattern of symptoms in response to anxiety and find some symptoms more distressing or unpleasant than others. In social phobia, blushing, sweating and shaking are often seen as the most troubling symptoms.

When anxiety becomes severe, most people try to escape the situation in order to prevent the feared consequences (the "flight" aspect of the flight or fight response). In other words, if an individual fears that their anxiety will cause them to look odd or say something inappropriate, they will try to escape the situation before this can happen. Once out of the situation, the anxiety usually settles quickly.

Most people rapidly learn to predict the situations in which the anxiety or panic is likely to occur. Some people quickly begin to avoid such situations altogether. Anticipatory anxiety can be a severe problem. Sometimes an individual really intends to go through with a social outing or performance situation but avoids it at the last minute because their anxiety has escalated to the point where they feel totally unable to manage the situation. Avoiding situations that cause anxiety may seem the only alternative to the negative evaluation that it is feared may result if social performance is adversely affected by anxiety.

But what if your performance wasn't as badly affected as you thought? You would lose the opportunity to learn this. Your anxiety would probably start spreading to other types of social situation. Meanwhile, your level of confidence and self-esteem would drop as you found yourself more and more restricted in what you felt you could cope with. Hence, you would become even more anxious about the situations you feared. When social phobia has been present for a long time the individual often structures his or her life around the need to avoid certain situations or expends considerable effort and anxiety planning what to do in case a panic should occur.

This program will teach you how to control your anxiety and panic and how to cope with situations in which anxiety is likely to occur.

Exercise: Make a list of situations in which you would feel very anxious

1. _____

2. _____

3. _____

4. _____

5. _____

2.1.1 The role of hyperventilation

We now turn our attention to one particular aspect of the flight or fight response, namely the increase in rate of respiration, or overbreathing.

Efficient control of the body's energy reactions depends on the maintenance of a specific balance between oxygen and carbon dioxide. This balance can be maintained through an appropriate rate and depth of breathing. The flight or fight response triggers an increase in the rate of breathing in preparation for taking flight. When this response is triggered by a social situation, you are unlikely to respond by running away – at least, not literally! The increase in oxygen intake is not matched by an increase in carbon dioxide production and an imbalance results.

Hyperventilation is defined as a rate and depth of breathing that is too much for the body's needs at a particular point in time. The imbalance that results can cause many physical symptoms, including:

- Dizziness
- Light-headedness
- Confusion
- Breathlessness
- Blurred vision
- Feelings of unreality
- Numbness and tingling in the extremities
- Cold, clammy hands
- Stiffness in the muscles (including the muscles of the chest, which can lead to a sensation of chest pain or tightness)

Hyperventilation also causes a heightened sense of anxiety, which in turn makes it increasingly difficult to think objectively. It may also be a factor in the experience of constant anxiety and edginess that some people describe.

You can demonstrate for yourself how an increase in breathing can affect the way you feel by deliberately overbreathing until you experience symptoms of overbreathing such as feeling dizzy and light-headed. Note that symptoms rapidly settle once you allow your breathing to return to normal.

2.1.2 Recognizing hyperventilation

One way to determine whether you are overbreathing is to count the number of breaths you take in a minute.

Exercise: Try monitoring your breathing rate now

For one minute (timed), count one breath in and out as 1, the next breath in and out as 2, and so on. It may be difficult at first, but don't try to change your breathing rate.

Time yourself for 1 minute and write the answer here ____.

If your rate was over 12 breaths per minute then you are probably hyperventilating.

A technique for controlling hyperventilation is described in Section 3.

2.2 What other factors contribute to anxiety?

Many individuals report an almost constant sense of anxiety, edginess or dread. There can be several reasons for this. One is chronic overbreathing as mentioned above. But many lifestyle factors also contribute to high levels of tension and anxiety.

Consider the following:

- *Are you feeling stressed or worried about something?* Are there situations in your life that are causing chronic unhappiness or anxiety? Can anything be done to improve the situation? If you don't know where to start, talk to your therapist about a structured problem solving approach.

- *Are you smoking too much or drinking too much tea or coffee?* Tobacco, tea, and coffee are all stimulants that increase your basic level of tension or arousal and accelerate the flight or fight response. Some individuals are particularly sensitive to caffeine.

- *Are you drinking too much alcohol?* Although alcohol has immediate anxiety-relieving properties that can make it seem attractive, when consumed in excess it has toxic effects on many organs, including the liver, heart, stomach, nerves and brain. Under the influence of alcohol you won't be yourself. You also won't be learning anything that will help you manage better in the future or to cope in situations where you can't drink. You will also tend to feel even more sensitive and prone to anxiety "the day after".

- *Are you using marijuana?* Many people believe that marijuana helps them relax. However, many also find that after the acute relaxation stage they find themselves feeling more sensitive than usual to others, and hence their anxiety levels rise. Again, you're not yourself, and you're not learning anything.

- *Are you getting insufficient sleep?* Excessive tiredness can reduce your coping reserves and predispose you to anxiety.
- *Do you have trouble being assertive?* Many people with social phobia have trouble getting their own needs met. Many have difficulty saying "No" to the requests and demands of others. This may leave the person feeling stressed and out of time for their own needs as well as resentful towards others for making these demands. Learning to be assertive will help to reduce your tension. This topic will be looked at in more detail later in the program.
- *Are you overly conscientious, working too hard or too fast, or trying to be perfect?* You will achieve more by staying calm and working at a reasonable pace. Have fair and reasonable expectations of yourself.
- *Are you getting regular exercise?* Exercise helps anxiety in several ways. In addition to its well-known physical benefits it also leads to better-quality sleep so you feel more rested. It improves mood and outlook. It also helps to reduce levels of tension and anxiety. You probably need to exercise at least every other day in sessions lasting 30 minutes or more in order to get most benefit.

It is impossible to eliminate stress altogether. Rather, the aim is to develop the best possible coping strategies and the confidence to use them in order to minimize the amount of stress and anxiety triggered by demanding situations. It is also important to reduce hypersensitivity and the tendency to misinterpret situations as more threatening than they really are.

Anxiety reduction will be most successful when an attempt is made to address all sources of stress and anxiety and introduce effective anxiety management strategies as a way of life.

2.3 The relationship of anxiety to performance

People who fear the consequences of anxiety become afraid of even small amounts of anxiety in case it escalates out of control. But anxiety can be useful. In the event of real danger the flight or fight response may save your life one day. The relationship between anxiety and performance is surprising. What would you predict it would be?

When this was first studied in a research experiment the researchers did not expect the results they found. In fact, the relationship between anxiety and performance was found to be as shown in the diagram.

Several important points arise from studying this diagram. First, it can be seen that an average performance can be obtained at two different levels of anxiety. A person who is reasonably calm will perform averagely well, as will a person who is very tense. However, should extra demands be placed on the reasonably calm

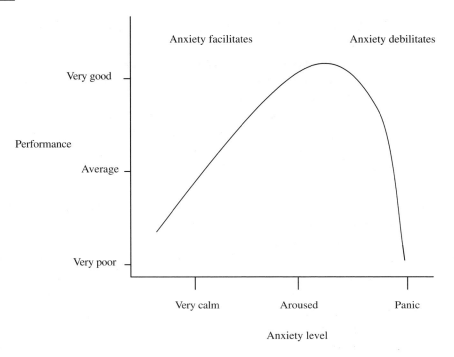

person, there is a wide margin for anxiety to increase without performance deteriorating. On the other hand, for the person who is already very tense, a further increase in anxiety is likely to result in deterioration of performance. But note that such deterioration does not occur until *very high* anxiety levels have been reached.

Ideally, then, we should aim for calmness as we go about our daily business. In this way, we will have larger coping reserves for times when we have to face stressful situations. Regular practice of a relaxation technique can help to achieve this.

Remember, however, that without some increase in tension or anxiety you will not do your best. Note, from the diagram, that the best performances come at higher levels of anxiety than those that produce average performances. The increase in mental alertness and ability to focus that anxiety produces is actually essential to achieving our best level of performance. You can probably think back to some situations in your own life where this was the case … Would you have done so well in a certain interview or in examination situations, for example, if you had not been more anxious than usual? This program does not aim to eliminate anxiety from your life. Rather, the aim is to learn to control unwarranted anxiety, and not get worried about appropriate and reasonable levels of anxiety.

Summary

Anxiety results when the flight or fight response is triggered by feeling threatened in some way. In social phobia, anxiety results when the fear of being negatively evaluated in a social situation triggers the flight or fight response. Hyperventilation occurring as part of the response can make symptoms worse but responds readily to controlled breathing. Moderate levels of anxiety actually enhance performance. It is probably best to aim to keep everyday levels of anxiety low by paying attention to lifestyle factors so that when faced with a demanding situation the resulting increase in anxiety will not be overwhelming.

SECTION 3

3 Anxiety-management strategies

Section 2 discussed the nature of anxiety and panic, and the situational and lifestyle factors that can contribute to generally heightened levels of stress and anxiety. By paying attention to these factors you can help to reduce your level of *arousal* – the degree of tension and alertness you feel – when this is excessive for your needs and your health.

Specific anxiety management strategies include:
- Hyperventilation control.
- Relaxation training.

3.1 Slow-breathing technique

It is known that even a slightly elevated rate or depth of breathing beyond what is required in the circumstances can contribute to feelings of anxiety. Many individuals do not have obvious hyperventilation, and currently it is not thought to play a major role in the anxiety experienced by most people with social phobia. It is more likely to be of importance if you noted an elevated breathing rate in the exercise above, or if you do actually suffer panic attacks.

The slow-breathing technique can be used as the foundation of your anxiety-management strategies, helping to calm you down so that you can think more clearly and apply the "straight thinking" strategies you will learn in the next part of the program. It can also be a useful strategy to shift your focus away from your anxious concerns, and many people over the years have found the technique helpful for these reasons. The best approach is to use the technique at the first signs of anxiety.

The slow-breathing technique will give you a breathing rate of 10 breaths per minute. It is best to use a watch in practice sessions initially to make sure that you get the feel for the right timing – when we feel anxious there is a tendency for us to feel a bit "speedy" and want to do everything too fast! Concentrate on making your breaths smooth and light. Breathe through your nose to help limit the amount of air you take in and thus prevent overbreathing. It should feel as though the air is just drifting lightly past your nostrils. Relax your stomach muscles. The breathing movement is so light that it is unnoticeable from normal breathing to anyone who may be watching. Ready? Now do the following:

Slow-breathing technique

1. Take a medium sized breath in, hold it and count to 6 (timing 6 seconds with your watch).
2. When you get to 6, think "relax" and breathe out. Try and feel as though you are releasing tension as you breathe out.
3. Next breathe in for 3 seconds and out for 3 seconds, in a smooth and light way.
4. At the end of each minute (after 10 breaths) hold your breath again for 6 seconds, think "relax", breathe out, and then continue breathing in the 6-second cycle for another minute.

Continue breathing in this way until you are feeling calmer. Sometimes, you will notice that symptoms of anxiety return after a short while. That's okay, just do your controlled breathing again for as long as it takes to settle. It is probably because you are still having anxious thoughts about the situation. As you develop your straight-thinking skills this should become less of a problem.

If you find it hard to do this in the anxiety-provoking situation, consider the possibility of taking "time out" to calm yourself. For example, at a party you might slip out to a quiet spot for a short time and do your breathing, then return to the party. With practice, you will find it easier to control breathing while you are actually in the situation.

3.1.1 Daily record of breathing rate

Instructions

It is important to practice this technique until you are able to use it automatically in anxiety-provoking situations. For the next 3 weeks at least it is recommended that you practice this slow-breathing technique for about 5 minutes at a time, four times a day. There are two reasons for this. The first is that frequent and regular practice will make the technique second nature to you. It will thus be more likely that you use it even when your mind is clouded by anxiety! The second reason is that regular practice will have the result that this healthy breathing style becomes your natural breathing rate and style. The chart on p. 212 is for you to record your breathing rates before and after each practice session.

Daily record of breathing rate

Date	Time 1		Time 2		Time 3		Time 4	
	Before	After	Before	After	Before	After	Before	After

Choose four convenient times spread through the day to monitor your breathing and do the practice. Wait for 20 minutes or so after any strenuous activity. Time yourself for a minute before you do your practice, without trying to modify your breathing rate. Then do your practice. After your practice, time your breathing rate for a minute, again without consciously trying to change your breathing. Your therapist will be able to use your records to monitor your progress. You may also learn more about your own patterns of anxiety and overbreathing from studying your chart.

Some people worry about the fact that counting their breathing rate makes them too conscious of it, and alters it somehow. This is probably true to a small extent, but not enough to really matter.

3.1.2 Problems with breathing control: troubleshooting

A small number of individuals report that they get symptoms of anxiety when they first start breathing retraining. This may happen as you become more aware of times when you are anxious as part of this program, which requires you to confront your anxiety rather than trying to avoid it. Most people find that if they persevere with the breathing practice it does begin to have a calming influence.

Other people report that when they first begin to practice this slow-breathing technique it feels unnatural. This is only to be expected if you have been habitually breathing at a higher rate, too deeply or too shallowly, or in some irregular fashion. As you practice the slow-breathing technique it will come to feel not only more natural, but also more comfortable.

Don't become too focused on your breathing. It's just one of the building blocks in your anxiety-management program. Do your practices, use it when you're anxious, and forget about it the rest of the time!

3.2 Relaxation training – progressive muscular relaxation

Progressive muscular relaxation is a specific technique for releasing tension from muscles. It is best seen as a skill which requires practice to master. The potential benefits include reduced feelings of overall tension, as well as the ability to better control acute rises in anxiety, especially with the technique of "applied relaxation". Applied relaxation is a follow-on skill to progressive muscular relaxation, which aims to provide a portable strategy that can be used in any situation to quickly reduce feelings of tension and anxiety. It has been shown to be useful in a number of anxiety disorders. Recommended reading for applied relaxation is included in Section 8 at the end of the Manual. It may also be possible to purchase audio tapes containing instructions for progressive muscular relaxation, and this is often a good way to start learning the technique.

Summary

The slow-breathing technique and the skill of applied relaxation can help to reduce acute symptoms of anxiety. Progressive muscular relaxation can help to reduce the overall level of arousal with frequent practice. Other strategies to help to reduce arousal levels include regular exercise, sufficient sleep, and reducing sources of stress and anxiety in the work and home environment.

SECTION 4

4 Cognitive therapy for social phobia

People with social phobia experience anxiety in the company of others. However, there are marked variations between individuals in terms of the degree of anxiety that is experienced, and the number and types of situations that provoke anxiety. In order to overcome social phobia it is important to develop an understanding of the general sorts of underlying thoughts and anxieties in this condition, and *your* specific thoughts and fears in particular. It will then become clearer to you why you are anxious in particular situations, and how you can begin to overcome your fears. We refer to these underlying thoughts as "cognitions", and learning to deal with them constructively is the "cognitive" part of the program, often referred to as "cognitive restructuring".

4.1 Cognitive therapy: the importance of the way you think

It may seem surprising, but no outside situation or event can directly cause feelings of distress. What does cause us to become upset? The answer is: it's our point of view!

Consider the following example. Three people are waiting at a bus stop. They see the bus approaching, hail the bus, and the bus just drives straight past without stopping. The first person in line begins to jump up and down waving her fists in the air and shouting: she seems angry. The second person in line bursts into tears, appearing distressed. The third person in line begins to laugh very heartily, seeming amused. Now, the same thing has happened to all of them, yet there were three different reactions. Clearly, it is not the event that caused the reactions. So what was it? To know why each person reacted as they did, we have to know what they were thinking. It turns out that the first person was thinking to herself, "How dare the driver go right past! I'm going to be late for an important meeting." Hence, she feels angry. The second person woke up feeling a bit blue that morning. When the bus goes past he thinks, "Oh no. Nothing is going to go right today, I feel so miserable." The third person thinks, "Hooray! The next bus is not for half an hour. I have a completely legitimate excuse to be late. I think I'll go have a cup of coffee."

A basic principle of cognitive therapy is that it is the interpretations we make of situations that determine our emotional response. These interpretations are influenced by our previous experiences of similar situations and by aspects of personality, including our general sensitivity, our feelings about ourselves and our relationships with others, and our worldview. Of course, some events may realistically be unpleasant, or situations uncomfortable, but they are rarely, of themselves, capable of causing us to feel extreme levels of anxiety, fear, depression, worthlessness, inferiority, anger, etc.

Hence, if you find yourself frequently feeling very anxious, angry or unhappy, it is likely that you may be making unhelpful or unrealistic interpretations of events or situations in which you find yourself. People tend to develop patterns of thinking about particular types of situation. One of the aims of cognitive therapy is to examine the ways in which we are thinking about ourselves and our world. If we identify some habitual unhelpful or unrealistic patterns of thinking about certain types of situations, the next goal is to identify more helpful ways of thinking about such situations. The ultimate goal is to create new habits of appraising situations that make our lives easier and happier. This will take a great deal of active practice.

4.2 Specific anxieties in social phobia

The predominant emotion in social phobia is anxiety. As we have seen, anxiety occurs in response to a perceived threat through activation of the flight or fight response. While this response developed in animals as an emergency response to physical danger, in humans it can also be triggered by the threat of some type of loss. It may be that a fear of losing our social standing with others may trigger the anxiety of social phobia. It may also relate to some deep-seated need to be accepted by others that could date from prehistoric times when an individual's survival in a harsh and dangerous environment depended on acceptance by the tribe. In any case, it is now clear that the anxiety in social phobia is triggered by a fear of being negatively evaluated. Underlying this is an excessive concern about the opinions of others.

You can compare your degree of concern about what others may think of you with the general population by completing the following questionnaire, developed by Watson and Friend.

FNE scales

In each case indicate whether or not the statement applies to you by writing either T for true or F for false. Please be sure to answer all the statements.

1. ____ I rarely worry about seeming foolish to others.
2. ____ I worry about what people will think of me even when I know it doesn't make any difference.
3. ____ I become tense and jittery if I know someone is sizing me up.
4. ____ I am unconcerned even if I know people are forming an unfavorable impression of me.
5. ____ I feel very upset when I commit some social error.
6. ____ The opinions that important people have of me cause me little concern.
7. ____ I am often afraid that I may look ridiculous or make a fool of myself.
8. ____ I react very little when other people disapprove of me.
9. ____ I am frequently afraid of other people noticing my shortcomings.
10. ____ The disapproval of others would have little effect on me.
11. ____ If someone is evaluating me, I tend to expect the worst.
12. ____ I rarely worry about what kind of impression I am making on someone.
13. ____ I am afraid that others will not approve of me.
14. ____ I am afraid that people will find fault with me.
15. ____ Other people's opinions of me do not bother me.
16. ____ I am not necessarily upset if I do not please someone.
17. ____ When I am talking to someone, I worry about what they may be thinking about me.
18. ____ I feel that you cannot help making social errors sometimes, so why worry about it.
19. ____ I am usually worried about what kind of impression I make.
20. ____ I worry a lot about what my superiors think of me.
21. ____ If I know someone is judging me, it has little effect on me.
22. ____ I worry that others will think I am not worthwhile.
23. ____ I worry very little about what others may think of me.
24. ____ Sometimes I think I am too concerned with what other people think of me.
25. ____ I often worry that I will say or do the wrong things.
26. ____ I am often indifferent to the opinion others have of me.
27. ____ I am usually confident that others will have a favorable impression of me.
28. ____ I often worry that people who are important to me will not think very much of me.
29. ____ I brood about the opinions my friends have about me.
30. ____ I become tense and jittery if I know I am being judged by my superiors.

Score this questionnaire by giving yourself one point if you said "True" to numbers 2, 3, 5, 7, 9, 11, 13, 14, 17, 19, 20, 22, 24, 25, 28, 29, 30. Score one point if you said "False" to 1, 4, 6, 8, 10, 12, 15, 16, 18, 21, 23, 26, 27. Your score gives an indication of how concerned you are to get the approval of others in your life. Approximately 75% of people in the general population score less than 19 on this scale. Scores higher than this indicate a level of over concern about others' opinions of you that is likely to cause distress – and result in anxiety in social situations.

That's not to say that others don't get any social anxiety. They do. Everyone would like to think that they are accepted and approved of by others they come in contact with. We all know the feeling of embarrassment when we make a silly mistake, say something inappropriate or draw attention to ourselves in an unflattering, and usually accidental, way. However, there are several differences between *normal social anxiety* and social phobia.

Normal social anxiety	Social phobia
Moderate desire for approval	Strong desire or perceived *need* for approval
Expectation of approval	Expectation of negataive evaluation
Reasonable tolerance for disapproval	Extremely distressed by disapproval
Easily forgets about social mistakes	Dwells on social mistakes, very upset by them
When in doubt interprets response as positive	When in doubt interprets reaction as critical

So, it is the fear of negative evaluation that is the core of the problem, but it is compounded by unrealistic beliefs about:

- How bad you think negative evaluation is, and what you believe the consequences will be for you.
- How likely you think it is that you will be evaluated negatively.

This explains why some people who show the apparent signs of anxiety that worry you – who blush or tremble, sweat or shake, appear lost for words or stumble over what they are saying – do *not* appear to worry about it. Indeed, many of the people we have treated in the past have commented that they have encountered people who did what they themselves feared without worrying about it, e.g., the person who shook when writing, yet seemed unconcerned, and certainly had not developed a fear of writing. Furthermore, most of our program participants report that they do not think any less of the person for showing these "embarrassing" behaviors. Nor do they feel that other observers at the time were critical of the person. It often seems that individuals with social phobia have one set of "rules" or standards for themselves – a very harsh and strict set – that they don't apply to others in their lives. This is despite the fact that they expect others to apply these rules to them.

Sometimes, though, people with social phobia apply the same unreasonable standards they have for themselves to everyone. Thus you may find yourself feeling sorry for someone who looks anxious or makes a mistake, or you may even judge them critically. It can come as a surprise to learn that others don't care nearly as much as you do about what others think of them, and probably wouldn't be overconcerned even if they knew you were critical of them! (But don't worry, they can't read your mind!) The range of behavior that is seen as acceptable and normal in social situations is almost certainly broader than you currently believe.

Common personal beliefs in social phobia	Common beliefs about what others think
"I have to appear competent!" "That person seems inept or silly."	"What a fool." "I must be entertaining or I'll be seen as a failure."
"If they see my anxiety, they will think me weak."	"What's wrong with them?"
"If I have nothing to say it will be a catastrophe."	"She seems a bit odd."
"They will start to dislike me."	"He can't control himself."

How does all this tie together with the material we have covered in previous sections, including your individual symptoms of anxiety and your own experience of what situations seem to trigger your symptoms? The diagram opposite is one model of social phobia that links all these elements.

As part of this program, we are going to examine the way you think about yourself and others. It is likely that you have some unrealistic and therefore unhelpful beliefs, and we now know that these are especially likely to revolve around the theme of negative evaluation from others. The aim of the program will be to reshape these views; to make them realistic and helpful to you in your daily life. We call this "cognitive restructuring" – or learning how to think realistically. Remember, however, that we are not aiming to eliminate all anxiety from your life, since there are times when such a reaction is perfectly reasonable, and helpful. Rather, we are aiming to reduce as much as possible unnecessary or extreme degrees of anxiety. We are also aiming to help you to learn to feel more comfortable with normal social anxiety.

The following sections will take you through a step-by-step, practical approach to making this happen.

COGNITIVE BEHAVIORAL MODEL OF SOCIAL PHOBIA

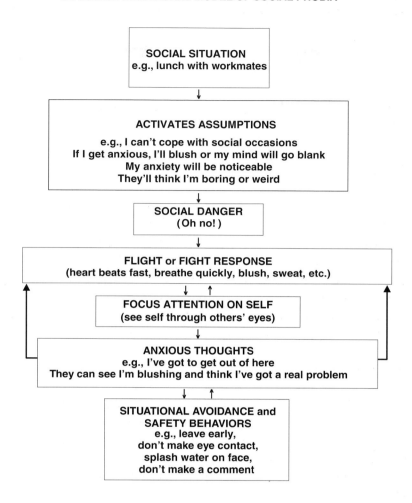

4.3 The ABCs of realistic thinking

The following boxes summarize what has been discussed previously.

A		C
The Activating event or Action	is presumed to lead to	The Consequences: your feelings and behavior
The bus not stopping for you	is presumed to lead to	*feeling angry, depressed, anxious or happy*

But thoughts intervene between A and C and thus the true association is:

A		B		C
The **Activating** event or **Action**	leads to	Your **Beliefs**, thoughts or interpretations	which results in	The **Consequences**: your feelings and behavior
The bus not stopping for you	*leads to*	*"I'll be late for an important meeting"* *or* *"Nothing goes right for me"* *or* *"This is a good thing to happen"*	*which results in*	*Feeling angry, or depressed or happy*

If you habitually tend to expect the worst, overreact when things don't go well, and worry too much about what others think, you will start to feel better if you can change these patterns!

4.4 Cognitive restructuring: changing the way you think

This will take some practice. It is best approached in a series of steps.

Changing the way you think

1. Learning to identify the thoughts that go through your head in response to events, and the interpretations you make of events and situations.
2. Learning how to look at each of these thoughts objectively, and decide whether they represent reasonable assessments of the situation (challenge them).
3. Restating any unrealistic or unhelpful thoughts in a way that better reflects the reality of the situation and is more helpful to you.
4. Putting the more helpful beliefs into practice by basing your behavior on them.

4.4.1 Step 1: Identify your thoughts

It is not easy at first to determine what you are thinking about any given situation. One reason for this is that many of our thoughts occur almost automatically in response to frequently encountered situations. For this reason they are sometimes referred to as "automatic" thoughts. Anxious individuals also develop habitual ways of thinking about the situations that worry them.

The following features are characteristic of habitual unrealistic thoughts. They are:

Automatic: They just pop into your head without any effort on your part.

Distorted: They do not fit all of the facts.

Unhelpful: They keep you anxious, make it difficult to change, and stop you from getting what you want out of life.

Involuntary: You do not choose to have them, and they can be very difficult to switch off.

Our appraisals of events and situations are made at lightning speed, and this is another reason why we are usually unaware of them and why, initially, they can be difficult to track down. But many people using these methods have demonstrated that it can be done. With sufficient practice it will begin to come naturally to you.

One way to get started is to use any feelings of anxiety, fear, or discomfort and work backwards. That is, if you feel uncomfortable, then there must be some underlying thought that caused the feeling. In any situation or interaction in which you find yourself unhappy with your feelings or actions, ask yourself:

- How do I feel?
- What has been happening recently?
- What do I think about myself?
- What do I think about the other person?
- What do I think about the situation?

To help you determine what you were thinking, you can also try asking yourself, "What could I just hear?" or "What might I have been worrying about?". With time, you will probably find that you have a small collection of particularly troublesome thoughts that occur in many situations. Once you know about these, you can have a high index of suspicion that they are also causing trouble in your current situation, and be sure to listen for them.

To practice this first step, think about a recent situation where you found yourself feeling more anxious or upset than you think was reasonable. In your workbook write down the situation which triggered the anxiety, think back to how you felt emotionally, then see whether you can work back to identify what might have gone through your head at the time. An example looks something like this.

A Activating event or situation	B Beliefs/interpretations	C Consequences: Emotional state and SUDs rating
Running into a colleague from work in the street at the weekend	I have to say something I don't know what to say I'll look awkward and uncomfortable They will wonder why I am looking so strange and . . . They will think less of me and might tell others at work who will laugh at me	Anxiety 80 (Ducked quickly into a shop to escape)

The "SUDs" rating is a way for you to estimate how strong or unpleasant the emotions that you experienced felt to you. "SUDs" stands for **S**ubjective **U**nits of **D**istress. You estimate the strength of the emotion according to the following scale:

x--------------------x---------------x-----------------------x---------------x				
0	30	50	80	100
Nil	Mild	Moderate	Severe	Worst ever

Keeping a diary in your workbook can help you to become aware of thoughts, or cognitions, that you get in particular situations, so that you can begin to see patterns emerging in the types of thought that are causing you to feel anxious and uncomfortable. It is important to record your challenges to these cognitions in your diary or workbook, too.

4.4.2 Step 2: Challenge your thoughts

You will now challenge your thoughts to meet the requirements of being helpful and realistic. In this step it is important to subject the beliefs and interpretations that you identified above to critical examination. Are your interpretations logical? Are they supported by the facts? If not, then you should not accept them as a true and accurate representation of the situation. You can ask yourself the following questions to help you challenge your thoughts:

- *What is the evidence?* Do the facts of the situation back up what you think, or do they contradict it? Imagine that you are presenting this evidence in a court of law: would it stand up to cross-examination? Would others probably make the same interpretation? It is important to be realistic about whether people really are looking at you, talking about you, judging what you do. You may be so anxious that you do not correctly interpret what is happening around you. Hence it takes a conscious effort to make interpretations of the environment, and your own performance, that are as objective as possible.
- *What alternative views are there?* There are many different ways to look at any experience. How else could you interpret what has happened? Think of as many alternatives as you can, and review the evidence for and against them. When you consider it objectively, which alternative is most likely to be correct?
- *How likely is it?* How likely is it really that what you fear will happen?
- *How much would it really matter?* If the thing you fear did happen, how much would it *really matter* in your life? Would it really be the worst thing you could ever imagine happening? Would it have to affect the rest of your life? Could you live with it? Be objective and realistic.

- *Are you making "errors" of thinking?* People with social phobia typically develop habitual patterns of interpreting information about their social environment. They may distort how they see their experiences in systematic ways. We call these "cognitive errors" or "cognitive biases". We now believe that these are very important in maintaining anxieties in social phobia. We also believe that they explain why, despite showing great courage and perseverance in "forcing" themselves to confront feared situations, many people only find things getting harder.

  Some of these types of cognitive biases have been given names to help you to remember them so that you can check for them in your own thinking. Particularly prominent are "mind reading", "fortune telling", "mental filtering", and "discounting". Which of these errors can you find in your own thinking?

Cognitive "errors"
All-or-none thinking

You see things in black-and-white categories. For example, because you felt uncomfortable at one stage during a dinner party you decide that the whole experience was a bad one. Or you think, "I made a mistake on that ... the whole job is ruined".

Overgeneralization

You see a single event as a never-ending pattern. For example, "I didn't handle that meeting very well ... I never cope in meetings".

Mental filter (focusing on the negative)

You pick out a single detail and dwell on it exclusively, or make unwarranted conclusions. For example, while talking to someone, you are momentarily at a loss for words at one point. Looking back on the whole experience, you think "I had nothing to say".

Discounting or disqualifying the positive

You reject successful experiences by insisting they don't count for some reason or another. In this way, you can maintain a negative belief that is contradicted by your everyday experiences. For example, you manage to take the bus all the way to work, but discount it by saying "It wasn't really full today, so it doesn't really count". Or you discount your achievements by saying something like "Even a baby could do that".

Jumping to conclusions

You make a negative interpretation even though there are no definite facts that convincingly support your conclusion. For example, after not receiving a promised phone call from a friend, you conclude "They don't really care about me".

Mind reading

You automatically assume that you know that someone is thinking negatively about you and you don't bother to check this out with them. "They thought I was boring ... I could just tell."

The fortune teller error

You anticipate that things will turn out badly, and you feel convinced that your prediction is an already established fact. For example, you worry about a presentation you have to give and think "I know I will make a fool of myself and they all will laugh".

Catastrophizing

You exaggerate the importance of your mistakes or someone else's achievements. You expect the very worst and tell yourself that things are extremely bad. "It was awful." "I can't stand it."

Emotional reasoning

You assume that your negative emotions necessarily reflect the way things really are: "I feel bad, so things must be going badly"; "I feel anxious so it must be obvious to others."

"Should" statements

You try to motivate yourself with shoulds, musts, and oughts. If you find yourself unable to do something, you then feel guilty and demoralized; for example, "I should be able to understand this the first time that I read it". If you direct these should statements towards others you feel anger, resentment, and frustration; for example, "They should have known how I was feeling".

Personalization and "omnipotence"

You see yourself as the cause of some negative external event, or as the center of attention. For example, you think "I always bring bad luck", or "Everyone was looking at me", or "I made them uncomfortable". Remember that just as you are responsible for your own thoughts and feelings, so are others responsible for themselves. You can't make anyone think or feel anything.

It is important to be realistic about how much attention people are paying to you, and how likely it is that you will be judged harshly. By and large, people who don't know you don't care about you and don't think about your behavior. They are much more interested in their own lives – the fight they had last night, the new car they just bought.

People who do know you would have already made up their minds about you. They are not going to make the extreme shifts in their opinions of you that you expect them to. They might think that you seem a bit stressed today. They *might* think of you as being a tense person, or even a nervous type, maybe even that you're shy – but that is about all they are going to think, and does it really matter? What things are most important to you in how you would like others to think of you? It is also important to be realistic about how much you need to have the approval of others.

A Activating event or situation	B Beliefs and interpretations	C Consequences	D Dispute (challenge) beliefs: record realistic thoughts
Drinking coffee in front of people at the railway café	Oh no! What if I shake and spill the coffee They will see me shaking and . . . They will think I am mad or crazy They won't like me and . . . They'll move or turn away They might even talk about me That would be awful because I can't stand to appear conspicuous, or tense, or nervous, because that means that I'm a failure as a person		I probably won't, as I usually cope okay They may, but they probably won't even notice me They probably wouldn't think anything of it Even if they did, it would probably be that I'm a bit tense They probably won't think that I'm mad or crazy – they might think I'm upset or physically ill They probably won't talk about me as they have much more interesting things on their minds
		Sadness 60/100 Anxiety 80/100	Sadness 0/100 Anxiety 45/100

4.4.3 Practice example

Write down an example of a situation where you may have overreacted. Choose some situation in which you recently felt panicky or uncomfortable. To begin with, choose a situation that was only mildly upsetting. As you become more familiar with the technique, you can work on situations that cause high anxiety. Record the details of this situation in the "A" column. It can be helpful to go next to the "C" column and write down how you felt about this situation at the time. For example, you may have felt anxious. You may also have felt disappointed, frustrated or angry. Write down all the emotions you can recall, and then give *each* emotion a SUDs rating to reflect how strongly you experienced it at the time. Next, try to recall what you were thinking, or would probably have been thinking, in that situation, and record these thoughts in the "B" column. Try to be as inclusive as you can – that is, try to catch *everything* that might have gone through your mind about the situation. If you are successful you will find that there is at least one thought that matches each emotion in an understandable way. In the fourth column, write down your realistic challenges to each thought. Rate the amount of anxiety you would experience if you were thinking in this more helpful and realistic way about the situation. Re-rate any other emotions you identified, too.

A Activating event or situation	B Beliefs and interpretations	C Consequences: emotions & SUDs	D Dispute (challenge) beliefs: record realistic thoughts
		Anxiety /100	

Realistic thinking does not reject all negative thoughts and it is not simply positive thinking. It is looking at yourself and your environment in a realistic way, a way that maximizes the chances of successful coping. It is important to distinguish realistic thinking from irrationally positive, or wishful, thinking.

Some examples of the difference between unrealistic, wishful, and realistic thinking are shown below. In each case, try to identify the type of cognitive distortion involved in the irrational thoughts.

Unrealistic thinking
"I didn't get the job, which proves that I am a failure. I'll never get a job or have things go right for me."

Wishful thinking
"I didn't want the job anyway."

Realistic thinking
"I am disappointed I didn't get that job, but I can cope."

Unrealistic thinking

"What if I can't cope with this? It will be absolutely disastrous."

Wishful thinking

"It'll be easy."

Realistic thinking

"I'll probably be able to cope. It doesn't have to be perfect: I'll give it my best shot."

It is often difficult to tell the difference between various forms of thinking. Here are some clues to what you might be saying:

Unhelpful or unrealistic thinking:

"I must..."
"I've got to..."
"What if... that would be awful/unbearable."
"I couldn't stand it if..."

Wishful thinking:

"It'll work out..."
"I don't care that..."
"It wouldn't have done any good anyway."
"I'll will it to happen."

Realistic and helpful thinking ("straight thinking"):

"I would like very much to..."
"I'd prefer not to..."
"I will do everything I can to..."
"If things don't go the way I want, I might be disappointed but I don't have to become overanxious or depressed."

4.5 Common problems challenging negative thoughts: troubleshooting

- *"I don't seem to have any thoughts."* If at first you find it difficult to pin down what you are thinking, ask yourself "What might I have been thinking about a situation like this?", "What would I be worried about?". If you can't identify your thoughts while you are in the situation, think about it immediately afterwards, once you are calmer. With practice, you will be able to identify and challenge your thoughts even when you are in a difficult situation.
- *"I can't think of any alternatives."* Standing back, questioning, evaluating, and challenging our thoughts is not something we normally do. You may well find it difficult at first to be objective and to find answers that affect your feelings to any great extent. Do not be discouraged if at first you cannot always find effective challenges. Would you expect to win the Wimbledon tournament after six tennis lessons?

- *"I don't really believe the realistic thought."* You don't have to be convinced. Treat the realistic thought as a hypothesis to be tested. Then act *as if* it's true, and see what happens. For example, to test the hypothesis that you are always the center of attention, try going for a walk down a busy street. As you pass people, glance at them to briefly make eye contact. What do you notice?
- *"I still feel anxious."* This feeling relates to the problem above. Since you don't yet fully believe that nothing terrible is likely to happen, you will not be free from anxiety. However, you know that you can cope despite feeling anxious, you know that some anxiety is a normal part of life, and as you collect evidence to support your rational views of social interaction you will believe these more and therefore gradually feel less anxious. Your graded exposure program is particularly helpful in this regard.

Do not get discouraged if you find the same thoughts occurring again and again. If you have been anxious for some time, these thought patterns have become a well-established habit. It will take time to break it. The more often a particular thought occurs, the more opportunity you will have to challenge and change it.

"Ten irrational ideas"

The following is based on Albert Ellis' work on rational emotive therapy and his book, *A New Guide to Rational Living* 1979; (see Section 8.1).

It is irrational to think that:
- You must have love or approval from all the people you find significant.
- You must prove yourself thoroughly competent and have talent at something important.
- You have to view life as awful, catastrophic, or depressing when things don't go the way that you want.
- People who harm you or do misdeeds are bad or villains and you should blame, damn, and punish them.
- If something makes you anxious, you should become terribly preoccupied with it and upset about it.
- People and things should turn out better than they do – if they don't, you have to view it as awful.
- Emotional misery comes from outside conditions and you have little ability to control your feelings and get rid of anxiety, hostility, and depression.
- You will find it easier to avoid facing difficulties and situations than to undertake rewarding forms of behavior that involve self-discipline.
- Your past is all-important, and because something affected you once it has to keep on determining your feelings and behavior.
- You can achieve happiness by being passive and uncommitted.

You may feel as though you disagree with some of these statements – it is often very helpful to discuss them with your therapist.

Do not expect your belief in the negative thoughts to disappear completely, all at once. They have probably been around for a long time, whereas the alternative thoughts may be quite new to you. It will take time and practice to build up belief in them, and you will need to test them out in action.

Summary:

Identifying and challenging unrealistic thoughts about situations and events is a key element in overcoming social phobia. By consistently challenging unrealistic beliefs and testing realistic beliefs in real life situations (through graded exposure), you will gradually develop habitually realistic and helpful ways of thinking about things.

SECTION 5

5 Graded exposure

Ultimately, a phobia can be overcome only when an individual confronts his or her fears. This is called "exposure" to the feared situation. The most commonly used technique is to start by confronting the *least* anxiety-provoking situations. As confidence grows, increasingly more difficult situations are tackled. This process is known as "graded exposure" and research has shown that it is a powerfully effective technique in overcoming phobias. The aim of this section is to help you to formulate a plan for confronting your fears that will be both tolerable in terms of the anxiety it causes you and effective in helping you to overcome your social phobia.

5.1 Why is exposure necessary?

In the section 2 of this Manual we discussed the development of situational fears; that is, fears of certain situations that the individual has learned to associate with anxiety or even panic. Being in such situations, or even thinking about being in such situations, triggers anxiety as part of the flight or fight response. The natural impulse is to escape or avoid the situation. This effectively reduces the anxiety.

Unfortunately, this natural tendency to avoid situations that provoke distress or uncomfortable degrees of fear or anxiety is one of the key factors which contribute to the development of a phobia in the first place, and then help to maintain it. For example, let's say you are asked to "say a few words" at a gathering of coworkers to say goodbye to a friend and colleague of yours who is leaving. You may immediately think "Oh no. There's no way I could do that. I wouldn't know what to say.

What if my mind went totally blank?".

This makes you feel so anxious that you devise some excuse so as to avoid having to make the speech. You then feel much calmer. You may be thinking something like "Phew! That was a lucky escape. I would have made a fool of myself." However, you probably also feel disappointed in yourself and perhaps even quite critical of yourself. This pushes your self-confidence even lower. You also lose the opportunity to discover that maybe you actually *could* have managed to say a few words that were well received by your audience and appreciated by your friend.

Several important consequences of avoidance are:
1. The original fear is strengthened or *reinforced* (that is, you strongly believe that had you not avoided the situation you would surely have embarrassed yourself because of your incompetence as a public speaker).
2. You miss the opportunity to have an experience that might disprove or *disconfirm* your negative beliefs about yourself and start to build some confidence.
3. You miss the opportunity to practice a social skill: most people only develop confidence in their social skills because of frequent practice, including learning from their mistakes.

Note, of course, the importance of *what you think* about these situations in determining your behavior and emotions. To mount a successful graded exposure program in social phobia it is essential to apply your cognitive challenging, or "straight-thinking", skills in every situation.

The other major problem with using avoidance to try to control anxiety is that fears often seem to spread or *generalize* across situations. For example, you might start out being anxious about speaking on the telephone only when someone who makes you nervous is close enough to overhear. You might then try to avoid that situation, but gradually you find that you're not really comfortable using the phone when *anyone* is nearby ... with time you find that you worry a lot about what the person on the other end might be thinking about what you have to say, too ... eventually you find yourself trying to avoid all phone conversations ... you don't make calls and you won't answer the phone... To relate this to the discussion above, about the importance of how you think about situations, it is likely that way back with that first element of avoidance the message you were unconsciously giving yourself was: "X might think what I have to say is foolish ... that would be awful ... I will make sure I don't say anything when he's/she's around". In other words "I can't trust myself" and "it is essential that others have a good opinion of me" or even "the opinions of others determine my worth as a person".

So, confronting feared situations is an absolutely essential part of the program.

What will make it bearable is taking a graded approach and applying your cognitive challenging skills to keep you realistic about the actual degree of risk.

5.2 Principles of graded exposure

There are several key features to a successful graded exposure program.

A moderate level of anxiety

Anxiety-provoking situations are listed, and the level of anxiety each might be expected to cause rated so that the situations can be ranked in order from least to most anxiety provoking, thus creating the *exposure hierarchy*. The individual chooses to confront a situation that is *moderately* anxiety provoking. It is better to err on the side of choosing a situation that is easier than expected, rather than choosing something daunting and feeling unable to proceed, or feeling over-whelmed. Fears can be made worse if a person suddenly forces himself or herself, without sufficient preparation, to confront something that has been avoided for years, or which is perceived as extremely threatening. In this situation, the anxiety produced by a sudden and overwhelming exposure can actually strengthen the association between the situation and the fear. This is known as *sensitization* and is the opposite of what we are trying to achieve!

Repeated exposure

Just confronting a situation once will not be enough. It takes many repetitions, in conjunction with consistent application of straight thinking techniques, to "wear down" the anxiety associated with a given situation. This is the process of *desensitization*, the desired outcome of a graded exposure program.

Frequent exposure

The more frequently a situation is confronted the sooner the degree of anxiety it is capable of provoking will begin to decrease.

No escape

It is very important to remain in the situation until the anxiety provoked by it begins to diminish. Many people initially feel anxious about this. "How bad could the anxiety get? What if I lost control?" are fears that many people report. First, remember that you are deliberately going to choose to tackle only those situations that are *moderately* anxiety provoking. Second, research has shown that anxiety increases only to a certain level – you have probably already had the worst panic or anxiety attack you will ever have, particularly now that you have already been practicing some anxiety-management strategies. Such research has shown that, even if an individual did not apply any breathing control or cognitive challenging strategies but simply stayed put in the situation, their anxiety would spontaneously diminish over the next 30 to 90 minutes. This makes physiological sense, since the flight or fight response is designed to be used as an *emergency* response. Anything that doesn't kill you within a half hour or so is reclassified by the automatic parts of our brains as not being a true emergency . . . and the response is switched off.

It is true that many individuals report experiences of anxiety that seem to last for hours at a time. However, in most instances the flight or fight response is waxing and waning in intensity in response to recurrent anxious thoughts about the situation. It's rarely maintained at a "full-blown" level for long. Once again, this illustrates the necessity of actively applying straight thinking techniques *while in the anxiety-provoking situation*. If our thoughts about a situation remain realistic and helpful, we will *not* suffer extremes of anxiety.

"No escape" also means not using alcohol or sedatives to control or avoid anxiety. Instead, choose a level of anxiety that you can manage without these unhealthy aids.

5.3 Planning your program

Step 1: Identify your problem situations and choose your goals to create your exposure hierarchy

In Section 2 you listed some situations in which you feel anxious. Add to this list any other goals of social interaction or performance that you would like to be able to achieve. At this stage it would be most helpful to identify very specific goals, such as the following examples:

> To be able to eat a meal with a couple of close friends at the local restaurant.
> To be able to sign credit card vouchers.
> To make a short announcement in front of 10 people at work.

It is helpful to have a range of goals that vary from relatively easy to very difficult. The more specific your goals are, the easier it is to formulate a program to achieve them. For example, "to enjoy going to parties" as compared to "to be able to go to Jane's party this Saturday night, stay for at least 20 minutes, and talk to two people for about 5 minutes each". Being specific also helps you to more accurately gauge the level of anxiety you feel and identify and challenge any unrealistic or unhelpful thoughts about the task.

Include both long-term and short-term goals. Some of your long-term goals may well be described in fairly broad terms, e.g., "to feel more comfortable socially". You will find it helpful to consider how you are actually going to achieve these goals, and devise some steps toward them. For example, if you chose "to be comfortable in social situations" you would have to decide how to define "comfortable", you would have to decide which social situations you want to be comfortable in, and then you would have to begin to practice exposure to each of these social situations, or groups of similar situations.

Do not aim to eliminate anxiety. For example, the goal "to go to Paul's dinner party and not feel anxious" will be very hard to achieve, since some anxiety in this situation is quite reasonable. A further problem with this approach is that the focus continues to be on the anxiety. The more you worry about trying not to get anxious, the more likely you are to actually get anxious. If you were told not to think about a pink elephant, how would you go about it? The goals "to go to Paul's dinner party" or "to go to Paul's dinner party and manage my anxiety" are much more reasonable.

Key points about setting social goals
- Make your goals realistic.
- Break difficult, broadly focused or long-term goals into specific steps.
- Do not aim to eliminate anxiety.

In the space below we would like you to work out five goals of your own choosing. These goals should vary in difficulty from those things that you hope to achieve in the next few weeks, to those that may take 6 months to attain.

My goals

1. _____

2. _____

3. _____

4. _____

5. _____

Step 2: "SUDs" ratings
Use the SUDs scale introduced in Section 4.4 to estimate the degree of anxiety each goal might cause. In this case, a SUDs rating of 100 represents the worst anxiety you have ever experienced, and 0 is no anxiety. We will also use SUDs ratings to monitor your progress.

Step 3: Breaking down your goals into steps

Any goal with a SUDs rating of more than 30 to 40 will need to be broken down into smaller steps to enable you to work up to the goal a little at a time. Take the example of the goal "to be able to eat a meal in the local restaurant". This comes from an individual with a fear of eating in public. In order to be able to work towards eliminating this fear you might start with (1) small amounts of food and (2) uncrowded restaurants. Then, gradually, you would increase the amount of food and the number of people.

Goal: To be able to eat a meal in the local restaurant

This goal could be broken down into the following steps:

	SUDs
Have a soft drink at the restaurant early in the morning	30
Have a soft drink at lunchtime	45
Have a cup of coffee and a sandwich early in the morning	50
Have a cup of coffee and a sandwich at lunchtime	65
Order a soup at dinner; stay at least 20 minutes then may leave even if not finished	75
Order a full meal at dinner and stay until it is all eaten	
With friend aware of problem	90
With friends not aware of problem	100

The task in planning steps to achieve an exposure goal is to think of ways in which you could do something similar to, but easier than, your goal task. Look at the example above and notice what changed at each step. The following are aspects of tasks or activities that can commonly be modified (you may think of others):

Who	is present when you are working towards your goal
What	behavior you set as your goal – exactly specified
When	you carry out the task
Where	you carry out the task
For how long (duration)	you perform the task or stay in the situation

The number of steps involved depends upon the level of difficulty of the task involved. Using the example above, for some people, some of these steps might be too easy. In that case, you would eliminate those that are too easy.

Be realistic in your rating – it's better to overestimate than underestimate the anxiety a given step might cause and work on tasks where you feel you have a reasonably good chance of being successful. Some people use the "75% rule". That is, you only set goals that you are about 75% certain you can achieve. If you use this rule you can determine whether you are going from one step to another with too big a jump; that is, attempting a level that you are not ready for. If you feel less than 75% certain of success, make that step easier so as to increase your confidence. But don't use the 75% rule as a reason for avoiding activities – you can always modify the activity in some way. (See Section 5.5 for imaginal desensitization for help in some situations.)

SUDs or confidence ratings can also be used to determine when you are ready to progress to the next step. Basically, you stay at a given level until either you are about 75% sure of being able to achieve the next step, or your anxiety ratings have fallen to 30/100 or less on the current step.

If anxiety becomes severe, don't panic or run away. If circumstances allow it, stop your activity temporarily. Find a place to sit down or rest, control your breathing and any unrealistic thinking, and wait for the fear to diminish, as it will within a few minutes. If circumstances prevent you from stopping an activity, consider allowing yourself to continue the activity with no pressure to perform. For example, if there are silences in the conversation, let them happen. It is not your responsibility to fill every gap.

Aim never to leave a situation out of fear: take time out if you need it, control your breathing, stay focused on the task at hand – not on yourself! Stay at least until you feel your anxiety level starting to decrease. Best of all is to remain for a time in the situation even after your anxiety has settled. If you do not stay until your anxiety has lessened, you will see it as a failure, lose confidence and your fear is reinforced.

Monitor your progress by keeping a diary of your exposure work that includes both the predicted and actual SUDs experienced. You may have to make running adjustments as you discover in the middle of a program that the next step is too easy or too hard. Your diary can include goals, steps and achievements, together with comments about how you felt and how you dealt with particular situations (coping strategies). This will help you to structure your progress and give you feedback as to how you are doing. You can learn as much from your difficulties as from your successes. Continued use of a diary is highly recommended.

Try to work on at least three goals at any one time. When you have achieved one step or goal, move on to a more difficult goal. It can be helpful to work on both short- and long-term goals at the same time. Remember that your long-term goals may require many steps.

Aim to do something every day.

5.4 Getting the most from your exposure program

Several thinking patterns that seem to develop commonly in those with social phobia can stop you from getting the benefit you deserve from all the hard work you put into exposure practice. These habits may be summarized as follows.

"Discounting" or minimizing

For example, "So I managed to ask a question in class. That's pathetic compared to what all the others can do." Or, "Yes, I caught the bus, but it wasn't very crowded and I only went a couple of stops so it hardly even counts. I should be able to catch the express at peak hour but I can't..."

Take one step at a time and give yourself credit! More is achieved by positive encouragement than by criticism. If you can be patient and keep taking the small steps you'll eventually reach your goal!

The video replay

Recent research has suggested that individuals with social phobia have quite a different perspective of social situations than those with only normal levels of social anxiety. When someone without social phobia attends a party or social gathering, they may be a little nervous and self-conscious initially, but after a few minutes their attention is focused firmly on what is happening around them – particularly other people with whom they are interacting, listening closely to what they say, and making eye contact. Their recollections will be as though they are watching a video that they themselves made.

In social phobia it is quite different. The anxiety and self-consciousness are probably worse to start with, particularly if there has been a lot of worry about the occasion in advance (we call this anticipatory anxiety). Unfortunately, it only gets worse for many. We now know that this is because their attention stays focused on themselves. It is as if they are watching a video of themselves taken by someone else. This is sometimes referred to as "self-focused attention" or as taking "the observer perspective". The person suffering with social phobia tries to imagine the image that others are getting of them – "Do I look relaxed? Do I sound anxious? Oh no, I can feel my face going red!" etc. Naturally, this constant monitoring is also very distracting, and sooner or later the person will miss some part of the conversation and possibly truly be at a loss as to an appropriate reply.

As if all this isn't bad enough, once safely home the "video replay" starts. As if watching a video of themselves the person replays every awkward moment, every sign of anxiety they felt they displayed – over and over. The video replay is often combined with "focusing on the negative" – positive achievements are over-looked. The net result can be that a person takes what was in fact a positive achievement of a planned goal and ends up interpreting it as a failure. This is the main reason why so many individuals who report having pushed themselves to do things describe it as having had a demoralizing effect rather than building their confidence.

Focusing on the negative

All positive elements are ignored and the person focuses only on perceived mistakes, the net result being a perception of failure.

Unrealistic expectations

Many people expect too much of themselves in too short a time. It takes time to overcome what may be close to a lifetime of anxiety. Additionally, it's important to know that improvement doesn't happen in a straight line. It's absolutely typical to find that something you did with relative ease last week causes unexpected difficulty this week, and to experience real setbacks from time to time. We devote a special section to this at the end of the Manual (see Section 7).

5.5 Imaginal desensitization

In a few instances, it may be difficult to approach your goal in a series of real-life steps. In such cases, some steps can be practiced in imagination. This type of desensitization is less powerful than real life exposure, but it does provide a way of adding in-between steps in some all-or-none or one-time-only activities. Imaginal desensitization is best limited to situations where you are unable to perform a step in real life. It should be used in combination with real life exposure to feared situations. Imaginal desensitization alone will not cure social phobia.

The following method can be used for imaginal practice:
- Specify in detail the situation to which you want to desensitize yourself.
- List all the steps involved in performing this activity, or devise versions of this activity that gradually increase in difficulty.
- Record these details on a card, or series of cards, that you will use to script your imagination sessions.
- Rank the examples in order of difficulty or anxiety that they provoke.
- Imagine each scene following a relaxation session. Do not imagine the scene when you feel tense or fearful: stop and relax.

For example, suppose that you wish to rehearse a job interview. This is a normal fear, but the person with social phobia may become so preoccupied about it that they are a nervous wreck by the time of the interview and thus more fearful about saying or doing something stupid, or being badly judged. Of course, you can always practice one or two of the steps associated with interviews in real life, e.g., getting a friend to be the interviewer, or actually visiting the interview building the day before the interview. However, there may be other factors that make it difficult for you to practice the situation.

You could proceed through the following in your imagination:

You arrive at the reception desk, and give your name.

You are seated waiting for the interview in a quiet room.

You are seated waiting in a room with three other candidates.

You are seated with three other candidates and about 10 office staff.

Your name is called and you have to stand up.

You are introduced to someone who gives his name.
You enter the interview room. There is one person to interview you.
You enter the interview room. There are three people to interview you...
and so on.

Begin by imagining yourself in these scenes operating in a competent manner. If you begin to feel anxious, don't go further until you have controlled your anxiety. In this way, you can rehearse competent behavior at the same time as desensitizing yourself to the fear. Only imagine one scene at a time. Move on to the next when you can imagine any given scene with little anxiety. Once you have mastered all your steps you can add some challenges to desensitize to. For example, if you have fears of particular things going wrong (e.g., your prepared speech blowing off the lectern if your feared situation is public speaking) imagine yourself coping with the challenge in a calm and competent way.

5.6 Exercises in planning activities

We would now like you to practice making a graded exposure plan for the following goals:

1. *Goal:*   Performing some task at work (e.g., filling out a form) while your boss is watching over your shoulder.

   Steps: 1. _____

   2. _____

   3. _____

   4. _____

   5. _____

2. *Goal:*   Giving a 5-minute speech at a friend's anniversary party.

   Steps: 1. _____

   2. _____

   3. _____

   4. _____

   5. _____

5.6.1 Achieving your own personal goals

From your list of five goals, select two that you would like to begin to work on first, and write these below. To get started, choose either something low on your anxiety hierarchy or else something that is a priority for you. Set out beneath each goal the steps you intend to take in order to achieve it.

1. *Goal:* _____

   Steps: SUDs

   • _____

   • _____

   • _____

   • _____

   • _____

   • _____

   • _____

2. *Goal:* _____

   Steps: SUDs

   • _____

   • _____

   • _____

   • _____

   • _____

5.7 Implementing your program

Use your diary to plan a week or so ahead. Even if you are having a bad day, try always to do something, but you need only go over the steps that you have already mastered. Confront a situation frequently and regularly until you overcome the fear. Many fears need to be confronted frequently (that is, three to four times a week) at first, otherwise your fear will rise again by the time you do it next. The general rule is: *the more you fear it, the more frequently you need to confront it.*

Repeat each step over and over until the SUDs it generates have dropped to 30 or less consistently (i.e., a few times in a row). An example of a diary is shown below.

Confront your previously feared situation regularly, even after you no longer fear it. This will make sure it stays under your control.

Practicing the steps

Use the standard relaxation and breathing control exercises before you go out. Think realistically and helpfully about the task you plan. Get yourself as calm as possible – but you don't have to be completely calm to cope.

Use your anxiety-management techniques while in the situation.

Concentrate on the task at hand, not on how you are feeling, how you look, or what others might be thinking about you.

Give yourself recognition for your efforts and plan rewards for achievements. Learn to congratulate yourself when things go well, and be supportive of yourself when you don't do as well as you'd have liked – learn to be a good friend to yourself.

Example of diary

This person is fearful of scrutiny and of interacting with others.

Date	Task	SUDs		Comments
		Predicted	Actual	
19 Mar	Sit with magazine in staff canteen for cup of coffee towards end of lunch (10 minutes)	40	50	It was more crowded than I expected; just kept my head down and tried to concentrate on magazine
20 Mar	Sit with magazine in staff canteen for cup of coffee towards end of lunch (10 minutes)	50	50	Quite difficult to walk in; reminded myself no-one pays much attention, really
21 Mar	Sit with magazine in staff canteen for cup of coffee towards end of lunch (10 minutes)	50	40	Seemed a bit easier today
22 Mar	Sit with magazine in staff canteen for cup of coffee towards end of lunch (10 minutes)	50	35	No-one really pays much attention
23 Mar	Sit with magazine in staff canteen for cup of coffee towards end of lunch (10 minutes)	50	30	Not as many people here on a Friday, maybe; looking forward to a break from this!
24 Mar	Go to movie with Sally at morning session; sit near exit	40	30	It was easier than I thought – cinema VERY quiet; Sally is really supportive; I actually enjoyed the movie! Will go more often.
25 Mar	Bus to local shops	40	40	Not busy on the weekend
	Try on 4 pairs of shoes at the shoe store where they have the assistants	60	80→50	Nearly couldn't go through with it as store was quite busy – felt sorry for assistant – but a few people left and assistant was very cheerful

Date	Task	SUDs Predicted	Actual	Comm
26 Mar	Sit with magazine in staff canteen for cup of coffee towards end of lunch (10 minutes)	50	50	Just as h... disappoi... – just har... break + ca... myself: no-... ~~cares~~
27 Mar	Sit with magazine in staff canteen for cup of coffee towards end of lunch (10 minutes)	50	30	Much more settled today
28 Mar	Sit with magazine in staff canteen for cup of coffee towards end of lunch (10 minutes)	50	30	No real problem: time to try the next step
29 Mar	Take late lunch & eat in staff canteen: join Trish if she's there or else sit with magazine (30 min)	60	40	Not much harder than the last step, really. Trish not there – read magazine. Will try this one a few more times to be sure
30 Mar	Take late lunch & eat in staff canteen: join Trish if she's there or else sit with magazine (30 min)	60	35	Feeling more confident. Looked up a few times and no-one was looking my way at all

Summary

An excessive fear of negative evaluation gives rise to anxiety in a range of social situations. The natural tendency is to avoid situations that make us anxious. Unfortunately, avoidance and escape only strengthen the underlying fears, and contribute to the spread of fear across more and more situations. In order to overcome anxiety it is necessary to confront feared situations. This can be done in a planned and graded way that builds confidence gradually without provoking extreme levels of anxiety. Anxiety-management skills and cognitive challenging techniques help to control the anxiety generated by confronting feared situations and help to reduce future anxiety. Success requires frequent and repeated exposure to feared situations.

SECTION 6

6 Assertiveness

6.1 What is assertiveness?

Healthy assertion – assertiveness – is about *choice* and *communication*. It is the making of active choices about what to do and say. It is the ability to communicate our opinions, thoughts, needs, and feelings in a direct, honest, and appropriate manner – when we choose. It is the ability to recognize our rights and make choices about exercising them. The principles of assertiveness hold that we all have rights and responsibilities. Being assertive means recognizing our rights and responsibilities and the rights and responsibilities of others, and making choices about how to manage interpersonal situations in a way that respects the rights of all concerned. Being assertive means taking care of ourselves – without trampling others.

Being assertive results in having more confidence and more control over your life, and taking responsibility to meet your own needs, which in turn leads to an increase in self-esteem. When you feel like this about yourself, you are more able to make closer and more satisfying relationships with other people. Being assertive includes the ability to choose how to relate in any type of relationship, having weighed the risks and benefits. Being assertive enables you to be flexible and modify your responses as the situation requires, rather than being locked in to one particular way of relating.

Being assertive includes:
- Valuing yourself and believing that you have the right to express your opinions and get your needs met.
- Being willing to share yourself with others, rather than holding everything inside.
- Respecting the rights and needs of others.
- Being able to choose how to respond to people or situations.
- Feeling okay about yourself, your needs, and actions.

6.2 What is faulty assertion?

There are two forms of faulty assertion: underassertion (passivity) and aggressiveness.

Underassertion

When you are underassertive you do not express your feelings, needs, and opinions to others. You deny your own rights to communicate. In practical terms, you often end up doing things that you can't really afford, don't enjoy, or haven't the time for. Emotionally, unassertiveness erodes your self-esteem as you criticize yourself for not having been able to say what you really thought, or what you really wanted. People who are unable to assert their own needs and opinions often bottle up feelings such as anger, resentment, and disappointment. Such feelings increase arousal and tension levels in the body, and make panic attacks and anxiety more likely. Often a point is reached where the feelings can't be controlled any more, and then the person explodes aggressively. Of course, after this, they feel guilty and go back to bottling their feelings up all over again. You can see that being underassertive can lead to more aggression than being assertive would!

Aggressiveness

Some people have a habit of reacting aggressively from the start in many interactions. There can be many reasons for this, including an underlying world view that others usually treat them unfairly or are out to make life difficult for them (another type of unrealistic, unhelpful thought). When people are aggressive, they are often left feeling guilty and ashamed of their behavior. Their victims often feel put down and want to get their own back. Aggressiveness leads to greatly increased arousal, and may leave a person always on the verge of anger and anxiety.

What is the difference between being assertive, aggressive, or underassertive? The following examples illustrate these different responses to various interpersonal situations.

Example 1: Your reckless brother wants to borrow your car. You don't want to lend it to him because you don't feel confident that he won't crash it. What do you say?

Nonassertive: Oh . . . all right, but please be careful.

Aggressive: You've got a nerve asking to borrow my car. I'm not that stupid.

Assertive: I don't feel comfortable about the way you drive, so I'm not going to loan it to you. That doesn't mean I don't want to help you. Have you thought of renting a car while yours is in for repairs?

Note that you may want to add a constructive suggestion to show that you are aware that the person has a problem that still needs solving. This is your choice and obviously will vary with circumstances. You could just say "No".

Example 2: The boss comes out of his office and puts your latest assignment down in front of you. "This is trash!" he tells you. How do you respond?

Nonassertive: I'm sorry is it that bad?

Aggressive: Well, if it's so bad, do it yourself then.

Assertive: I think it would be best if you could tell me what's wrong and how it can be improved.

Example 3: Waiting in line at the post office, Janice is about to be served when someone starts to speak and says "It's only a quick question." There are many people waiting, for various reasons. What would you do?

Nonassertive: Okay, go ahead.

Aggressive: Don't you think I've got better things to do than to wait here and listen to your problem?

Assertive: I've been waiting quite a while and it is my turn now. I don't expect to be very long either.

Being nonassertive is the most common assertiveness problem for individuals with social phobia or an avoidant personality style. The two most common reasons for this seem to be:

Fear of negative evaluation: The person with social phobia fears that if they say what they really think, or what they would like to happen, then others will reject them, criticize them, or think less of them.

Fear of upsetting others: In particular, you may believe that if you say "No" to someone, or disagree with their opinion, then you will be responsible for upsetting them and causing them distress. This involves cognitive errors such as omnipotence, personalization, fortune telling, and mind reading.

People learn faulty assertion from their experiences throughout their lives. Many people learned to make nonassertive responses because that's the way they saw their parents behave, or because that was the way their parents, teachers, or other authority figures expected them to behave. Once these patterns become established, they can be difficult to change because the thought of behaving in a more assertive manner provokes too much anxiety (How would the other person respond? What if they became angry or upset?). After many years, people act this way purely from habit. A new, healthier style of assertive interaction can be learned in place of these old habits. It is time for you to critically examine whether your current style of relating to others is most appropriate and helpful to you in your life now.

The principles of assertiveness hold that each of us is responsible for ourselves and our actions. It is up to us to choose how to respond to others, and up to them to choose how to respond to us. We have the *right* to make up our own minds about what to think and how to act. In reality, this makes life a lot easier! It means that we don't have to try to be a "mind reader" to know what others really want and thus try to "make them happy" – it's up to them to tell us what they want (or don't want). We don't have to feel that asking for something is an imposition on someone else – because they have the right to refuse us if what we ask is not convenient. The Bill of Assertive Rights, below, lists the basic rights of interpersonal interaction to which each of us have claim. Look carefully through each of these and note your reaction to them.

Bill of Assertive Rights
- You have the right to be the judge of what you do and what you think.
- You have the right to offer no reasons and excuses for your behavior.
- You have the right not to be responsible for finding solutions to other people's problems.
- You have the right to change your mind.
- You have the right to make mistakes.
- You have the right to say "I don't know."
- You have the right to make your own decisions.
- You have the right to say "I don't understand."
- You have the right to say "I don't care."
- You have the right to say "No" – without feeling guilty.

Many people feel somewhat shocked by some of these statements. It is important to note that this is a list of your *rights*. That is, not what you *should* do in any situation, but rather what you *could* choose to do. When you make your decision about how to respond in any given situation, you have these rights to take into consideration.

6.3 Choosing how to respond in any situation

When we feel uncomfortable in some interaction it is helpful to think through the situation and decide how to respond. This is particularly relevant in difficult interactions of a recurring nature – e.g., the colleague who is often rude, a demanding relative.

The first step is to use your cognitive challenging skills to identify your thoughts and feelings in the situation and check that they are realistic. For example, be sure that you are not misinterpreting someone's reaction, jumping to conclusions about things or taking things personally. Just because you have strong feelings does not mean that they give a true picture of what is happening – you might *feel* anxious and inadequate but it doesn't mean that you are coming across badly to others. There may be a problem, but you will deal with it most effectively if you are realistic about it. For example, there may be a colleague who says, "I'm busy. Come back later.", in a terse manner when you ask for some assistance that it is their job to provide. You might think, "They don't like me. They're always rude . . . I can't stand working with them." You might start to feel anxious and uncomfortable any time you have to interact with them and might try to put it off or avoid it. It would be important to be realistic about the situation:

- Just because the person was a bit short with you, does it mean they don't like you? What other explanations could there be?
- Are they only like this with you, or have you seen them behave this way with others?
- Are they always like this, or only sometimes? In what situations are they more likely to behave this way?

You could then consider ways you might resolve the situation without having to quit your job! The process of making sure that your interpretations about the situation are realistic helps you to clarify the problem, and it is usually now possible to state the problem more accurately. In this case, the problem might be expressed as: "X often refuses to help me when I need their assistance and does this in a manner which I find slightly aggressive." The next step in finding a solution to this problem is to consider each person's *rights and responsibilities* in the situation. For example, with the situation above, you might decide the following:

My rights	X's rights
I have the right to ask for what I need I have the right to be treated with respect	To be treated with respect To communicate their needs and wishes

My responsibilities	X's responsibilities
To get my job done – this means I need X's assistance at times – I may have to be prepared to negotiate about how this is best accomplished	To do their job – this means they need to assist me at times

It can then be helpful to use a technique called structured problem solving to help you choose the best solution to the problem.

6.4 Structured problem solving

Structured problem solving provides a framework for identifying and evaluating potential solutions to problems, and for planning the implementation of chosen solutions or problem-solving strategies. The steps in this process are summarized below.

Structured problem solving

Step 1: Identify the problem.
Step 2: "Brainstorm" potential solutions.
Step 3: Critically assess the pros and cons of each potential solution.
Step 4: Choose the best solution(s).
Step 5: Plan how to implement the solution(s).
Step 6: Review outcome.

In step 1 it is important to clarify the problem and state it as accurately as possible, trying to avoid being overly emotional about it or making "cognitive errors" about what is really happening.

In step 2 the aim is to think as creatively as possible about potential solutions. Don't be critical at this stage – just let the ideas flow. If there are people you would feel comfortable talking the problem over with, you can include on your list any suggestions they make. Make sure you also consider what *you* would like to happen – it might not prove the most feasible option, but you owe it to yourself to at least consider your own preferences.

Step 3 is where you critically evaluate the pros and cons of each potential solution. Be sure to be realistic in your assessments. For example:

- Would you have the resources to carry out this solution?
  - Time.
  - Money.
  - Personal resources and skills including ability to be assertive at this point in time (i.e., being mindful of what you can do now, not what you'd *like* to be capable of eventually).
- Would this solution be likely to solve the whole problem? Part of the problem?
- What problems might the solution itself lead to?
- How might the other person react to this solution?

It can be helpful to give a relative weighting to the pros and cons of each solution. It's important not to cut corners in this exercise – take the time to consider *each* solution in turn. You will usually find that the time you spend on this structured problem-solving exercise is a good investment. It helps to stop worrying in an unstructured, ultimately unhelpful way, and it helps you to feel comfortable that you considered every option that you could think of at the time. Your work sheet might look something like this:

Solutions

1. Speak to my superior about the problem with X

Pros	(weight)	Cons	(weight)
Don't have to confront X myself	***	X might be angry about not being approached directly – might hold a grudge	*
Superior is very approachable	**	I don't improve my assertiveness skills	**
		Superior may think less of me for not handling it myself – might count against me for promotion	**

2. Email X and suggest that I notify him/her when I need help so we can arrange a mutually convenient time

Pros	(weight)	Cons	(weight)
Don't have to speak to X directly about it	***	Means I have to wait for help until convenient for X	*
Likely to be an acceptable solution to X as allows him/her to help me at his/her convenience	***	X might be offended that I didn't speak to him/her directly	*
Gives X time to consider it & at his/her convenience	*		

List other possible solutions here:

1. _____

2. _____

3. _____

What might be the pros and cons of each?

In step 4 the best solution, or sometimes a combination of solutions, is chosen by reviewing the pros and cons of all the options.

Step 5 calls for a specific plan of action to be devised for implementing the chosen solution(s):

- *What will you say and to whom?*
- *When will you say it?*
- *How will you organize to meet or otherwise get the message to the person?*

Step 6 is equally important. By planning a review it helps you to recognize that it may not be possible to find the "perfect" solution no matter how hard you have tried. In some cases the review is best scheduled after you have carried out a specific planned behavior or intervention. In other cases, e.g., a situation where you decide to try out a new style of response or of relating to another person, you might decide to review the situation after a certain period of time has elapsed. When you perform your review, re-evaluate the problem, and decide whether it requires further action. If so, go through the above process once more, taking account of what you have learned and the changes that may have occurred.

6.4.1 Sending the message effectively

If you choose a solution involving direct discussion with another person, send messages effectively and without blame by:

- Careful timing.
- Using "I" rather than "you" statements. "I feel … when you … because…"
- Matching your spoken and nonverbal messages.
- Being specific about how others' behavior disturbs you.
- Acknowledging others' feelings when appropriate, "You seem upset by what I've said", and checking whether this is an accurate perception.

You can see from the examples throughout this section that in an assertive encounter no one should feel put down. If people choose to react badly to your assertion, then you can regard this as their problem and not some fault of your own. It is their choice how to respond. People who attempt to make you feel bad after a healthy assertive encounter are usually trying to manipulate you without concern for your wishes, often because of their own problems of low self-esteem. Such people would themselves benefit from an assertiveness training program.

A key word is *choose*, because you can be assertive, choose not to speak up for your rights, or choose to act more aggressively on occasions. This is quite different from continuously acting passively or aggressively without having any control over how you react. There may be times where you choose *not* to assert your rights. That's perfectly okay and quite normal: as long as it was an active choice. For example, you might choose to put yourself out for a loved one. You might choose not to assert your rights in a brief encounter where you judge it is not worth the energy and you will never have to deal with that person again. You also need to consider the long-term consequences to the other person and to the relationship of speaking up for yourself. Your partner, friends, and colleagues may need time to adjust to the positive changes in your behavior. In some relationships, your new assertiveness may challenge the current balance of power and you and the other(s) in the relationship will need to allow time for communication.

Choices

- To assert your rights or keep them in reserve.
- How much of your inner feelings to reveal.
- How much to tell people about yourself.
- How to respond in any situation.

Choosing the assertive option is often much more difficult than acting in an aggressive or underassertive manner. Try giving responses that illustrate the different styles of reacting in the following examples:

Example 1: You are just about to answer a question that your brother has asked you and your father answers for you. He has done this ever since you were young. You want to answer for yourself. Your response to your father is:

Nonassertive:

_____

_____

_____

_____

Aggressive:

_____

_____

_____

_____

Assertive:

_____

_____

_____

_____

Example 2: Your friend sees that you are just going shopping. She says, "While you're shopping, would you pick up my dry cleaning, please?" You are not planning to go anywhere near the dry cleaners and parking there is inconvenient, so you don't want to say yes.

Nonassertive:

_____

_____

_____

_____

Aggressive:

_____

_____

_____

_____

Assertive:

_____

_____

_____

_____

Example 3: When you took a new job 12 months ago, one colleague in particular was very welcoming, helping you to settle in by inviting you to sit with them at lunch, and introducing you to others. On a number of occasions this friend has asked you to loan them money to tide them over until pay day, and you did so as you felt you couldn't refuse. They have never paid any of the money back. Now they come to you for another loan. What do you do?

Nonassertive:

_____

_____

_____

_____

Aggressive:

_____

_____

_____

_____

Assertive:

_____

_____

_____

_____

6.5 Nonassertive myths

There are beliefs that many people hold that make it difficult for them to assert themselves. These beliefs are called myths because they are very rarely tested against reality. When they are, they are usually found to be untrue. The two most common myths that prevent people with excessive social anxiety from asserting themselves are:

1. *The Myth of a Good Friend.* You are following this myth if you say things like "He should have known that I didn't want that." or "She should have understood why I said that." What you are really saying is "He/She should have been able to read my mind." The assumption is that friends should know how you feel about everything at any given moment. It is also important to remember that other people do not always hold the same things to be important as you do. For example, you may believe that punctuality is important. If a friend is late for an appointment, you may say "If he took me seriously he would have been on time." Your friend, however, may see no relationship between how seriously he takes you and how punctual he is. Punctuality may simply be an unimportant factor in his life. In this case, he would not understand why you would be offended. The most sensible way to resolve this type of problem is by open discussion. You will not always get your own way, of course, but at least you will let your friends know what is important to you and you won't have to rely on their "reading your mind".

2. *The Myth of Obligation:* You believe in this myth if you say to yourself "If my friend asks me a favor, I have to agree if I am a true friend." Also, you are likely to believe the converse of this, i.e., if you ask a friend a favor, he or she has to agree if that person is a true friend. If you believe in this myth, you will never feel comfortable about asking or giving favors, because you will not see that there is a choice involved. That is to say, when someone asks you to do something you may feel resentful because you will not be able to say no. Also, you will not be able to ask anyone to do anything because you will believe that they cannot say no!

6.6 Protective skills

In some situations, your healthy assertion will be met by strong resistance. Others may act aggressively, irrationally, in an extremely emotional fashion, or refuse to listen to your point of view. In these circumstances, you may need to use protective skills. These are less than ideal in that they rarely resolve a situation in a mutually satisfactory way, but they can help you to deal with highly unsatisfactory situations where your assertive behavior is not reciprocated. Remember: first respond assertively. Only when this seems to be failing because of an unreasonable response from the other person should you use these "protective skills".

Protection 1: Broken record

When it is clear that another person is not prepared to accept your response or even consider your point of view, then it is time to give up on explanations, stop answering questions, and simply repeat your answer over and over again, without any further reasons or explanations. For example, saying "No", without explanation, over and over again to a pushy salesman or refusing an inappropriate request from a friend, over and over again. It is important to remain calm and not become aggressive yourself, as this can escalate the situation. The most common mistake that people make with this technique is not sticking to the same response, but allowing themselves to be drawn into making further explanations or answering questions that the other person raises.

Protection 2: Selective ignoring

With this technique you choose not to respond to the inappropriate aspects of another person's communication to you. Often this will lead them to give up on it. For example, someone continues to complain to you about some past event, despite the fact that you have discussed it many times with them in an effort to help them, and they never seem to listen to advice or try to get over it. When you fail to respond to their complaints, while continuing to respond to other topics of conversation, the lack of response will eventually make it too unrewarding for them to keep bringing it up. It may help to say once and for all: "I know you are still upset about that, but you know that I don't believe it is at all helpful to keep going over it. So, if you bring this up again, I will ignore it. I would much rather talk to you about other things." Selective ignoring can also be a helpful technique where you feel others are repeatedly criticizing you over something from the past (that you may or may not agree was deserving of criticism at the time). You might say something like: "I have listened to your point of view, and we have discussed this matter many times in the past. You know that I disagree with you. I don't want to talk about it any more and I am not going to respond to it from now on. If you bring this up again, I will ignore it. This doesn't mean that I'm not prepared to talk to you about other issues." Then make sure you do ignore it! Of course, it is often hard to ignore criticism, especially if we think it is unfair – but if you've not succeeded in changing their mind thus far you probably never will.

Protection 3: Disarming anger

When someone is being inappropriately aggressive towards you, it is sometimes possible to disarm his or her anger by refusing to carry on the conversation until the anger dies down. For example, you can say, "I can see that you're angry about this and I want to talk it over with you, but I don't feel that I can while you're angry. Let's talk later when we're both calm and ready to discuss it." Be prepared to listen and discuss their concerns when they do calm down. If you have both been arguing, and are both angry, it may be more appropriate to suggest that you both have "time out" – time to cool down – without blaming each other for the anger. "Look, we're both pretty worked up. Why don't we leave it for now and talk about it later when we're calmer?"

Protection 4: Sorting issues

Often people will confuse several issues. For example, someone close to you might say "If you really cared for me you would loan me that money." This can confuse us too, and make it harder to respond assertively. It is important to sort the issues here, e.g., "It is not that I don't care for you, it is just that I don't wish to lend money." You may need to combine the broken record technique with this technique to get maximum effectiveness.

Protection 5: Dealing with guilt

Some people have learned to try to get their needs met by making others feel guilty, rather than behaving assertively themselves. For example, a friend or relative may ask for a favor by saying "I helped you out by picking up the kids … you really owe it to me to help me move house." Does this accord with the Bill of Assertive Rights? Sorting the issues can be important here. For example, "I am grateful to you for having picked up the kids the other day. I'm sorry I can't help you move house on Saturday." Our susceptibility to *unreasonable* guilt can be increased if we have unrealistic expectations of our own behavior (to always do the right thing, never to upset anyone, to please everyone, to be perfect). If you find yourself feeling guilty, the first thing to do is ask yourself why are you feeling guilty, what have you not done that you told yourself you "should" have done?

Protection 6: Apologies

There are circumstances in which apologies are appropriate. We all make mistakes. For instance, it may be that you forgot to do something you said you would do. The person you said you would help complains about it but extends their complaint to a criticism of everything about you. You can see that the person may have been inconvenienced, and recognize their right to be annoyed or a bit upset by your forgetfulness, yet make it quite clear that, in apologizing for that, you do not accept everything else they say about you (sorting the issues). Note that a more assertive response from the person involved would have been to tell you how they felt about your forgetfulness, and what they might like you to do to rectify the situation. The words "I'm sorry" are frequently overused. Often, they are not genuinely meant. The person who is always saying he is sorry feels guilty when there is no need. She fails to recognize her right to her own opinions and her own life. It is useful to avoid saying "I'm sorry" unless you genuinely feel there are good reasons to apologize.

Protection 7: "I'll let you know"

For many of the reasons that underlie other forms of unassertive behavior in social anxiety disorders, sufferers often feel unable to say "No". Their first response to requests for assistance is always "Yes". This often leaves them over-committed and with no time for themselves. When such assistance is not reciprocated it can also lead to feelings of resentment. Many people are not quite ready to say "No" without feeling guilty or offering reasons or excuses. Or they never give themselves a chance because they say "Yes" right away! This protection is about learning to give yourself some time to think about it; time to consider your rights and your wishes and make a considered *choice* about how to respond; time to plan how to say "No" if you want to – it's not easy at first. Train yourself to say, "I'll need to check my diary." or "I need to think about it." or "I'll let you know tomorrow." (make sure you do).

6.7 Decision to change

In order to gain from an assertiveness training program, you have to be sure that there are some aspects about your normal way of responding that you wish to change, i.e., you have to make a conscious decision to change. You have to weigh up the costs and benefits of changing versus staying the same. The following questions can help you to make this decision. Add any other comments or dimensions that may apply to your particular situation.

What do I gain from staying nonassertive?

- Praise for conforming to others' expectations.
- Maintenance of a familiar behavior pattern.
- Avoidance of taking responsibility for initiating or carrying out plans.
- Avoidance of possible conflict.

- _____

- _____

- _____

What do I lose by being nonassertive?

- Independence.
- The power to make my own decisions.
- The opportunity to get my own needs and wishes met.
- Others' respect for my rights and wishes.

- The ability to influence others' decisions, demands, and expectations.

- _____

- _____

- _____

What do I gain by becoming assertive?

- Improved confidence and self-esteem.
- The opportunity to take control over my own destiny.

- _____

- _____

- _____

What do I lose by becoming assertive?

- If I try and fail I would be more upset than being able to tell myself that I failed because I didn't really try . . .
- My friends may not like the change in me.

- _____

- _____

- _____

Do the gains of becoming assertive outweigh the losses?

If not, why not?

If so, am I willing to make the change by acting assertively?

Can I enlist the support, understanding, and cooperation of others involved, either in the situation or in my life?

How will I begin to make these changes?

_____

_____

_____

_____

_____

6.7.1 Be prepared to negotiate

Keep the "we" in the relationship and be prepared to be flexible. You will feel more comfortable when you know what the other person's wishes are (because they have told you, rather than because of your mind reading!), they know what your wishes are, and you can begin to negotiate if these differ.

Try starting with a few assertive skills in a few situations and gradually build up your skills. It's often easier to begin with new acquaintances, then friends of longer standing. It's hardest of all to change long-standing patterns of interaction with family members. Give yourself, and others, time to adjust. You may find useful some of the books listed in Section 8.

Summary

Assertiveness is about making choices in your interactions with others and communicating with them in ways that are satisfying and effective. When you behave assertively you consider the rights of yourself *and* others, then choose how to respond. Healthy self-esteem requires the ability to be assertive. Behaving assertively builds self-esteem and confidence. Being assertive challenges many of the unhelpful beliefs that are part of social phobia.

SECTION 7

7 Coping with setbacks and difficulties

Setbacks are inevitable. They happen to *everyone*. When it happens, people often become alarmed or despondent, fearing they have gone back to their very worst. The setback is often viewed as devastating because it has a lot of emotional meaning for the person who has put considerable effort into recovering. No matter how badly you feel during a setback, no-one ever seems to go all the way back to their worst level of incapacitation or to totally lose their new skills.

Setbacks often occur at times when you face additional stresses in your life, such as job, family, or money worries, or ill health, or when facing some particularly challenging situation. For most people, the apparent setback is only a passing phase. After the stressors pass, you will find it easier to get yourself out and about again. You can help this process by actively working to resolve the problems that face you so that you can once again devote your energy to facing your fears. While you feel stressed, don't let your program go completely, but try to maintain the gains you have already made. However, even if you slip back a little, it is not a catastrophe: you moved forward before and you can do it again. Ups and downs in the recovery process are the rule rather than the exception. A typical pattern is illustrated in the diagram overleaf. Coping successfully with setbacks actually builds your confidence, and you are less likely to stumble over the same problem in the future.

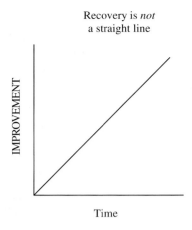

Recovery is *not* a straight line

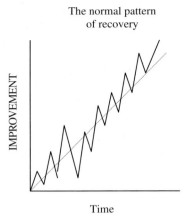

The normal pattern of recovery

7.1 Prolonged setbacks

Prolonged setbacks or difficulties in making progress are generally the consequence of not practicing your new skills! You will not get better just by thinking about it and hoping your anxiety will just go away. If you are experiencing difficulties, carefully read your Manual again (from the beginning) and follow the recommendations. Go back to basics with your anxiety-management strategies: practice the hyperventilation control and relaxation exercises – *every day*. Review your cognitive challenging skills and check for "cognitive errors". Be alert for "shoulds" and unhelpful expectations of yourself. Be honest about avoidances and safety behaviors: these stop you from really confronting and therefore mastering your anxiety. Set yourself realistic goals of graded exposure and give yourself plenty of support and encouragement.

Checklist

I am doing the following: .

- ☐ Using hyperventilation control at the first sign of anxiety.
- ☐ Exercising four times per week.
- ☐ Getting up at the same time every day.
- ☐ Keeping my nicotine, caffeine and alcohol intake nil or low.
- ☐ Abstaining from illicit drugs.
- ☐ Regularly *writing down* anxious thoughts and challenging them.
- ☐ Working to eliminate cognitive distortions and "shoulds".
- ☐ Setting realistic goals.
- ☐ Giving myself praise and encouragement.
- ☐ Confronting feared situations daily.
- ☐ Using graded exposure.
- ☐ Remaining alert for subtle avoidance and safety behaviors.
- ☐ Working to eliminate avoidance.
- ☐ Really confronting my fears.

7.1.1 Learn to be your own best friend

Many sufferers of social phobia have low self-esteem. They are highly critical of themselves when they fail to meet their own expectations. It is essential to learn how to give yourself support and encouragement – it means more when it comes from within. Be kind to yourself when you don't do as well as you'd have liked – how would you respond to someone else, or, especially, a child? Congratulate yourself on your effort as well as your successes. Consider setting yourself small rewards for meeting goals. Set your goals at realistic levels and learn to appreciate small successes. It may be only a small step, but if you keep taking small steps you will eventually reach your goals.

Mastering anxiety is going to take time. It is challenging and tiring and difficult, and no-one else *really* knows what it's like. Learn to be kind to yourself and you'll not only last the distance, but you'll find it a whole lot easier to challenge unhelpful beliefs about how much the opinions of others really need to matter.

If you are still having trouble, seek advice from your therapist.

Summary

Setbacks are inevitable. They can be a learning experience and result in greater confidence. Don't panic, but go back to basics – revise the work you have done in this Manual. The techniques work, but only if you use them. Get help if you need it. Learn to be kind to yourself.

SECTION 8

8 Recommended resources

8.1 Recommended paperbacks

The following books are on the shelves in many bookstores and libraries. If not, they can often be ordered. When you read these or any similar books on the management of anxiety, remember that they are best regarded as guidelines only. Be critical in both a positive and negative sense when reading these books, so that you get what is best for you out of them. Most of these books are fairly inexpensive.

Alberti RE, Emmons ML. (1978) *Your Perfect Right: A Guide to Assertive Behavior.* San Luis, CA: Impact Publishers.

Antony M, Swinson R. (1998) *When Perfect Isn't Good Enough: Strategies for Coping with Perfectionism.* Oakland, CA: New Harbinger.

Barlow D, Rapee R. (1997) *Mastering Stress: A Lifestyle Approach.* Killara, NSW: Lifestyle Press.

Burns D. (1980) *Feeling Good: The New Mood Therapy.* Melbourne: Information Australia Group.

Davis M, Eshelman E, McKay M. (1995) *The Relaxation and Stress Reduction Workbook.* Oakland, CA: New Harbinger.

Ellis A, Harper R. (1979) *A New Guide to Rational Living.* Hollywood, CA: Wilshire Book Company.

Greenberger D, Padesky C. (1995) *Mind Over Mood.* New York: Guilford.

Jakubowski P, Lange A. (1978) *The Assertive Option: Your Rights and Responsibilities.* Champaign, IL: Research Press Company.

McKay M, Davis M, Fanning P. (1995) *Messages: The Communication Skills Book.* Oakland, CA: New Harbinger.

McKay M, Fanning P. (1987) *Self-Esteem: A Proven Program of Cognitive Techniques for Assessing, Improving and Maintaining Your Self-Esteem.* Oakland, CA: New Harbinger.

Page A. (1993) *Don't Panic! Overcoming Anxiety, Phobias and Tension.* Sydney: Gore Osment.

Rapee R. (1997) *Overcoming Shyness and Social Phobia: A Step-by-Step Guide.* Killara, NSW: Lifestyle Press.

Tanner S, Ball J. (1989) *Beating the Blues.* Sydney: Doubleday.

8.2 Video

The following video provides a useful overview of social phobia and cognitive behavioral treatment of social phobia from the perspective of both sufferers and therapists:

Rapee R, Lampe L. (1998) *I Think, They Think: Overcoming Social Phobia*

Available through Monkey See Productions (PO Box 159, Blackheath, NSW 2785, Australia, or visit their website at: www.monkeysee.com.au).

8.3 Journal article

The following journal article provides a description of the technique of applied relaxation. It may be obtained with the help of your local librarian:

Ost L-G. (1987) Applied relaxation: description of a coping technique and review of controlled studies. *Behavior Research and Therapy*, **25**, 397–409.

8.4 Websites

Clinical Research Unit for Anxiety and Depression website. See Self-Help Clinic: www.crufad.org

Anxiety Disorders Foundation of Australia: www.geocities.com/adfanswinc

Mental Health website, Melbourne: www.sane.org

12

Specific phobias

Syndrome

There is broad agreement between ICD-10 and DSM-IV regarding specific (or isolated) phobias. Distilling from these two diagnostic systems, the major features of a phobia are:

1. A stimulus-bound fear reaction that is
2. distressing to the point of causing emotional, social, or occupational disruptions,
3. recognized as excessive or unreasonable, and
4. leads to avoidance or intense anxiety upon exposure to the feared stimulus.

From studies of the diagnostic reliabilities it is apparent that specific phobias are readily identified but it is difficult to determine the threshold of impairment to define when such fears become phobias (Di Nardo et al., 1983). One of the strengths of the DSM system is that it explicitly encourages subtyping of the specific phobias into four categories. It specifically identifies phobias as:

1. Animal.
2. Natural environment (e.g., heights, storms, water).
3. Blood, injection, and injury.
4. Situational (e.g., planes, elevators, enclosed places).

It also mentions (but includes in an "other" category) phobias of situations that may lead to choking, vomiting, or contracting an illness. At present, the prognostic value of subtyping is not clear. Although individuals with one subtype of phobia are likely to have other fears from within the same subtype, they are also likely to have other specific phobias (Hofmann et al., 1997). Nevertheless, the value of subtyping is not without its merits, and in the case of blood, injection, and injury phobia there are distinct treatment implications of the unique properties of this disorder (Marks, 1988; Page, 1994b). Kleinknecht and Lenz (1989) divided blood–injury phobics on the basis of fear and propensity to faint and were able to identify a subgroup who fainted in response to blood or injury but reported no significant fear. Interestingly, an association was found between parents and children for fainting but not for fear, suggesting separate etiologies. Presently, neither of the major diagnostic systems make mention of the role of fainting, even though this is an important consideration when tailoring treatment to the individual (Öst et al., 1984a; Öst and Sterner, 1987; Page, 1991a). In the majority of cases diagnosis is relatively straightforward but it is made easier by structured diagnostic interviews. The Anxiety Disorders Interview Schedule – Revised (ADIS-R) and the Composite International Diagnostic Interview (CIDI) both provide reliable assessments of specific phobias (Page, 1991b; Peters and Andrews, 1995).

Clinical presentation

Because specific phobias are a well-known diagnostic category, a case illustration may be considered redundant. However, blood–injury phobia is perhaps less familiar and will be illustrated. The individual, typical of the specific phobias, demonstrates an excessive fear-driven avoidance but also manifests the complication of fainting in the presence of the phobic situation.

Mr. B., a 32 year old solicitor, sought treatment because of fears that were preventing him from being present at the imminent birth of his child. He reports being terrified in situations even remotely associated with illness and injury. For example, he is unable to have injections, to have blood taken, or to even hear about sick people. He becomes very afraid in such situations, the fear being indicated by palpitations, sweating, dizziness, weakness in the muscles, nausea, and trembling. His primary concern when afraid is that he will faint. For this reason, he has avoided consulting a doctor for years even when sick. He also avoids visiting sick friends or family members, or even listening to descriptions of medical procedures, physical trauma, or illness. Recently, he has also started to decline legal cases that make mention of blood or injury. He dates the onset of his disorder to the age of 9 years, when his mother gave a detailed account of an operation to remove a skin blemish. He felt anxious and dizzy, he began to sweat profusely, and fainted. He recalls having great difficulty when receiving immunizations and other routine medical procedures through the rest of his childhood, as well as numerous fainting and near-fainting episodes throughout his adult years whenever he witnessed the slightest physical trauma, heard of an illness or injury, or saw a sick or disfigured person. He recently attempted to give blood, but while standing in the queue began to feel very warm, dizzy, and light-headed as he saw the people giving blood. He tried to distract himself but the next thing he remembered was waking disoriented upon the floor.

Differential diagnosis

In terms of differential diagnosis, other anxiety disorders and the psychoses need to be excluded. In panic disorder – and almost always in agoraphobia – the fear is of having a panic attack and not of some external stimulus. (However, the boundary between the disorders may not be as clear as previously thought;

Liebowitz et al., 1990; for a discussion see Chapter 4). In social phobia, the fear is of scrutiny and concomitant humiliation or embarrassment in defined social situations. In PTSD, the fear is often stimulus-specific, but the situations are related to a prior traumatic event outside the realm of normal experience. OCD can be distinguished from specific phobias primarily by the presence of the repetitive stereotyped behaviors (compulsions) and intrusive thoughts that are ego-dystonic (obsessions). Finally, a diagnosis of a psychotic disorder would be considered if the resistance of the fear to the possibility of correction was of delusional intensity.

Assessment

In addition to diagnosis, a thorough assessment is useful, primarily because assessment techniques are more sensitive to patient-specific characteristics relevant to treatment progress than are diagnostic labels. Since phobias may manifest in behavior (e.g., avoidance), cognitions (e.g., "the air might run out in a confined space"), and physiology (e.g., pounding heart), assessment devices have corresponded to these three domains. However, due to practical considerations, clinicians have tended to favor the cognitive and behavioral assessments.

Cognitive assessment

Frequently used cognitive measures have included self-ratings of fear and anxiety that have been found to be particularly sensitive to treatment changes (Sturgis and Scott, 1984). One way that self-reports have been formalized is with the Fear Thermometer (Walk, 1956) or a Subjective Units of Discomfort Scale (SUDs). The patient rates the level of subjective anxiety on a linear scale (e.g., 0 to 100). The ease with which this tool can be administered has meant that it has been readily incorporated into clinical practice. More formally, the types of fear a person has have been assessed with the Fear Survey Schedule (Bernstein and Allen, 1969), an instrument that provides an overall phobia rating, as well as an assessment of the different types of fear (e.g., agoraphobia, blood–injury, etc.).

While an examination of anxiety and tension are appropriate for most phobias, blood-injury phobia represents an exception because sufferers also experience feelings of faintness and may lose consciousness on occasions (Marks, 1988; Page, 1994b). To assess this pattern of symptoms the Blood–Injection Symptom Scale (Page et al., 1997) is a useful measure because it assesses the symptoms of faintness as well as two components of the construct of blood fear (i.e., anxiety and tension).

Behavioral assessment

Similarly, behavioral indices of anxiety have been found to be sensitive to treatment effects. The behavioral test most frequently used in clinical practice is some index of the person's ability to remain in the presence of the phobic object or situation. For instance, in a behavioral avoidance test, fear is assessed by measuring how close the person is able to get to the feared object, how long they can remain in the situation, and so on. This is usually combined with self-reports, such as the Fear Thermometer or a SUDs score. The cognitive assessment permits assessment of the perception of the amount of anxiety experienced during exposure tasks and behavioral avoidance tests. The combination of cognitive and behavioral indices in measuring specific phobias is important because the phobia may be associated with either avoidance (i.e., assessed via behavior), which may limit the experience of anxiety, or fear upon exposure to the object or situation (i.e., assessed via self-report). Obtaining cognitive and behavioral assessments will provide the clinician with important information for treatment. Following initial assessment, it will be clear what stimuli trigger the anxiety (both anticipating and during exposure) and what form the anxiety reaction takes. The treatment goal will be to reduce anxiety so that the person no longer meets diagnostic criteria for an anxiety disorder. The assessment information will provide quantitative feedback regarding progress towards that goal. However, etiology needs to be understood in order to identify which aspects of the disorder particular interventions target.

Etiology

Early conditioning and preparedness theories

Watson and Rayner (1920) reported that they were able to classically condition a fear in "Little Albert" by pairing a previously neutral stimulus (a tame white rat) with a loud noise. Their interpretation was that a neutral stimulus (the rat) was paired with an aversive stimulus (the noise). This produced a conditioned response (CR; a "fear" response) upon subsequent exposure to the rat. By extension, the obvious treatment implication was exposure to the feared stimulus in the absence of any aversive stimulus (i.e., extinction), or even in the presence of pleasant stimuli (i.e., counterconditioning). Cover-Jones extended these ideas in 1924 and successfully treated a phobia of rabbits using gradual in vivo exposure. Other successful exposure-based interventions were then developed (Wolpe, 1958). However, although theoretically consistent treatments were effective and theoretically consistent data became available, Seligman (1971) identified serious weaknesses in the simple conditioning account. Seligman noted that phobic fears were not evenly distributed across all possible stimuli. Phobias were most usually of the dark, water, heights, insects, or small animals. This clustering of fears would not have been predicted by a theory that all stimuli were equally conditionable. Since phobias tended to group around commonly feared objects and situations, Seligman searched for a common denominator. He suggested that typical phobic stimuli could all be considered a significant biological threat to the evolving ancestors of a species. Seligman (1971) suggested that certain associations were "prepared" – that is, they were more easily acquired than others. All associations can be placed on a continuum from highly prepared to highly contraprepared. For this reason, potentially phobic stimuli could be considered members of a class of highly prepared associations. They comprise a small nonarbitrary set of stimuli that signal the heightened probability of danger in a species' evolutionary history. Phobias and other instances of highly prepared learning would share similar characteristics. Phobic reactions: (1) would be out of proportion to the actual demands of the situation; (2) could not be reasoned away; (3) would be beyond voluntary control, rapidly acquired, and difficult to extinguish; and (4) would lead to actual or desired avoidance. Seligman's account inspired much research including that of Öhman and colleagues (Öhman et al., 1975a,b, 1976). In their human autonomic conditioning paradigm, Öhman et al. (1975a) paired two classes of stimuli with aversive stimuli. Their data suggested that physiological arousal conditioned to potentially phobic stimuli (e.g., snakes) was more resistant to extinction than physiological responses conditioned to neutral stimuli (e.g., flowers), paralleling the chronicity of specific phobias.

Difficulties with conditioning theories of phobias

Unfortunately, more recent studies have failed to demonstrate the increased speed of acquisition of fear to "prepared" stimuli that Seligman (1971) predicted. Furthermore, unlike the situation with a true phobia, informing participants that shocks were no longer to be delivered immediately abolished the conditioned response to fear-relevant stimuli (McNally, 1981). Another difficulty with the early and modified conditioning accounts is the incompatibility with retrospective reports of fear acquisition. For example, Di Nardo et al., (1988) reported that, while nearly two-thirds of dog phobics report a conditioning event, an equivalent number of nonphobics reported similar pairing of dogs with aversive events. Another serious difficulty with direct traumatic conditioning accounts is the data on vicarious acquisition of phobic fears (Rachman, 1990, 1991). For example, when a model is observed to react fearfully in the presence of an object, the observer may acquire the same fear reaction (Mineka, 1988). Direct conditioning accounts have difficulty explaining such findings (since the unconditioned stimulus is difficult to identify). One response has been to note that many of the criticisms of conditioning accounts (e.g., Menzies and Clarke, 1995) have been attacks on "stress-in-total-isolation" models (Mineka and Zinbarg, 1996). That is to say, the criticisms have been of a limited conditioning theory that fails to acknowledge the dynamic context within which organisms live. Outside the laboratory, organisms are rarely naïve with respect to threat-related stimuli, they have conditioning histories that influence subsequent learning, they respond to compound and contextual cues, and there are biological constraints on learning (see Mineka and Zinbarg, 1996; Forsyth and Chorpita, 1997). Mineka and Zinbarg (1996) argued convincingly that, when the dynamic context is taken into account, many of the apparent difficulties with conditioning theories disappear.

Another response to these difficulties has been to suggest that there must be a number of possible pathways to phobic fears. Rachman (1991) has identified three of these as conditioning, vicarious transmission, and verbal acquisition. The final common pathway in each of these three pathways is the acquisition of a representation linking the stimulus with a feared outcome or aversive event. Acknowledging such, it is possible to provide theoretical coherence by assimilating novel developments in conditioning theory.

Recent theories of phobias

Recently, some conditioning theories have undergone a conceptual shift (see Dickinson, 1980; Mackintosh, 1983; Rescorla, 1988). Classical conditioning was first conceptualized as a cortical process (Pavlov, 1927). The representation of a previously neutral or conditioned stimulus (CS) was activated simultaneously with a representation associated with some reflex. The previously neutral stimulus then came to elicit the CR. Classical conditioning was conceived as a simple, objectively defined, reflexive process. Recent evidence has challenged this position and provided a more useful picture of classical conditioning.

Two important findings challenged the simple idea of cortical coactivation as critical for classical conditioning. Rather than contiguity between stimuli, it is proposed that there must be a contingency (Rescorla, 1968) between the CS and the unconditioned stimulus (US), such that the former can be considered in some fashion to signal the occurrence of the US. By way of explanation, Kamin (1968) demonstrated that once an organism learns that one CS is predictive of a US, it fails to learn about other stimuli now equally predictive of the US. If, therefore, organisms are active information seekers determining probable causes of significant events by identifying plausible contingent relationships, then conditioning is a specific form of problem solving – solving the question "What 'caused' some significant event?".

By extrapolation, the three pathways to fear (Rachman, 1991) can be conceptualized as different ways to acquire belief about contingent relationships. First, the organism may acquire the knowledge of a contingent relationship via direct experience. Second, in vicarious acquisition the organism perceives the model reacting fearfully and learns that the stimulus is subsequently to be avoided and feared. Third, verbal transmission can likewise be considered to convey contingent relationships. Therefore, a more cognitive view of conditioning (Rapee, 1991a) permits speculation that each of the different pathways to fear shares the feature of permitting a person to acquire a belief about the existence of fear-relevant contingencies.

In addition to the cognitive shift in models of phobias, there has been a shift in emphasis within etiological models towards assimilating components from etiological models of panic disorder and agoraphobia. Panic attacks are now seen as the primary trigger for the development of agoraphobic avoidance (Clum and Knowles, 1991). Panic attacks themselves are believed to originate from a misfiring of an "alarm reaction" (i.e., the flight or fight response) in vulnerable individuals (Barlow, 1988; Andrews, 1991; Franklin, 1991). High trait anxiety decreases the threshold for the activation of the flight or fight response. Various other factors, such as stress and exposure to anxiety-provoking stimuli, likewise decrease the threshold of activation. As a consequence, the alarm reaction may be triggered by certain stimuli. When the stimulus signals a real danger, Barlow (1988) called the alarm a true alarm. When the stimulus does not signal a real danger, the stimulus is called a false alarm.

Consistent with these ideas, specific phobias show some similarities to agoraphobia. For instance, some specific phobias develop following the occurrence of an alarm reaction. Munjack (1984) noted that 20% of driving phobias followed a true alarm reaction (e.g., an automobile accident) and 40% followed a false alarm reaction (e.g., a panic attack while driving). That is to say, although having a panic attack while driving is doubtlessly a frightening experience, it is a false alarm in the sense that the initial occurrence of anxiety has not been triggered by a readily identifiable threatening stimulus, as in the case of an automobile accident. Consistent with the notion that some specific phobias are learned alarm reactions to particular objects and situations, panic control treatments appear to be useful in the treatment of phobias (Rygh and Barlow, 1986, and Zarate et al., 1988, both cited by Warren and Zgourides, 1991). Furthermore, animal phobics have been reported to fear the consequences of panic more than they fear the attack of the animal (McNally and Steketee, 1985).

Putting these various pieces of evidence together, specific phobias can be conceptualized as instances of the flight or fight response being triggered inappropriately or excessively in the presence of specific objects or situations. The fear may have its origins in an accurate appraisal of a past dangerous event (e.g., a car accident) or an inaccurate but threatening appraisal of an innocuous event (e.g., a panic attack). The direct (e.g., conditioning) and indirect (verbal or vicarious transmission) pathways involve a cognitive representation of the knowledge (not necessarily accessible to conscious awareness; Mattick et al., 1995) that certain stimuli will probably bring about (or predict) certain aversive – and, hence, feared – outcomes. The aversive outcomes, previously considered only as potentially painful events, can probably now be extended to include other aversive events, such as panic attacks.

The more recent conceptualization of specific phobias as a function of a tendency to have false alarms suggests that a component of the etiology may lie in a threshold to anxiety (e.g., elevated neuroticism). These questions have been addressed using methodologies in behavioral genetics. Various twin studies have merged on a common conclusion: there is good evidence that: phobias exhibit a heritable component (Torgersen, 1979; Phillips et al., 1987); the degree of heritability varies with feared stimulus (Rose and Ditto, 1983); and a single genetic factor accounts for most of the genetic covariance (Phillips et al., 1987). Consistent with this finding, Kendler et al. (1992a) have found evidence that, although specific phobias involve genetic factors predisposing an individual to all phobic disorders, unique environmental factors are particularly important in the etiology of some specific phobias to a greater degree than others.

In summary, a general neurotic predisposition may underly phobic disorders generally, but the specific phobias involve unique phobia-specific environmental factors to a greater degree than do other phobias. However, there are some recent data to complicate this picture. It has been found that, unlike inherited trait anxiety, the heritable component of the etiology of specific phobias does not increase the risk for other anxiety disorders (Fyer et al., 1990). This finding is consistent with the relatively low comorbidity with other anxiety disorders (see below) and suggests that, while a general anxiety proneness may predispose an individual to specific phobias, unique environmental factors and unique genetic factors may also contribute to the etiology. By way of speculation, it may even be the case that specific phobics who fear the anxiety response (McNally and Steketee, 1985) have relatively high trait anxiety (similar to agoraphobia), while specific phobias involving fear of the consequences of contact with the phobic object have a relatively greater share of the heritable component unique to specific phobias and the phobia-specific environmental experiences.

Course and complications

Most phobias begin in childhood and early adolescence (Öst, 1987a) and the general impression is that, untreated, specific phobias exhibit a chronic course.

The extent of disruption to lifestyle is usually a function of the ease with which the phobic situations can be avoided. However, the proportion of childhood phobias is much greater than that found in the adult population. As children mature, many phobias tend to remit without professional treatment. The typical age of onset varies across the different (adult) phobias. The most obvious difference is between claustrophobia and the remainder of the specific phobias (Öst, 1987a). Claustrophobia tends to develop after adolescence (age 20 years), whereas the other phobias tend to develop before or during adolescence. Animal phobias develop around age 7 years, blood phobia around age 9 years, and dental phobias around age 12 years. It has been suggested that the difference between claustrophobia and the other specific phobias reflects a descriptive and possibly functional overlap between claustrophobia and agoraphobia (Klein, 1981; Öst, 1987a). Claustrophobia may reflect a form of panic disorder in which the agoraphobic avoidance is limited to enclosed spaces (see Chapter 4).

Prevalence

The fears of a person with a specific phobia focus upon a specific object or situation: most typically animals, insects, confinement, water, heights, storms, or blood and injury. While the estimated prevalence varies with the feared situation (Agras et al., 1969; Myers et al., 1984; Öst, 1987a) and culture (Raguram and Bhide, 1985), it is approximately 8% (with a male/female ratio: 1 : 1.7; Burns, 1980), with less than 1% of these individuals seeking treatment (Agras et al., 1969; Regier et al., 1990).

Comorbidity

The general pattern among anxiety disorders is for individuals assigned a primary anxiety diagnosis to exhibit a number of additional anxiety diagnoses. Specific phobias exhibit this tendency to the smallest degree of all the anxiety disorders. For instance, Sanderson et al. (1990) found that their sample was split between those who had specific phobia alone and those who had one additional diagnosis. The most common additional diagnoses were social phobia and dysthymia. In contrast, individuals with a primary diagnosis of another anxiety disorder were likely to report a specific phobia as a comorbid diagnosis (Barlow et al., 1986b; de Ruiter et al., 1989). Therefore, individuals with specific phobias tend to report relatively few comorbid diagnoses, yet individuals with other anxiety disorders will tend to report comorbid specific phobias.

Summary

Specific phobias are fears of circumscribed objects or situations. The fear reaction is so distressing or the situation is believed to signal such danger that the individual avoids the phobic object. Such phobias are acquired early in childhood and – if they have not remitted by early adulthood – will tend to persist. The reasons for the phobia persisting may lie in the early traumatic learning experiences a person may have had or it may persist because the person becomes distressed by the fear reaction. Either way, if the phobic object cannot be easily avoided, the phobia will interfere with the person's life to a degree frequently underestimated by clinicians.

13

Specific phobias

Treatment

A successful treatment for specific phobias should decrease the fear-driven avoidance behavior. Coupled with reducing the avoidance are two related problems. First, some phobics do not avoid feared situations, but endure them with distressingly high levels of anxiety. More recent etiological accounts have suggested that some specific phobics fear the anxiety (and its imagined consequences) as much as others fear the phobic object (and its imagined consequences). The second difficulty in decreasing avoidance is that specific phobics typically exhibit anticipatory anxiety; either worrying about an inevitable contact with the feared object or situation or worrying about the possibility of contact with what is feared. Therefore, a successful treatment will also reduce the amount of anxiety experienced during exposure and in anticipation thereof. In summary, an effective treatment will reduce (1) the level of anxiety triggered by exposure to feared objects, (2) the level of anticipatory anxiety, and (3) the extent of avoidance.

Nondrug treatments

Nondrug treatments of the specific phobias can be divided into two categories: behavioral and cognitive treatments. Before discussing these empirically-validated treatments, it is worth addressing a treatment that has appeared recently in the literature. Eye Movement Desensitization and Reprocessing (EMDR) was initially developed in the context of PTSD, but it has been applied to specific phobias. Muris and Merckelbach have conducted three controlled trials of EMDR (Muris and Merkelbach, 1997; Muris et al., 1997, 1998). Despite some methodological concerns (Cahill et al., 1999) the strongest conclusions that can be supported from these studies are that exposure is an effective method for reducing self-reported fear and avoidance behavior, EMDR shows no evidence of being able to reduce avoidance behavior and there is occasional support that EMDR reduces self-reported fear. Thus, outside a research context, it would seem negligent to attempt a trial of EMDR for specific phobias before a comprehensive attempt at in vivo exposure has been conducted.

Returning to the behavioral and cognitive treatments, in clinical practice both components are combined to varying degrees. However, in order to evaluate the unique and combined contributions of each, it is useful to discuss the interventions separately.

Behavioral treatments

A learning-based etiological model suggests that treatment should involve extinction or exposure to the feared stimulus in the absence of the feared consequences. Such exposure has been widely demonstrated to be a rapid and effective treatment of specific phobias (Emmelkamp, 1979; O'Brien, 1981; Butler, 1989b). Exposure should be repeated as frequently as possible. Chambless (1990) suggested that sessions should be scheduled between daily and weekly, although Öst (1989) has found that treatment retains its efficacy if sessions are prolonged. The research literature also suggests that exposure exercises need to be clearly specified and of sufficient duration for anxiety to decrease substantially (Watson et al., 1971; Marks, 1975, 1978; Stern, 1978). Exposure in vivo is probably more effective than in imagination (Marks, 1978; Gelder, 1979), but both can reduce phobic concerns (Mathews et al., 1981). It is also preferable to use exposure exercises that are organized into a hierarchy of increasing difficulty, with each item being attempted as it becomes challenging but not overwhelming (Dryden, 1985). Although outcome studies comparing graded exposure and flooding (ungraded exposure) indicate similar effectiveness (Sturgis and Scott, 1984), clients appear more comfortable with graded exposure and are more likely to complete treatment (see Clarke and Jackson, 1983; Barlow, 1988).

Of the behavioral techniques available, each can be organized on a dimension reflecting the degree to which anxiety buffering is available. At one extreme is flooding. Flooding involves presentation of the most anxiety-provoking object or situation, usually with the therapist present (Sherry and Levine, 1980). This is continued until anxiety has dissipated. Implosive therapy can be considered similar to flooding except that it occurs in imagination. In practice, the therapist describes the feared scene as dramatically and vividly as possible, continuing until anxiety dissipates (for further details, see Levis and Hare, 1977). A technique involving greater buffering of anxiety is participant modeling (Denney et al., 1977). The therapist demonstrates approach and contact with the phobic object and subsequently encourages the patient to do likewise. The exposure tasks are ordered in a graduated manner. Finally, at the other end of the continuum to flooding, is systematic desensitization (Wolpe, 1958; Goldfried and Davison, 1976). The client is taught progressive muscle relaxation (Jacobson, 1962), hierarchy construction, and graduated imaginal presentation of scenes. The patient then engages in graduated imaginal exposure to feared situations, using relaxation to keep anxiety at minimal levels. Thus, potentially effective exposure-based treatments can be organized in terms of the amount of anxiety buffering included. A thorough assessment prior to hierarchy construction will indicate the amount of anxiety buffering necessary to optimize client participation and therefore which form of exposure to use.

Two issues of importance concern the type of exposure used and the duration of exposure. First, considering the type of exposure, systematic desensitization has a demonstrated efficacy in the treatment of specific phobias (Curtis et al., 1976), although there are suggestions (Barlow, 1988) that in vivo exposure is preferred to imaginal exposure. This conclusion is based on studies that have reported a superiority of performance-based treatments (Emmelkamp and Wessels, 1975). However, these data need to be interpreted in the light of other studies that failed to find such differences (Öst, 1978; Bourque and Ladoucer, 1980). A further difficulty with imaginal exposure is evidence that the transfer of learning to real-life situations is less than perfect. A second important issue is the duration of time spent in the presence of the phobic object or situation. Generally, it is found that longer exposures are preferred to shorter exposures, even though specific phobics' fears decrease faster than those of people with other anxiety disorders (Foa and Kozak, 1985). However, Rachman et al. (1986) compared the outcome of agoraphobics who remained in the presence of their phobic object with a group who were permitted to escape when anxiety reached a certain level. According to an operant conditioning account of the maintenance of phobic avoidance, it would be predicted that the anxiety reduction following escape would negatively reinforce avoidance and therefore be counterproductive. In fact, the escape did not appear to reinforce avoidance behavior, suggesting that alternative or additional mechanisms are operating during exposure. Rachman et al. (1986) suggest that the permission to escape and return provided a sense of safety and self-control that facilitated fear reduction. This process would be similar to systematic desensitization, where the person is allowed to resume relaxation whenever anxiety rises beyond a certain level. However, it is also possible that the exposure (with or without escape) is therapeutic because it serves to enhance self-efficacy (Williams et al., 1985; Hoffart, 1995). In support of this position, Penfold and Page (1999) found that a distracting conversation reduced within-session anxiety to a greater degree than did a conversation that focused on the feared stimulus, and that the therapeutic effect of distraction during in vivo exposure appeared to operate by enhancing the perceived control over anxiety. Although this effect was limited to within-session anxiety, Oliver and Page (2002) have replicated these effects across multiple sessions and found that the perceived control over anxiety continues to climb when the exposure sessions have been terminated, but only for people in the exposure plus distraction condition.

Dangers of behavioral treatments

There can be dangers associated with behavioral treatments. The chief pitfall, inherent in the procedure, is the possibility of sensitization. A conditioning account suggests that exposure to the feared stimulus accompanied by the reduction in anxiety will decrease the amount of fear experienced in the future. Brief exposure, when the level of anxiety is not decreased, may sensitize the person, thereby increasing future levels of fear. The data of Rachman et al. (1986) suggest that this danger may not be as serious as previously thought. Their data may be taken to imply that the critical danger to avoid is exposure that elicits fear when the person feels an absence of control. It may be speculated that short exposures could be counterproductive if the person tries but fails to remain in the presence of the phobic object because of the intensity of their fear. On the other hand, short exposures may reduce subsequent anxiety when the person faces the feared object and learns that control is possible. A second danger with behavioral treatments is one that is uniquely associated with blood–injury phobia. Sufferers not only experience fear in the presence of the phobic stimuli, but on occasions may also faint. The unsuspecting therapist may find such an outcome frightening, but it can be more serious for the patient who may be injured. This issue and methods for dealing with fear-related fainting will be discussed in more detail below, in the context of blood–injury phobia.

Cognitive treatments

Recently, with the rise of cognitive explanations in clinical psychology, cognitive therapies have been advocated as effective treatments for phobias in their own right or combined with exposure-based strategies (see Oakley and Padesky, 1990). Given the cognitive view of conditioning, it is necessary to modify any cognitions that lead to the perception of possible contingencies and enhance anxiety. Although these conceptual changes could be considered to have blurred the distinction between cognitive and behavioral treatments, Last (1987) concluded that cognitive treatments in specific phobias do not yet have clear empirical support. It was argued that while studies with analogue populations are encouraging, when clinical samples have been examined (Biran and Wilson, 1981; Ladouceur, 1983) cognitive techniques initially appeared to be ineffective relative to behavioral interventions and added nothing in combination (Last, 1987). These results are unexpected, first, because cognitive theories (see Beck et al., 1985) predict that the modification of maladaptive cognitions would be an effective therapeutic strategy. Second, cognitive therapy appears to augment treatment effectiveness in other anxiety disorders (Mattick et al., 1990). At this early stage, it would be unwise to rule out the possibility that cognitive techniques enhance exposure-based therapies. Indeed, Marshall (1985) has found that coping self-statements enhanced the efficacy of exposure-based programs. Similarly, Emmelkamp and Felten (1985) reported that training in adaptive thinking (i.e., relabeling and reappraisal of feared situations) enhanced the efficacy of exposure-based programs. Therefore, the principal theories of specific phobias provide reasons why cognitive therapies should enhance behavioral treatments. There are also some data that can be considered preliminary demonstrations that cognitive therapy can enhance exposure-based programs in some instances. For these reasons, it would be premature either to strongly support or to strongly reject cognitive interventions in specific phobias.

Drug treatments

No psychotropic drug can yet be recommended as the treatment of choice in specific phobias (Fyer, 1987). Bernadt et al. (1980) reported that diazepam decreased anticipatory anxiety and avoidance whereas beta blockers inhibited somatic symptoms of anxiety. However, the results did not generalize to the subjective components of the phobic's concerns. There are a variety of studies showing some beneficial effects of benzodiazepines and beta blockers (Whitehead et al., 1978; Campos et al., 1984), but there is no strong evidence of a long-term reduction in symptoms following such treatment. Further, Zitrin et al. (1983) reported that the tricyclic antidepressant imipramine did not enhance a systematic desensitization program. As Barlow (1988) noted, the absence of clear indications of efficacy for the tricyclics for specific phobias is surprising given the benefits noted in other anxiety disorders. Future research may lead to a different conclusion. However, reviewing the current literature (see also Fyer, 1987), we find that exposure-based and not pharmacological interventions are the treatment of choice.

Combining drug and psychological treatments

Given that exposure-based programs are the treatment of choice, the next question is "Can pharmacological and behavioral interventions be combined to enhance treatment success?". Providing initial support, Hafner and Marks (1976) reported that exposure at peak blood levels of diazepam inhibited extinction, but exposure when blood levels were waning was associated with the greater decline in anxiety than exposure among patients given a placebo tablet. However, a more recent study extinguishing conditioned fear in rats found a dose-dependent relationship between levels of benzodiazepines and extinction (Bouton et al., 1990). The higher the blood levels, the less well extinction transferred to a subsequent test session. Thus, at present, benzodiazepines should be used with caution among those with specific phobias who are concurrently undergoing exposure-based therapies. Nevertheless, the issue is an important one because when they come for behavioral treatment many patients have already been prescribed benzodiazepine tranquilizers.

Blood–injury phobia

While discussion of treatment has so far been generally applicable to all specific phobias, concerns about blood and injury warrant separate consideration. Although exposure-based interventions are effective and appropriate (Connolly et al., 1976; Öst et al., 1984a), the frequently concomitant fainting (see Kleinknecht, 1987; Steptoe and Wardle, 1988) requires additional treatment and has led some to consider a separate etiology (see Marks, 1988; Kleinknecht and Lenz, 1989; Page, 1994b, 1998b). Specific phobics during exposure exhibit sympathetic arousal in the form of the flight or fight response. Unique to blood–injury phobia about 80% (Connolly et al., 1976; Öst et al., 1984a; Thyer et al., 1985) of sufferers in treatment exhibit initial sympathetic arousal followed by a rapid switch to parasympathetic arousal (the rate appears lower in community samples; Page, 1996; Bienvenu and Eaton, 1998). The concomitant decrease in heart rate and blood pressure may lead to "emotional fainting" (i.e., vasovagal syncope).

The clinician has a number of options in overcoming the complications that fainting presents. Marks (1988) suggested that exposure should be conducted with the client lying down. Öst and Sterner (1987) have suggested an alternative and much more practical treatment. Assuming that a rapid shift to parasympathetic arousal mediates vasovagal syncope, they train clients to tense various muscle groups in response to the first indication of syncope. They reported success with clients that was maintained over 6 months. In a comparison between applied relaxation and applied tension during exposure, they found similar results at 6-month follow-up but favored the latter because treatment took half the time (Öst et al., 1989). In a process study, Foulds et al. (1990) confirmed that applied tension did increase cerebral blood flow and the mechanism suggested by Öst and Sterner (1987) appeared to have merit.

Summary

Specific phobias are characterized by an excessive and distressing stimulus-bound fear reaction that leads to avoidance. Many people have phobias, but relatively few have a phobic disorder (i.e., the avoidance handicaps them in some way). When avoidance produces handicap, treatment is indicated. The treatment of choice will involve exposure to the feared object or situation, in a manner that progresses as quickly as possible while maintaining patient compliance. Anxiety-buffering techniques are useful to achieve this balance. Treatment should then progress rapidly and a successful outcome should be observed within six to eight sessions.

14

Specific phobias

Clinician Guide

Issues in assessment

A behavioral analysis should begin with a description of the phobic behavior and an analysis of the anxiety response and the associated avoidance. Next, the antecedents to the anxiety and avoidance can be identified and will typically involve the phobic object and situations that increase and decrease the amount of phobic behavior (e.g., the proximity of the object, the ease of escape, etc.). Finally, the consequences of the behavior should be examined. Most obviously, the reduction in anxiety associated with avoidance requires attention, but it is also useful to examine the effects that the anxiety and phobic avoidance have upon the individual's life and relationships.

Format of treatment

Although self-help programs can be used (Page, 1993), the treatment outlined may be delivered individually or in a group context. The major difficulty with group treatment is that, while phobias may be restricted to one object or situation, rarely will it be possible to select a group of individuals who exhibit the same phobic concerns and, even if this were possible, it is not apparent that these would be representative of phobics (Hofmann et al., 1997). Data regarding the treatment of mixed phobias in a group context are not yet available. For practical reasons, it seems preferable to select individuals with similar fears. Our group treatment runs over eight 3-hour sessions. The therapist begins by teaching anxiety-management strategies. This process involves working through the relevant sections in the Patient Treatment Manual regarding the nature of anxiety, hyperventilation control, relaxation, graded exposure, and straight thinking. Once the skills have been taught, the patient is assisted in constructing graded hierarchies so that exposure to feared stimuli can begin. Since this is the core component of the program, the remainder of the time is spent working through the identified steps to achieve the desired goals. Individual treatment is usually scheduled over four to eight treatment sessions.

Treatment process

Conceptually, the treatment program contained in the Manual involves two stages. The first stage involves teaching anxiety-management strategies. The second stage involves exposure to feared situations. The anxiety-management strategies are included to facilitate exposure to the feared stimuli. Therefore, the main issue regarding treatment process is how exposure is conducted. First, and foremost, it is essential to expose individuals to what they fear. For instance, fear of flying can be due to quite different core fears – fears of heights, losing control when unable to escape, crashing and dying, fear of being out of control, and so on. While traveling in an airplane may be the ultimate goal of all sufferers, the steps will be quite different depending on the fear. For instance, someone who fears crashing may feel less anxious in a large jet, while someone who fears being out of control may feel less anxious in a small propeller-driven airplane where the pilot is visible. A thorough behavioral analysis of the situations that trigger the fear and an assessment of the cognitions in the various situations will assist in addressing this.

The second issue in terms of conducting exposure for phobias generally is eliciting and maintaining motivation. Anxiety-disordered individuals appear to be well motivated for treatment, yet they are also ambivalent. They are afraid to confront feared situations; most have tried to do so and have failed. The task of the clinician is to ensure that the person's motivation for treatment is maximized and remains sufficient to propel the individual to a successful completion of the treatment program. The present section will discuss the issue of motivation in phobic disorders in general. The most extensive discussion of empirically based techniques to enhance motivation has been offered by Miller (e.g., Miller and Rollnick, 1991). He identified five general principles of motivational interviewing that can be used to motivate patients to engage in and complete a cognitive behavioral treatment program. The five principles are expressing empathy, developing discrepancy, avoiding argumentation, rolling with resistance, and supporting self-efficacy.

Expressing empathy

People who suffer from anxiety disorders frequently complain of being misunderstood. For example, take the panic experienced while confronting a feared object or situation. When sufferers bring themselves to describe their terrifying experience to another, they may be frustrated with the responses. Trite advice may be forthcoming ("You must be uptight; why don't you just relax?"), or even worse, sympathy is offered ("I've been anxious and panicky too, I understand how you must feel"). It is imperative that the individual feels, from the therapist's first utterance, that their complaint has been heard. An accurately empathic response reacts to the meaning and emotion expressed in a communication, all the time accepting the validity of the person's experience. Someone describing the experience of panic is usually trying to communicate an occurrence of fear perceived to be qualitatively different from any anxiety, worry, tension, fear, or "panic" that they have experienced before. By extension, the person is communicating that, although they have previously been able to manage anxiety in all its forms using various coping strategies, this is different. An accurately empathic response accepts the validity of the person's experience, leaving the person with the perception that the listener has heard what has been said. Consider the following:

Patient: When I'm facing my fear, all my rational thoughts go out the window.
Therapist 1: But you know the spider isn't dangerous.
Therapist 2: It makes it difficult to stop the fear when the worry becomes so overpowering.

The first therapist jumps in to offer premature reassurance. The person is not saying that they really believe that they are in danger, but that the anxiety appears to rob them of their rational powers. The second therapist responds to this comment by reflecting the meaning conveyed. It is the second response that will lead to the patient continuing the interaction having accurately perceived that the therapist has heard the communication.

Developing discrepancies

Accepting the validity of a person's experiences does not necessarily involve accepting that patients stay as they are. In direct contrast, the purpose of offering empirically validated treatments is to modify maladaptive cognitions and behavior. Miller and Rollnick (1991) argued persuasively that vigorous confrontation leads to alienation of the patient. That is to say, while the goal may be to produce an awareness of the need for change, direct verbal challenges may not be the best way to achieve this (Miller and Page, 1991). Alternatively, they suggest developing a discrepancy between the person's current behavior (and its consequences) and future goals. By drawing attention to where one is – in relation to where one wants to be – it is possible to increase awareness of the costs of a maladaptive behavioral pattern. One satisfactory way to develop discrepancies between current behavior and future goals is to inquire about what the person would most enjoy doing when unshackled from his or her anxiety disorder. When this image (or images) has been developed, it can be contrasted with the person's present state. The resulting discomfort can then be used to motivate the person to engage in therapeutic exercises.

Avoiding argumentation

Once a person initiates treatment and begins to comply with the components of the program, setbacks invariably occur. Patients may refuse to engage in the next step on their hierarchy or they may not complete homework assignments. An unsatisfactory way for a therapist to respond is to harass the person to complete the exercise or berate their noncompliance. Miller and Rollnick (1991) suggested that it is more profitable to avoid argumentation. They encourage the perception that therapeutic resistance is a signal of therapist, rather than patient, failure. When a person refuses to complete an assignment, it is time to stop forcing the point and shift strategy. The therapist has a problem that they must take the responsibility to solve. The shift towards problem solving enables the therapist and patient to avoid argumentation and overcome the difficulty, and is a critical part of rolling with the resistance.

Rolling with resistance

Therapeutic resistance may signal a lack of understanding of the reason for part of the program or it may indicate a lack of success with one of the treatment components. Resistance may also indicate a weakening of resolve, indicating the need for the therapist to develop a discrepancy to once again enhance motivation. Whatever the case, the therapist must backtrack and solve the problem. Regardless of the origin of the difficulty, it is necessary to avoid argumentation and roll with resistance. The therapist can extract from the complaint or refusal a foundation of motivation upon which to rebuild the treatment. The best way to illustrate this otherwise vague concept is by example.

Patient: I'm having a bad day. I don't think that I can do today's assignment.
Therapist 1: You have to face your fears. Remember, avoidance makes fears worse. You will just have to go out and do it.
Therapist 2: When we planned the assignment yesterday, you felt that it was achievable. How are you going to get yourself to be able to achieve the task?

Both therapists have the same goal in mind – they want to motivate the person to complete the agreed assignment. The first therapist pursues this goal by reinforcing good reasons for attempting the assignment. Even though the reasons are valid, they are suboptimal for two reasons. First, they encourage refusal from the patient, leading to a possible confrontation. Second, the response indirectly encourages dependence upon the therapist for the recruitment of motivation necessary for task completion. The second therapist encourages the patient's autonomy by asking the person to find a solution. While the therapist would obviously provide assistance, the goal is for the patient to identify why the task is no longer achievable and how these obstacles can be overcome. As part of rolling with resistance, it is useful to implicitly convey the expectation that the patient has the resources necessary to achieve the task. For this reason, the second therapist did not ask how the task could be made more simple (which may implicitly convey that the task is too difficult), but shifts attention towards how the task can be achieved. While the latter approach may involve breaking the step into a series of graded easier steps, the therapist conveys an expectation that the task is achievable.

Supporting self-efficacy

Resistance in therapy for phobias often follows a setback. At such times, self-efficacy decreases as the person feels that successful mastery is no longer an achievable goal. In working with a patient to overcome fearful avoidance, it is particularly important to reverse decreases in self-efficacy. Central to supporting self-efficacy is conveying the principle that change is possible. This has already been alluded to in the context of rolling with resistance but there are three critical times when the possibility of change needs to be explicitly communicated. First, at the start of therapy it is essential to communicate a positive and realistic expectation of therapeutic change. The second time when self-efficacy must be supported is during setbacks. At these times, when the patient is demoralized and possibly resistant to therapeutic interventions, it is necessary to solve any problems while conveying the belief that change is still possible. The third time when self-efficacy must be particularly supported is at the termination of treatment. At these times clients are often worried about how they will fare without the support of the therapist and other group members. This difficulty can be tackled by reminding patients that the gains during treatment were due to their efforts. In addition, it is our practice to offer ongoing regular follow-up meetings.

Problem solving

Cognitive behavioral treatment of specific phobias involves encouraging patients to confront their fears until anxiety substantially decreases. To achieve this aim it is necessary to be able (1) to enhance motivation for treatment, (2) to enhance treatment comprehension and compliance, and (3) to successfully handle criticisms and difficulties presented by patients during treatment. The present chapter describes some ways to maximize compliance, and hence success, with cognitive behavioral treatment programs for specific phobias.

Enhancing motivation for treatment

It is very easy to underestimate the fear associated with the confrontation of phobic situations. Frequently, we are reminded of the difficulty when patients burst into tears when just asked to consider items to include in a graded hierarchy.

No matter how motivated the patient is upon presentation for treatment, confronting feared objects and situations erodes the best intentions. While motivational interviewing as applied to phobic disorders has been discussed above, a few points of particular relevance to specific phobias are in order. In terms of expressing empathy, people who suffer from specific phobias are ambivalent. They know their fear to be excessive, yet they simultaneously fear something about the object or situation. It is important to convey an understanding of the ambivalence. An accurately empathic response accepts the validity of a person's experience, leaving a perception that the listener has heard what has been said. For example:

Patient: Why can't I get into an elevator? Even kids can do it, but I just get scared.
Therapist 1: Phobias are irrational. There is no reason at all to be scared in elevators, is there?
Therapist 2: Although other people can travel in elevators without displaying anxiety, it is restricting when your worries stop you getting in the elevator.

The first response is not ideal because it dismisses any ambivalence. Elevators per se cannot cause anxiety; therefore, there must be a mediating variable. One plausible hypothesis is that catastrophic cognitions are important (Warren and Zgourides, 1991). It is this hypothesis that the second therapist pursues. The therapist acknowledges the anxiety and its incapacitation, but draws attention to the role of worrying thoughts. It would not be unusual for the patient to respond by identifying the worries that are harbored about elevators (e.g., it may break down, it may plummet to the ground, etc.). More importantly, the therapist has drawn attention to the ambivalence, that although the person knows the situation to be relatively safe nevertheless anxiety occurs.

Enhancing treatment comprehension and compliance

Once motivation for treatment has been recruited and the patient begins to learn, practice, and implement the treatment techniques, it is the therapist's task to ensure that obstacles to progress are managed effectively. Hindrances to treatment comprehension and compliance can be grouped according to (1) problems in education, (2) problems with slow breathing, (3) problems with relaxation, (4) problems with graded exposure, and (5) problems with cognitive restructuring. These issues have been discussed in Chapter 6 but problems with graded exposure and with relaxation require further discussion.

Problems with graded exposure

When patients are taught anxiety-management techniques, it is essential for them to be encouraged to face their fears as soon as possible. Without confrontation of feared situations, patients may accept the theory of the treatment program but remain skeptical about the ability of the techniques to help them to overcome their fears. It is only when an individual is successfully able to control anxiety that the treatment is perceived to be credible. In addition, the sooner the patient comes to this realization, the easier treatment becomes. No longer do therapeutic efforts need to be directed towards defending the treatment rationale; instead, therapy can be focused upon how the person can use the techniques to master fear as quickly as possible. The place to begin graded exposure to feared situations is with hierarchy construction, which in turn begins with a clear identification of the patient's fear. In order to expose an individual to their fears, it is essential that these fears are clearly identified. Only then can a series of ordered steps be developed to help the person to gradually face the fear. Unfortunately there are no shortcuts. The most helpful strategy is to allow patients to guide their own exposure tasks and construct their own hierarchies.

One common difficulty in constructing a hierarchy is the patient who wants to dispense with steps along the way, going immediately to the most feared situation. The patient may be impatient and therefore unwilling to "waste time" breaking down the goal. In contrast to our practice in panic disorder and agoraphobia, where we may encourage attempting difficult items of a hierarchy if the person has lost the fear of panic, our practice with specific phobias is different. If individuals have failed to conquer their fears in the past through self-directed flooding, we recommend a different approach. We draw attention to past failures and suggest that, in the long-term, graded exposure really will be the most time efficient. We make this choice because specific phobias sufferers have generally chosen flooding not because they believe that they can control their fears but in the hope that they can get it all over quickly. Nevertheless, we stress that this is our current clinical practice and we wait to be guided by data that may become available in the future. In contrast to these apparently fearless patients are the more common individuals who wish to progress too slowly. In fact, it has been found that the majority of phobic patients overestimate the amount of anxiety that they will experience in a given situation (Rachman and Bichard, 1988). In dealing with this difficulty there is no simple solution. The principle for handling the problem is to elicit from the patients reasons why they think they cannot achieve a more difficult step. They may be lacking resolve and commitment; therefore, motivational interviewing is necessary. They may lack confidence in the ability of the techniques to control fear; therefore, greater successful practice of the techniques is warranted. They may believe that the situation truly represents a danger; therefore, these thoughts need to be explored and modified using cognitive restructuring techniques.

Another difficulty, often encountered early in treatment, is the failure of fear to decrease despite repeated exposure to feared situations. Once again, this difficulty can be resolved only by examining the person's behavior and cognitions during the exercise. However, one common reason for the failure of anxiety to decrease is attempting a task that elicits too much anxiety. In such a situation, it will take a long time for anxiety to decrease, longer than most individuals are prepared to wait. We find that our patients are usually prepared to wait only minutes for anxiety to decrease. Therefore, if a less anxiety-provoking exercise is selected, the probability of anxiety decreasing in the time available is increased. In addition, if anxiety-management strategies (i.e., slow breathing, relaxation, and cognitive restructuring) are used, anxiety will decrease faster than it otherwise would, thereby assisting exposure.

Problems with relaxation

As a complement to slow breathing, the Patient Treatment Manual presents relaxation as an anxiety-management technique. We teach progressive muscle relaxation to help patients to recognize tension and to help them to relax their bodies totally. We teach isometric relaxation as a quick relaxation strategy to be used to reduce muscle tension in phobic situations when progressive muscle relaxation is not possible. As a result, people are encouraged to use progressive muscle relaxation to reduce general levels of tension before facing their fears and isometric relaxation to attempt to maintain a relaxed state (even during graded exposure). One frequently encountered difficulty with relaxation is relaxation-induced anxiety (Heide and Borkovec, 1984). While relaxing, some patients become very anxious and even panicky. Following such an episode, it is difficult to encourage patients to persevere with relaxation training. Therefore, it is useful to address the possible reaction before beginning relaxation exercises. Patients can be taught what may happen to them during relaxation and what feelings to expect so that the experience is less disquieting. One experience that frequently causes concern is the feeling that one's mind is wandering from topic to topic in a seemingly unbridled manner. It is helpful to reframe this experience as a sign that relaxation is occurring: during the flight or fight response the mind becomes focused; during relaxation, it becomes less focused.

Handling patient complaints and difficulties in treatment implementation

In addition to general difficulties during treatment, patients will often make statements about the treatment or their condition that require a response. Some common comments and possible answers are detailed in the following section.

"I have had cognitive behavioral therapy before." Consistent with a motivational interviewing approach it is best not to attempt to defend one's therapeutic skill or highlight how one's own therapy is different. If true, both of these will become evident as treatment progresses. It is more useful to express empathy and model a problem-solving approach. For example, the therapist can inquire

about why they believed that the treatment failed in the past, or what motivated them to seek further cognitive-behavioral therapy when it failed in the past.

"My fear is reasonable." It is not uncommon to find a patient refusing to expose themselves to a particular feared situation because they believe that their fear is reasonable. For instance, someone may refuse to enter a train because, if the air conditioning failed, the air would be unable to enter and they would suffocate. It is necessary to challenge these beliefs using the cognitive restructuring techniques described in the Patient Treatment Manual.

"Irrational thoughts come too quickly to challenge when anxious." This is one of the most frequently encountered difficulties with cognitive therapy with phobias. A technique useful in overcoming the problem is to encourage the person to write down their irrational and maladaptive thoughts after being in the situation and then to write down challenges to the thoughts. Writing the thoughts down enables the person to focus attention upon individual worrying thoughts rather than mentally hopping from one maladaptive thought to another. Each new thought can then be evaluated against the criteria: (1) is the thought believable? and (2) is the thought anxiety-reducing? Encouraging a post hoc analysis of thoughts develops a problem-solving approach to setbacks and allows the person to develop rational, accurate self-statements that can be used to tackle a re-emergence of the maladaptive thoughts.

"I am obsessed with anxiety management, I cannot do relaxation, slow breathing, and cognitive restructuring forever." In the early stages of learning to stop anxiety spiraling during graded exposure, patients become preoccupied with the various techniques. Frequently, they feel overwhelmed with the number of tactics they must use. It is useful to remind patients of times when they acquired other skills (e.g., driving). Progress was slow and required complete concentration. Managing anxiety is no different, but, in the same way as driving becomes automatic, with persistence patients will be able to learn to control anxiety with minimal effort.

"I have relapsed." Patients often fear, and are frequently troubled by, setbacks that occur after treatment has been terminated. We have resolved this difficulty by scheduling monthly evening follow-up meetings. These are open for any patient who has completed treatment to attend, at any time, without an appointment. There are various advantages to this procedure. Primarily, it is time efficient for therapists, since individuals who call at other times or seek additional appointments can be encouraged to attend the next follow-up meeting. Since follow-up meetings are conducted in groups, appointments are not necessary and patients are comforted with the knowledge of the permanently available "safety net". Being conducted in groups means that patients can benefit from the opportunity to talk to other people who have had similar

setbacks. The meetings serve to remind patients of what was taught in the program and motivate each individual to re-engage the treatment techniques.

General summary

Conducting treatment for specific phobias requires a thorough understanding of the science behind the disorder and its treatment. If individuals with phobic disorders are gently encouraged to face their fear, after being taught to manage anxiety, it appears that compliance increases and exposure to feared situations can reduce anxiety and provide a context in which maladaptive cognitions can be modified.

15

Specific phobias

Patient Treatment Manual*

This Manual is both a guide to treatment and a workbook for persons who suffer from specific phobias. During treatment, it is a workbook in which individuals can record their own experience of their disorder, together with the additional advice for their particular case given by their clinician. After treatment has concluded, this Manual will serve as a self-help resource enabling those who have recovered, but who encounter further stressors or difficulties, to read the appropriate section and, by putting the content into action, stay well.

Contents

SECTION 1

1 The nature of anxiety and phobias

A phobia is a particular type of fear. Just as people fear many things, there is a large range of things people can be phobic about. However, a phobia is different from a fear for three reasons. The first difference is that the fear is intense and includes many of the following sensations:

- Bodily sensations
  - Heart racing
  - Sweating
  - Trembling
  - Rapid breathing
  - Breathlessness or shortness of breath
  - Muscular tension
  - "Butterflies" in the stomach
  - Nausea
  - Weakness in muscles
  - Tingling in hands and feet
  - Hot and cold flushes
  - Tight or sore chest
- Actions
  - Feeling like fleeing or doing so
  - Feeling frozen to the spot
  - Crying or screaming
- Thoughts
  - Fear
  - Worrying "what if . . ." something terrible happened
  - Embarrassed or irritated
  - Shame
  - Confused thinking
  - "Something might happen"
  - "This is dangerous" or "I might act in a dangerous way"

All of these actions, thoughts, and feelings are signs of fear and anxiety. It is important to note that, while they are unpleasant to experience, on their own they are not dangerous or life-threatening. We will discuss later why these experiences occur, but before we do, the second feature of a phobia needs to be described.

Phobias involve avoidance of what is feared or the object or situation is endured with distress. Because anxiety is unpleasant and people worry what might happen when they confront what they fear, people with phobias avoid the objects or situations that make them afraid. This avoidance may take many different and subtle forms, such as:

- Not going near the feared object or situation
- Escaping the situation
- Making excuses for not doing what scares you
- Imagining yourself somewhere else
- Thinking about something else
- Looking the other way
- Drinking alcohol or taking other drugs
- Taking antianxiety medications
- Seeking the presence of others
- Talking to the people you are with about anything

The final important characteristic of a phobia is that it seems unhelpful. As you may have found, people who do not have phobias have difficulty understanding those who do; they may say that the fears are silly, childish, and nonsensical. And, while you also know that the situation does not always involve a real danger, at another level you may believe that it could do so. You may even be able to agree with your family and friends and say that "I know that nothing will happen" but it doesn't help. There is still this other part of you that is afraid of a nagging doubt that says "What if..."

To summarize what we have covered so far, three things characterize phobias.

- First, there is an *intense fear* and anxiety about some object or situation.
- Second, there is an *avoidance* of the feared object or it is endured with great difficulty.
- Finally, there is a *conflict* between the knowledge that the situation is relatively safe and the belief that it may not be.

1.1 Rationale of the program

The program will focus on the three aspects of the phobia and you will be given skills that specifically target each of them. As such, the treatment is like a tripod. It requires all three legs to be present to stand firmly. This means that you will need to learn, practice, and keep using all of the techniques to control your anxiety. The three strategies that this program covers are techniques designed to help you (1) to control your physical sensations, (2) to face the things that you currently fear and avoid more comfortably, and (3) to modify what you say to yourself. (An optional module will cover skills that are relevant to controlling the fainting in the presence of blood and injury.)

It is important to realize that achieving control of anxiety is a skill that has to be learned. To be effective, these skills must be practiced regularly. The more you put in, the more you will get out of the program. It is not the severity of your fear or avoidance, how long you have had your phobia, or how old you are that predicts the success of the program. Rather, it is your motivation to change your reactions. Using all three techniques, you will be able to master your fear.

1.2 Anxiety: the life-saving alarm

People who have suffered with a phobia often become afraid of even small amounts of anxiety. But anxiety is useful.

Consider the following: a person is walking across a field that seems to be empty. Suddenly, a bull emerges, sees the walker, bellows, and then charges. The walker realizes the danger and starts running for the fence some distance away. Automatically, changes occur in the body so that the walker is able to run very quickly towards the fence.

Your brain becomes aware of danger. Immediately, adrenaline (epinephrine) is released to trigger the body's involuntary nervous system, which causes a set of bodily changes. Every change enables you to act quickly, avoid injury, and escape danger. By examining each of the changes in turn, the advantages of this alarm response can be made clear.

- Breathing speeds up and the nostrils and lungs open wider, increasing the oxygen available for the muscles.
- Heart rate and blood pressure increase so that oxygen and nutrients needed by the body can be taken quickly to where they are needed.
- Blood is sent to muscles. Less blood goes to areas that do not immediately need nutrition. For example, blood moves away from the face and you may "pale with fear".
- Muscles tense, preparing you to act quickly.
- Blood clotting ability increases so that blood loss will be minimized.
- Sweating increases to cool the body.
- The mind becomes focused. It becomes preoccupied with the thought "Where is the danger and how can I get to safety?".
- Digestion is put on hold. Your mouth dries as less saliva is produced. Food sits heavily in the stomach and nausea or "butterflies" may occur.
- Glucose is released into your blood to provide energy.
- The immune system slows down. In the short term, the body puts all of its efforts into escaping.
- Sphincter muscles around the bowel and bladder constrict so that no trail is left by which a predator could track you down.

It is the automatic activation of this flight or fight response that allows you to run and escape. The flight or fight response is an automatic reaction that will first lead you to flee from danger. When escape is impossible you will turn and fight for your life.

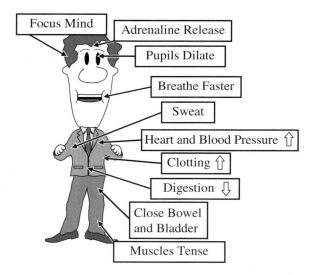

In contrast to this life-saving alarm, it is clear that not all anxiety is of the same intensity. The prospect of examinations or a job interview may increase anxiety but not usually to the same degree as if one were faced with a vicious dog. At these times the alarm is triggered, but to a lesser degree. Whatever the degree of anxiety experienced, it is controlled by the involuntary nervous system.

1.3 Anxiety: false alarms

Anxiety problems originate when the flight or fight response is too sensitive. Like an overly sensitive car alarm that goes off at the wrong time, when the body's anxiety alarm is too sensitive, the flight or fight response is triggered at the wrong times. If your anxiety alarm goes off too easily, you will be more likely to become anxious in situations where most other people would not feel anxious. If you have become anxious in situations in which other individuals would not be so anxious, it suggests that your anxiety "alarm" (the flight or fight response) is too sensitive. The alarm reaction, designed to protect you from charging bulls and other physical dangers, was triggered at the wrong time.

The flight or fight response is useful in the short term, especially if the danger can be avoided by physical exertion. But it is of no use in the long term and certainly of little use in most stressful situations in the modern world. It does not help to run when the traffic cop pulls you over and it doesn't help to fight physically when the boss threatens you. However, because the flight or fight response was useful when we were cavemen and cavewomen, it is still part of our bodily make up.

1.4 Why do I have false alarms?

If phobic fears are false alarms triggered because your flight or fight response is too sensitive, why do you have false alarms? Psychological research has revealed three causes of a sensitive anxiety alarm. The first is stress, which we all know can increase anxiety. The second is overbreathing (or hyperventilation), and we will discuss this soon. The third reason is your own history.

1.5 The effect of history and learning

One thing that stands out about phobias is the limited number of objects and situations that are feared when the total number of possible objects and situations is considered. Common phobias include:

- Fear of the dark
- Fear of heights
- Fear of animals (e.g., dogs, insects, and reptiles)
- Fear of enclosed spaces or being trapped
- Fear of blood and injury
- Fear of water

If you look over this list, one of the things that becomes obvious is that they are all sensible objects or situations to be wary of if one lived more as our predecessors did. For instance, those people who had a healthy respect for the dark would not venture into potentially dangerous caves, and so on. People who had these fears would be more likely to live to an age at which they could pass on the genes to their children. Over many years, human beings would all acquire a certain degree of fearfulness of these potentially dangerous objects and situations. In fact, children as a rule develop fears of the dark, heights, enclosed spaces, and so on. Thus humans seem to become afraid of objects and situations that have had the potential to be dangerous to humans for centuries. It is situations such as these that become the focus of a person's phobia.

Phobias then seem to arise in one of four ways. First of all, some people have terrible experiences with potentially dangerous objects and situations that cause them to develop a phobia. For instance, being bitten by a dog may be enough to cause a person to become afraid of dogs. Second, a person may witness a terrible experience happening to another and this may cause them to develop a phobia. For example, watching a person get bitten by a dog may be enough to start a phobia. Third, a person may acquire their fear by being given information. That is to say, being told about the terrible consequences that could arise from a dangerous object or situation may be enough to start a phobia. Finally, there are some people who find that their phobia has always been there. They cannot recall any event that started the phobia. Rather, for as long as they remember, they have always been afraid. It is possible that the trauma occurred at an early age and this explains the lack of memory. However, it is also possible that some people's fears have always been with them. Whichever one (or combination) of these causes started the phobia in the first place, what is now important is to identify what keeps the phobia going in the present.

We will discuss the factors that keep a phobia going as the program continues. However, by way of summary, it is clear that people with phobias worry more about the objects and situations that are the focus of their fear than others do and they worry more than is necessary. We will consider these worries and how to challenge them in Section 5. Another factor that maintains avoidance – fleeing from or never even facing what you fear. The problem is that avoidance helps in the short term, but in the long term it causes the phobia to grow. We will discuss avoidance and how to stop it causing phobias to grow in Section 4. Finally, phobic anxiety is excessive and unreasonable. Thus, by definition, the anxiety and fear is more intense than it should be. Two factors that we know can elevate anxiety and fear are muscle tension and overbreathing. We will consider muscle tension and how to combat it in Section 3, but for the time being we will turn our attention to overbreathing.

1.6 Role of hyperventilation

Having talked about why a phobia may have developed, we shall focus on one aspect of the flight or fight response of concern in phobias, namely overbreathing (or hyperventilation).

As we discussed in the context of the fight or flight response, the anxiety alarm involves an increase in breathing. This overbreathing can make many of the symptoms that occur in phobias much worse than they would be otherwise. These symptoms are important among people with phobias, because some people fear the occurrence of the anxiety reaction at least as much as they fear the danger in the feared situation.

Overbreathing has the power to make anxiety symptoms worse. Let us see how this can happen. The diagram shows how the major components of breathing link together.

Whenever we breathe in, oxygen goes into the lungs. The oxygen travels to the blood where it is picked up by an "oxygen-sticky" chemical. This oxygen-sticky chemical, called hemoglobin, carries the oxygen around the body. Oxygen is released by the hemoglobin for use by the body's cells. The cells use the oxygen and produce a waste product called carbon dioxide. The carbon dioxide is released back to the blood, taken to the lungs, and breathed out.

The puzzle is, if hemoglobin is "oxygen-sticky", then how did the oxygen become unstuck? What is the key that unlocks the oxygen? The key is carbon dioxide. Whenever the hemoglobin meets some carbon dioxide, the oxygen is

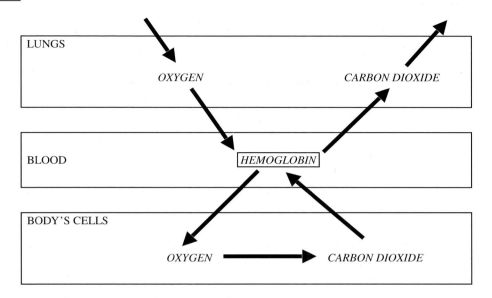

unlocked so that it can go into the body's cells. Therefore, while it is important to breathe in oxygen, it is just as important that there is carbon dioxide in the blood to release the oxygen. Overbreathing makes anxiety worse, not because you breathe in too much oxygen but because you breathe out too much carbon dioxide.

Breathing "too much" has the effect of decreasing the levels of carbon dioxide, while breathing "too little" has the effect of increasing levels of carbon dioxide. The body works best when there is a balance between oxygen and carbon dioxide. When you overbreathe, you end up with more oxygen than carbon dioxide in your blood. When this imbalance happens, a number of changes occur in the body.

One of the most important changes is a narrowing of certain blood vessels. In particular, blood going to the brain is somewhat decreased. Coupled together with this tightening of blood vessels is the fact that the hemoglobin increases its "stickiness" for oxygen. Thus less blood reaches certain areas of the body. Furthermore, the oxygen carried by this blood is less likely to be released to the cells. Paradoxically, then, while overbreathing means we are taking in more oxygen, we are actually getting less oxygen to certain areas of our brain and body. This results in two broad categories of sensations:

1. Some sensations are produced by the slight reduction in oxygen to certain parts of the brain. These symptoms include:
   • Dizziness
   • Light-headedness
   • Confusion

- Blurred vision
- Feelings of unreality

2. Some symptoms are produced by the slight reduction in oxygen to certain parts of the body. These symptoms include:

- Increase in heartbeat to pump more blood around
- Breathlessness
- Numbness and tingling in the extremities
- Cold, clammy hands
- Stiffness in the muscles

It is important to remember that the reductions in oxygen are slight and totally harmless.

Hyperventilation is also responsible for a number of overall effects. The act of overbreathing is hard, physical work. Hence, the individual may often feel hot, flushed, and sweaty. Because it is hard work to overbreathe, doing it for a long time can result in tiredness and exhaustion.

People who overbreathe often tend to breathe from their chest rather than their diaphragm. As the chest muscles are not made for breathing, they tend to become tired and tense. Thus these people can experience symptoms of chest tightness or even chest pains.

If overbreathing continues, a second stage of hyperventilation is reached. This produces symptoms such as:

- Severe vertigo
- Dizziness and nausea
- An inability to breathe freely
- A crushing sensation or sharp pains in the chest
- Temporary paralysis of muscles in different parts of the body
- Actual momentary loss of consciousness ("blackouts")
- Rising terror that something terrible is about to happen, for example, a heart attack, brain hemorrhage, or even death

The symptoms in the second stage of hyperventilation are produced by the body's automatic defence reaction to decreasing levels of carbon dioxide. This defence reaction forcibly restricts the person's breathing, allowing carbon dioxide levels to return to normal.

At the risk of repetition, the most important point to be made about hyperventilation is that it is not dangerous. Increased breathing is part of the flight or fight response and so is part of a natural biological response aimed at protecting the body from harm. Thus it is an automatic reaction for the brain to immediately expect danger and for the individual to feel the urge to escape.

Hyperventilation is often not obvious to the observer, or even to the persons experiencing it. It can be very subtle. This is especially true if the individual has been slightly overbreathing over a long period of time. In this case, there can be a marked drop in carbon dioxide but, because the body is able to compensate for this drop, symptoms may not be produced. However, because carbon dioxide levels are kept low, the body is less able to cope with further decreases and even a slight change of breathing (e.g., a sigh, yawn, or gasp) can be enough to trigger symptoms.

1.7 Types of overbreathing

There are at least four types of overbreathing that you should learn to recognize. The first three tend to be episodic and are probably more common among people with specific phobias. That is to say, they occur only during episodes of high anxiety, such as when you are exposed to what you fear. The other is habitual: it occurs most of the time and is essentially a bad breathing habit or style.

- *Panting or rapid breathing*: Such breathing tends to occur during periods of acute anxiety or fear. This type of breathing will reduce carbon dioxide levels very quickly and produce a rapid increase in anxiety.
- *Sighing and yawning*: Sighing and yawning tend to occur during periods of disappointment or depression and both involve excessively deep breathing.
- *Gasping*: Gasping occurs when people think of frightening things such as doing something that they have avoided for a long time.
- *Chronic or habitual overbreathing*: This type of breathing involves slight increases in depth or speed of breathing sustained over a long period. Generally, this happens during periods of worry. It is not enough to bring on a sense of panic, but leaves the person feeling apprehensive, dizzy, and unable to think clearly. If such people are placed in the presence of what they fear and increase their breathing even by a little, this may trigger panic.

The relationship between phobic triggers and hyperventilation is summarized in the diagram overleaf.

1.8 Common myths about anxiety symptoms

When fear is intense, people often worry about the possible consequences of extreme levels of anxiety. They may worry that anxiety will escalate out of control or that some serious physical or mental problem may result. As a result, the sensations themselves become threatening and can trigger the whole anxiety response again. This accounts for why many people with phobias fear being anxious as much as, and sometimes more than, the potential dangers in their feared situation. It is therefore important to review the common misinterpretations about anxiety that some people have.

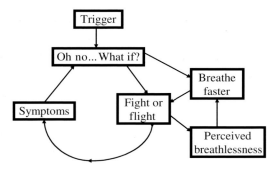

(Modified from Salkovskis, PM (1988) Hyperventilation and anxiety. *Current Opinion in Psychiatry*, **1**, 78.)

1.8.1 Going crazy

Many people fear they are going crazy when they experience the physical sensations of a panic attack. They may think they have the severe mental disorder called schizophrenia. However, schizophrenia and panic attacks are quite different. Panic attacks begin suddenly and tend to occur again and again. Schizophrenia begins gradually and once the symptoms are present, they do not come and go like panic attacks. The experience of panic is also quite different from that of schizophrenia. People with schizophrenia experience disjointed thoughts and speech, delusions or strange beliefs, and hallucinations. This is not the same as having your mind go blank or worrying about things that other people do not worry about. The strange beliefs might include the receiving of bizarre messages from outer space. Examples of hallucinations may be the hearing of voices that are not really there. Additionally, because schizophrenia runs strongly in families and has a genetic base, only a certain number of people can become schizophrenic and in other people no amount of stress will cause the disorder. Finally, people who develop schizophrenia usually show some mild symptoms for most of their adult lives. Thus, if this has not been noticed in you, then it is unlikely that you would develop schizophrenia. This is especially true if you are over 25 years of age, as schizophrenia usually first appears in the late teens to early 20s.

1.8.2 Losing control

Some people believe that they will "lose control" when they panic. Sometimes they mean that they will become totally paralyzed and not be able to move. Other times they mean that they will not know what they are doing and will run around wild, hurting people or swearing and embarrassing themselves. It is clear where this feeling may come from when you remember our discussion of the fight or flight response. Your body is ready for action when the anxiety response is triggered and there is often an overpowering desire to get away from any danger. The problem is that when you do not use the anxiety response to flee or fight, you may feel confused, unreal, and distracted. Nevertheless, you are still able to think and function normally. You are still able to decide what action to take in response to panic; that is, whether to stay or leave.

1.8.3 Heart attacks

Many people misinterpret the symptoms of the fight or flight response and believe that they must be dying of a heart attack. This is because most people have never experienced a heart attack and therefore never know how this differs from a panic attack. The major symptoms of heart disease include breathlessness and chest pain but these symptoms are generally related to effort and will go away fairly quickly with rest. This is very different from the symptoms associated with a panic attack that can happen at any time. Certainly panic symptoms can occur during exercise and feel worse with exercise, but they are different from a heart attack. Lastly, if a doctor has checked your heart with an electrocardiogram (a device that measures electrical changes in the heart) and has given you the "all clear", then you can safely assume that heart disease is not the cause of your attacks. Heart disease will produce very obvious changes in the electrical activity of the heart that are not produced during a panic attack.

1.8.4 Other fears

Another fear that individuals with certain types of phobia report is the fear of fainting. This is especially common among people who fear blood, injections, illness, and injury and will be discussed in greater detail later in the program.

SECTION 2

2 Control of hyperventilation

2.1 Recognizing hyperventilation

The first step in preventing and controlling hyperventilation is to recognize how and when you overbreathe.

Try monitoring your breathing rate now. Count one breath in and out as 1, the next breath in and out as 2, and so on. It may be difficult at first, but don't try to change your breathing rate voluntarily. Write the answer here ____. As part of treatment you will be required to monitor your breathing rate for 1 minute during various times of the day. The form in Section 2.3 should be used for this purpose. Now consider the following:

• Do you breathe too quickly? The average person only needs to take 10 to 12 breaths per minute at rest. If your rate of breathing is greater than this, then you must reduce it.

- Do you breathe too deeply? Does your chest sometimes feel overexpanded? You should breathe from the abdomen and through the nose, consciously attempting to breathe in a smooth and light way.
- Do you breathe from your chest? Sit with your arms folded lightly across your tummy and while breathing naturally observe your arms, chest, and shoulders. While all three will move, the main movement should be in your tummy if you are breathing correctly from your diaphragm.
- Do you sigh or yawn more than others? Become aware of when you sigh or yawn and avoid taking deep breaths at these times.
- Do you gasp or take in a deep breath when, for example, someone mentions what you fear? Taking one deep breath can trigger the hyperventilation cycle in many people.
- Do you breathe through your mouth? You are more likely to hyperventilate if you breathe through your mouth. Whenever you notice this, you should consciously revert to breathing through your nose.

2.2 Slow-breathing technique

This technique is to be used at first signs of anxiety or panic.

You must learn to recognize the first signs of overbreathing and immediately do the following:

- Stop what you are doing and sit down or lean against something.
- Hold your breath and count to 10 (don't take a deep breath).
- When you get to 10, breathe out and mentally say the word "relax" to yourself in a calm, soothing manner.
- Breathe in and out slowly in a 6-second cycle. Breathe in for 3 seconds and out for 3 seconds. This will produce a breathing rate of 10 breaths per minute. Mentally say the word "relax" to yourself every time you breathe out.
- At the end of each minute (after 10 breaths), hold your breath again for 10 seconds, and then continue breathing in the 6-second cycle.
- Continue breathing in this way until all the symptoms of overbreathing have gone.

If you do these things as soon as you notice the first signs of overbreathing, the symptoms should subside within a minute or two and you will not experience any panic attacks. The more you practice, the better you will become at using it to bring your phobic fear under control. Remember that your goal should always be to stay calm and prevent the anxiety and fear from developing into panic. You need to identify the very first symptoms of hyperventilation, and the moment you experience any of these, use the above slow-breathing techniques immediately.

2.3 Daily record of breathing rate

Instructions: Your breathing rate should be monitored at the times shown below unless you are performing some activity that will inflate your rate, such as walking upstairs. In this case wait for about 10 minutes. Try to be sitting or standing quietly when you count your breathing. Each breath in and out counts as 1: so, on the first breath in and out count 1; on the next breath in and out count 2, and so on. Count your breathing rate in this way for 1 minute, then do the slow-breathing exercise for 5 minutes. After this, count your breathing rate again for 1 minute. Your therapist will be able to check whether your breathing rate remains low following the exercise.

Date	8 a.m.		12 noon		6 p.m.		10 p.m.	
	Before	After	Before	After	Before	After	Before	After

SECTION 3

3 Relaxation training

3.1 The importance of relaxation training

Human beings have a built-in response to threat or stress known as the flight or fight response. Part of this flight or fight response involves the activation of muscle tension, which helps us to perform many tasks in a more alert and efficient manner. In normal circumstances, the muscles do not remain at a high level of tension all the time but become tensed and relaxed according to a person's needs. Thus a person may show fluctuating patterns of tension and relaxation over a single day according to the demands of the day, but this person would not be considered to be suffering from tension.

If you remain tense after demanding or stressful periods have passed, you remain more alert than is necessary and this sense of alertness ends up turning into apprehension and anxiety. Constant tension makes people oversensitive and they respond to smaller and smaller events as though they were threatening. By learning to relax, you can gain control over these feelings of anxiety. In this program, you will be taught how to recognize tension, how to achieve deep relaxation, and how to relax in everyday situations. You will need to be an active participant, committed to daily practice for 2 months or longer.

Since some tension may be good for you, it is important to discriminate when tension is useful and when it is unnecessary. Actually, much everyday tension is unnecessary. Only a few muscles are involved in maintaining normal posture, e.g., sitting, standing, walking. Most people use more tension than is necessary to perform these activities. Occasionally, an increase in tension is extremely beneficial. For example, it is usually helpful to tense up when you are about to receive a serve in a tennis game. Tension is unnecessary when (1) it performs no useful alerting function, (2) it is too high for the activity involved, or (3) it remains high after the activating situation has passed.

In order to be more in control of your anxiety, emotions, and general physical well-being, it is important to learn to relax. To do this you need to learn to recognize tension; learn to relax your body in a general, total sense; and learn to let tension go in specific muscles.

3.2 Recognizing tension

When people have been tense and anxious for a long period, they are frequently not aware of how tense they are, even while at home. Being tense has become normal to them and may even feel relaxed compared with the times they feel extremely anxious or panicky. However, a high level of background tension is undesirable, because other symptoms, such as hyperventilation and panic, can easily be triggered by small increases in arousal brought on by even trivial events.

Where do you feel tension? For the next 12 days we want you to monitor the tension in your body. Use the following form to indicate the location of your tension and the degree of tension. Always choose approximately the same time each day to monitor your tension. Before your evening meal is usually a good time for this.

In each box place the number corresponding to your level of tension

0	1	2	3
Nil	Low	Medium	High

Muscle tension rating

Location of tension	D1	D2	D3	D4	D5	D6	D7	D8	D9	D10	D11	D12
Around the eyes												
Jaw												
Side of the neck												
Top of scalp												
Back of neck												
Shoulders												
Top of back												
Lower back												
Chest												
Abdomen												
Groin												
Buttocks												
Thighs												
Knees												
Calves												
Feet												
Top of arms												
Lower arms												
Hands												

3.3 Relaxation training

3.3.1 Progressive muscle relaxation

Progressive relaxation means that the muscles are relaxed in a progressive manner. This section will outline how to use both progressive relaxation and "isometric" relaxation. You should master both forms of relaxation, because the progressive muscle relaxation exercises are useful for becoming relaxed (before you confront your fears) and the isometric relaxation is useful for remaining relaxed (while you confront your fears).

Relaxation exercises should be done at least once a day to begin with, preferably before any activity that might prove difficult. Select a comfortable chair with good support for your head and shoulders. If a chair does not provide good support, use cushions placed against a wall. Some people prefer to do the exercises lying down, but do not use this position if you are likely to fall asleep. These relaxation exercises are not meant to put you to sleep, since you cannot learn to relax while asleep. Sleep is not the same as relaxation. Consider those times when you have awakened tense. When possible, it is advisable that you use a relaxation tape as a preparation before you expose yourself to what you fear.

You will need to commit yourself to daily practice in order to achieve really longlasting effects. Some people continue daily relaxation many years after leaving treatment. If you can do this, we strongly advise it. However, not all people continue relaxation in this way. People who benefit most from relaxation either practice regularly or practice immediately after they notice any increase in tension or anxiety.

3.3.2 Isometric relaxation

Isometric relaxation exercises can be done when you experience fear. Most of the exercises do not involve any obvious change in posture or movement. This is because isometric refers to exercises in which the length of the muscle remains the same. Because it stays the same length, there is no obvious movement.

The most common mistake that people make with isometric exercises is putting the tension in too quickly or putting in too much tension. These are meant to be gentle and slow exercises. The aim of the exercise is to relax you, not get you even more tense. If circumstances do not allow you to hold the tension for 7 seconds, you can still benefit from putting in the tension slowly over some period of time and releasing it in the same manner.

When sitting in a public place:
- Take a small breath and hold it for up to 7 seconds.
- At the same time, slowly tense leg muscles by crossing your feet at the ankles and press down with the upper leg while trying to lift the lower leg.
  Or

- Pull the legs sideways in opposite directions while keeping them locked together at the ankles.
- After 7 seconds, breathe out and slowly say the word "relax" to yourself.
- Let all the tension go from your muscles.
- Close your eyes.
- For the next minute, each time you breathe out, say the word "relax" to yourself and let all the tension flow out of your muscles.
- Choose other parts of the body to relax, e.g., the hands and arms.
- Take a small breath and hold it for up to 7 seconds.
- At the same time, tense hand and arm muscles by placing hands comfortably in your lap, palm against palm, and pressing down with the top hand while trying to lift the lower hand.

   Or
- Place hands under the sides of chair and pull into the chair.

   Or
- Grasp hands behind chair and try to pull them apart while simultaneously pushing them in against the back of the chair.

   Or
- Place hands behind the head, interlocking the fingers, and while pushing the head backward into hands try to pull hands apart.
- After 7 seconds, breathe out and slowly say the word "relax" to yourself.
- Let all the tension go from your muscles.
- Close your eyes.
- For the next minute, each time you breathe out, say the word "relax" to yourself and let all the tension flow from your muscles.

   If circumstances permit, continue with various muscle groups.

   When standing in a public place:
- Take a small breath and hold it for up to 7 seconds.
- At the same time, straighten legs to tense all muscles, bending the knees back almost as far as they will go.
- After 7 seconds, breathe out and slowly say the word "relax" to yourself.
- Let all the tension go from your muscles.
- Close your eyes.
- For the next minute, each time you breathe out, say the word "relax" to yourself and let all the tension flow from your muscles.

   Other exercises for hand and arm muscles:
- Take a small breath and hold it for up to 7 seconds.
- At the same time, cup hands together in front and try to pull them apart.

   Or
- Cup hands together behind and try to pull them apart.

Or

- Tightly grip an immovable rail or bar and let the tension flow up the arms.
- After 7 seconds, breathe out and slowly say the word "relax" to yourself.
- Let all the tension go from your muscles.
- Close your eyes.
- For the next minute, each time you breathe out, say the word "relax" to yourself and let all the tension flow from your muscles.

3.3.3 Further isometric exercises

Various muscles can be tensed and relaxed in order to make up additional isometric exercises. You need first to decide which of your muscles tense up most readily. (If you have difficulty deciding, consider what people say to you: "Your forehead is tense"; "You're tapping your feet again"; "You're clenching your jaw.") Once you have decided on a muscle or muscle group, decide how you can voluntarily tense these muscles, and finally how you can relax them. In this way, you can design your own tailor-made set of isometric exercises.

Instructions: Some example exercises are given below. Complete the remainder by starting with those muscles that you rated as highly tense on the muscle tension rating form earlier in Section 3.2. Write down some suggestions for putting tension in the muscle area and then suggestions for relaxing that muscle. Give the suggestions a try, but remember to tense gently and slowly.

Site of tension	Manner of tensing	Manner of relaxing
Shoulders and neck	Hunching shoulders up towards the head	Letting shoulders drop and let arms hang loose
Hand tension	Make a fist	Let all fingers go loose. Place hands palm facing upward on lap

---

Important points about learning to relax quickly

1. Relaxing is a skill – it improves with frequent and regular practice.
2. Do the exercises immediately whenever you notice yourself becoming tense.
3. Develop the habit of reacting to tension by relaxing.
4. With practice, the tensing of your hand and leg muscles can be done without any movement that would attract attention. It helps to slowly tense and relax the muscles.
5. When circumstances prevent you holding the tension for 7 seconds, shorter periods will still help but you may have to repeat it a few more times.
6. Do not tense your muscles to the point of discomfort or hold the tension for longer than 7 seconds.
7. Each of these exercises can be adapted to help in problem settings such as working at a desk or waiting in a queue. Use them whenever you need to relax.
8. Using these exercises you should in a few weeks be able to reduce your tension, prevent yourself from becoming overly tense and increase your self-control and confidence.

3.3.4 Difficulties with relaxation

Some people report that they can't relax, or they can't bring themselves to practice relaxation. Since all human beings share the same biological make-up there is no purely physical reason why relaxation should work for some and not others. The reason relaxation may not work for some people is usually due to some psychological factor or insufficient practice. These problems can be overcome. If you are experiencing difficulty relaxing you should discuss this with your therapist. Some examples of difficulties are given below.

1. *"I am too tense to relax."* In this case the individual uses the very symptom that needs treating as an excuse for not relaxing. Relaxation may take longer than expected, but there is no reason why someone should have to remain tense. It might be useful to consider whether there is some other factor getting in the way of relaxation.

2. *"I don't like the feelings of relaxation."* About 1 in 10 people report that when they relax they come into contact with feelings they don't like or that frighten them. These feelings indicate you are coming into contact with your body again and noticing sensations that may have been kept under check for many years. You do not have to worry about losing control during relaxation sessions. You can always let a little tension back in until you get used to the sensations. As you keep practicing these sensations will pass.

3. *"I feel guilty wasting so much time."* You need to see relaxation as an important part of your recovery. Relaxation exercises take time, just like many other therapies.

4. *"I can't find the place or time."* Be adaptive. If you can't find 20 minutes, find 10 minutes somewhere in the day to relax. If you do not have a private room at

work, go to a park. You may need to consider whether other factors are preventing you from relaxing if you keep making the excuse that there's no time.

5. *"I'm not getting anything out of this."* Unfortunately, many people expect too much too soon from relaxation training. People often exaggerate the speed of recovery. You cannot expect to undo years of habitual tensing in a few relaxation sessions. Impatience is one of the symptoms of anxiety and often indicates a need to continue with relaxation training. Give the training time to take effect.

6. *"I haven't got the self control."* You need to realize that quick, easy cures for phobias calling for no effort from you do not exist. The longest-lasting treatment effects occur when an individual takes responsibility for his or her recovery. Responsibility means self-control, but self-control is difficult if you are not motivated.

SECTION 4

4 Graded exposure

One of the hallmarks of a phobia is that the feared object or situation is avoided or endured with considerable distress. Remember that the sorts of avoidance that we are talking about are not only the obvious ones (e.g., running away from or not going near what you fear) but also the more subtle ones (e.g., thinking about something else). However, avoiding the feared object or situation is good in the short term but its longer-term implications are not good. Whether you avoid in a subtle or obvious way, the result is the same. Each time a person with a phobia approaches some situation and then avoids it, in whole or in part, the fear subsequently increases because the drop in anxiety (which follows the "escape") is rewarding. Thus the avoidance is rewarded: after all, if you can avoid the fear by avoiding, why not do so? Unfortunately, the fear really doesn't stop, you just find more and more situations that could be "dangerous" and avoid them also.

What, then, is the way out? If leaving the situation strengthens the fear, what would happen if you stayed put? Actually, if you stayed in the situation for an hour or so, the fear would eventually go and the fear the next time you entered that situation would be less. But few people with situational fears can actually stay in the situation for the time required for intense fear to wear off. So they keep avoiding those situations.

The best remedy is to control the level of the fear using hyperventilation control, relaxation, and straight thinking (which will be discussed in Section 5), and then stay in a situation until you are calmer. Obviously, intense fear will take substantially longer to decrease than would lower levels of anxiety. For this reason, it is recommended that you begin with situations associated with small amounts of anxiety and work up to situations associated with higher levels of anxiety. In this way, you will experience anxiety, but only levels that you will be able to manage relatively quickly. As a result, you will have more successes in managing your fear.

But how do you organize such experiences? First, you make a list of all the situations in which you are likely to ever have your phobic fears. Next, you rank those situations in terms of the fear associated with them. Put them into a fear "stepladder", beginning with the least fear provoking and moving through to the most feared situations. Then, you work your way up the "stepladder", staying again and again in a situation at each level until the situation loses its power to evoke excessive anxiety. This procedure is discussed in more detail in the following sections.

4.1 Facing your fears

Situational fears are fears of places or situations that the person with a phobia thinks are dangerous or fear provoking. Once situational fears are established, avoidance often develops. It is the goal of treatment to have you overcome avoidances. The process is a gradual one, as fears can often be made worse if the person suddenly forces himself or herself, without sufficient preparation, to confront something he or she may have avoided for years.

If the associations are instead to be weakened, exposure to the feared situations is managed most easily when it is gradual. First, the person must learn to master situations associated with only mild anxiety and then progressively master situations associated with greater anxiety. It should be remembered that anxiety is different from fear and panic, and moderate anxiety in new or previously feared situations is a perfectly normal and reasonable response. Thus we do not expect you to wait until you have no anxiety at all to enter a situation. Instead, identify specific goals that you wish to achieve and then break them down into smaller steps. Each step is practiced and mastered before moving onto the next. The skills you have learned for the control of anxiety and hyperventilation are to be used in practicing each step.

4.1.1 Planning your program

1. Draw up a list of goals that you would like to be able to achieve. These should be specific goals that vary from being mildly to extremely difficult. You may have many goals but the ones that are relevant are those which involve anxiety in specific situations. Examples of general goals that do not lend themselves to graded exposure could include:

- "I want to get better."
- "I want to know what sort of person I am."
- "I want to have purpose and meaning in life."

Although they are appropriate goals to have, they do not allow you to work out practical steps by which such problems can be solved. Your goals should be precise and clear situations that you can approach in a series of graded steps. The following examples are based on fears that some individuals with phobias have:

- To travel to the city by underground train in rush hour.
- To be able to hold a nonpoisonous spider for 5 minutes.
- To swim out of one's depth for 15 minutes.

2. Break each of these goals down into easier, smaller steps that enable you to work up to the goal a little at a time. Note that the first goal comes from an individual with a fear of traveling by train. In order to be able to work towards eliminating this fear, you would need to start with (1) small trips by train, starting with traveling one station above ground, and (2) uncrowded trains. Then, gradually you would increase the number of stations, the number of people likely to be on the train, and eventually go under ground. The first goal mentioned above could be broken down into the following steps:

- Traveling one stop on an above-ground train, quiet time of day.
- Traveling two stops in an above-ground train, quiet time of day.
- Traveling two stops in an above-ground train, rush hour.
- Traveling one stop on an underground train, quiet time of day.
- Traveling two stops in an underground train, rush hour.
- Traveling five stops in an underground train, quiet time of day.
- Traveling five stops in an underground train, rush hour.

The number of steps involved depends upon the level of difficulty of the task involved. To make the above steps a little easier, you might wish to do them in the company of a friend or partner to begin with, and then do them alone. For other people, these steps might be too easy. In that case you would eliminate those that are too easy. You should always be working on those activities that you can perform, knowing you have a reasonably good chance of managing the anxiety that you experience. All of your goals can be broken down into smaller steps within your capabilities. Use this method to more easily achieve your goals.

3. You may also need to consider the practical aspects of how you are going to organize your exposure tasks. For example, if you need to be in the presence of a spider, how are you going to get one into a jar for the exercise if you have a spider phobia? Often a useful strategy is to recruit the assistance of someone without your phobia – maybe a partner or a reliable friend.

4.1.2 Implementing your program

- Make sure that you perform some activity related to your phobia every day. Avoidance makes fears worse. If you are having a bad day, you should always do something, but you need only go over the steps that you have already mastered.
- Confront a situation frequently and regularly until you overcome the fear. Many fears need to be confronted frequently (i.e., three to four times per week) at first, otherwise your fear will rise again by the time you do it next. Once you have largely overcome the fear, you need only do it less frequently.

    The general rule is: *The more you fear it, the more frequently you need to confront it.*

- Carefully monitor and record your progress. Keep a diary of your goals, steps, and achievements, together with comments about how you felt and how you dealt with particular situations. This will help you to structure your progress and also to give you feedback as to how you are doing.

4.1.3 Practicing the steps

- Use the progressive relaxation exercises before you perform the activity.
- Mentally rehearse successful performance of your activity. A good time is at the end of the relaxation session.
- Perform all activities in a slow and relaxed manner. This means giving yourself plenty of time.
- Monitor your breathing rate at regular intervals during the activity. This may be once every 5 or 10 minutes for an extended activity, or more frequently if it is shorter.
- When the circumstances allow it, stop your activity at the point at which you become anxious. Stop and implement the strategies you have learned to overcome your fear and then wait for it to pass.
- Do not leave a situation until you feel your fear decline substantially. This means you need to agree with yourself (and anyone who accompanies you) exactly how long or exactly how much your anxiety must decrease before you leave the situation. Never leave the situation out of fear. Face it; accept it; let it fade away; and then either move on or return. If you do not do this, you may see it as a failure and lose confidence.
- Try to remain in the situation as long as possible.
- Congratulate yourself for successful achievements.

4.1.4 Coping with difficulties

It is important to acknowledge that many phobic objects and situations are potentially dangerous or at minimum need to be dealt with effectively. You will need to work out the ways in which you can cope with various difficulties associated with what you fear. By way of illustration, consider a person who has a phobia about being trapped in elevators. Exposure to the elevator will reduce the anxiety associated with elevators but it is possible, though not very probable on any day, that the person could get trapped in an elevator. In such a situation, the person is faced with two difficulties. The first is coping with any anxiety and fear, which would involve breathing control, relaxation, and thinking straight. The second problem is how to get out of the elevator. Being prepared to cope with this eventuality will help to minimize worry about what may happen and also would make responding more efficient.

A planned coping strategy could include:
- Begin breathing control and isometric relaxation.
- Challenge any unhelpful thoughts (we will see how to do this later).
- Try pushing the "door open" button or the button for the level to which you wish to go.
- Look for the emergency bell and ring until someone responds.
- Use the emergency telephone if present.
- Continue using anxiety–management strategies where necessary.

Think about what you fear and how you may choose to cope with any possible difficulties. Remember, this is an exercise in planning helpful and effective coping strategies for possible eventualities, not a chance to worry about everything that you fear.

4.2 Facing fears in imagination

In a few instances, it may be difficult to approach your goal in a series of real life steps. In such cases, some steps can be practiced in imagination. This is slower than real-life exposure, but it does provide a useful way of adding in-between steps in some "all-or-none" types of activity. In order to use desensitization in imagination, you will need to specify the characteristics of the type of step you would ideally like to perform, write this on a card or series of cards, and then practice the activity specified on the card in your imagination after your next relaxation session. You will need to use cards so that you can read predetermined details about the situation that you are "rehearsing". We do not want you to let your imagination run riot. Simply imagine yourself performing the activity in a calm, collected manner. If you imagine yourself getting overly anxious or panicking, continue the session, using one of the various techniques outlined in previous sections to control anxiety.

Remember, you imagine yourself in these scenes operating in a competent manner. Even if you do not think you would, you imagine that you are. In this way, you can rehearse competent behavior at the same time as facing your fears.

Only imagine one scene at a time. You do not have to imagine all scenes in a single session.

4.3 Exercises in planning activities

An essential skill in overcoming situational fears is the ability to establish clear, helpful goals for yourself and to break these down into a number of smaller, easier steps through which you can progress. Nothing will encourage you like previous success.

A goal can always be broken down into a series of smaller, easier steps by varying the following:

- Whether you do the activity in company or with a companion.
- How far you are from help.
- How long you stay in the feared situation.
- How many things you do while you are there.
- How close you go to what you fear.

Using various combinations of these, you can easily build up a set of steps that enable you to more easily achieve your goals.

Practice examples

We would now like you to practice making out a similar set of steps for each of the following goals:

1. *Goal:*   Traveling up the tallest available building in an elevator.

   Steps: _____

   _____

   _____

   _____

   _____

   _____

   _____

2. *Goal:*   Picking up a spider and holding it for 5 minutes.
   Steps: _____

   _____

_____

_____

_____

_____

_____

In the space below, we would like you to work out up to 10 goals of your own choosing. These goals should vary in difficulty from those things that you hope to achieve in the next few weeks to those that may take longer to attain.

1. _____

2. _____

3. _____

4. _____

5. _____

6. _____

7. _____

8. _____

9. _____

10. _____

Now select three (at the most) of the above goals that you would like to work on first, and write these below. Set out beneath each goal the steps you intend to take in order to achieve it.

1. _Goal:_ _____

    Steps: _____

    _____

    _____

    _____

    _____

    _____

    _____

2. *Goal:* _____

    Steps: _____

    _____

    _____

    _____

    _____

    _____

    _____

3. *Goal:* _____

    Steps: _____

    _____

    _____

    _____

    _____

    _____

    _____

    _____

SECTION 5

5 Thinking straight

This part of the program is designed to help you to control the kinds of thoughts that occur when you are in the presence of something you fear. These thoughts not only accompany your anxiety reactions but can also promote them. You will achieve this control by learning procedures that reduce the frequency, intensity, and duration of upsetting emotional reactions by labeling the situation more appropriately and accurately. Simply put, the procedures you will practice involve learning how to "think straight."

5.1 The importance of the way you think

Humans are thinking, feeling, and behaving beings. These three aspects of our make-up interact with each other. However, thoughts can often go unrecognized.

Consider the following example:

Peter is on an errand from work and enters an office building. He approaches the elevator and thinks to himself, "Here we go again, another elevator. I hate elevators. Maybe if I got inside I may get anxious and panicky. What if someone saw me, I would be so embarrassed because they would see what a weak person I am. What if the elevator was to break down. I might get stuck in there for weeks. A few weeks without food, I am bound to die. Maybe it would be better to take the stairs." Peter then looks slightly anxious and turns around and climbs 15 flights of stairs to reach his destination.

Why did Peter become anxious and climb the stairs? The most accurate answer is "Peter made Peter anxious". To make this clear, consider another version of the same story:

Peter is on an errand from work and enters an office building. He approaches the elevator and thinks to himself, "The office is on the 15th floor. What if the elevator broke down? Chances are that it will not, and even if it did, I would be able to use the telephone in the elevator to call for assistance. There is no need to worry unnecessarily." He becomes less anxious and enters the elevator.

As you can see, the situation is exactly the same in the two stories except for two important features. First of all, Peter's thoughts have changed. Second, Peter's emotional reaction has changed: in the first scene he became anxious; in the second he remained in a pleasant mood. Peter's emotional reaction is no accident: the elevator hadn't made him afraid. Rather, it was the catastrophic thoughts that Peter had that caused him to feel afraid.

Putting this all together, there was an activating event, i.e., the elevator. This was presumed to lead to the consequence of Peter feeling afraid and later angry with his boss. However, in the expanded story, it was apparent that Peter's explanation was incomplete because there were a number of intervening beliefs or thoughts that he had. Thus, the way in which emotions are produced can be written as As, Bs, and Cs. **A** is the **A**ctivating event, **B** is the **B**eliefs or thoughts that a person has about the activating event and its meaning, while **C** is the emotional and behavioral **C**onsequence of having those beliefs and thoughts about the event. In other words, the activating event does not cause the consequence on its own, but, rather, it is the way we think about the activating event that causes the emotional consequence.

5.2 Misinterpretation and mislabeling

Many people realize that their emotional responses to various situations differ from others around them. This occurs because the people with phobias label some situations as threatening or dangerous, and therefore feel anxious. It is important to realize that it is appropriate to feel anxious in response to objectively threatening or dangerous situations. The problem in a phobia is that the label is incorrect and is based on an exaggerated estimate of the severity of danger or the probability of danger.

Individual with phobia	Individual without a phobia
Activating event Spider in a jar	*Activating event* Spider in a jar
Beliefs "What if it is poisonous?" "Any movement means that the spider is about to kill me "	*Beliefs* "I've been told it is harmless" "I've never been so close to one of these spiders before"
Consequences Anxious and refuse to touch it On edge and desiring to escape	*Consequences* Relaxed Settles down to study the spider

At its heart, the unhelpful thinking that makes the fears of people with phobias much more intense than they need to be involves overly pessimistic ratings of the *probability* and *cost* of danger. The greater the chance of something bad happening (i.e., the probability) and the worse that the event will be (i.e., the cost), then the more a person is going to worry about it. For example, a person with height phobia may start to climb a steep ladder and think that the probability that they will fall from the fifth step is about 80% (i.e., the probability is high) and that they will almost certainly die from the injuries (i.e., the cost is high). Quite reasonably, the person will be afraid of climbing the ladder.

Sometimes a person with a phobia will be afraid because their estimates of probability and cost are both high. Other times, the worry may arise because one or other is excessively high. For instance, a person who is afraid of flying may agree that the airplane they may fly in is less likely to crash than the car they drove to the airport in, but they may think that the cost of a crash is greater in an airplane because most car accidents are not fatal.

However, this isn't the whole story. Estimates of probability and cost change as a person gets closer to what it is that they fear. Interestingly, estimates of the probability and cost of danger are higher when people consider confronting what they fear than when they are actually in its presence. You may have noticed this yourself, that you can be more worried when thinking about facing your fears than when you actually face them.

These worries that are based upon overly high ratings of the probability and cost of danger can encourage a person to avoid fear-provoking situations. Avoiding situations only strengthens unhelpful and fear-producing thinking habits, as it prevents individuals from getting new, helpful information that the probability and cost are not as high as you may be thinking.

Given the thoughts a person with a phobia is having, the fear is reasonable. The problem is that the thoughts are not appropriate to the situation. They have labeled the situation as more threatening than they need to or they have worried that danger is more likely than it is. By changing the way a person labels or interprets events, a person can gain more control over their feelings in a more helpful and adaptive way.

It is important to recognize that unhelpful thinking patterns are habits, and that habits can be changed with effort and practice. Identifying unhelpful thoughts associated with anxiety is the first step in changing your thinking.

Step 1:	*Identify* anxiety-provoking thoughts.
Step 2:	*Challenge* unhelpful anxiety-provoking thoughts.
Step 3:	*Generate* helpful, more helpful alternatives.

Step 1: Identifying anxiety-provoking thoughts

It may be difficult to spot anxiety-provoking thoughts at first, especially if they have been around for a long time. In situations where you feel anxious or uncomfortable, ask yourself:

1. What do I think about myself?
2. What do I fear will happen?
3. What do I think about the situation?
4. How do I think I will cope?
5. What will I do?

Some common errors in thinking that produce anxiety in individuals with phobias include:

1. *Overestimating the chances or probability of danger:* Individuals with phobias often believe that danger is more likely to occur than it really does.
2. *Exaggerating the feared consequences (or cost):* Individuals with phobias often worry that the consequences of facing up to the feared object or situations are more serious than they are.
3. *Underestimating their own ability to cope:* Individuals with phobias often judge themselves as being unable to cope. For some people, it is the worry that they will be unable to control their own anxiety, while for others it is the worry that they will be unable to control the feared object or situation.

Individuals can also apply anxiety-provoking thoughts about one situation to other situations, and then start to become more anxious in those situations. This process is known as generalization. For example, an individual who is worried about panicking on a train may start to generalize this worry to being on buses and airplanes. This is understandable, because all three of the situations share some features: other people, limited opportunities to leave, and limited control over their direction.

Step 2: Challenging anxiety-provoking thoughts

It may be difficult to challenge anxiety-provoking thoughts, especially when they have been present for a long time. Some thoughts may even appear to be automatic. One of the best ways to challenge unhelpful thinking is to write them down, and replace the unhelpful beliefs with more helpful or helpful alternatives.

Some important questions to help you challenge unhelpful thoughts are:

1. What is the evidence for what I fear?
2. How likely is what I fear to happen?
3. What is the worst possible thing that will happen?
4. What alternatives are there?
5. How helpful is the way I'm thinking?

Step 3: Generating alternative thoughts

Through the process of challenging unhelpful thoughts, you may have started to generate more helpful thoughts. We will begin by starting with an example of unhelpful thinking. After this, we will look at specific examples from your own experience.

Consider the following example.

Description of situation	Anxiety-provoking thoughts and initial anxiety rating	Helpful thoughts and subsequent anxiety rating
Catching an express train, where I couldn't get off if I wanted to	I'll panic – being on a train makes be lose control and panic I'll go crazy if I can't get out What'll people think of me? If I can't get out I'll do something stupid or out of control I won't cope No-one else feels this way	I probably won't lose control; I'll just feel anxious Even if I do feel anxious and uncomfortable that doesn't mean the situation is dangerous I've never done something out of control on a train, and probably won't do something this time either I can use my techniques to manage my anxiety People won't notice me, and, even if they do, they'll just think I'm a little tense
	I must be loopy to feel this way	I'm not loopy, just anxious, and I'm doing something about that

Now think of a recent situation where you felt anxious because of your phobia. Write down a description of the situation and any anxiety-provoking thoughts that you may have had. Then write down some more helpful thoughts that could be applied to that situation, in order to reduce your anxiety. There is also space for an additional individual example.

Description of situation	Anxiety-provoking thoughts and initial anxiety rating	Helpful thoughts and subsequent anxiety rating

This technique should be used with the technique of graded exposure, to help you re-enter situations that you currently avoid because of anxiety.

Helpful thinking is not simply positive thinking; it does not reject all negative thoughts. It is looking at things in a way that is most helpful given the facts. It is therefore important to distinguish helpful thinking from unhelpful positive, or wishful, thinking.

Some examples of the difference between unhelpful, helpful, and wishful thinking are:

Unhelpful   What if I can't cope with this? I just know I'll do something wrong.

Wishful   It'll be easy this time.

Helpful   I'm going to give this a try. I'll do my best, and see how it goes.

If you have an unpleasant experience or event, go through the questions listed earlier in this section. At the same time, check whether your response is reasonable. If so, face your disappointment, but don't make a catastrophe of it either! It is sometimes difficult to tell the difference between unhelpful, wishful, and helpful thinking. Here are some clues to help clarify these:

Unhelpful thinking

> I must...
>
> I've got to...
>
> What if... [something happened] ... that would be terrible.
>
> > I couldn't stand it if...

Wishful thinking

> It'll work out.
>
> I don't care...
>
> It wouldn't have done any good anyway.
>
> I won't be anxious at all.

Helpful thinking

> I'd like to...
>
> I'd prefer not to...
>
> It's unlikely that ... [something] ... will actually happen.
>
> If things don't go the way I want, I might be disappointed, but I'll use my anxiety management skills to help me cope.

Troubleshooting

1. *"I don't know what I'm thinking – I'm too scared."* Ask yourself "What am I scared of? What am I scared might happen?". It is difficult to identify unhelpful fears, especially to begin with. It may help to wait until the anxiety has dropped, then think about the situation and associated fears. Re-entering a situation may make the fears clearer.

2. *"I can't think of alternatives."* After many months to years of having anxiety-provoking thoughts, it may be difficult to think up less threatening alternatives. Look at all available evidence, especially evidence that contradicts your thoughts. Ask yourself why others around you do not fear the situation, and try to consider what they might be thinking about the situation.

3. *"I'm doing it and it's not working."* Use all available techniques, including relaxation and slow breathing, to reduce your anxiety. Do not expect to be perfect at controlling your thoughts or expect the technique to work immediately. Changing well-established patterns takes time and effort.

4. *"I still feel anxious."* Straight thinking is designed to provide more helpful and appropriate responses to given situations, events or interactions. If the reality is that a particular situation is associated with some anxiety for most people, do not expect to use the technique to reduce all anxiety.

5. *"I don't believe my new thoughts."* This may occur if you have not addressed all of your anxiety-provoking thoughts. Go back and look at the original thought, and try to think whether there are any related thoughts that still cause anxiety. Also, you don't have to believe your new thoughts immediately, as part of the exercise is to disprove your old, unhelpful thoughts. Try to act as if your new thoughts are true, and see what happens.

Coping statements

There are times when you may need some shortcuts to coping with feelings. Here are a few:

1. Have a cue that makes you turn a potentially bad feeling into a coping one. For example, if you feel butterflies in the stomach, instead of saying "Oh no, I'm really getting anxious and upset" say "I know what these feelings mean. They mean I'm getting anxious. That means: slow down, regulate my breathing and do some isometric exercises."
2. Develop some personal self-statements, such as "Take this step by step", "Don't jump to conclusions" or "This fear can't hurt me – I can tolerate it". Make these statements up yourself so that they are relevant to your life.
3. Don't always put yourself down. Don't say, "A baby should be able to do this", "I'm hopeless" or "I'll never get the hang of this". As long as you say these sorts of things to yourself you make them come true (but only for as long as you say them, fortunately).
4. Praise yourself. Say things like "That was good" or "I felt I was having a bad day this morning, but I still managed to get on the crowded train." Remember the most important source of praise is from inside you, because you know yourself best and what your actions mean to you.

5.3 Putting it all together

Having discussed previously how unhelpful thoughts can be identified, challenged, and disputed we shall move on to see how you can use this to challenge your phobia. It is not enough to think helpful thoughts when there is nothing to be afraid of. You must be able to think helpful thoughts when you confront what you fear. In other words, it is not enough to engage in a mental exercise of weighing up the evidence, you must actively go out and seek evidence for and against the belief.

You now have three skills that you have been taught and now need to practice. You need to use the exposure tasks, working up the fear stepladder, to reduce your fear of the phobic situations. Relaxation will help to reduce your general levels of tension before the exposure task and the isometric exercises will regulate tension during exposure. The slow breathing will finally help you to keep control of any anxiety that you may experience during the exposure, and by thinking straight you will be able to wait in the feared situation until the anxiety levels have decreased significantly to levels that are mild to moderate.

Over the next few weeks you will need to keep a record of your daily activities. This will help you to remember what you did, the steps forward, and the difficulties. To help in planning, below is a schedule that you can complete. On the first page, you can plan what you are going to do. Remember that your aim should be to attempt a graded exposure exercise and a relaxation session every day. Following the plan is room for you to write any comments that you may have about the activities. On the pages after the plan are tables for you to write in the unhelpful thoughts and level of fear that occurs during your graded exposure exercises. You can then write down helpful thoughts so that you will be better able to manage your fear.

DIARY

Day: _____

Graded exposure exercise: _____

Time

7–8	
8–9	Breathing exercise
9–10	
10–11	
11–12	
12–1	Breathing exercise
1–2	
2–3	
3–4	
4–5	
5–6	
6–7	Breathing exercise
7–8	
8–9	
9–10	Breathing exercise

Graded exposure exercise

Exercise 1

Situation	Unhelpful thoughts and first anxiety rating	Helpful thoughts and second anxiety rating

Exercise 2

Situation	Unhelpful thoughts and first anxiety rating	Helpful thoughts and second anxiety rating

SECTION 6

6 Blood and injury phobia

6.1 Fear and fainting

Blood and injury phobias are relatively common, being found in about 4% of people. People with blood and injury phobias can be divided into two overlapping groups. On the one hand, there are those who experience fear when faced with blood or injury. On the other hand, there are those who faint when faced with blood or injury. Therefore, some people experience only fear, some only fainting, and others both.

The skills that have been covered in the Patient Treatment Manual so far have addressed fear and how to cope with it. These same skills are just as applicable for dealing with blood and injury fears as for any other phobia: you must continue to expose yourself to the distressing situations and wait for the discomfort to decrease. What has not been covered is how to control fainting when in the presence of blood or injury. This requires additional skills, but, before describing these, we shall consider why the fainting occurs.

Among individuals with blood and injury phobias, fainting is extremely common and is associated with a characteristic pattern of physiological responding. The particular pattern of responding has been called "vasovagal syncope". The vasovagal syncope involves a two-stage process. In the first stage, an increase in heart rate and blood pressure occurs. This happens because there is an increase in arousal caused by the sympathetic part of the involuntary nervous system. It is the sympathetic branch of the involuntary nervous system that is responsible for the flight or fight response and activation of it will trigger the fear reactions described in Section 1 of the Manual. However, the involuntary nervous system has another branch that opposes the sympathetic branch. This so-called parasympathetic branch of the involuntary nervous system serves to regulate the body and does the opposite to the sympathetic part of the nervous system. In people with a blood and injury phobia, this compensation is very rapid and tends to be an overcompensation. The heart slows too much and the blood pressure falls too low. Therefore the blood (obeying gravity) will run away from the brain, causing a deficiency in oxygen for the brain cells. If you do not lie down at this stage, the brain will shut down and you fall unconscious. This reaction, when you think about it, is really quite sensible because you are forced to lie down and the blood can return to your brain cells.

As you can see from this description, the fainting is beyond your control. The changes in heart rate and blood pressure are controlled by the autonomic part of the nervous system, which is not under direct conscious control. The reason why your brain responds this way is not entirely clear but some parts of the puzzle are available. It is now known that just under half the number of people with blood and injury phobias have other members of their family who faint. Interestingly, it was also found that while people who fainted were more likely to report a parent who also did, people who reported fear of blood and injury did not report that their parent did. This suggests that the fainting may be inherited but the fear is not. It has also been found that people who faint tend to be more empathic; that is, they are more able to see things from another person's point of view. It is possibly the ability to be able to "get inside another person's shoes" that leads to people fainting when they witness, think, or hear about injuries.

Hearing these facts about fainting may lead you to feel frustrated. "If I have inherited it from my family and it is controlled by the nonconscious part of my brain, what can I do?" The answer is that just because the fainting may be inherited and controlled unconsciously does not mean that you cannot control it. Think for a moment: can you increase your heart rate and blood pressure at will? If you run quickly up a steep flight of stairs, your heart rate and blood pressure will increase. If you sit down and do relaxation exercises, they will decrease. Thus you can engage in certain activities that can change these processes. Section 6.3 will therefore go on to describe what techniques you can do to avoid fainting. These activities are a little more practical and unobtrusive than running up stairs.

6.2 Fainting control skills

It is important to learn to control fainting because people with blood and injury fears often tend to avoid medical situations because of the possibility of fainting. You will learn two techniques that can help you to avoid fainting. The first we have already covered but a reminder is in order.

Slow breathing

People with blood and injury fears may increase their breathing rates when a needle is placed on their arm. As you will remember, overbreathing has a number of results one of which is feeling faint. You should monitor your breathing rate and check to see whether it is elevated before you start your "fear stepladder". Also check to see whether it is subtly increasing during exposure. In order to counter these experiences, you will need to use your hyperventilation control exercise.

The most important point to remember is that slow breathing will be of most use early in the physical reaction.

As the heart rate increases and the body prepares itself for danger, slow breathing will help to restore the normal level of arousal to the body. However, once you are aroused you need to stop the rapid decrease in heart rate and blood pressure. For this, a different skill is needed.

Applied tension

The second technique you will need to learn and master is "applied tension". The aim of applied tension is to counteract the drop in blood pressure so that you have control over your reactions. Essentially it aims to increase physical arousal, much the same as running up a set of stairs would do, in a manner that is appropriate to most medical settings. The steps involved require you to:

- Tense muscles in the arms, chest, and legs simultaneously.
- Continue to apply the tension until there is a feeling of warmth in the face (usually about 10 to 20 seconds).
- Release the tension and relax to starting level (without becoming too relaxed remember the technique is applied tension).
- Wait 20 seconds.
- Repeat the whole cycle a minimum of five times and always until the feeling of faintness has significantly decreased to manageable levels.
- You will need to be able to identify your particular signals of fainting, which may include light-headedness or dizzy feelings.

This technique will need to be incorporated into your exposure tasks and combined with relaxation and slow breathing. As you develop your skill with breathing control and applied tension, you will become able to discriminate when the best time is to apply the slow breathing and the applied tension. The rule of thumb is that you begin with slow breathing to keep you relaxed as you move into the situation but then switch (still keeping an eye on your breathing rate) as you approach the blood or injury stimulus or when you notice the very first signs of faintness. The first signs are different for different people, but some commonly reported ones include dizziness, a cold sweat (across the forehead), a queasy feeling in the stomach, or nausea.

A commonly reported problem with applied tension is headaches. This indicates that you are applying too much tension. This problem is solved by increasing the length of time between muscle tensions from 20 seconds to a time when the headaches do not occur. Also you can try to avoid tensing muscles in the face (e.g., the jaw and eyebrows) that constrict and cause pressure to be applied to the head. Another problem is difficulty in identifying the muscles to tense and how to make them taut. Looking back at the isometric exercises for some ideas may be helpful. Many people find it useful to imagine they are a bodybuilder and think about how a bodybuilder would tense those muscles. One other problem is that tensing muscles can make receiving injections more painful. You will need to be able to relax the muscle group in which the injection will be given (typically the non-dominant arm) while maintaining tension in your other arm, torso, and legs.

SECTION 7

7 Keeping your progress going

7.1 Coping with setbacks or difficulties in making progress

Setbacks or difficulties in making progress are generally the consequence of either poor management or poor planning of goals and steps. If you should experience such difficulties, you must carefully analyze the way in which you carry out these two exercises.

7.1.1 Managing anxiety and hyperventilation

- Are you regularly monitoring your breathing while performing activities?
- Are you using the isometric relaxation exercises and the slow-breathing technique when you experience the first signs of anxiety?
- Are you regularly practicing the progressive muscle relaxation exercises, especially prior to entering a situation?
- Are you too obsessed about having antianxiety medication with you?
- Are there mounting background stresses in your life that need to be defused, e.g., marital, family, or financial problems?
- Are you suffering from any form of physical stress, e.g., illness, premenstrual tension, poor diet, lack of sleep, or overwork?

7.1.2 Planning of goals and steps

- Are you trying to progress too quickly or too slowly?
- Is the difference between levels of difficulty at each step too great?
- Do you need to develop in-between steps of gradually increasing difficulty that lie between the last step you completed successfully and the step with which you are now having difficulty?
- Do you need to practice new steps more frequently and for longer periods before moving on to more difficult ones?
- If your objectives are too easy or too difficult, you will not make progress.
- Are you sure that you are not expecting too much of yourself? Make sure that you give yourself sufficient praise for your achievements. Remember that the key to success is gradual but regular progress.

7.2 Emotional problems during setbacks

Setbacks do occur occasionally, even in persons who are making excellent progress. When this happens, some people become alarmed and despondent, fearing they have gone back to their very worst. Remember, no matter how badly you feel during a setback it is very rare for you to go all the way back to your worst level of incapacitation. For most people, the apparent setback is only a passing phase, due to factors such as outside stressors, the flu, or school holidays. In such cases, the setback is often viewed as devastating because it has a lot of emotional meaning for the person, who has put considerable effort into recovering. This effort is not wasted, and after the stressors pass you will find it easier to get yourself out and about again. This pattern has been demonstrated again and again. Therefore, if you have a setback, don't add to the problem with all the old catastrophic, emotional, and self-destructive ideas. Keep practicing all the techniques you have been taught and you will be able to make progress. If you feel that you have genuinely lost the skills necessary to control anxiety and panic, then you may want to consider retreatment. Most people do not lose the skills but need some fine-tuning of their skills. "Booster" sessions or follow-up meetings are the best way to receive this form of assistance.

7.3 Expect a lapse occasionally

Here, a lapse means that you stop listening to your relaxation tape, start to worry about having a panic attack, or stop slow breathing. Most people will have some sort of lapse when they are trying to change their behavior.

The trick is not to turn a lapse into a relapse and exaggerate the lapse into being bigger than it really is. If you have noticed that you have stopped using your panic control skills, don't say things to yourself like: "I'm really hopeless; I'm right back where I started from; I'll never be able to change." Instead, you should view your lapse in the following light: "I'm disappointed that I have let things slip, but I can cope with that and I'm not going to turn it into an excuse for giving up altogether. Now I'll get out my Manual and start again."

Of course, some people do stop things like relaxation training or slow breathing when they have been feeling okay for some time. This is fine, as long as you keep aware of any stress or anxiety that may be creeping back into your life, and restart the training as soon as you become aware of any increase. Also, it will be important to reinstate such techniques if you have recently experienced any stressful life event.

7.4 Conclusion

You now have three skills that you have been taught and now need to practice. You need to use the various exposure tasks, working up the fear stepladder, to reduce your fear. Relaxation will help to reduce your general levels of tension before the exposure task, and the isometric exercises will regulate tension during exposure. Slow breathing will help to keep control of any anxiety that you may experience and by thinking straight you will be able to stop anxiety from spiraling out of control.

SECTION 8

8 Recommended resources

The following books are available from most large bookstores, many smaller ones, and some news-stands. If in doubt, ask whether the book can be ordered. We also suggest that you use your local library to gain access to many of these books. When you read these or any similar books on the management of anxiety, remember that they are best regarded as guidelines only. Be critical in both a positive and negative sense when reading these books, so that you get what is best for you out of them. Most of these books are inexpensive.

8.1 Books

Barlow D and Rapee R. (1997) *Mastering Stress: A Lifestyle Approach.* Killara, NSW: Lifestyle Press.

Burns DD. (1999) *The Feeling Good Handbook,* revised edition. New York: Penguin.

Copeland ME. (1992) *The Depression Workbook: A Guide for Living with Depression and Manic Depression.* New York: New Harbinger.

Davis M, Eshelman ER and McKay M. (1995) *The Relaxation and Stress Reduction Workbook,* fourth edition. Oakland, CA: New Harbinger.

Ellis A and Harper R. (1979) *A New Guide to Rational Living.* Hollywood, CA: Wilshire Book Company.

Emery G. (2000) *Overcoming Depression: A Cognitive-Behavior Protocol for the Treatment of Depression.* Oakland, CA: New Harbinger.

Greenberger D and Padesky C. (1995) *Mind Over Mood.* New York: Guilford.

Marks IM. (2001) *Living with Fear.* New York: McGraw-Hill.

McKay M and Fanning P. (1987) *Self-Esteem: A Proven Program of Cognitive Techniques for Assessing, Improving and Maintaining Your Self-Esteem.* Oakland, CA: New Harbinger.

McKay M, Davis M and Fanning P. (1995) *Messages: The Communication Skills Book.* Oakland, CA: New Harbinger.

McKay M, Davis D and Fanning P. (1997) *Thoughts and Feelings: Taking Control of Your Moods and Your Life.* Oakland, CA: New Harbinger.

Meichenbaum D. (1983) *Coping With Stress.* London: Century Publishing.

Page A. (1993) *Don't Panic! Overcoming Anxiety, Phobias and Tension.* Sydney: Gore Osment.

Walker CE. (1975) *Learn to Relax: 13 Ways to Reduce Tension.* Englewood Cliffs, NJ: Prentice Hall.

Weekes C. (1966) *Self-Help For Your Nerves.* Sydney: Angus and Robertson.

Weekes C. (1972) *Peace From Nervous Suffering.* Sydney: Angus and Robertson.

8.2 Video

Rapee R, Lampe L. (1998). *Fight or Flight? Overcoming Panic and Agoraphobia.* Monkey See Productions. P.O. Box 167, Waverley, NSW 2024 Australia.

8.3 Internet resources

Anxiety And Panic Internet Resource: http://www.algy.com/anxiety/

Clinical Research Unit for Anxiety and Depression: http://www.crufad.unsw.edu.au/

Internet Mental Health: http://www.mentalhealth.com/

Mental Health Net: http://mentalhelp.net/

Robin Winkler Clinic (Printable handouts on psychological problems): http://www.psy.uwa.edu.au/rwclinic/

16

Obsessive–compulsive disorder

Syndrome

Obsessive–compulsive disorder (OCD) was considered a relatively rare syndrome with a reputation for being a chronic, incapacitating, and intractable condition. Epidemiological studies have suggested that OCD is considerably more prevalent than was previously thought, with lifetime estimates ranging between 2% and 3%. More recent studies that have reassessed the diagnosed cases of OCD in epidemiological studies have suggested that the true rate of OCD may be somewhat less, with 1 month prevalence rates of 0.6% (Stein et al., 1997). Similar prevalence rates (0.7%) have been reported in a recent Australian Survey of National Mental Health and Well-being (Andrews et al., 2001a). The intractability of the disorder has been called into question, with the development of effective psychological and pharmacological interventions that mean that the majority of sufferers can be assisted in controlling their disabling symptoms. The following sections review the current state of knowledge regarding OCD and its treatment. Rather than attempt to be exhaustive in the areas covered, the aim has been to supply the practicing clinician with information that will be of use within clinical practice, particularly in terms of questions often asked by sufferers and significant others, as well as treatment issues and factors that may affect outcome.

Diagnostic criteria

Obsessions are defined as ideas, thoughts, images and impulses that enter the subject's mind repeatedly. They are recognized as a product of the subject's own mind, are perceived as intrusive and senseless, and efforts are made to resist, ignore or suppress such thoughts. Compulsions are repetitive or stereotyped behaviors that are performed in response to an obsession in order to prevent the occurrence of an unlikely event or to prevent discomfort. Resistance is often evident, but may be minimal in longstanding cases. The diagnosis of OCD is to be made if the individual experiences both obsessions and compulsions, obsessions alone or compulsions alone, given that such symptoms are time consuming or significantly interfere with the person's functioning. A comparison of ICD-10 and DSM-IV diagnostic criteria shows considerable agreement.

CASE VIGNETTE

Patient identification

Mr. P is a 30 year old father of two children who presents with a 9-year history of compulsive behavior. At the time of presentation, he was engaging in extensive checking behavior that significantly interfered with his life.

Presenting problem

Because of thoughts that something terrible may happen and he may inadvertently be responsible for harm befalling loved ones, neighbors, or other people, Mr. P states that he must check "dangerous" items repeatedly before being able to leave his home. He performs his checking in a ritualized manner, ensuring that electrical items are switched off and at times has to count to 4 as he stares at each item. If he is interrupted while completing these behaviors or feels under pressure, he must recommence his checking rituals. Similarly, if the thought that something may have been left on reoccurs while checking, the time spent ritualizing is considerably extended by his need to check repetitively. In addition to ensuring that possibly harmful events are unlikely to occur, Mr. P feels that he must check that all taps are turned off and has difficulty in writing and posting cheques and letters. He reports that he is consistently late in getting out of the house and was in fact asked to resign from his last two positions of employment as a result of his constant tardiness.

History of presenting problem

Mr. P reports that he has always been a worrier and that, as a teenager, he would occasionally phone home to ask family members to ensure that he had switched something off. When he commenced work at age 18 years, he would sometimes have to return to work from the train station to ensure that he had not left his computer or other electrical items switched on. Leaving the parental home following his marriage at age 21 years, he found that his checking behavior increased dramatically. He attributes this to no-one being at home when he and his wife left for work each morning. He found that he would check items repeatedly before leaving in the morning and at times have to leave work to go home to ensure that items were turned off. Despite his good work record, he was asked to resign due to his lateness and his having to leave work and return home on a number of occasions because of his concerns. He obtained temporary employment but was also asked to leave this position due to similar difficulties. At the time of presentation, he had been unable to work for 2 years.

Previous psychiatric history

Mr. P was referred to a psychiatrist at age 26 years because he became depressed after losing his job. He was commenced on a trial of clomipramine, both for his obsessional symptoms and his secondary depression, but was unable to tolerate the side-effects and consequently did not achieve therapeutic dosage. He continued to see his psychiatrist on a weekly or fortnightly basis over a period of 6 months for supportive counseling. He terminated the sessions as he felt his mood had improved and there was little further to be gained by continuing to attend. He remained handicapped by his obsessional behavior. There were no other psychiatric interventions until his current referral to a specialist unit.

Personal and social history

Mr. P is the youngest of three siblings, having two older brothers. He reports his family life and upbringing as strict but caring. Schooling was uneventful, with Mr. P having a number of friends. He had average academic abilities and completed school at age 18 years and then completed a 2-year accounting certificate course. He was subsequently employed by an accounting firm and he retained this position for a period of 6 years before resigning. He was then employed for a period of 6 months in a temporary position. He married at age 21 years to his girlfriend of 3 years standing. He has not sought employment since the birth of his second child 2 years previously. He describes his marriage as stable and his wife, a school teacher, as caring and supportive.

Differential diagnosis

The diagnosis of OCD should not be made if the thoughts or behavior are ego-syntonic or pleasurable, and resistance to such thoughts is primarily a function of deleterious consequences. Where the obsessional thought has developed into an overvalued idea, the diagnosis of OCD is still possible if the sufferer is able to eventually acknowledge that the belief is unfounded. The co-occurrence of depression in OCD is frequently noted in the literature. Where major depressive symptoms precede the onset of OCD symptoms or where both depressive and obsessional symptoms equally predominate, a diagnosis of depression may be indicated and the primary depressive disorder should be addressed. In making the differential diagnosis, a qualitative difference is often noted between obsessional and depressive thoughts, particularly with regard to the perceived senselessness and resistance to the thought. The absence of compulsive rituals in those suffering from depression also assists in making the differential diagnosis. Similar qualitative differences are evident in relation to stereotyped behavior in schizophrenia, where the behavior is often engaged in as a result of fixed beliefs or delusional ideas or in response to other psychotic symptoms.

The symptoms of generalized anxiety disorder (GAD) may be distinguished from OCD on a number of dimensions. In terms of content, the anxious cognitions of GAD are usually concerned with problems of everyday living (health, family, finances, work, etc.) as opposed to the frequently encountered themes of dirt/contamination, violence, sex, aggression and blasphemy in OCD sufferers. The absence of rituals – either overt or covert – in response to the worrying thoughts in GAD is another often noted difference and may well be a reflection of the degree of resistance to the thoughts. Differentiation may also be made in terms of "unacceptability" of the thoughts (i.e., obsessional thoughts are ego-dystonic), intrusiveness of the thoughts, and, of course, on the basis that GAD sufferers experience worrying thoughts about realistic concerns. In reviewing the differences between worry and obsessions, Turner et al. (1992a) suggested that compared to obsessions, worry appears less often to be experienced as being outside of personal control and that worry, particularly as associated with GAD, refers to substantially different cognitive processes than is characteristic of obsessional phenomena in OCD.

Spectrum disorders

A growing trend in the literature has been concerned with the classification of a variety of impulse control and other disorders as "obsessional". The notion that patients experience a subjective urge to complete behaviors – as well as anxiety relief upon their completion – has led some authors to speculate that a number of disparate disorders, such as trichotillomania, sexual compulsions, kleptomania, borderline personality disorder, or Tourette's Syndrome, may be related to OCD along an impulsive–compulsive continuum. Although individuals with a spectrum disorder may respond to thoughts, urges, or preoccupations with particular maladaptive behaviors, the relationship of their disorder to OCD is questionable at a number of levels. OCD is characterized by intrusive, unwanted thoughts while many of the spectrum disorders are characterized by thoughts or preoccupations that are perceived as appropriate and rational. As the content or cognitive component of their symptoms is markedly different from OCD, the reasons for engaging in the particular behavior are different. While behaviors associated with spectrum disorders may appear to have a sense of compulsion, important differences are noteworthy in that the behaviors themselves are gratifying or pleasurable (e.g., impulse control disorders), are in response to an urge rather than an intrusive thought (Tourette's syndrome, trichotillomania), or to a physical symptom or sensation (hypochondriasis), or are selectively purposeful (eating disorders) or in response to a delusional belief (body dysmorphic disorder). In contrast, rituals or behaviors in OCD are engaged in to reduce distress or anxiety associated with the perceived threat resulting from the intrusive thought. Cognitive factors involved in the mediation of OCD have been reported in a number of investigations and these further differentiate OCD from spectrum disorders. Inflated responsibility has been proposed by investigators as an essential element in the development of OCD (Salkovskis, 1989; Salkovskis and Kirk, 1997). Thought–action fusion interacting with inflated responsibility is also considered to be cognitive bias directly involved in the development and maintenance of OCD (Rachman, 1997). Danger expectancies rather than responsibility have been implicated in compulsive washing (Jones and Menzies, 1997a) and manipulation of such expectancies in washers, or responsibility in compulsive checkers has been shown to have a direct effect on symptoms (Lopatka and Rachman, 1995; Jones and Menzies, 1997b). The cognitive factors of responsibility, thought–action fusion, and danger expectancies have to a large extent been ignored by the proponents of the OCD spectrum, yet it is on the basis of such factors (i.e., the reason why someone engages in certain behaviors) that significant differentiation between superficially similar disorders can be made.

This is not to suggest, however, that obsessive–compulsive symptoms or the disorder itself does not co-occur with many of the conditions purported to be part of the OCD spectrum. Considerable research has been conducted into the relationship between OCD and Tourette's syndrome (TS) as OCD and OC symptoms have been noted to be relatively common in TS. However, important phenomenological differences have been noted between the obsessional symptoms evident in TS patients with or without comorbid OCD and those with OCD alone (George et al., 1993; Holzer et al., 1994; Cath et al., 1992; Miguel et al., 1995). While some family studies of OCD have found no relationship between OCD and TS (Flament et al., 1988; Black et al., 1992), others have tended to indicate some relationship between the two conditions. However, the relationship is anything but clear. Pauls et al. (1995) reported that some cases of OCD may be familial and related to TS or tic disorders, others cases were familial and unrelated to tics, and others were neither familial nor related to TS.

Sex ratio

Black (1974) summarized 11 studies of OCD and reported that of 1336 cases, 651 were male and 685 female, suggesting an almost equal sex ratio. Similarly, Yaryura-Tobias and Neziroglu (1983) reported an equal sex ratio in their review of six OCD studies, while another study reporting on a clinical cohort (Noshirvani et al., 1991) found a slightly higher proportion of women. Rasmussen and Eisen (1992) also reported a slightly higher proportion of women (53.8%) in a large cohort of 560 OCD patients. The opposite has generally been the case with child and adolescent studies, which have tended to indicate a predominance of males (Swedo et al., 1989, Rapoport, 1990). However, this may in part be due to an earlier onset in males than in females.

Age of onset

In reviewing a number of studies, Black (1974) found that the majority of cases had an onset of OCD between ages 10 and 40 years. The distribution, however, was skewed, with 21% beginning between ages 10 and 15 years. Mean age of onset was 10–15 years, with 10% having syndrome onset prior to age 10 and 9% after age 40 years. Noshirvani et al. (1991), reporting on a large clinical cohort (N=307), found a significantly earlier onset in males (5–15 years). The mean age of onset was 22 years, with the vast majority (92%) commencing between ages 10 and 40 years. Earlier onset for males was also reported in childhood onset OCD (Rapoport, 1990). Similarly, in another large clinical cohort of 560 individuals, Rasmussen and Eisen (1992) report, the mean onset age as 20.9±9.8 years. Males were reported to have a significantly earlier onset (19.5±9.6 years), as compared with females (22.0±9.8 years). Sixty-five percent of sufferers were found to have illness onset prior to age 25 years, and fewer than 15% reported onset after age 35 years.

Course of illness

Prior to the development of effective treatments of OCD, Ingram (1961) reported a constant worsening in 39% of 89 inpatients, a constant and static unremitting course in 15%, a fluctuating course with periods of worsening and relative improvement in 33% and a phasic course with periods of remission in 13%. An early follow-up study of OCD sufferers by Kringlen (1965) found that 5% had a constant worsening, 30% were constant and static, 20% fluctuating and 5% phasic. More recently, Rasmussen and Eisen (1992) reported that 85% had a continuous and fluctuating course, 10% had a deteriorative course and 2% were classified as episodic. More recently, Skoog and Skoog (1999), in a 40 to 50 year follow-up of OCD patients found that 83% of patients had improved over the follow-up period, and 48% showed clinical recovery. However, 37% still had diagnosable OCD after 50 years, and only 20% of the sample showed complete recovery. Overall, clinical and subclinical symptoms were still evident in two-thirds of the sample at follow-up, and 10% of the sample showed a deteriorating course.

Phenomenology and classification

OCD sufferers have traditionally been classified into three broad groupings. Those who experience both obsessions and compulsions represent the majority of sufferers, less frequent are those who experience obsessional thoughts alone, and those who engage in compulsive rituals without obsessional thoughts are relatively rare. Such a classification system, however, fails to acknowledge that individuals who experience obsessional thoughts alone will often engage in covert cognitive behavior in order to neutralize or suppress the obsessional thought, thus serving the same purpose as overt behavioral rituals. The presence of covert compulsions has been recognized for some time. Foa and Tillmans (1980) have suggested that the definition of compulsions be broadened to include both overt and covert behaviors. Further support for this notion is found in the work conducted by Salkovskis and Westbrook (1989), who differentiated between obsessional ideas and cognitive rituals. They defined obsessional ideas as the original anxiety-arousing intrusions. In contrast, cognitive rituals are defined as thoughts that the patients voluntarily initiate to attempt to reduce the anxiety or discomfort aroused by obsessional ideas. Within this approach, cognitive rituals are also often referred to as "neutralizing" thoughts. DSM-IV criteria now acknowledge the presence of covert compulsions and revision of the diagnostic criteria include neutralizing thoughts within the compulsion definition. Although obsessional ruminators are conceptualized as being similar to individuals with obsessions and overt compulsions, a number of differences have been noted by Arts et al. (1993), who, in comparing 26 ruminators to 48 patients with both obsessions and compulsions, reported that the former group were more depressed, were more often married, had achieved a lower level of education, were older at symptom onset and were more often on medication.

The types of obsessional thoughts and compulsive behaviors have been reported to be consistent across cultures (Tseng; 1973, Mahgoub and Abdel-Hafiez, 1991; Okasha et al., 1994) and time, with similar phenomenological reports and clinical descriptions appearing in medical writings of the last century (Berrios, 1985). Obsessional thoughts are often concerned with worries of contamination, harming others, or going against social mores such as swearing or making inappropriate sexual advances in public (Marks, 1987). Rasmussen and Eisen (1992) reported that 50% of 560 OCD patients had obsessions regarding contamination, 42% pathological doubt, 33% somatic obsessions, 32% need for symmetry, 31% aggressive, and 24% sexual. Compulsive behavior has generally been categorized as washing, checking, repeating and ordering, with both adult and child sufferers exhibiting similar phenomenology (Last and Strauss, 1989; Swedo et al., 1989). Washing or cleaning, which generally affects more women than men, is characterized by a fear of contamination and associated washing, decontaminating or cleaning rituals, with extensive avoidance of the contaminant. Washing/cleaning compulsions were evident in 50% of 560 OCD patients investigated by Rasmussen and Eisen (1992). Checking behaviors were evident in 61% of the their sample, with patients engaging in repeated checking in order to prevent a dreaded event or disaster from occurring. Counting was evident in 36%, a need to ask or confess in 34%, a need for symmetry or precision in 28%, and hoarding in 18% of the sample. In another large clinical cohort, Noshirvani et al. (1991) reported significantly more compulsive washing in females and significantly more checking in males. Compared with late onset cases, early onset cases exhibited significantly more checking and fewer washing rituals. Obsessional slowness without visible rituals has also been reported, though to a much lesser extent than other presentations, and is most likely a function of mental checking or the need to follow a meticulous preset order (Rachman, 1974; Marks, 1987; Ratnasuriya et al., 1991).

The utility of classifying subjects according to phenomenology is questionable, given that sufferers often have more than one obsession and more than one form of ritual. In a large cohort of 560 OCD patients (Rasmussen and Eisen, 1992), 72% experienced multiple obsessions and 58% experienced multiple compulsions. Other research suggests that phenomenology may change over time (Marks, 1987; Hodgson and Rachman, 1977). A more promising classification with implications for behavioral treatment was proposed by Foa et al. (1985), and is based on the presence or absence of external cues, disastrous consequences and either overt or covert anxiety-reducing responses. Classification according to these criteria hold implications for the cognitive behavioral treatment of the disorder and would therefore be of greater clinical utility to the practicing clinician. A comprehensive behavioral program should include exposure to all cues, both internal and external, as well as response prevention that focuses on overt and covert rituals in addition to avoidance.

Assessment instruments

A thorough assessment of OC symptomatology for the purposes of designing a behavioral program relies heavily on clinical interview. No instrument will provide the clinician with the detailed and often idiosyncratic information regarding the cues that create anxiety or discomfort, the responses (rituals) to those cues, and the avoidance that the patient often engages in to minimize their discomfort. Despite these limitations, it is good clinical practice to utilize assessment instruments that may provide an independent validation of treatment effectiveness. An often-used therapist-administered instrument utilized in both clinical practice and research settings that focuses on target obsessions and compulsions is the Yale–Brown Obsessive Compulsive Scale (Goodman et al., 1989). The Maudsley Obsessive Compulsive Inventory (Hodgson and Rachman, 1977) is a 30 item "true–false" self-report inventory that is also often used in the treatment of OCD. The major shortcoming of this instrument is that it asks the patient to rate the presence or absence of symptoms and therefore does not lend itself to changes in interference, severity or frequency as a result of treatment. A more comprehensive instrument, the Padua Inventory (Sanavio, 1988) consists of 60 items reflecting OC symptoms that the patient rates in terms of degree of disturbance. In its original version, the Padua Inventory was found to be significantly correlated with measures of neuroticism and trait anxiety. A revision of the Padua was undertaken by Burns et al. (1996) in order to delete items that overlapped with worry. This resulted in a 39 item questionnaire (WSUR revision) consisting of five subscales: obsessional thoughts about harm to self or others, obsessional impulses to harm self or others, contamination obsessions and washing compulsions, checking compulsions, and dressing or grooming compulsions.

Etiological and theoretical models of OCD

A variety of models and hypotheses have been put forward in recent years in an attempt to explain the development of OCD. Although such models may in part assist in our understanding of what remains a puzzling disorder, no single theory, either biological or psychological, provides a comprehensive explanation of the syndrome. Invariably, patients presenting for treatment will request some explanation of the symptoms. As this book is concerned with the cognitive behavioral treatment of anxiety disorders, the emphasis will obviously be on formulations that will assist the individual to implement their treatment. It is the clinician's responsibility to remain abreast of the latest findings and report these to patients and significant others.

The serotonin (5-hydroxy tryptamine; 5HT) hypothesis, which suggests that 5HT dysregulation may be etiologically linked to OCD, is doubtful. In summarizing the evidence from the various pharmacological challenge studies, Baumgarten and Grozdanovic (1998) concluded that the studies do not show support for a primary pathogenetic role of 5HT in OCD. Although the utility of certain 5HT reuptake inhibiting medications in the treatment of OCD is beyond doubt, it is only the manufacturers of these medications that continue to propose the notion of a serotonergic "imbalance" as being solely responsible for OCD.

Neuroimaging studies of OCD have shed considerable light on the neuro-anatomical structures involved in the expression of OCD. The most consistent finding has been increased activity in the orbito-frontal cortex in patients with OCD. A number of studies have also suggested the involvement of the anterior cingulate, caudate nucleus, and thalamus. On the basis of such findings some authors have proposed neuroanatomical models of the pathophysiology of OCD (cf. Saxena et al., 1998; Saxena and Rauch, 2000). Although presentation and explanation of such a model to patients is of limited utility, as it does not equip them with any direct skills to deal with their OCD, Schwartz (1998) suggested that teaching patients to relabel obsessions as "false messages" and that symptoms are the result of a "leaky gate" in the striatum assists them to distance themselves from the symptoms and make choices about their responses.

A number of behavioral theories also attempt to provide etiological and maintenance formulations of OCD. Mowrer's (1960) two-stage theory of fear acquisition and maintenance does well to explain the negative reinforcing properties of rituals but not the development of the disorder itself. Similarly, Foa and Kozak's (1986) reformulation of Lang's (1979) bioinformational theory assists in the differentiation of normal from neurotic fears but does not address the development of those fears in OCD. Nevertheless, both models have implications for the behavioral treatment of the disorder. In terms of Mowrer's formulation, rituals are seen to have anxiety-reducing properties. Engagement in these behaviors inhibits habituation to the feared stimuli from taking place. Similarly, Foa and Kozak's formulation suggest that, in order to modify obsessional fears, the fear network has to be accessed so that new information regarding the stimuli can be processed and the fear structure changed. Treatment with exposure and response prevention is implied in both models.

Salkovskis (1989; Salkovskis and Kirk, 1997) proposes a cognitive behavioral formulation for the development of obsessional disorders. A primary feature of this model is the notion that particular types of intrusive thought, upon appraisal, will interact with beliefs of responsibility in vulnerable individuals and lead to behaviors designed to neutralize the threat posed by the obsessional thought. Central to Salkovskis' hypothesis is the notion of responsibility – both in terms of having the thought as well as responsibility for the implications of the thought. Rachman (1993, 1997) elaborated on the mechanisms of appraisal at work in OCD and suggested that OCD patients tend to psychologically fuse thoughts and actions. Although such cognitive biases as thought–action fusion and negative appraisal of the content and occurrence of the intrusive thoughts are often evident in those individuals whose symptoms are concerned with harm to others (obsessional checking, obsessional rumination), there is little evidence to suggest that such factors are at work in compulsive cleaners who do not fear harm befalling others. Nevertheless, the implications for treatment are similar to those of the above-cited behavioral theories, i.e., exposure and ritual prevention, although for some patients cognitive interventions may be warranted to deal with the cognitive biases mentioned above.

Genetics

At the time of writing, there is growing evidence for a contribution from genetic factors in some OCD presentations. The evidence for possible genetic predisposition in OCD derives from two sources: twin studies and investigations of the first-degree relatives of OCD sufferers. Early twin studies reporting concordance may be criticized on the basis of failing to establish firm diagnoses of either zygosity or OCD (Hoaken and Schnurr, 1980). However, even in those studies where zygosity was established and diagnosis confirmed (Woodruff and Pitts, 1964; Marks et al., 1969; McGuffin and Mawson, 1980), the effects of social learning cannot be ruled out.

As with the twin studies, early investigations of first-degree relatives of OCD sufferers can be criticized on a number of grounds. The use of loose diagnostic criteria, confounding of obsessional symptoms and traits, absence of control data, as well as reliance on information provided by the proband rather than direct interview of the relatives renders the findings of early investigations, as well as some later studies (Insel, Hoover and Murphy, 1983; Rasmussen and Tsuang, 1986) difficult to interpret. However, more recent studies, have attempted to overcome such methodological flaws through the use of structured diagnostic interviews and direct relative interview. A study by Black et al. (1992) used the Diagnostic Interview Schedule to assess the prevalence of OCD in the relatives of OCD sufferers and normal controls. The authors found that, while first-degree relatives of probands with OCD were significantly more likely to develop anxiety disorders than relatives of the control group, the prevalence of OCD in both the index and control relatives did not exceed the estimated occurrence in the general population. Pauls et al. (1995), however, reported that the morbid risk for OCD was significantly higher in OCD proband relatives (10.3%) as compared with relatives of controls (1.3%). The addition of subthreshold OCD raised the morbid risk to 18.2%.

In contrast, studies that have utilized structured interviews to assess first-degree relatives of children and adolescent sufferers report a considerably higher incidence of diagnosable OCD. Riddle et al. (1990) directly interviewed parents of children with OCD using a standard clinical assessment. Results showed that 71% of 21 children or adolescents with OCD had a parent with OCD (*N*=4) or obsessional symptoms (*N*=11), indicating that 37.5% of parents had diagnosable or subthreshold OCD. Lenane et al. (1990) reported similar results, with diagnosable OCD being found in 25% of fathers and 9% of mothers of 46 children with OCD. With the inclusion of subclinical OCD, age-corrected morbidity risk was estimated at 35%, not unlike the findings of Riddle et al. (1990).

The discrepancy between the child and adult studies may be a function of differences between childhood/adolescent onset OCD and later or adult onset OCD. In one early study, Bellodi et al. (1992) reported a morbid risk of 3.4% in the first-degree relatives of 92 OCD patients. Separation of the probands according to age of onset, however, resulted in a morbid risk of 8.8% of relatives of probands with onset prior to age 14 years and 3.4% for relatives of probands with a later onset. More recently, Nestadt et al. (2000) reported that the lifetime prevalence in relatives of 80 OCD patients was significantly higher than controls (11.7% versus 2.7%). When the sample was divided into early onset (5–17 years) and late onset (over 18 years) groups, the prevalence of OCD in relatives was 13.8% and 0%, respectively.

To some extent, OCD is familial, particularly in early onset OCD. However, while the above studies indicate that familial factors may play a role in some forms of OCD, there are a significantly large proportion of probands in all of the cited studies that have no family history of OCD. Thus genetics, while important, do not provide a total answer.

Comorbidity

Depression

The occurrence of obsessional symptoms in depressive illness sufferers has been noted by a number of authors (Gittleson, 1966; Kendell and Discipio, 1970), as has the high incidence of depressed mood in OCD sufferers (Rosenberg, 1968; Goodwin, 1969; Rasmussen and Tsuang, 1986). However, the obsessional symptoms seen in patients with depressive illness are generally not of the intensity seen in patients with OCD, and recovery from depression has been shown to result in a reduction of obsessional symptoms. Other studies also indicate that obsessional features in depression appear to parallel the course of the primary illness and that, if present beforehand, will revert to their original intensity after resolution of the depression (Videbech, 1975; Marks, 1987).

The presence of depressed mood or depressive symptoms has consistently been shown to be a frequent complication of OCD (Rosenberg, 1968; Goodwin et al., 1969; Black and Noyes, 1990), and some authors have suggested a psychobiological link between depression and OCD (Hudson and Pope, 1990). Studies of child, adolescent, and adult OCD sufferers report high rates of depressed mood, with between 20% and 35% of OCD clinic attenders meeting criteria for major depression (Rasmussen and Tsuang, 1986; Swedo et al., 1989; Sanderson et al., 1990). Lifetime prevalence has been reported as affecting up to 67% of OCD patients (Rasmussen and Eisen, 1992). However, such clinical data need to be interpreted cautiously, as many OCD sufferers tend to seek help only when depressed (Marks, 1987). It is, moreover, important to carefully assess the severity of depression in OCD patients presenting for treatment – particularly as the presence of severe depression hinders the effectiveness of behavioral interventions in OCD (Foa et al., 1983a,b). Aside from improving less than sufferers with mild or moderate depression, OCD sufferers with severe depression also tend to have a higher relapse rate. Where such patients present for treatment, the possibility of combining behavioral treatment with antidepressant medication, preferably with antidepressant medication which has 5HT reuptake inhibiting properties, needs to be carefully considered.

Anxiety disorders

The co-occurrence of anxiety disorders in OCD sufferers is considerable. Similar results are reported in both epidemiological and clinic samples for adults, adolescents, and children (Rasmussen and Tsuang, 1986; Flament et al., 1988; Karno et al., 1988; Swedo et al., 1989; Brown and Barlow, 1992; Crino and Andrew, 1996a). Severity of co-occurring anxiety disorders should be assessed by the clinician, as these conditions may require intervention after, or even before, the obsessional problems have been addressed. Alternatively, these "conditions" may be secondary to the obsessional complaints, so that what appears to be agoraphobic avoidance or social phobic concerns may be the direct result of the obsessional fears or attempts by the sufferer to keep their rituals hidden from others. For example, a patient with contamination concerns may experience difficulty in using public transport, eating or drinking away from home, or other situations that may expose the individual to contamination and therefore be wrongly identified as suffering from a phobia. If there is a clear co-occurring anxiety disorder, it should be the patient's decision as to which disorder should be dealt with first, and such a decision should be made on the basis of level of interference with their life.

Personality disorder

The relationship between OCD and axis II diagnoses have generated considerable interest among researchers. Findings suggest that anywhere from 48% (Jenike et al., 1986) to 87.5% (Black et al., 1993) of OCD patients have one or more personality disorders, as diagnosed by a variety of instruments. The results of many of these studies are questionable on a number of grounds. First, the validity of the instruments is uncertain, particularly as there is no "gold standard" against which to compare the various questionnaires. Second, the confounding of state and trait is certainly an issue worthy of consideration when effective treatment of the obsessional symptoms in OCD subjects results in a marked lowering of personality disorder diagnoses (cf. Joffe and Regan, 1988; Mavissakalian et al., 1990). One would expect the enduring maladaptive traits that constitute personality disorder should persist after the Axis I condition is treated. Effective treatment of OCD and other anxiety disorder patients, however, results in the majority of patients leading essentially normal lives, uncomplicated by any obvious Axis II pathology. Results from our clinic (Crino and Andrews, 1996b) suggest that the rate of personality disorders in OCD and other anxiety disorders is relatively low, and that minor but important differences between the anxiety disorders exist when one takes a dimensional rather than categorical view of personality disorder.

Conclusion

Many facts regarding OCD and its possible causes remain unknown despite the extraordinary burgeoning of research in this area in recent years. While there is general agreement of the diagnostic criteria across the two major classification systems as well as acknowledgment of the frequently encountered complication of depression in OCD, much still remains to be learned of the etiology, comorbidity, and other complications of what remains a puzzling and, if left untreated, crippling disorder. One important question that continues to re-occur in the recent literature is the possibility that OCD is a heterogeneous disorder. Taking such a view would go part of the way to explain some of the disparate findings noted above (e.g. genetics, relationship to TS, differing cognitive styles, etc.) Nevertheless, effective treatments for OCD are available and, either alone or in combination, will result in the majority of patients gaining control over their disorder.

17

Obsessive–compulsive disorder

Treatment

Although OCD has been recognized for centuries, effective treatment for this condition has been available only for the past four decades. The treatments of choice for OCD are behavior therapy, consisting of exposure and response prevention, and selective serotonin reuptake-inhibiting medications. Recent studies have also included specific cognitive techniques targeting the appraisals of intrusive thoughts, responsibility for harm and threat estimates. Whether the addition of such techniques results in superior efficacy is yet to be demonstrated in further trials. Nevertheless, the use of cognitive techniques to challenge the dysfunctional appraisal of intrusive thoughts is warranted in individuals with cognitive styles that interfere with treatment. Cure of OCD is not commonplace. The primary goal of treatment in the majority of cases is to have the individual control the disorder rather than the obsessional disorder control the individual. Achievement of this goal allows the patient to minimize the impact and effects of the disorder on their daily life and enhances their ability to reach their full potential.

Behavioral therapy

The basic principles of exposure and response prevention include the deliberate exposure to obsessional cues and prevention of the behaviors that the sufferer typically engages in to lessen the anxiety, discomfort, or distress associated with the feared stimuli. Repeatedly employing prolonged exposure (45 minutes to 2 hours) to the obsessional cues, with strict response prevention, allows habituation to take place. Exposure tasks are arranged hierarchically, with treatment commencing with the least anxiety-provoking situation and progressing rapidly through the hierarchy.

In reviewing the results of more than 200 OCD patients treated with behavior therapy in several countries, Foa et al. (1985) reported that 51% of sufferers achieved at least a 70% reduction in symptoms. Thirty-nine percent of patients achieved reductions ranging from 31% to 69%, and 10% were considered failures, failure being defined as patients with an improvement of 30% or less. At follow-up (mean duration 1 year), the number of failures increased from 10% to 24%. However, 76% of patients remained improved to a degree rated as moderately improved or better.

Further evidence for the efficacy of exposure and response prevention is reflected in a long-term follow-up of nine cohorts from five countries conducted by O'Sullivan et al. (1991). Both self- and assessor ratings were used, and two cohorts had received exposure plus either clomipramine or placebo. The overall dropout rate was reported at 9% and – of a total of 223 patients – 87% were followed up for a mean of 3 years (range 1 to 6 years). All studies reported a significant improvement at posttreatment, which remained evident at follow-up, with 78% of individuals remaining improved. On average, there was a 60% improvement in target rituals as compared with pretreatment. These findings need to be tempered with the fact that approximately 25% of patients refuse behavior therapy when offered, because of the time commitment, or because of fears of overwhelming anxiety when confronting their triggers, or because they fear that the dreaded outcome from not performing their ritual will eventuate (Greist, 1998). In our experience, motivational interventions may assist in those who do not wish to make the time commitment, cognitive techniques may assist those who fear the dreaded outcome, while a more graded approach to exposure may assist those who fear overwhelming anxiety or panic.

Although the utilization of exposure and response prevention techniques have had a significant impact upon the treatment of individuals with compulsive rituals, the efficacy of behavioral techniques in the treatment of obsessional thoughts has, until recently, been considered problematic. However, Salkovskis and Westbrook (1989), employing revised habituation procedures in which the subjects were exposed to obsessional thoughts via loop tapes and avoided cognitive neutralizing, reported a favorable outcome in four subjects. More recently, Freeston et al. (1997) randomly assigned 29 OCD patients without overt rituals to a wait-list control condition or a comprehensive cognitive behavioral program that involved a cognitive model of obsessions, cognitive restructuring of the dysfunctional assumptions, loop tape and in vivo exposure and response prevention, and relapse prevention. Significant improvement was reported in Yale–Brown Obsessive Compulsive Scale (YBOCS) scores, self-report of OCD symptoms and self-reported anxiety, with 77% of treatment completers ($N = 22$) showing clinically significant changes.

Cognitive therapy

The efficacy of cognitive interventions in the treatment of OCD has been investigated by a number of researchers. The contribution of self-instructional training (SIT) to exposure and response prevention was examined by Emmelkamp et al. (1980). Fifteen patients received either self-controlled exposure or exposure combined with SIT. No group differences were found at posttreatment or 1- or 6-month follow-up. Emmelkamp et al. (1988) compared self-controlled exposure and response prevention to rational emotive therapy (RET) in 18 OCD sufferers and reported that cognitive therapy was as effective as exposure and response prevention. In a replication, Emmelkamp and Beens (1991) compared six sessions of RET to six sessions of exposure followed by a 4-week waiting period and six further sessions of exposure for both groups. Although no difference was found between the RET condition and exposure condition, there was no indication that RET enhanced outcome when combined with exposure and response prevention. In a larger study, Van Oppen et al. (1995) randomly allocated 71 patients to either self-controlled exposure or a cognitive therapy condition on the basis of work of Beck (1976) and Salkovskis (1989). Both conditions led to significant improvement and there were some indications that cognitive therapy may have been superior; however, the differences were not significant when initial differences between conditions were taken into account. Effect sizes tended to be larger in the cognitive therapy condition and there were significantly more patients rated as recovered in the cognitive condition. Although the authors discuss the results in terms of the efficacy of cognitive techniques, the addition of behavioral experiments to test the empirical basis of dysfunctional assumptions (exposure) after six sessions of cognitive therapy would tend to confound the observed outcome. No study directly comparing cognitive techniques alone, cognitive techniques combined with exposure, and exposure alone has yet been conducted.

Factors affecting outcome with behavioral treatment

Despite these impressive outcome results, behavior therapy has not been of benefit to all patients. To begin with, it is estimated that 25% of patients do not comply with treatment (Foa et al., 1985), and of those who do comply and complete treatment 10% do not respond, increasing to 24% of treatment completers at follow-up. A number of factors that may affect the outcome of behavioral treatment have been delineated.

Factors affecting treatment drop out were examined by Hansen et al. (1992), who approached 15 patients who had terminated treatment and compared their response with that of individuals who had completed treatment. Dropouts differed significantly from treated patients in five areas: they were less obsessive compulsive, they had more discongruent treatment expectations, they were more critical of the therapist, they experienced less anxiety in homework exposure, and they were less often pressured by significant others to continue treatment. Foa et al. (1983a,b), attempting to determine predictors of outcome, found that significant depression may affect outcome when exposure and response prevention is used by influencing reactivity and habituation between sessions. Similarly, the presence of overvalued ideation has been noted to affect outcome negatively (Foa, 1979). In contrast, Lelliot et al. (1988) found that patients with bizarre and fixed beliefs responded well to treatment. While there was a significant correlation between clinical improvement on a number of measures and the reduction of fixity of obsessional beliefs, the fixity of such beliefs did predict severity of target rituals at 1-year follow-up (Basoglu et al., 1988). More recently, Ito et al. (1995) reported that reduction in fixity of OCD beliefs parallelled improvements in other measures of OCD symptoms.

Other factors that may affect the success of treatment include excessive behavioral or cognitive avoidance and excessive arousal in the presence of feared stimuli (Foa et al., 1983a). In the first case, attention-focusing techniques while using in vivo exposure may assist in promoting habituation. Excessive arousal may be a function of the program design, and require a reanalysis of the fear-evoking potential of the stimuli so that arousal is kept at moderate levels, thereby promoting emotional processing and habituation. Clinical factors not found to influence treatment include age at symptom onset. In fact, Foa et al. (1983a) reported that the younger the individual was when symptoms began, the better maintained was the improvement at follow-up. Similarly, neither duration of symptoms nor symptom severity was associated with poor outcome. The types of ritual (washing versus checking) were also not predictive of outcome with exposure and response prevention. In contrast, Basoglu et al. (1988) reported that severe rituals and social disability predicted poorer outcome in patients treated with clomipramine and exposure. Similarly, Cottraux et al. (1993), in examining predictors of treatment outcome in 60 patients treated with behavior therapy, fluvoxamine or a combination, found that high avoidance was the best single predictor of poor outcome. While depression was not a significant predictor of outcome in a number of other studies (Basoglu et al., 1988; Hoogduin and Duivenvoorden, 1988; O'Sullivan et al., 1991; Riggs et al., 1992), depression predicted failure in Cottraux et al.'s (1993) study. Severe depression was also associated with poorer outcome in a follow up of 72 OCD patients treated with behavior therapy (Foa et al., 1981).

More recently, Castle et al. (1994) examined outcome predictors for 178 outpatients with OCD. Forty-one patients who dropped out of treatment did not differ significantly in terms of demographic or illness variables or initial rating scale scores. As with data from Foa et al. (1983a), age, age of onset, and illness duration were not significantly associated with outcome, nor were meticulous or anxious personality traits. Patients living alone were significantly less likely to be classified as "much improved". The "much improved" group had significantly lower initial scores on global phobia as well as ratings of work and home impairment, and were more likely to have had a co-therapist. While gender was not a predictor of outcome, predictors of outcome differed between the sexes. Factors associated with a good outcome for women were being in paid employment, having a co-therapist (relative, friend or appropriate other), and low initial severity ratings of global phobia, impairment of work and home activity, and compulsion checklist. For men, however, the only factor to approach statistical significance was living alone, which was associated with less improvement.

Keijsers et al. (1994) also reported greater initial severity of obsessional complaints to be associated with poorer outcome but also reported that poorer motivation, dissatisfaction with the therapeutic relationship and longer duration of complaints predicted poorer immediate (posttreatment) outcome for "obsessive fear", while higher pretreatment levels of depression predicted poorer outcome of compulsive behavior.

In summary, the most consistent outcome predictor appears to be symptom severity, with the more severely symptomatic patients tending to have a poorer outcome. The role of depression as a predictor of outcome remains unresolved, with some studies reporting less improvement in depressed patients (e.g., Foa et al., 1983b; Cottraux et al., 1993) while others report no association (e.g., Basoglu et al., 1988; Hoogduin and Diuvenvoorden, 1988; Castle et al., 1994). Overvalued ideation and fixity of beliefs have also been delineated as possible predictors of outcome.

Pharmacotherapy

Although a wide variety of medications have been utilized in the treatment of OCD, there is little doubt as to the consistent efficacy of serotonin reuptake inhibitors (SSRIs), of which clomipramine is the most widely researched. Placebo controlled trials have in general attested to its efficacy and comparison to other antidepressants have also demonstrated its superiority in decreasing obsessional symptoms (Greist, 1990a; Jenike, 1990a). Average symptom reduction, however, is only moderate (Zak et al., 1988; De Veaugh-Geiss et al., 1989; Greist, 1990a).

Although not as extensively researched as clomipramine, other more potent SSRI appear to be of equal benefit in the treatment of OCD, and in general have the added benefit of a lower side-effect profile. The efficacy of fluoxetine at three fixed doses (20, 40, and 60 mg) was examined in a multicenter trial by Tollefson et al. (1994), who reported symptom reduction of 32.1%, 32.4%, and 35.1%, respectively, as compared with 8.5% for placebo after a 13 week trial. Pigott et al. (1990) in a randomized double-blind crossover design compared clomipramine to fluoxetine and reported similar therapeutic effects. Fluvoxamine has also been shown to be superior to placebo in the treatment of OCD in a number of double-blind studies (e.g., Goodman et al., 1990; Perse et al., 1987; Jenike et al., 1990b) and in a multicenter trial (Goodman et al., 1992). Fluvoxamine was also compared with desipramine in a study by Goodman et al. (1990) and was found to be superior in reducing the severity of OC symptoms. A direct comparison of fluvoxamine with clomipramine by Lorin et al. (1996) reported similar levels of symptom reduction in a similar proportion of patients in both groups. Sertraline, another SSRI, has also had mixed results initially, with one placebo controlled study finding no effect in a small number of patients (Jenike et al., 1990a). Other studies have attested to the efficacy of sertraline in OCD. Chouinard et al. (1990) reported that sertraline resulted in significant decreases in OCD symptoms on three of the four measures used. Greist et al. (1995) reporting on a large multicenter placebo controlled trial of fixed-dose sertraline (50, 100, 200 mg) found that doses of 50 mg and 200 mg were significantly more effective than placebo in reducing obsessional symptoms. More recently, Kronig et al. (1999) found sertraline at varying doses from 50 to 200 mg per day to be significantly more effective than placebo on all measures used. Paroxetine has also been reported to be more effective than placebo in a multicenter trial but only at doses of 40 mg and 60 mg per day, with 20 mg being no different from placebo (Hollander et al., 2000). There also is growing evidence concerning the effectiveness of citalopram in the treatment of OCD (Kopenon et al., 1997). Mundo et al. (1997) reported equal effectiveness of fluvoxamine, paroxetine and citalopram in a single-blind comparative trial of 30 patients with OCD.

The issue of treatment-refractory OCD patients has been addressed by a number of authors, and several pharmacological agents (e.g., lithium, buspirone, haloperidol, olanzapine) have been suggested as possible augmenting strategies. Few controlled trials of such substances have been reported. However, in a recent placebo controlled trial, McDougle et al. (2000) found augmentation of SSRIs with risperidone to be of assistance in patients who did not respond to SSRI monotherapy. The issue of how to define a treatment-refractory patient was addressed by Rasmussen and Eisen (1997), who suggested that the emerging consensus is "someone who has failed both adequate trials of an SSRI and exposure with response prevention" (ibid., p. 11), rather than monotherapy with either exposure or SSRIs.

Perhaps the major difficulty with the use of SSRIs in the treatment of OCD is the high relapse rate with medication discontinuation. For example, Pato et al. (1988)

reported that 89% of patients treated with clomipramine over a 5- to 27-month period experienced substantial recurrence of OC symptoms. Significant worsening of depression was reported in 11 of the 18 subjects. Estimates of relapse following discontinuation of medication range from 65% to 90% (Rasmussen and Eisen, 1997). Such findings have resulted in some authors suggesting that the addition of behavior therapy to medication may prevent relapse and assist patients to discontinue medication (March et al., 1994; Greist, 1998). No study has as yet specifically addressed the issue of medication discontinuation following behavior therapy, though a number of studies have compared the effects of combining SSRIs and behavior therapy with either monotherapy. A number of studies have suggested that combining SSRIs with behavior therapy may be useful for depressed OCD sufferers in the short term, with behavior therapy an effective and sufficient treatment for nondepressed OCD sufferers (e.g., Marks et al., 1980, 1988; Cottraux, 1989; Hohagen et al., 1998), while others have found no difference in outcome when comparing combined SSRI and behavior therapy to behavior therapy alone (de Haan et al., 1998; van Bolkom et al., 1998). Kobak et al. (1998) conducted a meta-analytic study that examined the efficacy of SSRIs and behavior therapy. From the medications that included clomipramine, fluoxetine, fluvoxamine and paroxetine, for clomipramine the effect size at 1.02 was largest; however, the difference as a whole was not statistically different from the other SSRIs. Although the effect size for exposure and response prevention was not significantly different from clomipramine, it was significantly larger than the effect size for the SSRIs as a whole; however, the result was nonsignificant when methodological variables were controlled. The effect size for exposure was not significantly different from the effect size for combined exposure and SSRIs. Interestingly, dropout rates from behavior therapy were similar to those of any individual SSRI.

The decision as to whether OCD sufferers are best treated with behavior therapy alone or in combination with pharmacological agents rests with the clinician and the sufferer. A number of reports in the literature suggest that a combined approach is the most favorable. There is, however, little evidence to support such recommendations for the majority of sufferers. As stated earlier, the notion that the addition of behavior therapy to pharmacological treatment may prevent the relapse associated with cessation of medication has not been specifically addressed in any study to date. Gradually tapering the medication as a method of reducing the high relapse rate has also not been tested in any controlled fashion. However, anecdotal evidence from our clinic suggests that medication reduction and eventual discontinuation is possible in individuals who have had a good response and remained stable for a 6-month period. Any attempt at reduction of medication is undertaken very gradually (over a 6- to 8-month period) and patients are carefully monitored so that emergence of symptoms can be dealt with in behavior therapy booster sessions. Nevertheless, given the current absence of knowledge regarding the possible superiority of a combined versus individual approach as well as the side-effects that, although variable across the medications, are nonetheless present, the decision to include medication as part of treatment should be made on the basis of such factors as severity of associated depression, the patient's willingness to undertake a behavioral program, failure to respond to exposure techniques, or the patient's choice on the matter.

Psychosurgical techniques, such as anterior cingulotomy, anterior capsulotomy, or subcaudate tracheotomy procedures that interrupt connections between the basal ganglia and frontal cortex have been shown to be of benefit in the treatment of severe, intractable OCD that has not responded to traditional treatments (Greist, 1998). However, it is recommended that following such intervention a comprehensive program of behavior therapy and pharmacotherapy be utilized, as surgical intervention, rather than being curative, tends to restore the patient to a status that is more amenable to such techniques (Greist, 1990b).

Conclusions

The effective cognitive behavioral treatment of OCD requires intensive intervention on the part of the therapist and strong motivation on the part of the patient. The decision as to whether to combine pharmacological and behavioral treatment should be made in consultation with the patient. In the presence of a severe major depressive illness, the decision is clear: a combined approach may be the most effective. If the patient is drug naïve, hesitant about taking medication, or cannot tolerate the side-effects, then behavior therapy alone may well be the treatment of choice. Given the high relapse rate associated with medication discontinuation, pharmacotherapy in the absence of behavioral therapy does not constitute an adequate or appropriate treatment of OCD.

18

Obsessive–compulsive disorder

Clinician Guide

The principles of exposure and response prevention are relatively straightforward. Rarely are there any major difficulties in their application as long as the groundwork is completed competently. However, as noted by Marks et al. (1975), "This treatment requires a good patient–therapist working relationship, and a sense of humor helps patients over difficult situations." The cognitive techniques that can be used to supplement the exposure-based treatment are not as straightforward as the behavioral procedures, and require some level of expertise in the use of cognitive therapy. Often, patients report that previous treatment has involved clinicians attempting to challenge the rationality of the intrusive thought itself. Needless to say, such an approach has led to difficulties, particularly as it is the appraisal of the intrusion that needs to be challenged rather than the intrusion itself. The following sections will refer to aspects of treatment and patient preparation that will facilitate the implementation of exposure and response prevention as well as address common difficulties in the application of these procedures in the treatment of obsessional disorders.

Common questions

Patients referred for treatment will often ask a number of questions about their condition and the proposed treatment. As much as possible, individuals are encouraged to ask questions, and answers are given on the basis of available knowledge regarding OCD. Common questions include those relating to the cause of their condition. Apart from discussing the research findings to date, it is pointed out that there is no one cause of OCD: it is not as simple as a "biochemical imbalance", nor genes, nor individual psychological factors, nor environment but a complex condition due to a combination of a variety of complex factors. Educating the patient about OCD, its many causal factors and its treatment is an important step in bringing about a cognitive shift from the helpless attitude of many sufferers to having a good understanding of the condition, its maintaining factors, and what patients can do to assist in their own treatment.

Assessment

Perhaps the most important aspect of the cognitive behavioral treatment of OCD is the detailed assessment of the problem behaviors. Because of inadequate assessment, many difficulties commonly arise in the treatment of the condition. While standardized assessment forms may yield information and clues as to symptoms that may have been missed on initial interview, the assessment process is interactive. The therapist tests hypotheses with the patient not only on the basis of information obtained in the initial stages of treatment but more importantly on information gained throughout the treatment process. In other words, assessment is an ongoing activity. It is rarely the case that sufferers will be able to elucidate all of the necessary information in the first one or two sessions. In addition, a proportion of patients will be reticent in giving full details of their symptoms because of embarrassment. In the first instance, it is a matter of modifying the program as more information is made available. Where embarrassment plays a role, it is important to reassure the patient that, as an experienced therapist, you have seen similar symptoms in OCD sufferers. It may be worthwhile offering examples of obsessional symptoms in order to allay any anxieties that the patient may have about being negatively evaluated by the therapist or others because of their symptoms.

Assessment should focus on the presence or absence of internal cues (e.g., images, thoughts, urges), and external cues (contaminants, situations, etc.) that elicit the urge to ritualize. Rituals, particularly covert rituals or cognitive neutralizing, need to be carefully assessed. Reasons for ritualizing should also be noted, as they may have implications for the exposure program and provide clues in relation to avoidance and therefore to further exposure tasks. Avoidance of situations by OCD sufferers is often considerable, relating to situations, objects, and so forth, that the sufferer knows will provoke discomfort and the urge to ritualize. In addition to discussing avoided situations with the sufferer, it is often worthwhile discussing the patient's obsessional symptoms with a significant other, who can provide further information relating to triggers, rituals, and avoidance. Assessment of individuals presenting with obsessional thoughts and no overt rituals requires close attention. It is essential that the intrusive thought be identified correctly in order for exposure to be effective. Similarly, it is necessary to identify cognitive neutralizing of the obsessional thought. While sufferers are often able to verbalize the intrusive cognition, it is sometimes difficult to identify the covert neutralization of the thought, as it may be a repetition of the thought itself – or perhaps even an image of the actions involved in the thought – both of which may be anxiety-provoking and therefore difficult to distinguish from the original anxiety-arousing intrusion. For example, one sufferer presented with intrusive thoughts and images of harming a loved one while asleep. The intrusions appeared to take the form of verbal thoughts – "I will kill him" – as well as images of the actions being carried out. Detailed questioning of the sufferer indicated that the "intrusive" image, while anxiety provoking, was in response to the thought and was voluntarily produced because it served to reassure the sufferer that she could never perform such a terrible act. It may be helpful to define the neutralizing behavior for the sufferer in terms of any cognitive behavior in which they voluntarily engage as a response to their intrusive thought. Recording of the thought on a loop cassette tape and playing the same back to the patient may also yield important information as to neutralizing cognitions.

Cognitive assessment is equally important when dealing with individuals who present with obsessional thoughts and no overt rituals or those who present with thoughts of harm to others through some act of their own or through their own negligence. Such assessment is focused on the appraisals and beliefs the individuals have of their thought ("I may act on the thought"), as well as the occurrence of the thought ("having this thought means that I want it to happen", or "having the thought means I'm an evil person", etc.). Freeston et al. (1996b) proposed five groupings of beliefs and appraisals commonly present among OCD patients: (1) overestimating the importance of the thought through thought–action fusion, magical thinking and distorted Cartesian thinking; (2) exaggerating responsibility for events that are beyond the person's control and the consequences of being responsible for harm; (3) a need to seek absolute certainty or completeness or complete control over thoughts and actions; (4) overestimating the probability and consequences of negative events; and (5) beliefs that the anxiety caused by the thoughts is dangerous or unacceptable (Freeston et al., 1996b). As patients may have one or a series of beliefs regarding the intrusions as well as differing dysfunctional assumptions of the same thought, the individual examples of cognitive styles are by no means mutually exclusive. The authors give excellent descriptions of specific interventions that may be utilized to challenge the beliefs and assumptions associated with the thoughts and the reader is encouraged to obtain the journal article.

Treatment process

It is essential that the patient has a good grasp of the treatment rationale. Taking time to explain graded exposure, response prevention, and habituation – using examples from daily life – will help to ensure that the sufferer has a good understanding of the procedures without engendering further anxiety and pre-cipitating a flight from the clinician's office. A typical example one might give to patients is that of learning to drive a motor vehicle. The majority of people upon entering a car for their first driving lesson will feel quite anxious and uncomfortable, trying to remember all of the basic things to look out for as well as control the motor vehicle. However, with repeated exposure, the anxiety gradually subsides to the point that, after performing the driving behavior innumerable times, the driver feels no anxiety and doesn't even have to think about their routine behavior. Clinical examples of exposure and habituation from previously treated cases will also serve to reinforce the principles for the patient.

When discussing the treatment rationale with the patient, a graded approach should be emphasized. Often, patients envisage being asked to do the impossible: not ritualizing at all when exposed to the most "noxious" stimulus. Unless clarified and explained to the patient, such a misconception will place the clinician in the same position as many "helpful" friends and relatives who have suggested to the sufferer that, if he or she does not like being the way they are, they should just put a stop to their behavior. By explaining the fact that exposure will be graded, with the patient and therapist working through a graded hierarchy of stimuli and the patient being asked to refrain from engaging in rituals to a gradually increasing number of stimuli, the task does not seem as insurmountable as being told that total exposure will take place and absolutely no rituals are allowed. As part of the rationale, it is imperative that the sufferer is made aware that they will be taking a very active part in their own treatment and should in fact take on the role of co-therapist in the treatment program.

Program design and implementation

Assuming a thorough assessment has been conducted and that the patient is well aware of the rationale for the graded exposure and response prevention program, the design of the treatment program should take place with the cooperation of the patient. For those sufferers who experience intrusive thoughts with behavioral rituals, this process primarily involves the listing of the cues or triggers that provoke discomfort and the urge to ritualize, as well as the associated responses to such stimuli. The sufferer's subjective ratings of discomfort if they were to encounter such stimuli and be unable or disallowed to ritualize are also noted for each of the stimuli. The role of anticipatory anxiety should be discussed thoroughly, emphasizing the fact that anticipation of the encounter is often more anxiety provoking than the actual physical confrontation. Demonstration of this phenomenon is usually conducted within the treatment session, with a mild to moderate anxiety-provoking situation being confronted.

It is important for the clinician to be aware of any anxiety-reducing responses, apart from overt or covert rituals in which the individual may engage during exposure sessions and that will interfere with habituation. Patients may distract themselves from the anxiety-inducing stimulus (e.g., looking away from the stimulus object) or they may attempt to cope by delaying their rituals (e.g., "I will wash my hands later today and touch as little as I can in the meantime"). While such techniques may lead to a reduction in distress during the session, habituation or decreases in discomfort between sessions will not occur. Again, in such circumstances, it is important to remind the sufferer of the treatment rationale and reinforce the notion that there is little to gain by utilizing such methods. If, however, such methods are being utilized by the patient because the distress associated with the stimulus is greater than expected, then it is likely that a more detailed behavioral assessment is required and a more gentle rate of progress implemented.

Where the sufferer experiences obsessional thoughts without overt rituals, program design and implementation follow lines similar to the treatment of sufferers with behavioral rituals. Intrusive thoughts are identified, as are the covert neutralizing responses to such thoughts. Obsessions are rated hierarchically and the patient is requested to refrain from engaging in covert neutralization. Exposure consists of having the patient record their least anxiety-engendering or distressing thought on a loop cassette tape. On replay, anxiety or discomfort ratings are noted. Replaying of the taped thoughts in the early stages of treatment may also assist in the identification of any covert neutralizing responses. Patients are requested to refrain from any neutralizing behaviors and are required to listen to the tape and allow the recorded thoughts to guide their thinking. For example, a sufferer with intrusive blasphemous thoughts who prays in response to those thoughts is asked to listen to the taped blasphemous thoughts and not engage in prayers. As with compulsive ritualizers, it is often useful to allow the sufferer to experience anxiety or discomfort reduction within the initial treatment sessions and set similar tasks as homework assignments. As habituation to each thought takes place, variations in procedures such as listening to the tape in previously avoided situations or varying the tone or loudness of the recorded thoughts should be implemented. In the case of the individual described above, for example, this may involve having the patient listen to the recorded blasphemous thoughts while sitting near or in a church, and so forth.

An alternative method to loop tape exposure, which has led to equal success at our unit, follows the same principles without the taped exposure and relies on spontaneous thought occurrence and voluntary cessation of cognitive neutralizing. Avoidance of situations that may trigger the intrusive thought is often considerable. For example, intrusive sexual thoughts will often result in the person avoiding to look at, or be near, triggering stimuli such as same-sex individuals, children or animals; intrusive blasphemous thoughts will often result in avoidance of anything of a religious nature; and intrusive thoughts about harm will often result in avoidance of objects with which to cause harm, especially in the presence of the loved ones or persons involved in such thoughts. Individuals are given a thorough rationale for the maintenance of the intrusion and the associated worry. This is followed by identification of all intrusive thoughts as well as the associated neutralizing or avoidance. Dysfunctional beliefs are challenged, and the patient is encouraged to passively accept the thought whenever it occurs, live with the anxiety until it fades, while exposure to previously avoided situations is conducted in a hierarchical fashion. To some, such exposure may be viewed as behavioral experiments aimed at testing the patient's beliefs and assumptions rather than exposure per se, but what's in a name?

Whether the clinician decides on a loop tape or relies on spontaneous exposure, the challenging of dysfunctional assumptions in obsessional ruminators and those who fear causing harm to others by their thoughts is an essential step in ensuring the success of exposure treatment. For example, a 23-year-old female was referred to our unit after having failed in treatment at another clinic. The primary concerns were intrusive thoughts of molesting children. There was considerable avoidance of children and places where children could be encountered (e.g., friends' homes, shopping centers, schools, parks, etc.). Specific neutralizing strategies included trying to push the thoughts out of her head, arguing with the thoughts in order to reassure herself that her sexual preference was for adult heterosexual relationships, telling herself that she would never act on the thoughts and that she would commit suicide if there was ever any chance of acting on the thoughts. Although she had undergone a well-designed treatment program that included exposure to the thought as well as previously avoided situations and prevention of the neutralizing responses, few gains were made. On assessment, it became apparent that treatment gains were minimized by the fact that her beliefs about the intrusive thoughts had not been addressed. Her underlying assumptions regarding the thoughts included the notion that only very disturbed individuals would have such thoughts, that she did not have OCD, and that perhaps she was a sexual deviate after all. Challenging these assumptions at a number of levels included education about the fact that intrusive thoughts are common human phenomena and that what differentiates OCD from normal intrusive thoughts is the meaning and importance individuals attach to intrusive thoughts. The notion that having an inappropriate thought directly reflects on the individual's nature was challenged by having her examine other inappropriate thoughts to which no meaning was attached, as well as having her discuss with significant others (family who were aware of her concerns) the nature of inappropriate thoughts that they had experienced. Such techniques, aimed at changing her appraisal of the intrusive thoughts, led to significant improvement with exposure-based treatment.

Unlike overt rituals, cognitive neutralizing is considerably more difficult to identify and control. Consequently, the clinician is much more reliant on the self-reported resistance to the covert neutralizing. Failure to habituate to the thought would tend to indicate that the neutralizing response is continuing or that some other coping technique (e.g., distraction) has been implemented by the sufferer and more detailed assessment and further discussion of the rationale may be warranted. Alternatively, as noted above, it may be the case that the beliefs and appraisals associated with the intrusive thought have not been adequately challenged, or are still adhered to despite cognitive interventions. Consequently, it is important that both cognitive and behavioral assessment is an ongoing process during treatment. Other strategies that may be employed to enhance the tape exposure, or as alternative treatments, involve the repeated writing of the intrusive thought combined with prevention of the covert neutralizing response.

Whether the sufferer presents with obsessional thoughts associated with behavioral rituals or obsessions with covert rituals, basic behavioral principles apply. The hierarchy is completed at the patient's pace. The role of the clinician is to actively encourage the patient to move through the steps as quickly as possible. Habituation is the key to successful treatment and, as such, progress is determined by the patient's self-reported decreases in anxiety or distress associated with the stimulus rather than with the passage of time.

Homework assignments

Homework assignments in which the patient is required to perform the exposure tasks conducted during the treatment session are an integral part of treatment. Little is to be gained if the patient engages only in exposure and response prevention in the clinic setting. In order to ensure habituation to the anxiety-evoking stimulus, exposure and self-directed response prevention need to be conducted repeatedly and such tasks should be included as part of the homework assignments. Diary notes of each assignment should be kept by the sufferer and ratings of discomfort and urge to ritualize (overtly or covertly) included in the diary. Involvement of significant others, such as partners or family members, as co-therapists will assist in ensuring that the required tasks are carried out as instructed. However, at all times it is emphasized that the sufferer himself or herself is responsible for the implementation of the program.

Follow-up

It is essential that OCD patients be seen on a regular basis for at least 12 months following intensive treatment. Invariably, sufferers will experience short-term difficulties in maintaining their gains, particularly as novel situations or thoughts provoke the urge to ritualize. The clinician needs to encourage the adoption of the principles of exposure and response prevention for each of the novel as well as the familiar stimuli. Although total cures are relatively rare, the goal of controlling the disorder rather than the disorder controlling the sufferer is both realistic and achievable in the majority of cases.

Problem solving

When using any cognitive behavioral procedure, it is important for the sufferer to be aware that they will be taught skills with which to deal with their own disorder. That is to say, they will not be "treated" in the traditional sense of the word and be passive recipients of the techniques that will alleviate their distress. This is much more the case in the treatment of obsessional disorders, particularly as ritual prevention must be self-directed and voluntary. As part of the treatment rationale, the patient should be made aware of the expectation that they will take an active part in their own treatment, being primarily responsible for the proper implementation of the techniques and therefore directly responsible for their own treatment gains. The role of the therapist is described as that of an instructor or teacher whose principal task includes encouraging the sufferer to face the various anxiety-provoking situations in a planned and systematic fashion. At all stages, the patient is encouraged to assist in their program design and he or she should be encouraged to take on the role of co-therapist in the assessment phase, for without total cooperation in the assessment of obsessional symptoms, program outcome will be less than satisfactory.

Reassurance

Invariably, OCD sufferers will request reassurance from their treating clinician. While this reassurance is confined to possible outcome of treatment or the rationale for exposure, the clinician is on safe ground in reassuring the patient about the techniques being used. However, reassurance relating to the possibilities of danger or harm must be diligently avoided by the therapist. If one considers that in the majority of cases, the OCD sufferer engages in repetitive ritualized overt or covert behaviors in order to minimize the risk of harm to themselves or others, reassurance of the lack of danger by the therapist will serve only to replace one anxiety-reducing behavior (washing, checking, praying, etc.) with another, i.e., checking with or gaining reassurance from the therapist. Once given, the patient will constantly seek the clinician's reassurance that the behavior engaged in poses no threat to the sufferer or significant others. Needless to say, the exposure program will then be confronted with major difficulties, as it becomes the clinician's permission that allows the behavior to be performed rather than the patient taking the risk in performing the behavior. Another pitfall in treating some patients is that the clinician inadvertently reassures the patient by setting the exposure task. Responsibility for any disastrous consequence is transferred from the patient to the clinician, as the task was conducted only at the clinician's request. In such cases, it is always helpful to have the patient select the exposure task without input from the clinician. Similarly, some individuals with intrusive unpleasant thoughts or images will, in each treatment session, insist on giving the clinician a detailed account of each occurrence of the intrusive thought and image, the content of the thoughts/images and every situation in which they occurred. This need to "confess all" is a more subtle way of gaining reassurance, for as the clinician sits impassively listening, the patient knows there is nothing to be concerned about because the clinician has not reacted in shock or horror by falling out of the chair. In such cases, it is better for the session to focus on more general issues such as frequency of the thoughts, intensity of anxiety, duration, neutralizing, etc. rather than specific individual instances of intrusive thought occurrences. In general, reassurance-seeking behavior should be dealt with by explaining to the patient that assurances regarding the lack of possible harm from any action is an impossibility, and that, in order to effectively overcome OCD, the patient must learn to live with the doubt.

19

Obsessive–compulsive disorder

Patient Treatment Manual*

This Manual is both a guide to treatment and a workbook for persons who suffer from obsessive–compulsive disorder. During treatment, it is a workbook in which individuals can record their own experience of their disorder, together with the additional advice for their particular case given by their clinician. After treatment has concluded, this Manual will serve as a self-help resource enabling those who have recovered, but who encounter further stressors or difficulties, to read the appropriate section and, by putting the content into action, stay well.

Contents

*Gavin Andrews, Mark Creamer, Rocco Crino, Caroline Hunt, Lisa Lampe and Andrew Page *The Treatment of Anxiety Disorders* second edition © 2002 Cambridge University Press. All rights reserved.

SECTION 1

1 The nature of obsessive–compulsive disorder

Obsessive–compulsive disorder (OCD) is an anxiety disorder that, until quite recently, was regarded as a rare condition. Recent studies have shown that OCD is considerably more common than was previously thought and as many as 2 in every 100 people may suffer from the condition.

OCD is characterized by persistent, intrusive, unwanted thoughts that the sufferer is unable to control. Such thoughts are often very distressing and result in discomfort. Many OCD sufferers also engage in rituals or compulsions that are persistent needs or urges to perform certain behaviors in order to reduce their anxiety or discomfort or to prevent some dreaded event from occurring. More often than not, the rituals are associated with an obsessional thought. For example, washing in order to avoid contamination follows thoughts about possible contamination. For some, there is no apparent connection between the intrusive thought and the behavior, e.g., not stepping on cracks in the sidewalk in order to avoid harm befalling one's family. Others have no compulsive behaviors and suffer from obsessional thoughts alone, while still others do not experience obsessions but have compulsive rituals alone.

The one common element to the various symptoms in OCD is anxiety or discomfort. For those suffering both obsessional thoughts and compulsive rituals, it is the anxiety or discomfort associated with the thought that drives the ritual. In other words, the ritual is performed to reduce the anxiety produced by the thought. For those suffering from obsessional thoughts alone, anxiety is often associated with the thought, and mental rituals, distraction, or avoidance may be used to lessen the discomfort and ensure that the fearful event does not occur. It's much the same for those with compulsive rituals alone in that the behavior is performed in order to lessen the urge to ritualize. The role of anxiety is important in OCD and will be discussed in much greater detail in subsequent sections.

Most OCD sufferers can see the uselessness and absurdity of their actions but still feel compelled to perform their various rituals. They know that their hands are not dirty or contaminated and they know that their house will not burn down if they leave the electric kettle switched on at the wall. Because they are aware of how irrational their behavior is, many sufferers are ashamed of their actions and go to great lengths to hide their symptoms from family, friends, and, unfortunately, even their doctors. It is extremely important that your therapist is aware of all of your symptoms no matter how embarrassing or shameful they may be, as this is the only way that a suitable treatment program can be designed for you. Rest assured that a therapist experienced in the treatment of OCD will have heard of symptoms worse than yours many times over.

1.1 Symptoms of obsessive–compulsive disorder

Obsessional thoughts are usually concerned with contamination, harm to self or others, disasters, blasphemy, violence, sex or other distressing topics. Although generally called thoughts they can quite often be images or scenes that enter the sufferer's mind and cause distress. For example, one sufferer may have the thought "My hands are dirty" enter his head. This thought will trigger washing rituals. Another sufferer will actually have enter her head the scene of her house burning down. This scene will trigger checking rituals. Individuals who suffer obsessions alone may also experience thoughts, images, or scenes. For example, someone who has obsessions about harming his or her children may have the thought of harming them or have a frightening scene of hurting them or an image of the children already hurt.

As was pointed out earlier, many obsessions produce anxiety or discomfort that is relieved by performing rituals. The most common rituals are washing and checking, although there are many others, e.g., counting, arranging, or doing things such as dressing in a rigid, orderly fashion. Although rituals are performed to alleviate the anxiety or discomfort that is produced by the obsession, the anxiety relief is usually short lived. An individual who washes in order to avoid or overcome contamination will often find himself or herself washing repeatedly, because either he or she was uncertain whether a thorough enough job was done or because the obsessional thought of contamination has recurred. Similarly, someone who checks light switches, stoves, and so forth in order to avoid the house burning down, often has to repeat the behavior over and over, because he may not have done it properly or the thought or image of his house being destroyed has recurred. Even individuals who have obsessional thoughts alone may find that they have to repeat the cognitive rituals such as counting or praying many times over as they may not have done them *perfectly* in the first place.

An important point to keep in mind is that many sufferers have more than one type of symptom so that individuals may engage in more than one type of ritual or have more than one type of obsessional thought. Another point to note is that symptoms change over time and someone who is predominately a washer may, over time, develop checking rituals that eventually supersede the original complaint. In addition to changes in symptoms, the course of the disorder may also fluctuate over time, with periods of worsening and periods of improvement. Other sufferers may find that their symptoms remain static, while yet others may find a gradual worsening of symptoms since the onset of the disorder.

For many sufferers of OCD, these symptoms take up a great deal of time, often resulting in their being late for appointments and work and causing considerable disruption and interference with their lives. Apart from disrupting their own lives, it also frequently interferes with the lives of family members, as the typical sufferer often asks the other members to do things a certain way or not to engage in certain behaviors, as this may prompt the sufferer to engage in rituals. Thus the symptoms are controlling, frustrating, and irritating not only to the patients, but also to their families, friends, and workmates.

Avoidance of certain situations or objects that may trigger discomfort and rituals is also quite common among OCD sufferers. It seems logical to avoid contact with contaminants if you are a person who washes compulsively, or to avoid going out of the house if you must check all the electrical equipment, the doors, and windows. While this seems like a reasonable way of coping, it actually adds to the problem, as the typical sufferer avoids more and more situations and gradually the problem comes to rule their life. Moreover, avoidance does little to deal with the problem as it serves only to reinforce the idea that such situations are dangerous. Because the situation or object is constantly avoided, there is no opportunity for the individual to learn that there is no danger.

SECTION 2

2 The causes and treatment of obsessive–compulsive disorder

At the time of writing, no one is certain of the causes of OCD. Though there are a number of theories that attempt to explain the development of the condition, in general there is little evidence to support any one of them exclusively. In fact, it may be best to consider OCD as a complex problem with complex causative factors. It is most likely that a combination of psychological, biological, environmental and other factors result in the development of the disorder. We do know that for some the onset is during childhood, while for others the onset may be during adolescence or early adulthood. We also know that in some cases the onset is sudden, while others have a slow, insidious onset. Some of the theories that have been proposed to explain the development of OCD follow and are for information purposes only.

2.1 The biochemical theory

This theory was put forward after it was found that certain medications were of benefit in the treatment of OCD. These drugs affect mainly one type of chemical in the brain, called serotonin. Consequently, it was hypothesized that a problem with serotonin could be the cause of OCD. Although the drugs are indeed effective in the treatment of this condition, there is little hard evidence to indicate that sufferers have a deficit of serotonin in their brains. As medications have become more specific and selective in their effects on OCD, there has not been any difference in outcome to those medications that did not have such specific effects.

2.2 The genetic theory

This theory was put forward to explain the finding that OCD can sometimes occur in families. Although a genetic predisposition may account for some sufferers developing the condition, there is also the possibility that the OCD behavior was learned from the parents or siblings. It is extremely difficult to differentiate between OCD behavior that may be the result of genetics or OCD behavior that may be the result of the environment. Nevertheless, emerging evidence tends to suggest that early or childhood onset OCD subjects are more likely to have close relatives with OCD than those who have a later onset. This, however, is by no means always the case as many childhood onset subjects have no relatives with OCD.

2.3 Learning theory

This model suggests that obsessive–compulsive behavior has been learned through a process of conditioning. Put simply, this theory states that a neutral event becomes associated with fear by being paired with something that provokes fear, anxiety, or discomfort. This fear then generalizes so that objects as well as thoughts and images also produce discomfort. The individual then engages in behaviors that reduce the anxiety and, because the behavior is successful in reducing anxiety, even if only for short periods of time, it is performed each time discomfort or anxiety is felt. The problem with this theory is that it fails to explain why particular fears such as those of contamination or of harm to oneself and others commonly occur in OCD. Another problem is that many sufferers do not recall any significant precipitating event that can explain the onset of their symptoms. However, this theory does explain how obsessive–compulsive symptoms are maintained, and, as a result, this issue will be dealt with in much greater detail in subsequent sections.

2.4 Cognitive theory

This theory is one of the more comprehensive theories put forward and suggests that intrusive thoughts are experienced by all people. Individuals with OCD, however, attach negative meanings to their intrusive thoughts or images and feel personally responsible for having the thoughts, as well as responsible for the possible outcome of the thoughts. For example, someone who has thoughts of harming a loved one may believe that they are a bad person for having such thoughts and that they should also be very careful to ensure that the thought of harm does not become a reality. They do so by ritualizing. What maintains the OCD is the meaning they attach to the thought as well as their responding to the thought through rituals or other attempts to neutralize the thought. Treatment focuses on challenging the beliefs about the thoughts as well as exposure and response prevention.

2.5 Psychoanalytical theory

This theory basically states that obsessive–compulsive symptoms are attempts to keep unconscious conflicts and impulses from conscious awareness. Unfortunately, there is little evidence to support this theory and psychoanalysis is of little value in the treatment of the majority of OCD sufferers.

As can be seen, no theory is able to adequately explain the development of OCD but that does not mean that there are no effective treatments. In fact, the cause, though of considerable interest, has little bearing on treatment outcome. It is important to note, however, that in some cases symptoms that resemble OCD may be the result of other illnesses such as depression and schizophrenia. Effective treatment of these conditions will generally result in a decrease in the OCD-like symptoms. Other conditions that may result in symptoms that resemble OCD are Tourette's syndrome, dementia, brain trauma, or other neurological disorders.

2.6 The treatment of obsessive–compulsive disorder

There are currently two effective treatments available for OCD that may be used separately or together. One is drug treatment, with medication that increases the availability of serotonin in the brain; the other involves the use of behavior therapy techniques. At present, it appears that they are both effective and there is little in the scientific literature to suggest that combining the two results in a better outcome than using them individually. However, some sufferers who find behavior therapy too difficult initially may benefit from a course of medication so that effective behavior therapy can be undertaken.

2.6.1 Medication

The medications that have been found to be particularly helpful in the treatment of OCD come from the antidepressant family of drugs and include clomipramine, fluoxetine, fluvoxamine, and sertraline. They have specific effects on serotonin levels in the brain. Serotonin is the biochemical substance that some researchers believe is involved in OCD. In general, these medications have been shown to be effective for some OCD sufferers and assist them in bringing their symptoms under control. If one of these medications is prescribed for you, you should be made aware of possible side-effects and report their occurrence to your therapist. It is important to remember that these medications are not a cure for OCD. In addition, research indicates that ceasing the medication in the short term generally results in a return of symptoms. It could be that sufferers need to remain on the medication for long periods of time or that behavior therapy should be used in conjunction with the drug.

2.6.2 Behavior therapy

The rationale for using behavioral techniques is explained briefly under learning theory (Section 2.3) above but it is important enough to state again in greater detail. Typically, the OCD sufferer has intrusive thoughts that generate anxiety, discomfort, or an urge to carry out a ritual in order to lessen anxiety or prevent some dreaded event. Performing the ritual results in a decrease in anxiety or discomfort, and is actually reinforcing through its ability to reduce these negative feelings. For example, an individual has the thought that his or her hands may have touched something dirty or contaminated. This thought produces anxiety in that the person feels uncomfortable about the possibility of being contaminated or contaminating someone else. This unpleasant anxiety or discomfort is relieved by washing of the hands or other contaminated objects and it feels good to rid oneself of such negative feelings, so it feels "good" to wash. In the same manner, an individual who must check the stove and heaters prior to leaving home in order not to cause a disastrous fire will feel some relief after checking these items many times to ensure they are off. Thus the anxiety-producing thought is temporarily minimized by checking, and it feels "good" to check.

This anxiety- or discomfort-reducing quality that the rituals possess is shown in the following graph. Patients were asked to rate their levels of discomfort and urge to ritualize (1) before being exposed to an anxiety-provoking stimulus, (2) after being exposed, and (3) after performing their rituals. As can be seen, exposure to the stimulus results in a marked increase in discomfort and urge to ritualize.

Engaging in the ritual brings about an immediate and dramatic decrease in both these measures.

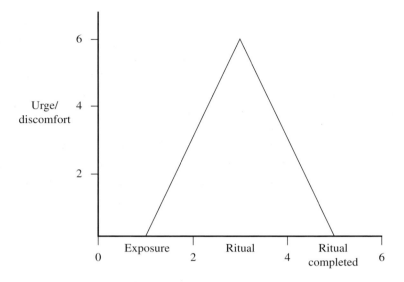

Though the decrease may be short lived, the individual very quickly learns that the discomfort may be reduced again by performing the ritual. The more anxious the individual feels, the more ritualizing they engage in. This is further worsened by their inability to concentrate on what they are doing to the extent that they are unsure that the ritual was conducted properly. This adds to their anxiety, which they try to bring under control by ritualizing further. For example, an individual who checks electrical equipment, doors, and windows prior to leaving home learns very quickly that checking alleviates the discomfort associated with the thought that the house may burn down or be broken into. The individual may have to perform the checking rituals a number of times in order to gain some relief. If he or she is under pressure from other sources and is preoccupied or distracted by these other worries, then they will have to engage in the rituals many more times because they may not have been done "correctly" the first few times. Having seen how compulsive rituals are maintained, the important question is what can be done to break the vicious cycle between the discomfort-producing thought and the anxiety-reducing rituals. Again, research into the condition provides the answer.

SECTION 3

3 Exposure and response prevention

Investigators looking at the phenomenology of OCD examined what happened when sufferers were exposed to stimuli that triggered rituals and were asked not to engage in their rituals. Initially, there was a significant rise in anxiety, discomfort, and urge to ritualize. Rather than continue to get worse, however, this rise remained quite steady and then gradually decreased so that by the end of the session, the level of discomfort had almost returned to normal. When this process was repeated again and again, the surprising finding was that the initial discomfort and anxiety was less with each exposure and the time taken to return to normal was shortened so that eventually exposure to the stimulus would result in a "hiccup" in anxiety that would then quickly settle. The initial findings of this research are demonstrated in the following diagram.

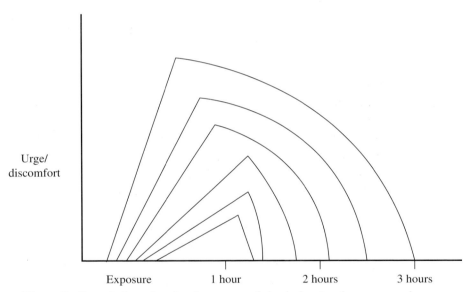

These findings led to the development of the behavioral treatment known as exposure and response prevention. As the names suggest, the two elements of this treatment are:

- Exposure to the cues or triggers of the compulsive rituals
- Prevention of the ritualized response

Prevention does not mean that the person suffering from the condition is restrained or held back from performing the ritual but rather that the individual, with the help of the therapist, voluntarily does not engage in the ritual.

In repeating this process of exposure combined with response (ritual) prevention, the end result is one of perhaps mild discomfort when the sufferer is confronted with triggers for the rituals, but the most important change is that the individual is now in a position to control the problem rather than be controlled by it.

When sufferers are made aware of this form of treatment, the initial reaction is either one of disbelief that such simple methods may work or, alternatively, that it appears extremely difficult. First, this form of treatment is *not* as simple as it seems. The approach must be structured, planned, and systematic in order to have maximum benefit. The individual needs to be motivated and consistent in his or her efforts to overcome the problem and faithfully follow all homework and clinic assignments. Approaching the problem in a haphazard manner will invariably result in a less than optimal outcome, with sufferers feeling disappointed, frustrated, and hopeless. A consistent and planned approach ensures that the problem is dealt with in a systematic manner. Any difficulties encountered can be quickly dealt with by the patient with the assistance of the therapist. Second, for those who see this approach as too difficult, the fact that the treatment program is planned by you in conjunction with the therapist ensures that the pace is at a level you are capable of mastering and the various steps can be graded to maximize your chances of success.

3.1 Obsessional thoughts

The principles of exposure and response prevention are also applied to the treatment of obsessional thoughts and images, except that there are no obvious behavioral rituals to work on. This does not mean that someone who has intrusive thoughts does not engage in rituals to reduce anxiety and discomfort; it is just that the rituals may also be thoughts. If, for example, an individual with OCD experiences frequent blasphemous thoughts, he or she may attempt to reduce the discomfort by saying a short prayer to himself or herself. Similarly, individuals who have thoughts of harming their children will often deal with the anxiety that such a thought produces by trying to push it out of their heads or by desperately reassuring themselves that they love their children and would never harm them.

Other sufferers with obsessional thoughts alone often have more elaborate and definite rituals. For example, having to mentally retrace their steps to ensure that they did not harm anyone while driving to their destination, or having to remember whether anything sharp stuck into their body because they fear contracting AIDS, or having to say something a certain number of times in order to avoid some disaster. When the problem of obsessional thoughts is conceptualized in this way, the treatment for the condition is readily apparent and involves exposure to the anxiety-provoking thought while, at the same time, not engaging in cognitive or mental rituals to lessen the discomfort.

There are, however, some important differences in the treatment of obsessional thoughts, especially considering that exposure to thoughts is not as easy as exposure to concrete objects: treatment involves confronting the thought or image until it no longer causes the individual distress or discomfort. For those who suffer from obsessional thoughts, this may seem to be an impossible task, but when you consider that everyone experiences unpleasant, strange, or bizarre thoughts at some time, then the goal of treatment appears more realistic. The major difference between obsessionals and everyone else is the meaning they attach to their intrusive thoughts. An individual who does not suffer from OCD will experience an intrusive thought but will dismiss the thought as silly and it will be gone. If it does recur, then it is again regarded as silly and meaningless and dismissed. Someone suffering from OCD, however, may experience the same thought and will desperately try not to think about it or will try to think of something to negate or cancel the thought. In other words, they react with fear, dread, and anxiety, so that the chances of the thought recurring and causing further distress is greatly heightened. Attempts not to think about the thought is like trying not to think of a pink elephant, whereas attempts to negate it through mental rituals only serve to reinforce the thought's apparent power. Put simply, it's your fear of the thought and the meaning you attach to the thought that ensures its continued return and your continued distress. The object of treatment is to disengage the emotional meaning of the thought from the thought itself so that it becomes "just another thought". This result is achieved through the exposure program, which should be designed to provide you with specific disconfirmations about the thoughts and their meanings. In cases where there are quite strong beliefs about the thoughts and their meaning, cognitive techniques aimed at challenging the beliefs about the intrusive thoughts may help to change your beliefs and assist you to more readily engage in exposure. It is important to discuss these techniques with your clinician.

Exposure should not only involve the obsessional thoughts but also must include any situations that the individual has been avoiding because of the possibility that the thoughts may be elicited. For example, a sufferer who fears harming his or her children may avoid contact with knives or other sharp objects while the children are around, or someone with blasphemous thoughts may avoid going to church for fear of bringing on the thoughts while there. Avoidance of such situations needs to be overcome in order to maximize and maintain the gains made from treatment.

3.2 Basic rules for success

The first requirement for the success of this treatment is motivation. Overcoming OCD is difficult and requires persistent effort on the part of the sufferer. Obvious-ly, there will be periods when treatment is going smoothly and others when the progress is slow and difficult. The important points to bear in mind are that the problems have been with you for a considerable period of time and are probably well ingrained in your daily routine. Overcoming these difficulties will most certainly take time and you should allow yourself as much time as it takes to get yourself better. You don't need to add to your difficulties by being impatient. Second, progress is not in a straight line but tends to be fluctuating so that having occasional bad days is the rule rather than the exception. The two graphs below are to demonstrate the difference between what people expect to happen and what actually happens.

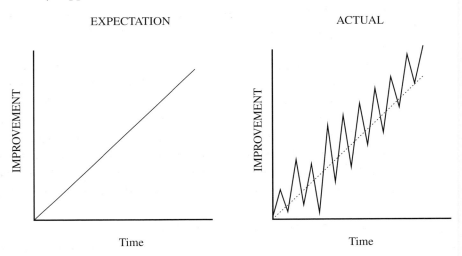

Most people expect the response to treatment to be linear, i.e. they start treatment and expect to get better and better. What actually happens, however, is that there are fluctuations from day to day, with some days being worse or better than others. When the fluctuations in the right-hand graph above are evened out (dotted line), it becomes obvious that the individual is improving, even though at times it may not feel as though they are getting better. They may even feel as though they are slipping back. It is important to reassure yourself that having a bad day does not mean that the situation is hopeless or that you are back to square one. In fact, the only individuals sure to return to square one are those who lose their motivation and no longer persist with the program.

Another basic requirement for a positive outcome is, for want of a better word, honesty. You need to be honest with yourself and your therapist in terms of your fears, avoidance, rituals, and thoughts. At times, individuals who know they have to be exposed to situations that they have avoided for long periods of time will avoid telling the therapist about similar situations or will not complete homework assignments. This does nothing to help the sufferer overcome the problem in any way. Telling yourself that the problem will be dealt with later is just another form of avoidance. It is important that you keep your therapist informed of your progress, difficulties, and fears at all times so that, if need be, the program can be modified to suit your needs. Others may avoid telling the therapist important information because they are embarrassed by the content of their thoughts or the nature of their rituals. Keeping this information to yourself means that the treatment program will not be comprehensive and ensures that the outcome will not be as successful as it could have been. As mentioned at the start of this Manual, your therapist will have dealt with many OCD sufferers and no doubt will have heard of problems such as yours many times over. These types of thoughts and rituals are quite common among sufferers, even though they may seem bizarre or strange to you.

Another important issue ties in with motivation. By attending the clinic, you have decided that it is time to work on your OCD problems. That is exactly what you should focus on doing to the exclusion of all else except the essentials. Your progress will be impeded if you have to deal with other issues such as moving to another house, leaving your partner, starting a new job, and so forth. It is essential that you set aside the time to work on your problems without the distraction posed by these other issues. If distractions are pressing, deal with them before commencing treatment and allow some time for yourself to come to terms with the changes.

The final important issue is that of self-mastery.

As you progress through the program, you will gradually gain confidence in dealing with the OCD problems. In order to gain this sense of mastery over the problem, it is essential that you do not use anxiety-reducing drugs, illegal drugs, or alcohol while participating in the program, as use of such substances results in your attributing positive changes to the drugs rather than to yourself.

SECTION 4

4 The treatment program

In previous sections an outline of the rationale and principles of treatment have been discussed. This section will review some of the important points and discuss the design of your treatment program. As mentioned above, treatment consists of repeatedly exposing the individual for prolonged periods (45 minutes to 2 hours) to circumstances that produce discomfort. In the initial sessions, such exposure will be under the supervision of your therapist, who will be with you throughout the task. Sessions may be conducted at the clinic, at your home, or in other settings where the rituals are a problem. The exposure is graded so that moderately disturbing situations are effectively dealt with before you proceed to more difficult ones. By breaking down the problems into steps and mastering each step before moving on to the next, you will find that what may seem like insurmountable problems become manageable. The sessions are held daily, with daily homework tasks being set during each session.

The importance of homework tasks cannot be overestimated, as it is with performance of these tasks that most of the treatment gains will occur. It is of little use to engage in the exposure and response prevention only while at the clinic. By completing your homework tasks faithfully, you are ensuring that what is being achieved at the clinic will transfer to the outside environment as well as reinforcing what has been learned during each session. Throughout the exposure, individuals are requested to refrain from ritualizing, regardless of the urges to do so. You should be prepared to experience some discomfort but you can rest assured that it will be considerably less than what you will anticipate. In fact, this is one of the major difficulties when describing this type of treatment to patients. Most sufferers fear that when exposed to a stimulus that evokes discomfort their anxiety will continue to rise for as long as they do not perform the ritual, until it eventually becomes unbearable. This is not the case. As described in previous sections, the discomfort will peak and then gradually decay, and each subsequent exposure will be less distressing and the decay will occur more rapidly.

4.1 Program design

The first step in designing your individual program is to conduct a thorough analysis of your difficulties by breaking down the problem into its various components.

Rituals are often triggered by thoughts, images, situations, events or feelings. In the sections below, you need to list your mental or behavioral rituals and the thoughts, situations or cues that trigger the urge to perform the ritual or lessen the anxiety. Some examples are listed to help you determine the triggers to the rituals and the rituals themselves. Your treating clinician will assist in your ratings of discomfort for each of the items. SUDs stands for subject units of discomfort.

Example 1

Cue or trigger:	Touching a cup or plate that someone else has used at my home	
Ritual:	Washing my hands with disinfectant repeatedly until they feel clean	SUDs

Example 2

Cue or trigger:	*Having an image of harming my child*	
Ritual:	Telling myself I love my child and would never harm it and making sure my partner is around when I'm near the child	SUDs

Example 3

Cue or trigger:	Closing the front door when I leave home	
Ritual:	Listen for the click of the lock and return six times to make sure the door is firmly locked	SUDs

Cue or trigger:		
Ritual:		SUDs

Cue or trigger:		
Ritual:		SUDs

Cue or trigger:	
Ritual:	SUDs

Cue or trigger:	
Ritual:	SUDs

Cue or trigger:	
Ritual:	SUDs

Cue or trigger:	
Ritual:	SUDs

4.1.1 Avoidance

Individuals with OCD will often avoid situations that will provoke the thoughts or urge to ritualize. For example, someone with intrusive blasphemous thoughts may avoid church or anything of a religious nature. Someone with a fear of being contaminated may avoid hospitals, doctors' surgeries, people who are ill, etc. In this section, please list all situations, objects, etc. that you avoid because they will cause you discomfort.

	Avoidance	SUD
1.		
2.		
3.		
4.		
5.		
6.		
7.		
8.		
9.		
10.		

4.2 Exposure tasks

The next phase in developing your program is to determine the exposure tasks and timetable them according to your ratings of discomfort so that, to begin with, you will be exposed to the least anxiety-provoking situation. Once this is mastered, you will move on to the next more difficult item.

Before moving on to this next phase, it is important to establish some ground rules with your therapist. The purpose of these rules is to ensure that you gain maximum benefit from treatment.

First, there need to be some limits set on your ritualized behaviors. If you wash compulsively, then certain limits will be set as to when you can wash, for how long, how much soap can be used, and so forth. If you check compulsively, there will be limits put on what you can check, how often, and so forth. These limits are to be in force 24 hours per day. The reasons are really quite obvious. If you are exposed to a situation or object that causes you discomfort and then resist the urge to ritualize for the required period, there is little gained if you subsequently engage in rituals because you have come in contact with some other stimulus. These rules will be set each week in consultation with your therapist.

Second, there is to be no enlisting of family members to perform your rituals, e.g., having them wash clothes or floors, or check doors, the stove, and so forth. By getting family members to do such things for you, you are in fact feeding the problem rather than overcoming it. Members of the family can certainly be enlisted to help you with your exposure tasks and your response prevention, but they should not be used to maintain the problem.

In the following forms, you and your therapist can list the ground rules for the planned daily tasks and the homework assignments. There is also the opportunity for you to make note of any difficulties encountered during the program.

Towards the end of the program, a new phase called overlearning will be introduced. This phase is an important part of treatment during which the exposure tasks are designed to ensure the consolidation of what has been learned during treatment. Your therapist will discuss this process with you when the time arises.

Permanent ground rules

1. _____

2. _____

3. _____

4. _____

5. _____

Exposure session

Session number: _____   **Date:** _____

Exposure task 1:

_____

_____

_____

Time spent in task:

_____

Difficulties:

_____

_____

Exposure Task 2:

_____

_____

_____

Time spent in task:

_____

Difficulties:

_____

_____

Comments:

_____

_____

_____

_____

SECTION 5

Recommended reading

5.1 Recommended paperbacks

The following books are available from most large bookstores, many smaller ones, and some newsstands. If in doubt, ask if the book can be ordered. We also suggest that you use your local library to gain access to these books. When you read these or any similar books on the management of anxiety, remember that they are best regarded as guidelines only. Be critical in both a positive and negative sense when reading these books, so that you get what is best for you out of them. These books are inexpensive.

Foa E, Wilson R. (1991) *Stop Obsessing! How to Overcome Your Obsessions and Compulsions.* Bantam Books.

Steketee G, White K. (1990) *When Once Is Not Enough: Help for Obsessive Compulsives.* Oakland, CA: New Harbinger.

20

Generalized anxiety disorder

Syndrome

Recent population-based studies of generalized anxiety disorder (GAD) have shown it to be prevalent, chronic, and associated with significant disablement. Two surveys, the National Comorbidity Survey (NCS) in the USA using DSM-III-R and ICD-10 diagnoses (Wittchen et al., 1995) and the National Survey of Mental Health and Wellbeing in Australia, using DSM-IV and ICD-10 diagnoses (Hunt et al., 2002) have provided the most recent and comprehensive information about the epidemiology of this disorder. Prevalence rates were found to be 1.6% for current GAD, 3.1% for 12-month, and 5.1% lifetime prevalence in the US population (Wittchen et al., 1994). GAD was shown to be a relatively rare current disorder but common if assessed over a person's lifetime. Lifetime prevalence rates were higher (8.9%) with the use of ICD-10 diagnostic criteria. In the Australian survey, the DSM-IV prevalence rates were 2.8% for 1 month and 3.6% for 12 months, somewhat lower than the ICD-10 rates of 3.6% for 1 month and 5.1% for 12 months (Hunt et al., 2002). These results provide somewhat lower lifetime prevalence rates as compared with earlier prevalence estimates using DSM-III diagnoses, possibly due to changes in the diagnostic criteria and differences in the study methods. For example, the Epidemiologic Catchment Area (ECA) study reported a lifetime prevalence of 4.1–6.6% in the three sites that assessed for GAD, but unlike the more recent surveys excluded cases with comorbid major depression or panic disorder (Blazer et al., 1991).

GAD is reported to be a common clinical diagnosis at the primary care level (Burvill, 1990; Goldberg and Lecrubier, 1995), yet it appears to be under-represented at specialist treatment centers. The comparatively low proportion of individuals with GAD who present to specialist services may indicate that the majority of these individuals are not sufficiently distressed to seek specific treatment or may consider their anxiety as part of their nature and hence not amenable to treatment (Rapee, 1991b). Furthermore, individuals with GAD tend to present later for initial treatment in comparison with panic disorder sufferers (Nisita et al., 1990). There may also be a problem with a lack of recognition and slowness to refer at the primary care level. The World Health Organization (WHO) primary care study surveyed 15 primary care sites in 14 countries. The prevalence of ICD-10 GAD was 7.9%, which was second only to major depression (Goldberg and Lecrubier, 1995). In a separate analysis of access and the provision of care, the general practitioners recognized only 46.1% of the identified cases as having a psychological disorder (Ustün and Von Korff, 1995).

GAD exhibits a chronic course, with patients reporting a duration of illness that spans the majority of their lifetimes (Anderson et al., 1984; Barlow et al., 1986a; Yonkers et al., 1996). Woodman et al. (1999) have recently reported a 5-year follow-up study of patients with GAD and panic disorder who had originally participated in drug trials but who had since received routine care in the community. They found that while the GAD sample had milder symptoms than the panic disorder at intake, fewer patients with GAD were in remission from their disorder at follow-up (18% versus 45%). Half of the GAD sample remained moderately impaired at the follow-up.

Data from the NCS has also shown that GAD is associated with significant disability, particularly if comorbid with a mood disorder (Judd et al., 1998). A diagnosis of GAD was found to be associated with significant health care utilization and role impairment (Wittchen et al., 1994), again an association that was strengthened by the presence of comorbidity with other mental disorders. While the presence of comorbid psychiatric disorders with GAD has routinely been associated with high levels of disability, findings from the WHO primary care study indicate that even "pure" cases of GAD show significant disablement relative to individuals with chronic somatic disease (Maier et al., 2000).

Wittchen et al. (1994) showed that a diagnosis of GAD was twice as common among women than among men, and was associated with being older than 24 years, separated, widowed, divorced, unemployed or a homemaker. Interestingly, the only previous major epidemiological study to investigate the correlates of GAD (the ECA study using DSM-III criteria) reported that GAD was more common in women, in African-Americans, and in persons younger than 30 years (Blazer et al., 1991). The discrepant findings with regard to age as a risk factor may be due to changes in the required duration of the disorder between DSM-III and DSM-III-R, with younger adults more likely to experience short episodes (less than 6 months) that meet criteria for DSM-III.

A number of descriptions of the clinical presentation of this disorder suggest a gradual onset ranging from the late teens to late 20s (Anderson et al., 1984; Rapee, 1985a; Thyer et al., 1985b; Cameron et al., 1986; Noyes et al., 1987b; Rickels and Schweizer, 1990; Yonkers et al., 1996). However, data from the National Comorbidity Survey (Wittchen et al., 1994) suggest that GAD is relatively less common in adolescence and the early 20s than in adults. Wittchen et al. suggested that younger people may be more likely to have shorter episodes that do not meet the

6-month duration requirements of DSM-III-R and DSM-IV. The course of the disorder can be either constant or waxing and waning in nature (Rickels and Schweizer, 1990). Noyes et al. (1987b) reported that most patients described being symptomatic for the majority of time since onset, with only 25% of patients describing episodes of remission, defined as 3 months symptom free.

Clinical description

GAD is characterized by generalized and persistent symptoms of anxiety, which are driven by worry. The worry is out of proportion to the feared event, pervasive, and difficult for the individual to control. The content of these worries usually covers several domains, primarily concerns for one's family, finances, work and personal health. Individuals with this disorder usually describe themselves as sensitive or nervous by nature, and their tendency to worry is usually longstanding, or at least of several months duration. The symptoms of anxiety usually involve motor tension (such as restlessness, trembling, or muscle tension) and overarousal (feeling keyed up or "on edge", irritable, or experiencing difficulty concentrating). Longstanding worry and anxiety may contribute to excessive tiredness, tension headaches, epigastric disturbances, and insomnia.

CASE VIGNETTE

Patient identification

Ms. G is a woman in her mid 30s. She is married with two children now aged 4 and 7 years.

Presenting problem

Ms. G had been troubled by worry for many years. She described herself as "a born worrier". Recently she had particularly worried about her family's health – fears that had been exacerbated by her husband suffering a serious illness several years previously. She stated "since then every time he mentions something, however minor, feeling tired, not eating as much as I think he should, I worry that he's getting sick again. And I won't stop worrying until he's been to see the GP and I'm convinced that it is nothing serious. And the kids too, I know it's ridiculous, but I'm constantly thinking about what might happen to them, even to the point of thinking how I would cope, and having to visit them in hospital, and worse...". She had tried to deal with these worries by seeking reassurance from family, friends and her general practitioner. Other worries included what other people thought of her, whether she might have said something to upset them. If her husband was late home – or even if he wasn't late – she worried that he had been in an accident. Some time ago she became concerned about global warming and the possibility that she might lose her house to flooding.

In regard to associated symptoms of anxiety, Ms. G reported feeling jumpy and nervous for much of the time. She said "I've never really been able to sit still, I always have to be on the go". She also described significant muscle tension that sometimes resulted in aching and stiffness in her neck and shoulders. During periods of increased worry she reported difficulty getting to sleep and a loss of appetite.

Previous psychiatric history

Ms. G has two previous major depressive episodes, the last of which required a course of antidepressant medication. She has been free from significant depression for the past 6 months but remains on this medication. She does not experience panic attacks, phobic avoidance or obsessions.

Personal and social history

Ms. G attended Arts College on leaving school and taught for a number of years at the local Further Education College before having children. Over the past several years she has worked on her own art from home, selling works through galleries and the local markets. She describes a very happy childhood and a stable family life. She also says that she may have "learnt to worry" from her mother. She does not smoke, drinks a small amount of alcohol occasionally, and does not use illicit drugs. She has avoided strong coffee and chocolate for the past few months, as she noted that they increased her anxiety symptoms.

Diagnosis

Prior to DSM-III-R, GAD had the status of a residual diagnostic category. Partly as a result of this residual position, the validity of the disorder has been brought under question. However DSM-III-R and DSM-IV no longer describe GAD as a residual category, consistent with evidence that it can exist independently of anxiety that is related only to the anticipation of panic or exposure to phobic or obsessive concerns (often simply referred to as anticipatory anxiety) (Barlow et al., 1986a). Thus a diagnosis of GAD can be made in a person with panic disorder provided that the worry is unrelated to having a panic attack. Likewise, GAD and social phobia can coexist if anxiety is not only related to a fear of negative evaluation but also results from the presence of pervasive worries about day-to-day concerns.

An additional change to DSM-IV has been the exclusion of autonomic symptoms from the list of required somatic symptoms. The low rate of endorsement of autonomic symptoms by GAD patients (Marten et al., 1993), together with the finding that symptoms within the motor tension and scanning and vigilance clusters are more closely associated with independent measures of GAD than symptoms from the autonomic activity cluster (Brown et al., 1995) support this change. Data from a nonclinical population using the Depression, Anxiety and Stress Scale (Lovibond and Lovibond, 1995) also supports the notion that worry is more closely associated with tension or stress symptoms than with the autonomic cluster of symptoms (Lovibond, 1998). Similar findings in a nonclinical sample, where only muscle tension across a number of somatic symptoms showed a unique relationship to worry, has been reported recently (Joorman and Stober, 1999). Physiological studies suggest that there is a diminished range of autonomic reactivity in response to psychological stress in GAD, although this pattern is not specific to GAD (Connor and Davidson, 1998; Hoehn-Saric, 1998). There appears to be a diminished vagal (or parasympathetic) tone associated with worry, rather than the sympathetic activity (dry mouth, sweating, urination) that is usually classed under the construct of autonomic activity (Thayer et al., 1996).

Unlike DSM-IV, ICD-10 requires the presence of symptoms of autonomic overactivity (e.g., light-headedness, sweating, tachycardia) and also imposes a diagnostic hierarchical structure. The diagnosis cannot be made if there is concurrent panic disorder, phobic disorder, OCD or hypochondriasis. A recent report of high levels of concordance between the two diagnostic systems is therefore surprising. These findings may need to be tempered by the fact that the patients studied had comorbid panic disorder (perhaps accounting for the high frequency of autonomic symptoms reported) and that critical DSM criteria (such as the excessive and uncontrollable nature of worry) were not assessed (Starcevic and Bogojevic, 1999).

Differential diagnosis and assessment

Physical factors that may initiate and maintain anxiety-like somatic disturbances include chronic use of drugs (e.g., stimulants such as amphetamines or caffeine) or withdrawal syndromes (e.g., from alcohol, benzodiazepines, or opiates). The exclusion of general medical conditions such as hyperthyroidism is given specific mention in both the ICD-10 and DSM-IV diagnostic criteria.

DSM-IV requires that an assessment of the specific cognitive focus of an individual's anxiety be made in order to obtain an accurate differential diagnosis from other anxiety disorders. Furthermore, DSM-IV requires exclusion of the anxiety about gaining weight observed in the disorder anorexia nervosa, the fear about having a serious illness observed in hypochondriasis, or the fear of being away from home or close relatives as observed in separation anxiety disorder. However, epidemiological research suggests that in community samples it is rare to exclude GAD as a diagnosis on the basis of the worry being related to another disorder or initiated or maintained by physical factors (Wittchen et al., 1995). DSM-IV also specifically excludes the diagnosis of GAD if the disturbance occurs only during the course of a mood disorder, PTSD, a psychotic disorder, or pervasive developmental disorder. ICD-10 does not allow the diagnosis to be made if criteria for a depressive episode are met.

The differential diagnosis of GAD and major depression is of some theoretical and clinical interest, as there is considerable overlap between these two disorders. Breslau and Davis (1985) argued that – given the scant evidence of temporal separation of episodes in patients who meet criteria for both GAD and depression – either the designation of residual status to GAD is justified or GAD may constitute a subtype of major depressive disorder. The lack of specificity of response to pharmacotherapy across GAD and major depression has also led to speculation that GAD may be a prodromal or residual entity of a mood disorder (Casacalenda and Boulenger, 1998). On the other hand, there are studies that suggest that GAD and major depressive disorder can be discriminated significantly in terms of scores on the Hamilton Depression and Anxiety Rating Scales (Riskind et al., 1987; Copp et al., 1990) or the Depression Anxiety Stress Scales (Lovibond and Lovibond, 1995; Brown et al., 1997). A large study of female twins assessing the role of genetic factors in the etiology of GAD has found that these genetic factors were completely shared with those for major depressive disorder (Kendler et al., 1992b). The findings suggest that, in women, the genetic vulnerability to GAD and major depression is likely to be the same, but whether one or the other disorder develops is likely to be a result of environmental experiences.

A more difficult differential diagnosis may occur in the case of GAD and dysthymia. In a review of the relationship between these two disorders, Riskind et al. (1991) pointed out that both disorders are characteristically low grade, cross-situational, and chronic. They concluded, on the basis of a systematic search of the literature and unpublished data sets, that support for the differentiation between GAD and dysthymia is equivocal.

OCD is commonly comorbid with GAD (Sanderson and Wetzler, 1991) and hence may pose another differential diagnosis dilemma. While the worry shown by GAD patients may often appear to be obsessive and ruminative in nature, it is possible to clinically differentiate between the worry observed in GAD and the obsessive thoughts observed in OCD. Turner et al. (1992a) first reviewed these two types of thinking process, and noted that while there are shared features, the two can be differentiated. GAD worries are typically self-initiated (as opposed to the unwanted and intrusive nature of obsessions), are ego-syntonic (as opposed to ego-dystonic), and are related to an undefined set of ongoing concerns in an individual's life (as opposed to being confined to a specific set of concerns, such as contamination, violence, or blasphemy). Likewise Abramowitz and Foa (1998) argued that worry in GAD and obsession in OCD are distinct phenomena. They found that the presence of comorbid GAD in patients with OCD was not associated with severity of obsessions or compulsions, but rather with greater levels of indecision, an excessive sense of responsibility, and excessive worry about everyday concerns. Langlois et al. (2000a,b) found a number of differences, but also some overlap, between worry and obsessions in a nonclinical population and confirmed the ego-syntonic/-dystonic distinction. Subjects reported to be less disturbed by intrusive ego-dystonic thoughts, found that they caused less interference, and found them more easy to dismiss than worries. However, it is unlikely that this difference would hold up in a clinical population where, by definition, the obsessions cause significant distress and are difficult to dismiss.

The assessment of GAD has traditionally focused on measures such as the Hamilton Anxiety Scale (Hamilton, 1959) or the State–Trait Anxiety Inventory (Spielberger et al., 1983). The Hamilton Anxiety Scale is primarily a measure of somatic anxiety while the State–Trait Anxiety Inventory includes both somatic and cognitive items. Other measures that will tap symptoms of anxiety are the Beck Anxiety Inventory (Beck et al., 1988) and the Depression, Anxiety Stress Scales (Lovibond and Lovibond, 1995), the latter being particularly useful in assessing only symptoms that are specific to depression, anxiety, and tension/stress and omitting symptoms that do not differentiate between these three syndromes. The Penn State Worry Questionnaire (Meyer et al., 1990) is widely used as a measure of pathological worry, and a reliable and valid version has been adapted for use with children and adolescents (Chorpita et al., 1997). Other questionnaire measures assess diagnostic criteria of GAD (Generalized Anxiety Disorder Questionnaire, Roemer et al., 1995), the content of worry (e.g., Worry Domains Questionnaire, Tallis et al., 1992; Anxious Thoughts Inventory, Wells, 1994) or theoretical constructs thought to contribute to the development or maintenance of the disorder (e.g., Intolerance of Uncertainty and Why Worry Questionnaires, Freeston et al., 1994, 1996a).

Comorbidity

Since GAD has been able to be diagnosed independently from other disorders, the problem of high comorbidity with other anxiety and depressive disorders has become apparent. Studies of both clinical and community samples have shown that "pure" cases of GAD are rare (Sanderson and Wetzler, 1991; Brown and Barlow, 1992; Brawman-Mintzer et al., 1993; Wittchen et al., 1994; Yonkers et al., 1996). Using NCS data, Wittchen et al. (1994) reported comorbidity with another mental disorder in 90.4% of the sample with a lifetime history of GAD. The most frequent comorbid disorders were major depression, panic disorder, and (for current comorbidity only) agoraphobia. The odds ratios reported were not strongly affected by the use of diagnostic hierarchy rules. Judd et al. (1988) reported that 84% of the NSC GAD sample had a comorbid lifetime mood disorder.

Even when other diagnoses are not met, a large proportion of GAD patients report experiencing at least one panic attack (73%; Sanderson and Barlow, 1990) and experience social phobic concerns (75%; Rapee et al., 1988). Moreover, Rapee et al. (1988) found that 79% of patients with a primary diagnosis of GAD reported at least one moderate fear, and 61% of patients report sometimes avoiding at least one social situation.

Construct validity of the diagnosis

The construct validity of GAD has been called into question in a number of areas, quite apart from its close relationship with major depression. For instance, reports of the reliability of the diagnosis of GAD prior to DSM-IV have proved disappointing. The relatively poor interrater agreement from earlier studies (e.g., Di Nardo et al., 1983; Riskind et al., 1987) may well be explained by the DSM-III diagnostic criteria that relegated GAD to a residual category and did not include worry as a defining characteristic of the disorder. Unlike the somatic symptoms of GAD, worry can be assessed with good reliability (Sanderson and Barlow, 1990). A later study that used DSM-III-R criteria produced disappointing agreement statistics, but was based on a small sample size (Mannuzza et al., 1989). However, recent data from field trials of the Composite International Diagnostic Interview (CIDI) produced excellent interrater agreement ($\kappa = 0.96$) for the diagnosis of GAD, which was as high or higher than other anxiety disorders, based on a sample of 575 patients across 18 centers (Wittchen et al., 1991). While these data are more promising, the diagnostic reliability of GAD may well be compromised by high rates of comorbidity.

Furthermore, GAD possibly constitutes a "basic" anxiety disorder, or a vulnerability to the development of additional anxiety or depressive disorders (Barlow and Wincze, 1998; Maser, 1998). Breier et al. (1985: 793) concluded that GAD may have been a "prodromal, incomplete, or residual manifestation of other psychiatric disorders". Their conclusion was consistent with evidence of a generalized anxiety prodrome in panic disorder (Garvey et al., 1988) and the notion that generalized anxiety may constitute the initial emotional disturbance in patients with agoraphobia (Roth and Argyle, 1988). Rapee (1991b) has also drawn attention to the trait-like nature of the anxiety in GAD, citing as evidence its temporal stability, insidious onset, and the lack of specific focus to the anxiety. GAD is the most "normal" anxiety disorder, given the normality of worry in the general population and the fact that it seems to lie along a continuum of trait anxiety. Akiskal (1998) has argued that GAD may be better classified as a life-long temperamental predisposition to worry, and thus an exaggeration of a normal personality disposition. However, GAD differs in quantity, if not quality, from the worry and anxiety that most of us experience from time to time, and once symptoms are of sufficient duration or severity to have interfered with lives or activities, a "disorder" exists.

Maser (1998) has argued that the high rates of clinical or subclinical GAD comorbid with other anxiety or depressive disorders may be responsible for the broad occurrence of worry across these other disorders, and a resulting lack of specificity of this feature. Using ECA data, Bienvenu et al. (1998) compared the demographic and comorbidity profiles across five samples comprising patients with a DSM-III-R diagnosis and four subthreshold groups. They found groups were comparable in respect to the demographic and comorbidity variables whether or not the worry criterion was met or whether the anxiety and associated symptoms were of 1 month or 6 months duration. The only group that differed from the GAD diagnosis group was that which had less than the required six associated symptoms. These authors argue against the construct validity of the DSM-III-R diagnostic criteria for GAD.

The associated somatic symptoms also suffer from a lack of diagnostic specificity. Brown et al. (1995) reported that, while most of a sample of patients with GAD endorsed the three of six symptoms required in DSM-IV, a large proportion of patients with other anxiety or mood disorders also fulfilled this criterion. However, not all patients with a principal diagnosis of another anxiety disorder meet diagnostic criteria for GAD (Sanderson and Wetzler, 1991), suggesting that, while symptoms of generalized anxiety are common to other anxiety disorders, these symptoms are not synonymous with the syndrome of GAD.

But there is also evidence supporting the validity of GAD as an independent diagnostic construct. An assessment of the genetic and environmental contributions specific and common to GAD and panic disorder in a cohort of male–male twin pairs has shown a genetic liability that is specific to panic disorder, suggesting that the two disorders are at least partially etiologically distinct (Scherrer et al., 2000). Breitholtz et al. (1999) found significant differences in the content of thinking between GAD and panic disorder patients, hence supporting the cognitive specificity of the two disorders. Likewise, Abramowitz and Foa (1998) have argued that worry in GAD and obsessions in OCD are distinct phenomena. They found that the presence of comorbid GAD in patients with OCD was not associated with severity of obsessions or compulsions but rather with greater levels of indecision, an excessive sense of responsibility, and excessive worry about everyday concerns. Brown et al. (1993) found that, while many of a sample of OCD patients endorsed worry symptoms, OCD and GAD patient groups could be reliably distinguished diagnostically by clinical interview. Lastly, an examination of the construct validity of diagnoses across the anxiety and depressive disorders showed that patients with a diagnosis of GAD had a unique score profile across a number of self-report measures, and that profile significantly differentiated patients with GAD from other diagnostic groups (Zinbard and Barlow, 1996).

The phenomenon of worry

The designation of worry as the definitive feature of GAD has led to the suggestion that this disorder is a largely cognitive anxiety disorder (Rapee, 1991b) and has focused new attention onto the validity and reliability of the worry construct. Descriptions of the nature and process of worry have tended to focus on the uncontrollable nature of worry and its possible role in avoiding negative outcomes of anticipated events. What makes the worry pathological in GAD is not its content or the degree to which the worry is recognized as unreasonable but rather the perception that the worry is excessive and uncontrollable (Barlow and Wincze, 1998). There has been a notable increase in investigations into the process of worry in both GAD patient and non-clinical samples, and in the development of theoretical models to understand worry as it relates both to GAD and to nonclinical populations.

Features of worry in nonclinical populations

Worry is a cognitive activity concerned with negative views of future events. Worry, relative to other cognitive activity, has been shown to be characterized by a decrease in present-oriented statements, an increase in anxious and depressive affect, a predominance of thoughts over images, fewer shifts in content across topics and a predominance of words implying catastrophic interpretation (e.g., always, never, awful, terrible) (Molina et al., 1998). It is also characterized by a disruption of attention-focusing ability. Worriers report more negative cognitions and less control over these cognitions than nonworriers during an attentional task (Borkovec et al., 1983).

Borkovec et al. have recently emphasized the distinction between mental imagery and the "predominance of negatively valenced verbal thought activity" of worry (Borkovec et al., 1998: 562). The distinction is important, as, while verbal thoughts elicit little cardiovascular response, images of the same material evoke greater response. Borkovec and his colleagues have hypothesized that worriers use verbalization as a strategy to decrease sympathetic arousal to threatening material and that the process of worry may account for the reduced autonomic variability found in GAD. While the verbalization strategy may be adaptive in many contexts, especially those that are interpersonal, the inhibition of emotional processing may be maladaptive in that it maintains negative emotional meaning and prevents extinction of the fear response. Stöber (1998) has investigated one possible mechanism for the link between worry and reduced somatic arousal, and argued that the abstract concepts that characterize worry may contribute to the lack of accompanying mental imagery and also contribute to the inability to engage in effective concrete problem-solving steps. Borkovec et al. also discussed the role of worry as an attempt to avoid negative events or prepare for the worst; because the worst rarely eventuates, the function of worry is negatively reinforced. Lastly, worry about relatively unimportant day-to-day concerns may function as a distraction from more emotionally laden topics.

Davey and Levy (1998) have investigated the process of catastrophic worry, typically associated with a "What if..." questioning style, where worriers adopt progressively worse and worse outcomes related to a specific topic. Of prime interest was the question of what caused worriers to continue to generate catastrophic steps despite increases in subjective discomfort. During a "catastrophizing interview", chronic worriers displayed a general perseverative iterative style in that they were more willing than nonworriers to catastrophize across a range of topics, including those that were novel or pleasant. They also found that chronic worriers tended to couch their catastrophizing in terms of personal inadequacies, perhaps stemming from dysfunctional beliefs. Davey and Levy hypothesized that core beliefs of self-doubt might make it difficult for individuals to obtain closure on their problems, leading to more catastrophizing steps, and hence greater opportunity to perceive the negative consequences that might result from personal inadequacies.

Worry in generalized anxiety disorder

The investigation of the phenomenology of worry in individuals with DSM-III-R- and DSM-IV-diagnosed GAD has yielded support of its relevance to the disorder. Patients with GAD spend over half of their average day worrying, with the majority (over 90%) recognizing that they worry excessively about minor things. Sanderson and Barlow (1990) have reported that while an affirmative response by patients to the question "Do you worry excessively about minor things?" did not necessarily ensure a diagnosis of GAD, given the presence of worry in other anxiety disorders, a negative response to the question virtually excluded such a diagnosis. The worries reported by GAD patients can be categorized into four spheres with high reliability (family, finances, work, and personal illness, in decreasing order of frequency), and interrater agreement of the excessive and/or unrealistic nature of the worries is high ($\kappa=0.9$; Sanderson and Barlow, 1990). Not surprisingly, the worries of adults in later life reflect their changing life circumstances, with a greater emphasis on health concerns, and a lessened emphasis on worries about work (Stanley and Novey, 2000).

While most reports of the content of worry have been derived from retrospective reporting, Breitholtz et al. (1999) asked patients with GAD or panic disorder to monitor their thoughts prospectively during episodes of anxiety. GAD patients had significantly greater numbers of thoughts in the categories of interpersonal conflict, competence, acceptance, concern about others and worry about minor matters than the panic disorder patients. Conversely, the panic disorder patients had more thoughts of physical catastrophe. Across worry topics, patients with GAD worry more about remote and future events than do anxious control patients (Dugas et al., 1998).

The level of perceived control over worries can discriminate GAD patients from nonanxious controls: GAD patients perceive less control over their worries and report a greater proportion of unprecipitated worries (Craske et al., 1989). Butler and Booth (1991) have pointed out additional features that tend to characterize the cognitions of patients with GAD. Accordingly, the worries of these patients tend to reflect a perceived vulnerability and threat (e.g., "Something will go wrong") and a perceived lack of personal coping skills (e.g., 'I won't be able to manage").

Etiological and theoretical models of generalized anxiety disorder

Barlow's (1988) model of GAD provides a comprehensive framework for understanding the biological, psychological, and environmental factors involved in the etiology of this disorder. Barlow's depiction of GAD as the "basic" anxiety disorder results from the view that GAD demonstrates the basic processes in anxiety in the absence of panic as a central feature. In short, a pattern of biological and psychological vulnerabilities provide the background from which negative life events produce negative affect. Negative affect includes "physiological arousal associated with stress-related neurobiological reactions and a sense that events are proceeding in an unpredictable, uncontrollable fashion" (Barlow, 1988: 579). The resulting shift in attention to being more self-focused (and less focused on more important ongoing activities) and increased vigilance to further threat causes further increases in arousal, and entry into the cycle of anxious apprehension.

An increased risk for GAD following life events has been found in a large community sample (Blazer et al., 1987). This survey also found that life events led to a greater increased risk for GAD in men as compared with women. In terms of early life events, there is some evidence, albeit weak, that the loss of or separation from a parent in early childhood is more common than one would expect in individuals with GAD (Raskin et al., 1982; Torgersen, 1986; Tweed et al., 1989). Nisita et al. (1990) reported that life events were linked to the onset of disorder in 30% of a group of 40 patients with GAD, significantly more so than is found in other anxiety disorders. They concluded, however, that GAD patients may overestimate work difficulties and interpersonal losses in order to explain the onset of symptoms, and hence a causal relationship is difficult to assess retrospectively. More recently Brantley et al. (1999) found that patients with GAD identified in a primary care setting reported a greater number of minor stressful events than a nonanxious control group. Even when the number of events were controlled, the GAD patients perceived minor events to be significantly more stressful. This finding is in keeping with Barlow's model that predicts that an increasing vulnerability to anxiety guarantees that the relatively minor events or disruptions to one's life become the focus of worry.

Drawing from evidence of the nature of worry in GAD and data from information-processing paradigms in anxious individuals, Rapee (1991b) has developed a model of the maintenance of GAD from an information-processing perspective. In summary, individuals with high levels of generalized anxiety have been shown to allocate extensive attentional resources to the detection of threatening information and hence have a "lower threshold" for threatening information (e.g., MacLeod et al., 1986; Dibartolo et al., 1997). There is evidence that threat-related information may be more accessible in memory to these individuals, resulting from selective encoding of further such information (e.g., Butler and Mathews, 1983; MacLeod and McLaughlin, 1995). Drawing on models of semantic networks, Rapee (1991b) proposed that once threat-related information has been accessed, there is activation of the anxiety node, which in turn will further lower the threshold for threat-related material. Activation of the anxiety node will also elicit information about potential responses to the threat, and the likelihood that these responses will successfully deal with the threat. It is argued that, if the information is consistent with successful control of the threat, then the activation of the anxiety node will be inhibited. Patients with generalized anxiety report that they lack control over threat and hence are less likely to experience this inhibition. Rapee has further argued that worry is a conscious and attention-demanding process that, through its hypothesized activity in working memory, may have an inhibitory effect on anxious affect. The resulting reduction of anxiety may thereby reinforce the role of worry.

Dugas et al. (1998) have developed a cognitive behavioral model of GAD in which a primary role is given to the concept of "intolerance of uncertainty", contributing to the typical "What if..." questioning style of these patients. Some preliminary support has been given to the role of this construct in worry. An experimental study that aimed to manipulate the level of intolerance of uncertainty in a nonclinical sample indicated that greater levels of intolerance of uncertainty led to reports of increased worry (Ladouceur et al., 2000b). Second, beliefs about worry such as "worry helps to avoid disappointment" or "worry protects loved ones", like Borkovec et al.'s "worry to avoid negative events", may be negatively reinforced by the nonoccurrence of the feared event central to the worry. Third, GAD patients lack confidence in their own ability to solve problems rather than lack problem-solving skills per se (Ladouceur et al., 1998). Lastly the model incorporates the role of cognitive avoidance, which, in keeping with Borkovec et al.'s concept of "worry as fear avoidance", hypothesizes that worry as a semantic cognitive process has the effect of decreasing the somatic arousal that is activated primarily by fearful imagery. Thus worry is negatively reinforced by a decrease in somatic symptoms. Preliminary support has been shown for this model. For example, questionnaire measures of each of the four contributing factors were able to discriminate GAD patients from nonclinical controls (Dugas et al., 1998). Furthermore, when tested across three samples of worriers (nonclinical worriers, individuals with GAD from a nonclinical population, GAD patients), measures of problem orientation, intolerance of uncertainty, and beliefs about worry were associated with GAD symptom level but not clinical status (seeking help for GAD) (Ladouceur et al., 1998).

Some individuals with GAD appear to intentionally initiate worry "with an almost superstitious assumption that, by doing so, they can avert the threat" (Rapee, 1991b: 426). For example, a mother may constantly worry about the safety of her child, with the expectation that if she stops worrying, some harm might indeed occur. The role of such beliefs about worry is central to the cognitive model of GAD developed by Wells and Carter (1999). While worry is a normal process, it becomes pathological in GAD when elicited as a coping strategy in response to threat-related triggers. Wells and Carter argued that GAD patients make use of worry as a coping strategy because of rigid beliefs that they hold about the usefulness of the worry. The initial worry (type I worry) – featuring concerns directly related to a feared event – increases anxiety symptoms in the short term, yet in the longer term may provide potential solutions that decrease anxiety, hence providing negative reinforcement of the worry. This assertion that worry will increase anxiety in the short term appears to contradict the models proposed by Borkovec et al., Dugas et al. and Rapee, who all say that worry decreases anxiety symptoms in the short term. Furthermore it is unclear how rigid beliefs about worry as a coping strategy develop, and there is no evidence that worry – even if extended over time – generates potential solutions to threat-related events. More support is, however, evident for the role of type II worry, or "worry about worry". Wells has shown that "worry about worry" beliefs are independent and stronger predictors of the severity of pathological worry than type I worry in a nonclinical sample (Wells and Carter, 1999).

Conclusions

The concept of worry and the associated somatic symptoms of motor tension and vigilance are central features of GAD. Little is known about specific etiology, but GAD is likely to share a common vulnerability with other anxiety and depressive disorders. A number of theoretical models have been developed and the research they continue to generate will add greatly to our understanding of this disorder. The weak evidence of diagnostic reliability, the high rates of comorbidity and the need for greater specificity of certain features of GAD are some of the issues that require further investigation. Even if GAD comes to hold a unique position within the anxiety disorders – as the "basic" anxiety disorder – it is unlikely that it will disappear from the diagnostic classification systems. Epidemiological surveys have shown that GAD is prevalent, chronic, and largely unremitting. Despite the disability associated with the disorder, the majority of sufferers do not receive treatment. However, Chapter 21 will demonstrate that treatments are available that produce clinically significant and long-lasting improvement.

21

Generalized anxiety disorder

Treatment

The goal of the treatment of GAD is the reduction of impairment that results from both cognitive and somatic symptoms of anxiety: the worry or anxious expectation, and the accompanying symptoms of tension and overarousal. This chapter aims to summarize the evidence for the effectiveness of psychological and pharmacological treatments for GAD.

Psychological treatments

Since the first edition of this book was published, five reviews of the psychological treatment of GAD have been published (Barlow et al., 1998; Borkovec and Whisman, 1996; Fisher and Durham, 1999; Gale and Oakely-Browne, 2000; Gould et al., 1997). All agree that a cognitive behavioral approach is effective for this disorder, a finding that is consistent with previous quantitative and qualitative reviews (e.g., Marks, 1989; Butler and Booth, 1991; Hunt and Singh, 1991; Durham and Allan, 1993). Hence, there is general agreement that cognitive behavioral therapy yields statistically and clinically significant improvement for the majority of patients, and that this change is maintained for up to a year following the end of treatment.

However there is less agreement on the extent to which different therapies produce differential effects. For example, Barlow et al. (1998: 311) stated "Until recently, most studies have not demonstrated differential rates of efficacy for active treatment techniques, although most studies have shown that active treatments are superior to non-directive approaches and uniformly superior to no treatment". Fisher and Durham (1999) applied Jacobson's criteria for clinical significance to six randomised controlled trials using the State–Trait Anxiety Inventory, Trait Version (STAI-T) as an outcome measure and showed that both cognitive behavioral therapy and applied relaxation produced recovery rates at 6-month follow-up of 50% to 60%. On the other hand, their results indicated that some individual therapies (behavior therapy and analytical therapy) were ineffective, with recovery rates of 11% and 4%, respectively. Of further interest was the finding that individual therapy produced higher recovery rates than the same treatment delivered in a group format. Fisher and Durham (1999) concluded that while cognitive behavioral therapy may not be the only treatment to deliver reasonable treatment outcome effects, it is unlikely that the effects observed were solely due to spontaneous remission, regression to the mean, or placebo factors.

Gould et al. (1997b) reported the results of a meta-analysis of 22 controlled trials of broadly defined "cognitive behavioral therapies". They concluded that there were no significant differences between the eight trials of cognitive and behavioral techniques (mean anxiety effect size of 0.91) and the three trials of relaxation training (mean anxiety effect size of 0.64). Of note was the finding that the mean effect size for measures of depression was also substantial across the "cognitive behavior therapies" (mean depression effect size of 0.77). In the trials where follow-up data were available, the analysis confirmed that the beneficial effects of therapy were maintained over time. Analyses were conducted to statistically assess the influence of a range of variables – including sex, duration of disorder, use of concurrent medication, group versus individual format, or treatment duration – but no variable was found to be significantly associated with outcome.

Combining information from a range of available evidence, Gale and Oakely-Browne's (2000) contribution to the *British Medical Journal* Clinical Evidence series concluded that the only intervention likely to be effective with a high degree of reliability is cognitive behavioral therapy. The approach used in this review grades intervention studies in their ability to predict treatment effectiveness (with systematic reviews with meta-analysis of randomized controlled trials seen to provide the most reliable evidence and expert opinion as the least reliable). Cognitive behavioral therapy was deemed to be effective on the basis of two systematic reviews of randomized controlled trials that found it to be more effective than remaining on a wait-list, anxiety-management training alone, or nondirective therapy. However, applied relaxation was deemed to be of unknown effectiveness as one systematic review had not established or excluded a clinically important difference between applied relaxation and cognitive therapy.

In conclusion, the reviews are largely in agreement despite the use of different methods to summarize the treatment outcome results. Cognitive behavioral therapy is certainly superior to no treatment and appears to be superior to nondirective treatments. Of interest, however, is a recent trial in adults over 55 years of age that found no differences between group-based cognitive behavior therapy or supportive psychotherapy at posttreatment and at the 6-month follow-up across all measures of anxiety, worry, and depression (Stanley et al., 1996). As Stanley et al. pointed out, it remains to be seen whether potential differences in the phenomenology of GAD in older adults or the use of a group-based program account for this finding.

The evidence is less strong that cognitive behavioral therapy is superior to other active treatments, specifically applied progressive muscle relaxation. Six published controlled treatment studies comparing active treatments have used patient samples meeting DSM-III-R criteria, hence providing a closer match than earlier studies to current diagnostic criteria. Consistent with the conclusions of the reviews, all studies showed that the treatment conditions produced significantly greater improvements than wait-list or nondirective therapy controls.

Barlow et al. (1992) compared applied progressive muscle relaxation, cognitive restructuring, and a combination of relaxation and cognitive restructuring treatment conditions. Over the 2-year follow-up there was no significant difference observed between the three treatment groups, and, while medication use was substantially reduced, the patients remained considerably anxious. However, the results must be tempered by the high rates of drop out from the active treatments and high attrition at follow-up. As only 10, 13 and 11 patients completed treatment in the three conditions, there may have been insufficient power to detect significant group differences. White et al. (1992) compared a didactic "stress control" group therapy that was cognitive, behavioral (relaxation, exposure and respiratory control) or cognitive behavioral in focus. A placebo treatment (subconscious retraining) and a wait-list control were also employed. All treatment sessions were conducted in large groups (20 to 24 participants in each group) at a local health center. All groups with the exception of the wait-list showed improvements over the treatment duration, and with the exception of the placebo condition, showed further improvements over follow-up. No significant differences were found between the active treatment groups. Borkovec and Costello (1993) compared applied relaxation and cognitive behavior therapy (which included a substantive applied relaxation component and therefore relatively brief cognitive therapy) and found no difference in outcome between the two treatment groups at posttreatment or the 6 month follow-up. Lastly, Öst and Breitholtz (2000) compared 12 sessions of weekly cognitive therapy against applied relaxation. There were significant improvements on most indices across treatment and 1-year follow-up, but no differences between the two treatments. When there is a failure to find a statistically significant difference between treatment conditions, it is useful to consider whether studies have had adequate power to detect a clinically significant different treatment effect. The sample sizes in each treatment condition required for the detection of a large effect size (say 0.40) as statistically significant are 26 for two-group and 21 for three-group comparisons (given a significance criterion of 0.05 and power of 0.80) (Cohen, 1992). Only White et al. (1992) had sample sizes in each treatment condition large enough to detect such differences; it may be possible that the conduct of the therapy in such large-sized groups may have diluted the treatment effects.

Two studies have demonstrated that cognitive or cognitive behavioral therapy produced significantly greater improvement than the other active treatments tested. Butler et al. (1991) compared cognitive behavioral therapy to behavior therapy and found at the 6-month follow-up that cognitive behavioral therapy produced significantly greater improvements than behavior therapy on measures of anxiety, depression and cognition. Furthermore, there were fewer dropouts from therapy in the cognitive behavioral condition. Durham and colleagues compared cognitive therapy, analytical therapy (delivered by experienced therapists across two levels of intensity) and anxiety-management training (delivered by inexperienced therapists) (Durham et al., 1994, 1999). At the 1-year follow-up cognitive therapy was significantly more effective than analytical therapy or the anxiety-management training. The results suggested that cognitive therapy delivered weekly showed greater improvement over the follow-up on some measures than when delivered fortnightly. The authors suggest that a higher intensity treatment may be important in a disorder that is often characterized by high rates of comorbidity and disablement, which in themselves appear to influence prognosis following treatment (Durham et al., 1997).

As worry has been given a central role in GAD, it seems important that specific therapeutic strategies be directed towards the cognitive aspects of this disorder. In Chapter 20, we saw that individuals who suffer from GAD describe their worries as difficult to control, excessive and hence out of proportion to the actual reality of the feared outcome. The characteristics of these cognitive aspects are amenable to cognitive therapy that aims to address unrealistic and erroneous beliefs, attitudes, and expectations. The efficacy of cognitive behavioral treatment packages for this disorder tend to support the case for such an approach to the amelioration of worrying thoughts, particularly in studies in which the measurement of worry has been included (e.g., Lindsay et al., 1987; Butler et al., 1991). In further support is the finding from one study that higher levels of apprehensive expectation or worry prior to cognitive behavioral treatment was significantly predictive of greater anxiety symptoms following treatment, irrespective of the level of anxiety symptoms prior to treatment (Butler, 1993).

More recently there has been an emergence of treatment packages specifically designed to address worry, with the rationale that a decrease in worry will produce concomitant changes in related subsystems (such as a decrease in somatic symptoms of anxiety) without these subsystems being specifically targeted (such as by relaxation training). Such treatments have been derived directly from research into the psychopathology of worry and conceptual models of GAD. Ladouceur et al. (2000a) conducted a wait-list controlled trial of a cognitive behavioral treatment that specifically targeted intolerance of uncertainty, erroneous beliefs about worry, poor problem orientation and cognitive avoidance. The treatment group showed significantly greater improvement than the wait-list group on all outcome measures that included self-report, clinician-rated and significant other ratings of GAD and associated symptoms. Furthermore, the treated sample showed statistically and clinically significant improvements following treatment, which was maintained at the 6- and 12-month follow-ups. Another specific approach to worry has been that of "worry exposure" (Craske et al., 1992) in which the worry is targeted using an exposure-based paradigm. In short, repeated and controlled exposure to the imagery and thoughts associated with the "worst possible outcome" in each worry domain allows habituation of the anxiety associated with that worry. The results of clinical trials of this approach are eagerly awaited.

These newer approaches to the treatment of GAD are particularly important, given that the size of treatment effects and indices of clinically significant change have been modest for GAD, at least compared with the outcome for psychological treatment of other anxiety disorders. In discussing these modest treatment outcomes, Öst and Breitholtz (2000) pointed out that treatments that were developed for other disorders (such as cognitive therapy for depression and applied relaxation for panic and phobias) may not have specific relevance for GAD. Further research into the psychopathology of worry will help to further develop treatments that specifically target worry and hence improve the effectiveness of current treatments for this disorder.

Commenting on the high proportions of individuals with GAD failing to achieve high end-state functioning following treatment, Newman (2000) has argued that more attention needs to be paid to the predictors of treatment nonresponse, including symptom severity, comorbid depression, interpersonal problems, and avoidance of emotional processing. Newman has argued for the need for outcome studies to incorporate strategies aimed at interpersonal difficulties or depth of emotional processing within cognitive behavioral treatments. These strategies might be specifically targeting individuals who, because of these additional difficulties, may not fully respond to standard cognitive behavioral intervention. At the other end of the spectrum, the evaluation of low-cost minimal interventions will be important to determine whether there are a significant number of individuals who can learn to control their symptoms without specialist-level care. While yet to be compared with an active treatment condition, a self-help package requiring individuals to examine what was important in their lives has been found to produce significant improvement in anxiety symptoms in GAD compared to a wait-list control (Bowman et al., 1997). Findings such as these may be particularly important in providing treatment options for a disorder that is common in primary care and whose sufferers tend not to reach specialist treatment programs.

Pharmacological treatments

For many years, benzodiazepines were the preferred pharmacotherapy for GAD and considered the treatment of choice (e.g., Rickels, 1987; Dubovsky, 1990; Gorman and Papp, 1990). There is ample evidence to conclude that the benzodiazepines are safe and provide effective symptomatic relief for the majority of patients. Furthermore, numerous trials have shown that all benzodiazepine groups appear to be equally effective (Gould et al., 1997b; Roy-Byrne and Cowley, 1998). In their meta-analytical study, Gould et al. (1997b) reported a mean anxiety effect size of 0.70 across 23 controlled trials of benzodiazepine therapy, equivalent to that calculated across all the "cognitive behavioral" therapies included in that study. While benzodiazepines undoubtedly produce good short-term treatment effects, side-effects include impaired cognitive performance, drowsiness and lethargy with high doses, and physical and psychological dependence following prolonged use. Discontinuation of benzodiazepine treatment can result in rebound anxiety or an intensification of previous symptoms in 25% to 75% of individuals, in a withdrawal syndrome in 40% to 100%, and a relapse of original symptoms in 63% to 81% of individuals (Dubovsky, 1990). Few pharmacotherapy studies address long-term outcome, but in one study using DSM-III-diagnosed patients, discontinuation of diazepam (when provided as the sole treatment) resulted in a reversal of treatment effects (Power et al., 1990). Although there is little research on long-term pharmacotherapy, some patients will have taken benzodiazepines for many years without tolerance to their anxiolytic effects (da Roza Davis and Gelder, 1991). However, medical, ethical, and legal concerns surrounding the long-term use of these drugs, particularly in regard to the potential for dependence, have led to recommendations of intermittent usage, using the lowest effective dose for the shortest possible time (Rickels, 1987; Gorman and Papp, 1990). Gale and Oakley-Browne (2000) have concluded in their evidence-based review that, although benzodiazepines are, compared with placebo, an effective and rapid treatment for GAD, they are not a beneficial treatment because of the trade-off between benefits and harms. In particular, they state that benzodiazepines have been found to increase the risk of dependence, sedation, industrial accidents and road traffic accidents. Furthermore, benzodiazepines have been associated with neonatal and infant mortality when used in late pregnancy or while breastfeeding (Gale and Oakely-Browne, 2000). Benzodiazepines should be used particularly cautiously in older adults because of the greater sensitivity to adverse effects (Sheikh and Cassidy, 2000).

The nonbenzodiazepine anxiolytic buspirone appears to be equivalent to the benzodiazepines in efficacy (Roy-Byrne and Cowley, 1998) but unlike the benzodiazepines produces virtually no sedative effects and no withdrawal syndrome or rebound anxiety following discontinuation. Gould et al. (1997b) reported a mean anxiety effect size of 0.39 from nine controlled trials of buspirone, apparently lower than that calculated from the benzodiazepine trials, but with equivalent dropout rates. Like the benzodiazepines, discontinuation of buspirone can lead to the return of original symptoms (Rickels and Schweizer, 1990). Its effects are likely to be mediated primarily through the dopaminergic neurotransmitter system, there is no cross-tolerance with benzodiazepines or alcohol, and the onset of anxiolytic effect may take several weeks. Some (e.g., da Roza Davis and Gelder, 1991) have suggested that buspirone may be useful for long-term use, given its lack of dependence potential, but its long-term effects are largely unknown.

Gale and Oakely-Browne (2000) have concluded that the antidepressants paroxetine, imipramine, trazadone, venlafaxine and mirtazepine are "likely to be beneficial" treatments for GAD on the basis of randomized placebo-controlled trials. The three controlled trials of antidepressant medication included in the Gould et al. (1997b) meta-analysis yielded a mean anxiety effect size of 0.57, and a high dropout rate of 33.5%, arguably due to the greater side-effects for these medications. Hoehn-Saric et al. (1988) found alprazolam and imipramine to be equally effective in reducing anxiety symptoms over 6 weeks in patients with DSM-III GAD without comorbid major depression or panic disorder. Rickels et al. (1993a) compared imiprimine, trazodone and diazepam over 8 weeks of treatment in a similar sample of patients. During the final 2 weeks of treatment, only imipramine produced significantly greater improvement in anxiety symptoms than placebo. The results also showed that, compared with the antidepressant medication, diazepam produced greater change in the first weeks of the treatment, had a greater effect on somatic symptoms, and fewer side-effects. However, the antidepressant medications were more effective in reducing psychic symptoms of anxiety. An 8-week trial of the specific serotonin reuptake inhibitor (SSRI) paroxetine in patients with DSM-IV GAD showed paroxetine to have equivalent treatment outcome to imipramine and the benzodiazepine 2-chlorodemethyldiazepam (Rocca et al., 1997). Most recently, venlafaxine was found to provide significantly greater symptomatic relief than placebo after 6 weeks and then 6 months of treatment (Gelenberg et al., 2000). Across the trial, a 69% response rate was achieved for the treatment group, compared with a 42–46% response rate for the placebo condition. Other medications have been studied in patients with GAD, such as abecarnil (Lydiard et al., 1997; Pollack et al., 1997), gepirone (Rickels et al., 1997), and hydroxyzine (Lader and Scotto, 1998). Where controlled trials have been conducted, treatment effects have tended to be significantly greater than placebo-treated groups and equivalent to the other active medications studied.

The treatment literature confirms that benzodiazepine treatment is effective in the short-term treatment of generalized anxiety. However the high risk of dependence and the common return of symptoms following discontinuation preclude the usefulness of these drugs in a chronic disorder. Buspirone, with equal effectiveness and an absence of dependence, may well provide a better treatment option, but tends not to be widely prescribed. This may be due to the lag in effect, so that neither patients nor their doctors may be prepared to tolerate the several weeks that may occur before a decrease in anxiety is experienced. In many of the earlier pharmacological studies reviewed, it is unknown how many patients would have fulfilled DSM-IV diagnostic criteria. Furthermore, there is a paucity of long-term data for any pharmacotherapy, despite epidemiological evidence that for most individuals GAD is a chronic disorder. Given the increased importance of the concept of worry in the disorder, particular attention should be paid to the measurement of the cognitive components of anxiety. It is of interest that most studies that compared anxiolytic and antidepressant medications concluded that while overall the outcomes were equivalent, the antidepressant medication produce greater improvements in measures of psychic symptoms of anxiety.

Combining psychological and pharmacological treatents

The common finding of relapse following discontinuation of benzodiazepine therapy has led some authors to address the issues of long-term use of benzodiazepines and adjunctive teaching of behavioral and cognitive coping strategies. Rickels and Schweizer (1990) have speculated that constant use of benzodiazepines may preclude patients from developing their own coping skills for anxiety relief, and suggest the concurrent use of such interventions as behavior modification or cognitive therapy. The treatment study of Power et al. (1990) tended to support the view that psychological and pharmacological treatments can be combined without a reduction in effectiveness. Power's study included a trial of combined cognitive behavioral therapy and fixed low dose (3×5 mg daily) diazepam. They found no significant differences posttreatment between the combined treatment and cognitive behavioral therapy alone or with placebo on a number of symptom measures of anxiety. No significant withdrawal symptoms or re-emergence of anxiety symptoms were reported following careful and gradual withdrawal from the diazepam. At 6-month follow-up over 85% of the combined group showed "clinically significant change" (greater than 2 standard deviations from the pretreatment mean) and 84% had not sought further treatment. This group made an interesting contrast from the diazepam-alone group, which showed higher rates of subsequent treatment (54% of the group) and lower rates of "clinically significant change" (30% to 70%) at 6 months following treatment.

While the findings of Power et al. (1990) require replication, they do suggest that the judicious use of long-acting benzodiazepines may not significantly interfere with cognitive behavioral therapy in individuals who have sought treatment for GAD. However, the cognitive behavioral treatments achieved similar clinical change in the absence of active pharmacological treatment. Therefore, while the use of benzodiazepines may not interfere with cognitive behavioral therapy, they do not appear to add to the treatment effect and the potential for adverse effects must be taken into consideration. In contrast, a review of psychological treatments in GAD (Durham and Allan, 1993) found that, across a number of studies, outcomes indicating above-average improvement in symptom measures and clinically significant changes were associated with patient samples that were free from anxiolytic medication. No data appear to be available concerning the combined use of psychological treatment and antidepressant medication. Clearly, the role of pharmacotherapy as an adjunct to psychological treatment in GAD has yet to be established.

Conclusions

The cognitive behavioral therapies appear to be at least as effective in the short term as pharmacotherapy, cause no adverse effects in terms of side-effects and withdrawal syndromes, and aim to increase coping skills, and hence increase the sense of control and mastery in patients. In other anxiety disorders, the same strategies have been shown to bring about long-term changes in measures thought to represent vulnerability to neurosis (Hunt and Andrews, 1998). Our present knowledge suggests that treatment should include, at the very least, education about the nature of the disorder and should address the beliefs, attitudes, and expectations relevant to an individual's worries and fears.

Despite the existence of efficacious treatments, there is still much to be done. For example, it will be important to replicate many of the reported treatment effects in DSM-IV samples and in the delivery of treatment in routine care. Furthermore, the development of treatments appropriate to the primary care setting will be important for the majority of GAD sufferers who will never reach specialist treatment settings. It will also be important for future outcome studies to target the prominent feature of worry in terms of assessment and treatment.

22

Generalized anxiety disorder

Clinician Guide

The present chapter aims to guide clinicians in the principles of treatment and the use of the treatment Manual, as well as highlight some of the more common problems encountered in therapy. While further studies are needed to identify the active components of effective treatment for generalized anxiety disorder, it appears that two core elements are:

- An underlying rationale, based on the "coping skills" model of cognitive behavioral therapy, where patients are taught skills to manage their anxiety and to take responsibility for change and control over their thoughts, feelings, and behavior.
- Cognitive therapy with the goal of bringing the process of worry under the patients control.

Relaxation training, usually a form of progressive muscle relaxation, is a useful adjunct to treatment, particularly where the effects of chronic and high levels of muscle tension trouble an individual.

Assessment

It is assumed that before the commencement of treatment, a clinical assessment will have ruled out comorbid diagnoses in need of immediate specific treatment, such as a major depressive episode. Where depression is present, it becomes the treatment priority and the need for further treatment of anxiety symptoms reviewed when the depression is resolved. Given the phenomenological similarities between the two disorders, it is often necessary to establish from historical information whether GAD existed before the onset of a major depressive episode, or to assess whether a GAD continues to exist following effective treatment of the depressive disorder.

While patients with a primary diagnosis of GAD will not always meet criteria for another diagnosis, they will often have concerns and behaviors that are characteristic of other anxiety disorders. Panic attacks, social anxiety, phobic avoidance, obsessions, and illness anxiety are common. The treating clinician will therefore need to be able to recognize these different features and address these in the course of treatment. For example, some time can be spent focusing specifically on fears of scrutiny and negative evaluation or fears that a physical sensation is really a sign of a serious, life-threatening illness within the framework of the cognitive behavioral approach. The use of a slow-breathing exercise (possibly due to its meditation-like features) can provide temporary control over acute episodes of high anxiety for many individuals. Hence patients can be relatively quickly provided with an increased sense of control that allows them to recognize the triggers of their anxiety and implement cognitive strategies. The differentiation between obsessive thoughts and worries or ruminations has been outlined in Chapter 20, and careful assessment may be required to differentiate these types of thinking. It will also be important that the individuals themselves are taught to recognize the difference between obsessions and worries/ruminations and then implement the appropriate management strategy (see treatment of obsessive thoughts in Chapter 17).

The relationship between different thoughts, feelings, or behaviors may require a certain amount of detective work between the patient and the therapist. Like-wise, the formulation of strategies to deal with such difficulties may not be entirely straightforward. A collaborative approach with the patient is vital, with interven-tion often framed in the following way: "I wonder whether these factors could be causing this problem? What strategies do you think would be useful, given our understanding of anxiety and the strategies we have learned about so far? How about we put them into practice and see whether they make a difference?" Therapists should help patients to use any problems or setbacks that occur during the course of treatment to provide them with more evidence to refine problem formulations and treatment strategies. For example, a thorough behavioral for-mulation will help to identify situations, events, thoughts, feelings, or behaviors that continue to trigger or maintain anxiety and hence provide a guide for improving intervention strategies.

Format

It is likely that most clinicians using this Manual will be seeing patients on an individual basis. Although the group versus individual format has not been studied directly, it appears that there is some advantage in an individual approach. While the structure of treatment can be flexible, treatment should begin with a discussion of the goals of treatment for each individual. Between-session monitor-ing of situations that trigger anxiety, avoidance, and worries can begin from the first sessions and will help the individual to develop a greater awareness of the incidence and impact of their worry. The presentation of information and skills as laid out in the Patient Treatment Manual is a good guide for the order in which topics can be covered, beginning with the presentation of information about the nature of the disorder and the rationale for treatment. Butler and Booth (1991) suggested that a treatment formulation should be developed at approximately the fourth treatment session. Further sessions can then be spaced on a weekly (or 2-weekly) basis, over which time skills are consolidated and applied in the patient's ongoing life and problems in progress pinpointed and solved. At the Anxiety Disorders Unit, Sydney, individuals are seen on average for 1 hour weekly for 8 weeks, then again at a 1-month follow-up session. Later sessions focus on review and practice of the skills, tailored to each individual's needs. Appropriate sections can be used from the Patient Treatment Manuals provided in this book for the other anxiety disorders if necessary (e.g., dealing with social anxieties from the Social Phobia Patient Treatment Manual).

The pace of change in individuals in treatment is variable. An expectation of complete absence of anxiety and worry by the end of treatment is unrealistic for the majority of individuals. However, it will be important that patients exhibit evidence that they can successfully apply the skills that are being taught and that they have consolidated their skills and are able to continue to apply these without regular therapist contact. Evidence should be sought for such progress, including the spontaneous and successful use of cognitive strategies outside of the sessions or the completion of graded exposure tasks.

The treatment process

Initial sessions

Following assessment, there are a number of important issues that should be raised with patients early in the treatment process. Individuals will often present for treatment after having suffered generalized anxiety for many years, sometimes for most of their lives. It is therefore likely that they will see their difficulties as longstanding, if not an integral part of their personality. Months or years of dealing with fluctuating levels of anxiety may well have left them feeling despondent and pessimistic about the possibility of change. Therefore it is important to convey the message early in treatment that real changes in longstanding patterns of thinking and reacting are indeed possible.

It is also important to make it very clear at the beginning of treatment that patients will be expected to take responsibility for changes in their own behavior and hence will need to practice the skills that they are taught. In other words, it is important to dispel any myths that patients may hold about treatment providing an easy answer to their anxiety difficulties. From the outset, it should be made clear that they will have to make a commitment to work on management of their anxiety on a daily basis, both during the course of treatment and for some months to come. It may be important to point out that years of habitual thinking and behaving will not change overnight. It will be critical to ensure that clinicians' and patients' goals and expectations of therapy are matched. For example, if the patient's goal is to "get rid of the anxiety", the clinician should present a realistic alternative such as "to better manage anxiety (which is an inevitable part of human existence) so that it ceases to interfere with functioning and cause undue distress". An adequate discussion of such issues, outlining the goals of therapy, and the provision of information about the nature of anxiety will account for at least the first session of treatment.

General issues

An emphasis on regular homework is as important in the treatment of this disorder as in all other anxiety disorders. Patients will soon learn that the strategies must be well practiced if they are to be successful, particularly in the face of high levels of anxiety. The importance of regular between-session practice of techniques when anxiety is relatively low may need to be addressed throughout treatment. Butler and Booth (1991) outlined the shared characteristics of successful treatments, which include:

- A treatment goal of increased self-control and independence on the part of the patient.
- The use of Patient Treatment Manuals, the provision of information about the nature of anxiety, and a rationale for treatment, record keeping, and homework.
- A collaborative relationship between the patient and therapist.
- A structure to treatment so that efficient use is made of time and the important points of therapy are salient.

Butler and Booth (1991) also suggested that therapists make use of "formulations" and "blueprints" in their treatment programs. Formulations of patients' problems provide a framework to clarify understanding of symptoms and the factors maintaining those symptoms in the context of a cognitive behavioral model of anxiety. These formulations aid in the generation of hypotheses from which treatment strategies are planned. Blueprints, or detailed plans of work to be done, that explicitly outline aspects of treatment that have been useful during treatment can be generated and kept for future reference so that future anxiety problems can be dealt with efficiently should they arise. The core specific treatment strategies are covered in detail in the Patient Treatment Manual. The material covered is relatively straightforward for a clinician with a good grounding in cognitive behavioral theory and techniques.

Relaxation therapy

It is unclear that progressive muscle relaxation per se is critical to the amelioration of GAD symptoms, particularly given the apparent efficacy of treatments that do not contain this component (e.g., Durham et al., 1997; Ladouceur et al., 2000a). Furthermore, it is possible that the efficacious effects of applied relaxation as a treatment package may be due to the consequence of providing an alternative strategy to engagement in worry in the face of triggers of worry. However, because many patients complain of high levels of tension and its effects, it is a useful skill that will help individuals to bring their somatic symptoms under control. Regular practice of relaxation exercises is always encouraged, but it is not recommended that a large proportion of treatment contact time be spent on this component. Used alone, relaxation appears to be no more effective than a placebo (see e.g., Hunt and Singh, 1991).

Cognitive therapy

One of the core features of GAD is the pervasive nature of the worry or concern, unlike the concerns of patients with other anxiety disorders that tend to be fairly discrete or limited to one general domain. The wide range of worries, beliefs, and expectations found in patients with GAD will require flexibility on the part of the therapist, who may need to address unhelpful thinking over a number of domains. Worry in generalized anxiety disorder is certainly characterized by catastrophic interpretations, often couched in terms of personal inadequacies (Butler and Booth, 1991; Breitholtz et al., 1999; Davey and Levy, 1998; Molina et al., 1998). These catastrophic interpretations are particularly amenable to standard cognitive interventions that aim to address unrealistic and erroneous beliefs, attitudes, and expectations. More often than not, the thinking of individuals with GAD will be colored by a general perception of threat and they will react with alarm to a multitude of cues in their day-to-day lives. Such threats can include the telephone ringing (bringing news of some disaster), meetings with work colleagues (who will finally discover the individual's incompetence), or symptoms of the flu (a deadly virus that the doctors will again ignore).

Often, individuals will feel overwhelmed when they become more aware of the pervasiveness of their unhelpful thinking. It is then useful to look for general patterns or themes that can then be targeted. For example, a belief that one is incompetent can drive a multitude of smaller crises whenever performance is required or decisions are to be made. Addressing the broad fear (e.g., "I'm incompetent, it's just that nobody has noticed yet") and getting individuals to consider the objective evidence (e.g., "I'm still employed; nobody has ever complained about my work; my friends all seem to like me; I always manage to get done what needs to be done") may circumvent a number of day-to-day anxieties. This approach will also serve to make vague and abstract worries more concrete (see below). However, the individual will need to regularly challenge and dispute their unhelpful thinking whenever in the presence of cues that may trigger it. Completing cognitive exercises in writing early in treatment is vital for the success of cognitive therapy for these individuals, providing an element of distance and control over thoughts that otherwise appear uncontrollable.

The *process* of worry requires further consideration. While the nature of worry in GAD is that it is unreasonable and excessive, its content differs little between individuals with and those without the disorder. Davey and Levy (1998) have investigated the "What if..." statements typical of worry and found an underlying general perseverative, iterative style of thinking. Furthermore, individuals with GAD may well see their worry as excessive and causing undue anxiety, but would often disagree that it is wholly irrational. For example, a mother who had been told by her 7-year-old son that he had been crossing a busy road without supervision during school would be unlikely to see her worry about his safety as unreasonable. However, she may be able to see that the effect of worrying about her son's safety throughout the day was unreasonable and caused unnecessary anxiety. In this case, a problem-solving exercise that resulted in the mother talking both to her son and to a teacher at the school, and reminding herself that "I have done all I can to ensure my son's safety, continuing to worry will not change what happens at school, I will get on with my usual activities" was more successful than trying to challenge the content of the worry itself. In other words, these strategies can help individuals to decide not to engage in the process of worry.

A characteristic of pathological worry is the relative lack of present-orientated statements and over concern about future events that are unlikely to happen (Borkovec et al., 1998; Dugas et al., 1998). Thus an important goal of therapy is to help patients to focus on concrete components of problems when they arise and help them to differentiate between problems that require immediate resolution and those that are distant or unlikely to occur. Strategies within cognitive therapy that require patients to realistically evaluate the probability of a feared event ("How likely is it really?") are important in this regard. Again, it is important to establish whether the fears underlying the worry are unrealistic (e.g., "I just know that I'm going to fail that exam"), whether there is a problem to be solved (e.g., "How shall I best prepare for the exam") or whether the concern is reasonable but excessive or unproductive (e.g., worrying about an important exam at 3.00 a.m., or at a time when it would be more productive to be studying).

The predominance of thoughts over images in worry provides the basis of Borkovec et al.'s avoidance theory of worry (1998) and also features in the model of Dugas et al. (1998). In these models, worry allows an avoidance of aversive imagery associated with the subject of the anxiety, and hence reduces the somatic anxiety associated with such imagery. There is now some preliminary evidence that worries can become more concrete following a cognitive behavioral approach that employs imagery exposure to the feared content of worry (Stober and Borkovec, 2000). It is again argued that identifying the components of worry that are more concrete or specific may also aid the identification of solutions to potential problems or help to invalidate those worries that are abstract in nature (e.g., "I won't cope" or "I'm incompetent").

A key component of the cognitive behavioral model of GAD proposed by Dugas et al. (1998) is an intolerance of uncertainty. It follows that an important aim of treatment will be to teach patients to become more tolerant of uncertainty in the face of ambiguity, both by directly challenging beliefs that certainty is either achievable or necessary, and indirectly through the use of behavioral experiments. For example, individuals can be encouraged to undertake activities or make decisions without the need for excessive amounts of information or reassurance from others and thus test whether the potential negative outcomes do in fact occur. Unhelpful beliefs about worry that may serve to maintain worry (Dugas et al., 1998; Wells and Carter, 1999) can also be challenged directly (e.g., "What evidence is there that worry is helping you solve your problems?") or more indirectly (e.g., "Can we stop the worry and see if the feared event actually eventuates?").

Lastly, because an important goal of treatment is for patients to function independently of the therapist, the use of reassurance that may in fact discourage patients from evaluating and challenging their own unhelpful thoughts should be avoided. While the therapist should provide accurate information about the disorder, its treatment, and prognosis, one should be wary of providing answers for patients who continually ask questions such as "Is this pain really just anxiety?" or "Will I ever get over this?" Such reassurance seeking is best redirected back to the patient to be dealt with using cognitive techniques. For example, "I can't answer that question. What do you think, given the evidence and our discussions about anxiety?".

Graded exposure

Many individuals with GAD have avoidance of certain situations that will need to be addressed during the course of therapy, using the principles of graded exposure. However, it is widely acknowledged that much of the avoidance behavior of these individuals can be quite subtle, and can include things such as avoiding any stimuli that might be a reminder of their fears (e.g., reading newspapers, talking to certain people, thinking about certain issues), avoiding interactions that might cause conflict with others, avoiding solving certain problems, or even forms of "internal avoidance" to prevent full engagement in certain activities (e.g., using distraction methods, such as counting or singing to oneself). Distraction will not be a useful anxiety-management technique if it prevents individuals from disputing core beliefs, solving problems, or exposing themselves to what they fear. Most subtle avoidance can be addressed using the basic principles of graded exposure:

setting specific behavioral goals that can be broken down into smaller steps if necessary.

Many patients engage in a range of other unhelpful behaviors in an attempt to relieve anxiety and distress in the short term (e.g., reassurance seeking, checking) and these may need to be addressed using the principles of exposure and response prevention. For example, individuals who worry constantly about the safety of a loved one may contact them frequently when separated, just to reassure themselves that the loved one has come to no harm. Dealing with this worry will necessarily involve exposure to the cues that may trigger the worry (e.g., separation from the loved one) and prevention of the reassuring behavior.

Structured problem solving

The method is very straightforward. Patients have little difficulty in understanding the six-step method. In practice, few patients with GAD have difficulty in solving their problems once their anxiety is at manageable levels, and in many cases there is little point in devoting much time to this strategy. Research evidence supports the notion that these individuals have difficulty in poor problem orientation, rather than skills in problem solving per se (Ladouceur et al., 1998). However, in cases where problems appear overwhelming or insurmountable, structured problem solving provides an excellent framework for solving problems or achieving goals. Furthermore, patients can be encouraged to apply problem solving to a wide variety of circumstances, not just the obvious day-to-day practical problems that they encounter. For example, it can be used as a framework to aid in the planning of exposure tasks, achieve short- and long-term goals, and help in making decisions.

The final session

The final session should be used to lay the groundwork for treatment gains to be consolidated and enhanced. The following points are worth covering:

1. Reinforce the idea that the end of treatment does not mean the end of regular and systematic practice of the anxiety-management strategies.
2. Remind patients that anxiety is a normal part of human existence and that there is no such thing as a "cure". However, they can aim to successfully control anxiety.
3. Overview the treatment goals as outlined at the beginning of treatment: establish what goals still need to be achieved and ensure that the patient is able to plan how they are to attain these.
4. Ensure that each patient has formulated a "blueprint" for managing anxiety for the future. Some discussion of the cues that may be likely to trigger further

episodes of anxiety, tension, or worry can be useful (based on prior experience) and should become part of the "blueprint".

5. Remind patients that it is unrealistic to believe that years of habitual worry and irrational thinking can be completely overcome over a number of weeks.

Solving difficulties in treatment

Because of the often longstanding nature of these patients' difficulties, and probably due to current public perceptions about what therapy may entail, there is often an expectation that events or relationships that occurred in the distant past require resolution if current difficulties are to be dealt with effectively. It is natural that patients will ask the question "Why am I like this?" and it is important to spend some time addressing current theories of how anxiety disorders develop and are maintained, not only to satisfy patients' understanding but also to lay a foundation and rationale for intervention. Information on the history of the presenting complaint gathered at the initial assessment may have brought to light major life events that may have played a role in the development of anxiety problems, but can also be uncovered during the process of therapy. In particular, maladaptive schemas become apparent in the process of identifying unhelpful thoughts, attitudes and beliefs in cognitive therapy.

It is important to remind patients that cognitive behavioral therapy deals with changing thoughts, feelings, and behavior in the here and now. Whether or not the development of the disorder has been attributed to a life event or factors in an individual's upbringing, the approach to the resolution of the anxiety in the majority of cases will remain the same. The focus of treatment will be on factors that currently trigger or maintain maladaptive responses. It is often important, however, to consider the role of past experiences in the development of schema so that the individual can more easily challenge an unhelpful belief. For example, an individual who has core beliefs of personal incompetence or inadequacy that appear to be based in messages received as a child can challenge automatic thoughts of incompetence (not only through direct evidence relating to current competence) by recognizing "I think I'm incompetent because I was always told so as a child – it doesn't have to be true".

Another expectation sometimes held by patients is that, following treatment, anxiety will be eliminated from their lives. If patients continue to believe this, then they will hold unrealistic expectations about their progress and will be unlikely to develop a plan to be set in motion should they become anxious again later in their lives. This point may be particularly important for individuals with GAD, whose anxiety is arguably more akin to a personality- than a symptom-based disorder and who therefore may take some time to change the traits that make them vulnerable to anxiety. The reasonable goal that anxiety is to be controlled rather than "cured" can be reinforced when providing information about anxiety, making it clear that it is a normal physiological response that may in fact be useful in a number of situations in an individual's everyday life.

Conclusions

In conclusion, to return to the advice of Butler and Booth (1991), two of the most important skills that a clinician can have in dealing with GAD patients are clarity and creativity. Following latest developments in regard to the psychopathology of the disorder (in particular worry) will help clinicians to develop more specific, and we hope effective, treatment strategies for their patients. It is likely that a cognitive behavioral framework provides clarity and direction to the treatment process, while the scientist-practitioner approach allows flexibility and creativity in dealing with individuals with GAD.

23

Generalized anxiety disorder

Patient Treatment Manual*

This Manual is both a guide to treatment and a workbook for people who suffer from generalized anxiety disorder. During treatment, it is a workbook in which individuals can record their own experience of generalized anxiety disorder, together with the additional advice for their particular case given by their clinician. After treatment has concluded, this Manual can serve as a self-help resource when challenges or difficulties are faced.

Contents

*Gavin Andrews, Mark Creamer, Rocco Crino, Caroline Hunt, Lisa Lampe and Andrew Page *The Treatment of Anxiety Disorders* second edition © 2002 Cambridge University Press. All rights reserved.

SECTION 1

This program will aim to teach you to manage your worry and anxiety by learning to change the way you think and the way you react to your thinking and other events. In essence you will be learning new methods of control.

It is important to realize that achieving control of worry and anxiety is a skill that has to be learnt. To be effective, the skill must be practiced regularly and you will need to take responsibility for change. The more you put into the program, the more you will get out of it. It is not the severity of your anxiety, or how long you have been anxious, or how old you are that predicts the success of this program, but rather it is your motivation to change your reactions.

1 What is generalized anxiety disorder?

Generalized anxiety disorder is characterized by persistent feelings of anxiety and worry. The worry is typically out of proportion to the actual circumstances, exists through most areas of a person's day-to-day life, and is experienced as difficult to control. The anxiety and worry are described as generalized, as the content of the worry can cover a number of different events or circumstances, and the physical symptoms of anxiety are not specific and are part of a normal response to threat.

Individuals with generalized anxiety disorder describe themselves as sensitive by nature and their tendency to worry has usually existed since childhood or early adolescence.

The symptoms of anxiety typically experienced by individuals with generalized anxiety disorder are:
- Feeling restless, keyed up, or on edge
- Being easily tired
- Having difficulty concentrating, or having your mind going blank
- Feeling irritable

- Having tense, tight or sore muscles
- Having difficulty sleeping; either difficulty falling or staying asleep, or restless unsatisfying sleep

Generalized anxiety disorder is one of the more common anxiety disorders in the community. A recent Australian survey has suggested that, in a 12-month period, 3 in 100 people will have a generalized anxiety disorder.

1.1 Generalized anxiety disorder and everyday worry

Everybody worries or gets anxious at some time in their lives. The worry in generalized anxiety disorder is identical in nature to that experienced by anybody else, but it tends to be out of proportion, pervasive, and difficult to control, unlike the worry most people experience. Hence it significantly interferes with an individual's functioning. The constant anxiety-provoking thinking and the accompanying physical symptoms of anxiety can be disabling, particularly if experienced over a long period of time.

Another feature of generalized anxiety disorder is that it has usually been present for much of an individual's life. From time to time, people may become unusually stressed, because of a physical illness or a life event such as divorce, bereavement, or loss (or threat of loss) of employment. During these times people may worry and become significantly more anxious, but after the stress resolves, the person can usually return to their usual functioning. This is not generalized anxiety disorder, but a temporary period of difficulty adjusting to stress.

1.2 Medication

You may be taking medication to help you cope with anxiety. If you are taking medication, you may need to talk about the issues discussed below with your therapist.

1.2.1 Antidepressant medication

Many of the medications that are useful to treat a depressive disorder are also useful in helping to control anxiety. If your doctor has prescribed you this type of medication, particularly if you have been depressed, it is important that you continue to take the medication for several months, and stop taking it only in consultation with your doctor. This medication typically has few side-effects, it is safe, and will not cause you to build up tolerance or become dependent.

When you are ready to stop this medication (usually after you have been feeling calm and in control for a number of months), it is very unlikely that you will experience a relapse of your anxiety if you have been able to learn and put into practice the strategies taught on this program.

1.2.2 Sedatives, tranquilizers, and sleeping pills

This class of medication is the benzodiazepines. They can block the feelings of anxiety very effectively, but also produce the following problems:

- They can interfere with thinking and your ability to remember new information.
- They can make you feel drowsy and sleepy.
- They can interfere with your natural sleep cycle and rhythms.
- They can produce tolerance, so that you might need bigger and bigger doses for the same effect.
- They can produce dependence, so that you come to rely on them and experience an increase in anxiety without them.
- They can produce withdrawal symptoms when you stop or cut down, producing unpleasant anxiety-like feelings.
- They can make it easier for you not to use the strategies taught in this program.

If you are taking this type of medication you would already have been asked to cut down gradually, with the aim of stopping completely. If you are experiencing any difficulties with this process, please discuss it with your therapist, who can then work with your doctor in achieving the goal of successfully stopping the medication.

SECTION 2

2 The nature of anxiety and worry

2.1 The nature of anxiety

Anxiety is a normal and healthy reaction. It describes a series of changes in the body, and in the way we think and behave, that enable us to deal with threat or danger; changes that can be very useful if you have to respond very quickly.

Consider the following: You are crossing a wide and busy road at a pedestrian crossing. You suddenly notice a truck that has failed to slow down and will probably not stop, and it is heading in your direction. You start running for the safety of the sidewalk some meters away. The brain becomes aware of danger. Automatically, hormones are released and the involuntary nervous system sends signals to various parts of the body to produce the changes listed below.

- The mind becomes alert.
- Blood clotting ability increases, preparing for possible injury.
- Heart rate speeds up and blood pressure rises.
- Sweating increases to help to cool the body.
- Blood is diverted to the muscles, which tense, ready for action.
- Digestion slows down.
- Saliva production decreases, causing a dry mouth.
- Breathing rate speeds up. Nostrils and air passages in lungs open wider to get in air more quickly.
- Liver releases sugar to provide quick energy.
- Sphincter muscles contract to close the openings of the bowel and bladder.
- Immune responses decrease, which is useful in the short term to allow massive response to immediate threat, but can become harmful over a long period.

And so you are able to run very quickly to the side of the road and escape being knocked down by the truck.

As you can see, this series of reactions, known as the "fight or flight" response, account for the many and varied feelings you can experience when you are anxious. In your mind you feel fear and apprehension; you are "on edge", "keyed up", and worried.

In your body, you may experience one or a number of the following sensations:
- Trembling or shaking
- Restlessness
- Muscle tension
- Sweating
- Shortness of breath
- Pounding or racing heart
- Cold and clammy hands
- Fast breathing
- Dry mouth
- Hot flushes or chills
- Feeling sick or nauseated
- "Butterflies" in the stomach

This fight or flight response is useful in the short term, especially if the danger can be dealt with by physical exertion. But it is of no use in the long term and certainly of little use in most stressful situations today – it does not help to run when the traffic cop pulls you over and it doesn't help to fight physically when you are threatened by the boss. However, because the fight or flight response was useful when, in the distant past we regularly had to deal with physical danger, it remains part of our physical make-up. It is no wonder that when we are threatened, we can't get enough air, our hearts pound, we feel nauseated, and our arms and legs tremble and shake, as all these responses would be useful if we could flee or fight.

2.1.1 The anxiety cycle

All of these changes in the body can be quickly reversed once vigorous physical activity has been carried out. This explains why many people report the desire to run or in some other way expend physical energy when placed in stressful situations. However, we are not often able to immediately engage in physical activity and therefore are less able to reverse the changes. For people who are prone to worry excessively, these changes can be quite disturbing and a new source of threat. This, of course, leads to further activation of the "fight or flight" response and the whole cycle is continued.

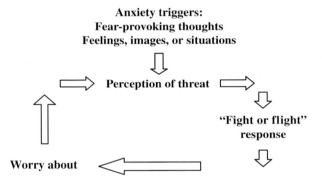

2.1.2 Anxiety and performance

Anxiety can become a problem if it occurs in situations where there is no real danger. The only part of the fight or flight response that is of use today when handling most stresses is the increase in mental alertness that it provides. It is very important to understand that, while increased awareness can be helpful, anxiety in some situations can be unnecessary or inappropriate.

Anxiety helps you to perform any skilled activity. If you are totally relaxed when you take an exam, play a sport, or discuss a problem with your colleagues, you will not give of your best. To do anything really well you need to be alert, anxious to do well, or "psyched-up", in present-day terms. Anxiety in moderation is a drive that can work well to make you more efficient.

People with anxiety disorders often become afraid of the healthy anxiety that aids performance – they fear it might become uncontrollable and hence avoid using anxiety in this healthy way. Thus they limit their ability to give of their best.

This reaction is understandable, for if you don't know how to control anxiety, it is probably better to have too little than too much. When people do get too anxious, their skill at problem solving, managing children, or meeting deadlines at work declines rapidly. Extreme anxiety interferes with the ability to think clearly and act sensibly. This, as everyone knows, is the sort of anxiety that robs us of our capacity to do things as well as we are able. In fact, the more difficult the task, the more important it is to manage anxiety carefully; ideally, one should be mildly anxious, alert, tense, and in control, for maximum efficiency.

The relationship between anxiety and skill is shown in the diagram. It is, therefore, important to learn strategies for remaining calm when appropriate, and alert, tense, and in control in difficult situations.

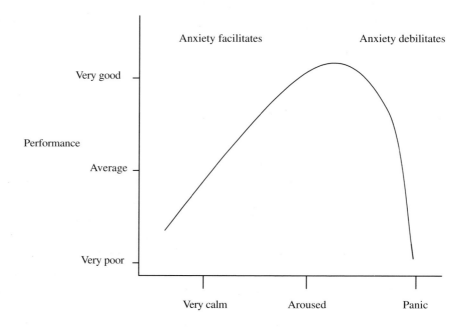

2.1.3 Chronic anxiety

If individuals find it difficult to break the anxiety cycle, the problems can become chronic. It is very likely that individuals with generalized anxiety disorder have had longstanding difficulties with managing anxiety, sometimes for months or even years. Some of the results of feeling anxious over a long time include:

- Feeling restless or keyed up or on edge
- Being easily tired
- Difficulty concentrating or mind going blank
- Irritability
- Muscle tension
- Trouble falling or staying asleep
- Restless unsatisfying sleep
- Feeling overwhelmed or unable to cope
- Feeling depressed or demoralized

When you experience these problems, the anxiety has begun to interfere with your everyday life. Because anxiety is a normal, *in-built*, and at times useful response, you will never banish it completely from your life, but the good news is that you can learn to manage and control it.

2.1.4 Why do the symptoms of tension and anxiety begin?

The reason why you have become anxious is probably due to a combination of causes. We will briefly consider some possible causes.

The effect of personality

Personality refers to the usual way we react, feel, and behave year in and year out. Most people who seek treatment for an anxiety disorder have come to regard themselves as nervous, not just because of their high levels of anxiety, but because they consider themselves to be people who are usually sensitive, emotional, and worry easily. There are advantages to being like this, for the sensitivity means you can understand other people quickly and hence are often liked in return. It also probably means that you like to do things properly and treat other people well. But the emotionality and the proneness to worry are the seeds from which anxiety can grow.

The various strategies that we will teach you will aid you to control this aspect of your personality. If you do become upset and worry easily, then you'll need to become particularly expert in remaining alert, tense, but in control to prevent you becoming too anxious in the face of difficulties.

The effect of life events and stressors

Anxiety may begin at a time when you are experiencing a high level of stress. Throughout our lives, we are constantly adjusting to demands placed upon us by changing circumstances. Making an important decision, meeting a deadline, changing jobs or routines, dealing with others in our lives all require constant adjustments. However, at times you may experience a single major problem, or several smaller problems, that may exceed your normal powers of adaptation. When high levels of stress occur, anxiety can result if they produce in you a sense of threat and lack of control.

The effect of your view of the world

Individuals with generalized anxiety disorder have an increased tendency – compared to individuals without an anxiety disorder – to automatically interpret information in their lives as threatening. For example, the ringing telephone is less likely to be considered with pleased anticipation of a friend ringing for a chat, but more likely to be viewed with alarm as news of an accident. Or a frown on the face of a supervisor at work is less likely to be viewed as the supervisor's personal problem, but more likely to be viewed as a sign of disapproval. This view of the world is thought to develop from previous life experiences, which might include the impact of stressful life events, or the messages received from parents and other important people in your life.

2.2 The nature of worry

Worry is a central feature of generalized anxiety disorder. Most people can identify with the idea of "worry", but scientists have defined the following features in the worry of individuals with generalized anxiety disorder:

- It is usually a stream of thoughts or ideas.
- It is accompanied by feelings of apprehension or anxiety.
- It concerns future events and catastrophes.
- It interferes with the ability to think clearly.
- It is very difficult to control.

Research has shown that the typical person with generalized anxiety disorder can spend over half of their waking hours worrying. In most instances, the individual can recognize, with hindsight, that the worry was excessive and out of proportion to the actual event that triggered the worry.

A large number of worries tend to focus on day-to-day concerns, most typically:

- Family and home life
- Relationships
- Work and study
- Illness or injury
- Finances

Common themes of worry in generalized anxiety disorder can include:

- Problems arising in the future
- Perfectionism and a fear of failure
- Fear of being negatively evaluated by others

It is clear that individuals with generalized anxiety disorder worry largely about events that are remote (as opposed to in the immediate future) and which are unlikely to happen. This sort of worry is rarely helpful as it is unlikely to promote effective problem solving. For example, worrying that a relative might develop a life-threatening illness in the absence of any risk factors (a remote and unlikely event) will not affect the likelihood of it happening. However, adaptive worry might take place prior to an important exam if the worry led to a good problem-solving behavior – a time-table of study.

2.2.1 Worry about worry

A second level of worry has been identified in individuals with generalized anxiety disorder and includes thoughts such as:

- "I can't control my worry."
- "Worry is bad for me."
- "My worry will never end."
- "I will go mad with worry."

These worries may increase the sense of threat and therefore symptoms of anxiety can rise even further.

Sometimes people come to believe that their worry might be useful. They might think:

- "If I worry about the worst possible outcome I can be better prepared for the worst possible outcome."
- "Worrying about an outcome will stop it from happening."
- "If I stop worrying and something bad happens, I'd be responsible."
- "I can sort it out if I keep worrying about it."
- "I'd have nothing to think about if I didn't worry."
- "My worry helps me to keep control of my anxiety."

These beliefs are rarely confirmed, are rarely put to the test, and the individual continues to worry. If you hold any of these beliefs, it will be important to challenge them in order to be able to let go of the process of worry and its negative consequences. For example, if you did stop worrying about a particular event, would it really make it more likely to happen? But more about strategies to combat worry later.

2.2.2 Behaviors that can maintain worry and anxiety

A number of things you do to deal with the worry in the short-term may actually cause the anxiety and worry to continue in the longer term.

- *Reassurance seeking*, or needing to check with others that things are going to be okay. For example, telephoning your partner frequently to make sure nothing bad has happened to them, or visiting your doctor any time you notice a sign or bodily sensation that might mean you are ill. Continually seeking reassurance from others might relieve the anxiety in the short term, but the relief is usually only temporary. Because you are never really allowed to deal with the initial worry yourself, you can come to depend on this reassurance, and unfortunately come to need it more and more to relieve anxiety.

- Other forms of *checking* include obsessively reviewing the report for work or study to make sure that it is perfect, or not being able to take a break until all the tasks for the day are complete (and we all know how likely that goal is to be achieved!!). While there is not a lot of evidence that this type of checking ensures that work is perfect, or that everything gets done, the individual never learns that their work can be acceptable without the checking or that they can take breaks and still get things done. Instead, goals are set too high, and the individual becomes upset, anxious, and demoralized when he or she doesn't achieve what has been planned.

- *Avoidance* of situations or events that are thought to produce anxiety. For example, avoiding listening to the news because stories of disasters or illness will trigger worry about personal disaster or illness. Or avoiding people because of what they might say to you. Or avoiding any situation in which the chances of danger have been overestimated. Avoidance can seriously limit your life and the possibility of enjoying a range of activities that are so much a part of everybody's life. When avoidance is based on an overestimation of danger, it is unnecessary and the belief of danger is never disconfirmed.

- *Procrastination*, a special form of avoidance, which involves not beginning a task because of the anxiety associated with a possible negative outcome. Many times tasks are started only when the negative consequences of not starting outweigh the negative consequences associated with completing the task – some tasks never get started at all! For example, consider a dressmaker who can never start on special orders because of her fear that her client would not like the finished product and therefore think less of her both professionally and personally. In most cases, the feared consequences are overly negative, usually catastrophic, and not based on reality.

- Another form of avoidance is trying to *suppress or control worry*. Unfortunately, the worry might well be made stronger by attempts to suppress it, possibly just because you are purposefully focusing your attention on it. Some research has suggested that the process of deliberately suppressing thoughts can cause them to intrude into your mind more forcefully when the thoughts are no longer being actively suppressed. This process has been called a rebound effect.

Alternative strategies for dealing with worry that do not maintain the anxiety and worry are covered in later sections of the Manual.

2.2.3 Keeping a record of your anxiety or worry

Identification of the thoughts, feelings and behaviors that contrib[utes ...] an important part of the program. This information will help [... your] therapist to plan the best strategies to manage problems with generalized [...]

Monitoring progress also allows us to see what works well and what doesn't work so well, and so the plan can be adapted on that basis. The monitoring will also make sure that you are aware of the progress you are making, even if in small steps.

In particular we will be asking you to:

- Identify the content of your worry.
- Identify the beliefs you hold about worry ("worry about worry").
- Identify behaviors that may be maintaining your worry.

Each time you have an episode of anxiety or worry we will be getting you to complete a "Record of worrying thoughts" listed at the end of this section.

Using the information in these records we will be able to identify:

- Situations or circumstances that trigger worry or anxiety.
- The situations that you avoid because of anxiety or worry.
- Behaviors in response to your worry.

1. Situations or circumstances that trigger worry or anxiety

_____

_____

_____

_____

_____

_____

_____

_____

_____

_____

_____

2. Situations you avoid because of anxiety or worry

_____

_____

_____

_____

_____

_____

_____

_____

_____

_____

3. Behaviors in response to your worry or anxiety

_____

_____

_____

_____

_____

_____

_____

_____

_____

_____

Record of worrying thoughts

Date: _____

Describe the situation	What triggered the worry?	Describe the worry	Describe worry about worry	What did you do?
		How did you feel:		How did you then feel:
		How strong was that feeling: ___ %		How strong was that feeling: ___ %

SECTION 3

3 Relaxation strategies

3.1 What is relaxation training?

Relaxation is the voluntary letting go of tension. This tension can be physical tension in the muscles or it can be mental, or psychological, tension. When we physically relax, the impulses arising in the various nerves in the muscles change the nature of the signals that are sent to the brain. This change brings about a general feeling of calm, both physically and mentally. Muscle relaxation has a widespread effect on the nervous system and therefore should be seen as a physical treatment, as well as a psychological one. Section 3 will discuss how to recognize tension, how to achieve deep relaxation, and how to relax in everyday situations. You will need to be an active participant in relaxation, committed to daily practice for 2 months or longer.

3.2 Importance of relaxation training

Part of the fight or flight response involves the activation of muscle tension, which helps us to perform many tasks in a more alert and efficient manner. In normal circumstances, the muscles do not remain at a high level of tension all the time but become activated and deactivated according to a person's needs. Thus a person may show fluctuating patterns of tension and relaxation over a single day, according to the demands of the day, but this person would not be considered to be suffering from tension.

When people have been anxious for long periods of time or when people have not taken time off from work or other activities, they seldom allow the muscle tension levels to become deactivated, and the tension tends to stay with them for longer and longer periods. Eventually, these people cannot recognize tension or are unable to relax the tension away. The tension no longer helps them to perform their daily tasks, and may even hinder normal activities. Because of the tension, these people may feel jumpy, irritable, or apprehensive. This may be why many people often report feeling slightly unwell much of the time, with headaches or backaches, or they feel slightly apprehensive all the time, worrying about things unnecessarily. Constant tension can make people oversensitive and they respond to smaller and smaller events as though they were threatening. By learning to relax, it becomes easier to gain control over these feelings of anxiety.

Since some tension may be good for you, it is important to learn to discriminate when tension is useful and when it is unnecessary. Actually, much everyday tension is unnecessary. Only a few muscles are involved in maintaining normal posture, e.g., sitting, standing, or walking. Most people use more tension than is necessary to perform these activities. Occasionally, an increase in tension is extremely beneficial. For example, it is usually helpful to tense up when you are about to receive a serve in a tennis game. Likewise, it is probably helpful to tense up a bit before a job interview. This tension keeps you keen and alert. Do not become frightened of this type of tension.

The tension is unnecessary when:

- It performs no useful alerting function.
- It is too high for the activity involved.
- It remains high after the activating situation has passed.

What physical changes occur during the relaxation response?
- The mind becomes more tranquil.
- Hormone production decreases.
- Breathing rate decreases as less oxygen is needed.
- Heart rate decreases and blood pressure drops.
- Sweating decreases markedly.
- Muscles relax.

Note that these responses are opposite to the "fight or flight" response.

3.3 Components of relaxation training

In order to be more in control of your anxiety, emotions, and general physical well-being, it is important to be able to relax. To do this you need to:

- Recognize tension.
- Relax your body in a general, total sense.
- Let tension go in specific muscles.

3.3.1 Recognizing tension

When people have been tense and anxious for long periods, they are frequently not aware of how tense they are, even while at home. Being tense has become normal to them and may even feel relaxed compared with the times they feel extremely anxious. However, a high level of background tension is undesirable, because worry or other anxiety symptoms can easily be triggered by small increases in arousal brought on by even trivial events.

Consider the following:

- Where do you feel tension?
  - Do you notice tension in your face and jaw?
  - Do you clench your fists?
  - What other parts of your body feel tense?
  - Are there parts of your body where tension goes unnoticed until you feel pain?

- What are the characteristics of the tension?
  - Do the muscles feel stretched and sore?
  - Do the muscles feel hard and contracted?
  - Do the muscles feel tired?
  - Does there appear to be effort involved in maintaining normal posture?
- Which events lead to an increase in tension?
  - Anger?
  - Worry?
  - The way people speak to you?
  - Having to wait in lines or at traffic lights?
  - Being watched while working?
  - Your relationships?

3.3.2 Relax your body in a general, total sense: achieving the relaxation response

Progressive muscle relaxation means that the muscles are relaxed in a progressive manner, usually starting with the hands and arms and ending with the leg muscles. Relaxation exercises should be done at least once a day to begin with, preferably before any activity that might prove difficult. Initially, do the exercises in a quiet room, free from interruption, so that you can give your entire concentration to relaxation. Explaining the exercises to those you live with will generally lessen any embarrassment and aid in cooperation in minimizing interruptions. Select a comfortable chair with good support for your head and shoulders.

If a chair does not provide good support, use cushions placed against a wall. Some people prefer to do the exercises lying down, but do not use this position if you are likely to fall asleep. These relaxation exercises are not meant to put you to sleep, since you cannot learn to relax while asleep. Sleep is not the same as relaxation – consider those times when you have awakened tense. If you do want some method to put you to sleep, go over the relaxation exercises in your mind or keep a relaxation tape specifically for that purpose. As you master the relaxation exercises, try inducing deep relaxation in various postures and situations.

It is usually not a good idea to practice progressive muscle relaxation while performing activities that require a high degree of alertness, e.g., driving a car or operating a machine. Instead, use one of the specific muscle exercises described further on.

When possible, it is advisable that you use the relaxation exercises as a preparation for some activity over which you anticipate difficulty. Decide which form of relaxation you will use, arrange your seating appropriately, finish all you need to do, and then start the exercises. It is important that you have nothing external to think about while you are relaxing. Therefore, if you are expecting a phone call, leave the phone off the hook; likewise, don't start cooking just before relaxing if something might boil over. When you are relaxing, you can be comfortably aware that any distractions that occur are not important and don't require your attention.

During the relaxation avoid tensing the muscles too tightly or they may become overly tense and then difficult to relax, or you may even cause cramping. About 60% to 70% of your maximum tension is usually recommended.

After you have finished the relaxation, don't jump up right away. First, you might feel momentarily dizzy and misinterpret this normal reaction as a sign of some other problem. Second, you might get straight back into the old habit of tensing. Get up slowly and try to preserve the state of relaxation for as long as possible. Set about your activities in a slow and peaceful manner.

Remember, relaxation is a skill and, as such, improves with practice. Do not despair if you do not reach deep levels of relaxation during your early sessions. The more frequently you practice relaxation, the deeper the relaxation will be, and the longer lasting the effect.

You will need to commit yourself to at least 8 weeks of daily practice in order to achieve really long-lasting effects. Naturally, longer is even better. Some people continue daily relaxation many years after leaving treatment. If you can do this, we recommend it. However, not all people continue relaxation in this way. It is our experience that people who benefit most from relaxation either practice regularly or practice immediately when they notice any increase in tension or anxiety.

3.3.3 Let tension go in specific muscles: isometric relaxation

Isometric relaxation exercises can be done in everyday situations. Most exercises do not involve any obvious change in posture or movement. Others involve some movement and are best reserved for doing in some place where movement or stretching isn't likely to draw too much attention.

In the early stages of training, you may have to do these exercises several times a day to counteract tension and maintain a relaxed state, particularly when anxious. As you improve, they will take less time and become easier. Eventually, you will find that you are doing them without thinking – i.e., they may well become a habit that you will use automatically to counter tension.

There are some important points that need to be remembered when you are doing the isometric exercises. You are asked to hold your breath for 7 seconds while you hold in tension, but some people occasionally find this too long. Don't become obsessive about holding your breath – try to hold it for 7 seconds if you can but this is not crucial. The most important thing is to concentrate on putting the tension in slowly over approximately 7 seconds and releasing the tension slowly over approximately 7 seconds. The most common mistake that people make with isometric exercises is putting the tension in too quickly or putting in too much tension. These are meant to be gentle and slow exercises. The aim of the exercise is to relax you, not to get you even more tense. If circumstances do not allow you to hold the tension for 7 seconds, you can still benefit from putting in the tension slowly over some period of time and releasing it in the same manner.

Some example exercises
When sitting or lying down in private:
- Take a small breath and hold it for up to 7 seconds.
- At the same time, straighten arms and legs out in front of you and stiffen all muscles in the body.
- After 7 seconds, breathe out and slowly say the word "relax" to yourself.
- Let all the tension go from your muscles.
- For the next minute, each time you breathe out say the word "relax" to yourself and let all the tension flow out of your muscles.

Repeat if necessary until you feel relaxed.

When sitting in a public place:
- Take a small breath and hold it for up to 7 seconds.
- At the same time, slowly tense leg muscles by crossing your feet at the ankles and press down with the upper leg while trying to lift the lower leg.
    Or
- Pull the legs sideways in opposite directions while keeping them locked together at the ankles.
- After 7 seconds, breathe out and slowly say the word "relax" to yourself.
- Let all the tension go from your muscles.
- For the next minute, each time you breathe out say the word "relax" to yourself and let all the tension flow out of your muscles.

Shoulders and neck:
- Hunch shoulders up towards the head.
- Let shoulders drop and let arms hang loose.

3.4 Important points about learning to relax quickly

- Relaxing is a skill – it improves with frequent and regular practice.
- Do the exercises immediately whenever you notice yourself becoming tense.
- Develop the habit of reacting to tension by relaxing.
- It helps to slowly tense and relax the muscles.
- When circumstances prevent you from holding the tension for 7 seconds, shorter periods will still help but you may have to repeat the exercise a few more times.
- Do not tense your muscles to the point of discomfort or hold the tension for longer than 7 seconds.

- Each of these exercises can be adapted to help in problem settings, such as working at a desk or waiting in a line. Use them whenever you need to relax.
- Using these exercises, you should in a few weeks be able to reduce tension and prevent yourself from becoming overly tense.

3.5 Difficulties with relaxation

Some people report that they cannot relax or that they cannot bring themselves to practice relaxation. Since all human beings share a similar biological make-up, there is usually no purely physical reason why relaxation should work for some people and not others. The reason that relaxation may not work for some people is usually due to some psychological factor or insufficient practice.

I am too tense to relax: In this case, the individual uses the very symptom that needs treating as an excuse for not relaxing. Relaxation may take longer than expected, but there is no reason why someone should have to remain tense.

I don't like the feelings of relaxation: About 1 in 10 people report that, when they relax, they come into contact with feelings that they don't like or feelings that frighten them. These feelings indicate that you are coming into contact with your body again and noticing sensations that may have been kept under check for many years. You do not have to worry about losing control during relaxation sessions. You can always let a little tension back in until you get used to the sensations.

I feel guilty wasting so much time: Relaxation is an important part of your recovery. Many therapies take time, e.g., physiotherapy. You do not have to be openly productive to be doing something useful.

I can't find the place or time: Be adaptive. If you can't find 20 minutes, find 10 minutes somewhere in the day to relax. If you do not have a private room at work, go to a park. Relax during the evening, while your partner is reading the newspaper – you do not have to be alone to relax. Don't choose a time when you would rather be elsewhere. For example, don't choose to relax at lunchtime if you would prefer to be with friends.

I'm not getting anything out of this: Unfortunately, many people expect too much too soon from relaxation training. You cannot expect to undo years of habitual tensing in a few relaxation sessions. Impatience is one of the symptoms of anxiety, so you need to understand that this reaction is a sign that you actually need to continue with relaxation training. Give the training time to take effect. Set long-term goals, rather than monitor your improvement day by day.

I haven't got the self-control: You need to realize that quick, easy cures for longstanding tension that call for no effort from you do not exist. The longest-lasting treatment effects occur when an individual takes responsibility for his or her recovery and commits to daily practice of a relaxation strategy.

SECTION 4

4 Thinking strategies

Humans are thinking, feeling, and behaving beings. These three aspects of our make-up interact with each other. However, thoughts can often go unrecognized and we fail to realize the important role they play in the way we feel and behave. People often presume that events lead directly to feelings.

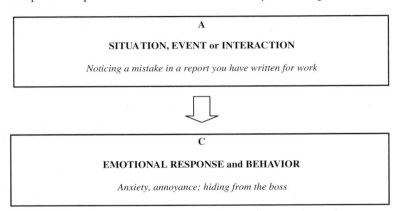

This presumption is important because it may lead people to believe that they have no influence over the way they think, feel or behave. But thoughts intervene between A and C, so the true association is:

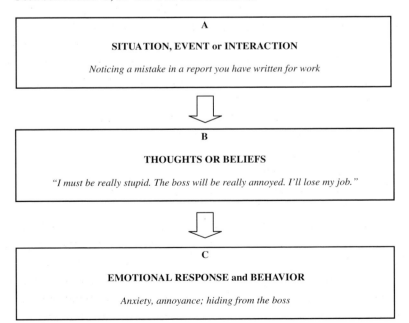

Another important point is that different people will often have very different thoughts, and therefore very different reactions, in response to the same event. Consider the following example. Three people are waiting at a bus stop. They see the bus approach, hail the bus – and it just drives past without stopping.

- The first person gets angry and clenches their fists.
- The second person gets anxious and their heart starts to pound.
- The third person shrugs their shoulders and gets on with reading the newspaper.

The *same* event produced three *different* responses, because it is not the event that directly produced the feelings and behavior, but rather the thoughts the three people had about the event.

- The first person might have thought, "That driver should have stopped! Now I'm going to be late for an important meeting!".
- The second person might have thought "I'm going to be late, I'll never get everything done in time, and the rest of the day will be a disaster!".
- The third might have thought "I might be late, but there's not much I can do about it right now".

So people can respond differently to the same situation. Their emotional response and behavior (C) is related to the way they think about or interpret (B) any given situation or event (A).

If you are like the first or second person in the example above you might tend to see things as worse than they need be, and you may be causing yourself unnecessary anxiety. All people who have suffered anxiety for many years develop habitual and unhelpful ways of thinking about situations. They often tend to expect the worst; often so much so that they bring the "worst" on. The way an individual reacts to events and to people is largely tied into the expectations and assumptions that that individual holds about particular situations and their self. Some of these expectations and assumptions may not be particularly helpful.

Expectations such as:

- "I know that something dreadful is going to happen."
- "I can't concentrate and it's affecting my whole life."
- "I'll always be anxious."
- "My worry will drive me crazy."
- "Everyone will see that I'm not coping."

... are likely to increase anxiety.

Typically, these expectations and assumptions have been built up over a number of years, so much so that they at times seem automatic. They do, however, have significant implications for how upset you feel and how you actually behave.

It is important to recognize that unhelpful thinking patterns are habits, and that habits can be changed with effort and practice. Identifying unhelpful thoughts associated with anxiety is the first step in changing your thinking.

nxiety-provoking thoughts.

unhelpful anxiety-provoking thoughts.

ore helpful alternatives.

4.1 Identifying anxiety-provoking thoughts

In any situation or interaction in which you find yourself unhappy with your feelings or actions, ask yourself:

- What do I think might happen?
- What do I think about myself?
- What do I think about the other person?
- What do I think about the situation?
- How do I think I might cope?
- What will I do?

Individuals with generalized anxiety are often preoccupied with worries, ruminations, and catastrophic thoughts. This "doom and gloom" type of thinking is centered on anticipated consequences (what might happen) or unreasonable self-expectations.

Hence individuals will often predict the worst outcome, overestimating the chance that it will happen:

"I'm not going to have enough time to prepare properly." "It'll be wrong." "I'll fail the test." "I'll develop a fatal illness."

or may underestimate their own ability to cope:

"I'm just not good enough to succeed at this." "I'll just fall apart."

In some cases, the personal consequences of an event will be greatly exaggerated:

"It will be a disaster if this doesn't work out right." "I'll never get another job." "I'll be a social outcast."

The thinking behind much anxiety is usually based on an extreme statement of what *might happen* rather than a realistic appraisal of what *probably will happen*. People are capable of taking a potentially unpleasant event and making it worse than it has to be by dwelling upon it, and by thinking in intricate detail of all the things that could potentially go wrong. If you have come to think about certain events or situations as dangerous or awful, then indeed you will be upset in direct response to your interpretation of "dangerous" or "awful".

You quite obviously don't do this deliberately, but over the years you may have developed patterns of thinking about the situations that upset you that are unhelpful and have become largely automatic. For example, the physical sensations of anxiety can be very frightening. Someone who is worried that their anxiety symptoms may really be signs of an underlying and yet unrecognized serious physical illness would be said to be responding reasonably to their label, or interpretation, of their experiences. They believe the symptoms to be dangerous, even though they are objectively harmless. The problem is that the label applied is wrong! Worrying that one may be ill will cause more anxiety, and bring on even more of the unpleasant bodily feelings that caused the worry in the first place.

Once you have been able to identify what you have been saying to yourself, determine whether it was helpful in the situation. The following guide should help. Helpful thoughts are generally:

Reasonable	not	Catastrophic
Self-enhancing	not	Self-defeating
Logical	not	Illogical
Accurate	not	Inaccurate
Flexible	not	Rigid

4.2 Challenging anxiety-provoking thinking

Identifying and challenging your unhelpful automatic thoughts is not always that easy. To give you some extra help, there are four types of question that you can ask yourself that may make the unhelpful aspects of the thoughts more clear.

- What is the evidence for what I thought?
- What alternatives are there to what I thought?
- What is the effect of thinking the way I do?
- What thinking errors am I making?

4.2.1 What is the evidence for what I thought?

Ask yourself if the thought would be accepted as correct by other people. From your or other people's experience, what is the evidence that what you believe is true? Ask yourself if you are jumping to conclusions by basing what you think on poor evidence. How do you know what you think is right?

As well as engaging in a mental exercise of weighing the evidence, you can actively go out and seek evidence for and against the belief.

Examples of anxiety-provoking thoughts could include:
1. "If I'm anxious, they'll think I'm stupid and never want to talk to me again."
2. "Worrying it through might stop the worst from happening."
3. "If I were to slow down for even one minute, I'd never achieve anything."

Each of the above thoughts may be unrealistic. If you had these thoughts, you could argue with yourself about their truth. However, the best test would be to see:

1. If people still spoke to you after you were anxious when you went out with them.
2. If the feared event happened if you stopped worrying about it.
3. Whether or not you still got things done if you did slow down.

In weighing up the evidence, ask yourself:

- How likely is what I fear to happen?
- What is the worst thing that will realistically happen?
- How bad would that be, really?

4.2.2 What alternatives are there to what I thought?

Is the thought the only possible one that you could have? Perhaps there are alternative interpretations of an event or ways of thinking about something. What might someone else say about the situation. Determine whether any of these alternative views have better evidence for them or would be more helpful in managing your feelings.

For example, you feel uncomfortable when talking to someone on whom you'd like to make a good impression. You notice yourself stammer slightly and are acutely aware of silences. You might think "They must think I'm acting weird, they'll see I'm weak and anxious and won't want to know me."

But how do you know?
They might be thinking
"She (he) seems a bit tense today, I hope nothing's the matter..."
"...maybe they're not feeling well."
"I wonder whether they'd like to see a movie tonight."
"Will I have enough time to get to the shops on the way home?"

4.2.3 What is the effect of thinking the way I do?

Another way of disputing your thoughts is to ask yourself what are the advantages and disadvantages of thinking that way. If you can think of an equally valid way of thinking that brings more advantages, why choose the one that brings disadvantages?

Perfectionism, or having to get it right all the time, is a common theme of worry in generalized anxiety disorder.

Advantages of having to get it right all the time	Disadvantages of having to get it right all the time
I can produce really good work	I get so anxious, I can't do my best
I try that much harder to do well	I don't take risks, and so miss many experiences
When I get it right, I feel really good	I don't allow myself to make the mistakes that are necessary for learning
	I can't let anyone notice my mistakes, so miss out on valuable advice
	When others criticize my work, I get defensive and angry
	My successes are ignored because being less than perfect wipes out their importance
	I don't have any constant idea of myself, just of how well I am doing at any given moment
	I can never think well of myself because it is impossible to get it right all the time
	My mistakes and failures are catastrophic

4.2.4 What thinking errors am I making?

Some examples of common thinking errors include:

Thinking in all-or-nothing terms: This is black-and-white thinking in which things are seen as all good or all bad, either safe or dangerous – there is no middle ground.

"I am totally hopeless if I am less than thoroughly competent or achieving in everything I do."

Using ultimatums: Beware of words like always, never, everyone, no-one, everything, or nothing. Ask yourself whether the situation really is as clear-cut as you are thinking.

"Things never go right for me. No-one else has problems like me."

Condemning yourself on the basis of a single event: Because there is one thing that you can't do or have not done, you then label yourself a failure or worthless.

"I made a mistake today; I am a complete failure."

Concentrating on weaknesses and forgetting strengths: Try to think of other times you have attempted or even been successful at something and think about the resources that you really do have.

"My anxiety is taking so long to get over, I haven't made any progress and that's just typical of me."

Blaming yourself for what is not your fault: This will only make things worse, so think through the arguments for and against. If it is not your fault, stop blaming yourself (even if you cannot think of anyone or anything else to blame).

"I'm too weak to deal with my worry."

Taking things personally: Are you "personalizing" everything so that it has relevance to you or caused by you when in fact it has nothing to do with you?

"That woman in the magazine with cancer is the same age as me, I could get cancer."

Expecting perfection: People invariably make mistakes. Accepting imperfection does not mean accepting low standards but it means acknowledging mistakes and learning from them rather than being paralyzed by failure.

"It's got to be exactly right, or it is not even worth starting."

Using double standards: Many people expect of themselves what they would not expect of others. Ask yourself, "How would I react if it was someone else in my situation? Would I be so hard on them?"

"I can't possibly say that I disagree with them; they'd be annoyed and dislike me."

Overestimating the chances of disaster: Things will certainly go wrong and there *is* danger in the world, but are you overestimating these? How likely is it that what you expect will really happen?

"I might lose my way; my car will break down; I'll be stranded, or bashed or raped."

Exaggerating the importance of events: Often we think that some event will be much more important than it turns out to be. Ask yourself, "What difference will it make in a week or 10 years? Will I still feel this way?"

"That fight we had yesterday has ruined everything."

Fretting about the way things *ought* to be: Telling yourself that things *should* be different or that you must act in a certain way indicates that you may be worrying about how things "ought" to be rather than dealing with them as they are.

"I must get rid of this worry. It's not normal."

I can do nothing to change the situation: Pessimism about a lack of ability to change a situation leads to feelings of depression and lowered self-esteem. There may be no solution, but you will not know until you try. Ask yourself whether you are really trying to find answers and solutions.

"I can't help the way I think. I can't change or control my feelings."

Predicting the future: Just because you acted a certain way in the past does not mean that you have to act that way forevermore. Predicting what you will do on the basis of past behavior means that you will cut yourself off from the possibility of change.

"I usually get anxious at parties, so I know I won't enjoy the next one."

Blaming the past: Just because certain things happened in the past doesn't mean that significant changes cannot be made by you for the future.

"My past is the cause of all my problems. It will continue to affect me and I will never change."

4.3 Generating alternative thinking

Changing the way you think sounds easier than it is. Having identified the automatic and unhelpful thoughts that contribute to anxiety, you will need to learn to look at each of these thoughts objectively and then say what a realistic view of the situation is. This process is going to take time and effort on your part.

If your thinking pattern is well-learned and practiced until it becomes habitual, it can become difficult to shake. You will need to *write down* your worries and what you fear and then evaluate whether the fear is justified or whether it is an unrealistic view of a situation. The objective in learning how to change the way you think is not to try to convince yourself that things are better than they are; rather, the aim is to be able to recognize when your thinking is unhelpful.

Following are some examples of such unhelpful thinking, together with some alternatives for each of the situations involved.

Anxiety-provoking thoughts	Helpful thoughts/alternative interpretations
What if everything goes wrong?	Its unlikely that everything will go wrong. Worrying about something that may go wrong won't stop it from happening. I will only plan for things that are likely to happen
I couldn't cope	I wouldn't like it, but if anything went wrong I will survive it. I always have done so in the past.
I'm not good enough to do this well	I like to do things well most of the time but like everyone, I will occasionally make a mistake. I may feel bad, but I can handle that. I will try my best
Surely these feelings really mean that I have a serious illness	I am feeling symptoms of anxiety, which I know cannot harm me. I am unlikely to have anything seriously wrong with me that all the doctors have missed
I keep thinking that something dreadful will happen to the people close to me	There is no evidence that anything bad is about to happen. I won't dwell on future events that are unlikely to happen

Helpful thinking does not reject all negative thoughts; it is not simply wishful thinking. It involves looking at things in a way that is most realistic, given the facts. For example:

Unhelpful thinking

"I didn't get the job, which proves that I am a failure. I'll never get a job or have things go right for me."

Helpful thinking

"I am disappointed I didn't get that job, but I can cope."

Wishful thinking

"Who cares! I didn't want the job anyway."

Unhelpful thinking

"What if I can't cope with this? It will be absolutely disastrous."

Helpful thinking

"I'm going to give this a try. I'll give it my best shot and see how it goes."

Wishful thinking

"It'll be easy!"

All our thoughts do not necessarily have to be centered on disappointments, but it is often in such situations that you can feel anxious or hopeless. If things do not go as you would hope or if people do not behave as you would like, check whether your disappointment is reasonable. If so, face your disappointment, but do not make a catastrophe out of it!

4.4 Assumptions and core beliefs

While automatic thoughts are usually easy to recognize as verbal messages in your conscious mind, it may be important to learn to understand the assumptions or core beliefs that lie behind the thoughts.

Assumptions operate as rules that guide our daily actions and expectations, and are usually "If ... then..." or "should" statements. Some examples of assumptions are "If I don't get things right all the time then people will think that I am stupid" or "If I let other people see what I'm really like then they might not like me" or "Others mightn't like you if you disagree with them".

The deepest level of thinking is the *core belief*. Core beliefs are absolute statements about yourself, other people, or the world. Some examples of core beliefs are "I am stupid" or "Others will reject the real me" or "It is wrong to disagree".

Many people would have held these assumptions and core beliefs since their

Record of attempts to change unhelpful thinking

Date: _____

Describe the situation	Identify and list automatic thoughts	Objective reappraisal
	How did you feel:	How did you feel:
	How strong was that feeling ___ %	How strong was that feeling ___ %
	How strong is your belief ___ %	How strong is your belief ___ %

childhood. Young children develop rules to make sense of their experiences ("dogs bite", "dogs are friendly") and to guide their behavior ("stay away from dogs", "play with dogs"). Children also learn rules from the things others tell them and from observing the way others behave. These rules are not necessarily true and, in childhood, may not be very flexible ("all dogs bite", "all dogs are friendly"). As people grow older they tend to be able to develop more flexible rules as they learn that everything is not black and white. However some beliefs may remain inflexible, even into adulthood, and will continue to dictate how you interpret and react across various situations. If the assumptions or core beliefs are unrealistic and unhelpful then they may lead to intense or long-lasting levels of anxiety or depression. Luckily, assumptions and core beliefs can be changed in much the same way as automatic thoughts.

- Identify beliefs.
  - Look for repeated themes in your thought monitoring or diary.
  - Ask yourself "If that were true, what would it mean about me?".
- Test beliefs.
  - Gather evidence that the belief may not be 100% true.
  - Critically examine your beliefs and their effect on your feelings and behavior.
- Consider the advantages and disadvantages of holding the belief.
- Allow more time for change in assumptions and beliefs than in automatic thoughts.
- Record evidence that a belief may not be 100% true all of the time.
- Identify alternative helpful beliefs.

Through the program, you will be asked to write down your thinking for each situation or circumstance where you find yourself anxious or worrying. Use the "Record of attempts to change unhelpful thinking".

SECTION 5

5 Managing worry

Individuals with generalized anxiety worry a lot. These worries tend to center on everyday things; we all worry to some extent about problems that might arise at home or at work, about illness or injury afflicting ourselves or our family, about difficulties in our relationships with others, or even financial pressures. Individuals with generalized anxiety will recognize that they worry *excessively* about these things, that the worries are often unrealistic, and that the worry takes up a large part of their typical day. Unfortunately, it is this type of worry that can interfere with daily functioning, and can increase anxiety and tension levels.

Excessive worry or ruminating about events that are unlikely to happen can make you feel worse than you need to and may even increase feelings that you cannot cope. It may feel as though by worrying about things you might anticipate and avoid future catastrophes, but in reality the worry does n[ ] productive or constructive action. Instead, problems remain unsolved, t[ ] not confronted, and the unhelpful beliefs about events or situations co..tinue unchallenged. In the following sections more practical steps for helping to deal with worry are described.

5.1 Problem solving

Determine whether there is a real problem that requires solving. Ask yourself:
- Is the feared event likely to happen?
- Is it imminent?
- Is there anything you can do about it?

If you answer yes, deal with the problem using an efficient problem-solving strategy (covered in Section 6). For example, you might be in a situation where you need to find a new job, move house, or put up an unexpected and unwelcome house guest. Rather than worry about how you will cope, you can short-circuit the worry by planning how to solve the problem – then make sure the plan is put into action!

5.2 Indecision

Determine whether the worry is driven by indecision. Many individuals with generalized anxiety disorder are anxious that they might do something wrong or make the wrong decision. They may be overly perfectionistic. The anxiety may cause these individuals to procrastinate or continually put off making a decision, or they may deliberately continue to "worry through" the decision in an attempt to ensure that they don't make a mistake. For example, people may find themselves going through a lengthy series of questions and answers about major life decisions such as "Am I in the right job?", "Am I in the right relationship?". Or there may be a series of day-to-day decisions that cause worry, such as "Should I go to that party?" "What present should I buy my partner?" or "Which task should I start first?"

Unfortunately this "worrying it through" process does not usually help to find the "right" decision (as there may not be such a thing as the "right" or "wrong" answer) but instead increases and extends feelings of anxiety and uncertainty, thereby feeding the indecision. Furthermore, this process may cause you to come up with a wider range of catastrophic consequences that you would otherwise have come up with. In other words, the more you worry, the more and more negative you may become.

Sometimes people will not want to make a decision until they believe they have *all* the information relevant to that decision. For example, every travel agent will need to be contacted to check out every deal before the holiday can be booked, or every consequence has to be thought out before a plan embarked upon. Unfortunately it is rarely necessary to have this level of certainty before making a decision, and impossible to be free from *any* doubt.

If your worry is driven by indecision:

- Determine whether there is any unhelpful thinking that lies behind your worry. For example, "Is there really a 'right' answer to your decision?" "Realistically, what would really happen if you made a decision one way or the other?" "What's the worst that could happen?" "What evidence is there that you are unable to make a decision?"

- If there is a decision to be made, set a reasonable amount of time to reach a decision, and then *act on it*! The problem-solving strategy described in Section 6 can be helpful here.

- Then make sure that you *don't engage in any further worry* about the decision (see Section 5.4).

5.3 Worry about worry

A number of examples of *worry about worry* can be challenged using the strategies covered in the previous section.

> Worry is really bad for my health.
> Worry will drive me mad.
> I can't control my worry.
> I will worry like this for the rest of my life.

Ask yourself:

- "What is the effect of thinking this way?"
- "What is the evidence to support these beliefs?"
- "What alternative explanations might there be?"
- "What is more likely based on past experience?"

For example, if you worry that you will be unable to control your worry, ask yourself what typically happens when you do worry. Are you really never able to stop it? What eventually stops the worry? So next time, how likely is it that the worry will go on and on forever? What do you think would happen if you tried to postpone the worry by telling yourself that you will give yourself time to think about it later in the day? Why don't you try this and see what happens? What would happen if you deliberately tried to lose control through worry?

Positive beliefs about worry can be challenged using similar strategies. For example, ask yourself when worrying about the worst possible outcome has actually helped you to cope with the outcome? It is likely that the answer to this question would be that the worst possible outcome has never come about! Would you really be increasing the chances that a bad thing would happen by not worrying about it? Why don't you stop worrying about it and see if it really happens?

5.4 Letting go of worries

Once you have reached the stage when you are able to effectively challenge catastrophic and unhelpful worries, and you are able to dismiss the notion that worry might be helpful, it is time to stop the worry process itself. In order to do this, you will need to say: "It may never happen I just don't need to think about it!"

It may be helpful to think of times when you have not been troubled by worry and rumination. Probably during these times you were involved intently in an activity that you enjoyed a lot or that took up all of your attention. It is very difficult to think properly about more than one thing at the same time.

Thus it is sometimes useful to have a strategy to draw your attention away from worrying thoughts – once you have decided that it is appropriate not to continue to think about them. You have probably already noticed that it is extremely difficult to stop such thoughts just by trying to push them out of your mind. A better solution is to acknowledge the worry, and then focus your attention on something else. For example,

"That's a worry. It's not worth my thinking about it. I'll get on with my work."

"I can't determine exactly what will happen in the future, I will focus on what I'd like to do today."

If stuck, here are some examples of things to do:

- *Concentrate on what is happening around you:* Get involved in the moment. Choose something that is likely to interest you and engage your attention. Give yourself a specific task: listen carefully to the conversation; begin the next task at work; make that telephone call.
- *Engage in some form of mental activity:* Read a magazine or book; complete a crossword puzzle; watch a movie.
- *Engage in some form of physical activity:* Do some exercise; wash the car; take the dog for a walk.

SECTION 6

6 Structured problem solving

Our lives are full of problems to be solved, ranging from major life crises to the more mundane hassles of our day-to-day lives. However, no matter how small or trivial the matter, if problems remain unsolved, or if the way they are resolved is unsatisfactory, they can lead to feelings of uncontrollability or the perception of threat, which are major contributors to anxiety.

Structured problem solving is a useful strategy for anyone with problems, whether those problems are related to anxiety, or other personal matters, such as dealing with a difficult colleague at work. The approach can also be used by groups of people, such as families, friends, and workmates. For example, your family may be facing financial difficulties and may need to cut expenses, or they may have a problem in that nobody is prepared to do the dishes in the evening. Problem solving can also be applied to achieving goals, such as getting a job, planning a social activity, or improving one's fitness.

There are no perfect or ideal solutions to problems, but the structured problem-solving approach aims to lead you to the most effective plan for action.

6.1 Setting up a problem-solving session

Because this structured approach is best suited to problems that are difficult, serious, or capable of causing anxiety and worry, problem solving should occur only in certain settings and at times specifically set aside for that purpose. For instance, do not try to do problem solving while watching TV or cooking the dinner. There should be no competing jobs or distractions: take the phone off the hook, or, if you have young children, plan to hold your problem-solving session after they have gone to bed.

Do not attempt to solve more than two problems in the one sitting. It is useful to plan an agenda in advance. In this way, you will more likely avoid unrelated worries or ruminations that will interfere with the problem-solving process. It is often useful to write down all of your problem-solving exercises. Use the same structure as the problem-solving sheet provided in Section 6.10. Writing things down will often put problems and solutions into better perspective and ensure that a record of the decisions you make is always available.

6.2 Identifying problems

Most people will have no difficulty in recognizing where their problems lie, but to help you in this task, the following points may be helpful:

- Use your feelings as a cue for recognizing problems. Rather than viewing your feelings as the problem, consider what may be causing the way you feel. If you have interpreted the circumstances correctly, then the event itself may be a problem that needs to be addressed, changed, or resolved.
- Use your behavior as a cue for recognizing problems. If you continue to make mistakes, or things don't work out as you would like, the situation itself may be the problem and you may be able to manage it more effectively.

- Consider the content of your worries. Is there a problem tha
  behind these worries?

6.3 Step 1: Defining problems and goals

A clear definition of a problem or goal is the next step in problem solving. Goals should be realistic and fairly easy to attain. Defining problems or goals helps to focus thinking on the issue at hand and minimize the possibility of getting sidetracked onto other issues. Also, it makes it easier to know when the goal has been achieved or the problem solved.

At this stage of problem solving, there are some "rules" that will make the definition of a suitable goal or problem more likely.

- Do not get sidetracked into attempting to solve the problem at this stage. This attempt will not help to define the problem and may only lead to increased worry or anxiety.
- Be specific. The more specific the goal or problem, the easier it will be to solve. For example, avoid vague statements along the lines of "I want to feel better", or "My boss is inconsiderate". Rather, redefine the problem in terms of the actual feelings or behaviors, such as "I want to reduce my headaches" or "I am unhappy about my boss expecting me to work on weekends without extra pay".
- Focus towards the future. Because problem solving aims to provide a plan to deal with present or future events, don't focus on past occurrences of the problem or distant causes underlying the problem. For example, "I would like to go out to lunch with my work colleagues and feel comfortable", is better than "I avoided lunching with my work colleagues last week because I was too anxious".
- Some difficult goals may need to be broken down into smaller goals that can be achieved more easily and in a shorter period of time. For example, if a goal involves finding a new job, the first step may be to decide what sort of job to look for.

Write down some of your problems and goals in the spaces below

_____

_____

_____

_____

_____

_____

Step 2: Generating solutions through brainstorming

Brainstorming is a method by which we come up with as many alternative solutions as possible. Rather than try to think of the best or ideal solution, we list any ideas that come into our minds, including those that we may think are not useful or even absurd. In fact, some of the proposed solutions should deliberately be absurd – use your imagination! Even though a solution may at first seem ridiculous, it may help to generate better solutions than those that are more obvious.

At this stage of problem solving, there is no discussion of the solutions. They are just listed.

Select a problem that you can work on and try to define it so that it is specific, concrete, and attainable. As an exercise in brainstorming, try to come up with as many possible solutions for this problem. Try also to think of a few ridiculous solutions.

What is the problem? _____

List all possible solutions:

1. _____

2. _____

3. _____

4. _____

5. _____

6. _____

6.5 Step 3: Evaluating the solutions

This step involves a brief discussion of the advantages and disadvantages of each solution. Do not write these down, just quickly run through the list of solutions, noting the strengths and weaknesses of each. No solution will be ideal, as every good idea will have some faults. However, most bad ideas will also have some advantages as well, e.g., they may be easy to apply and provide some short-term relief, but not really solve the problem in the longer run.

Briefly run through the solutions you generated to the problem above.

6.6 Step 4: Choosing the optimal solution

In this step, the aim is to choose the solution (or combination of solutions) that will solve the problem or achieve a goal.

It is often helpful to choose a solution that can be readily applied and not too difficult to implement, even though it may not be the ideal solution. At least, you can get started right away. The problem may not be solved immediately, but you might have made a difference, and what you learn by trying might be useful the second time around. This is preferable to choosing a solution that is doomed to failure because you have been overly ambitious.

Outline the solution (or combination of solutions) you have agreed upon in the space below.

_____

_____

6.7 Step 5: Planning

A detailed plan of action will increase the likelihood that the problem will be solved. Even if your solution is excellent, it will not be of any use if it isn't put into practice. The most common reason why solutions fail is through a lack of planning. Be sure to spend some time on this planning stage.

Imagine that you are planning the solution for the problem you have solved. Outline the steps you would plan in the space below

1. _____

2. _____

3. _____

4. _____

The following checklist applies to any problem and is helpful to see whether you have planned properly.

- Do you have the necessary resources available (time, skills, equipment, money) or are you able to arrange the necessary resources or help?
- Do you have the agreement or cooperation of other people that might be involved in the plan?
- Have all the steps been examined for possible difficulties?
- Have any strategies been planned to cope with likely difficulties? Setting specified times or deadlines will minimize the risk of procrastination.
- Have any strategies been planned to cope with any negative (or positive) consequences?
- Have difficult parts of the plan been rehearsed, e.g., a telephone call, conversation, interview, or speech?
- Has a time been set for a review of the overall progress of the plan?

6.8 Step 6: Review

Problem solving is a continuing process as problems are often not resolved or goals not attained after only one attempt. Because not every possible difficulty is considered at the planning stage, ongoing reviews are necessary to cope with unexpected set-backs. Steps may need to be changed or new ones added.

It will also be important to praise all efforts that have been made. If you reward yourself and others for the work that has been done, it is more likely that the successful process will be followed and that problems will be solved in the future.

6.9 When things don't go as planned

- What went right?
- What went wrong?
- What alternative strategies could be used?
- Acknowledge feelings of disappointment, but do not allow any unhelpful thinking to turn the disappointment into a catastrophe. Difficulties are usually due to a poorly planned strategy rather than personal inadequacy. Everyone does as best they can.
- Label any attempt as partial success rather than failure. Consider partial success as practice and a useful learning experience.
- Try again as soon as possible.

6.10 Problem-solving practice

From now on, whenever you are faced with a difficulty or problem that appears difficult to resolve, use the following six-step method of structured problem solving. For many problems, there are no easy answers or ideal solutions, but at least you will know that you have tackled your problem in the most effective and efficient manner.

Structured problem solving

Step 1:   *What is the problem/goal?* Think about the problem/goal carefully, ask yourself questions.

Then write down *exactly* what the problem/goal is.

_____

_____

Step 2:   *List all possible solutions:* Put down all ideas, even bad ones. List the solutions *without evaluation* at this stage.

1.   _____

2.   _____

3. _____

4. _____

5. _____

6. _____

Step 3:   *Assess each possible solution: Quickly* go down the list of possible solutions and assess the *main* advantages and disadvantages of each one.

Step 4:   *Choose the "best" or most practical solution:* Choose the solution that can be carried out most easily to solve (or to begin to solve) the problem.

Step 5:   *Plan how to carry out the best solution:* List the resources needed and the major pitfalls to overcome. Practice difficult steps, make notes of information needed.

_____

_____

_____

_____

_____

_____

Step 6:   *Review progress and be pleased with any progress:* Focus on *achievement first.* Identify what has been achieved, then what still needs to be achieved. Go through steps 1 to 6 again in the light of what has been achieved or learned.

SECTION 7

7 Dealing with behaviors that maintain anxiety or worry

When anxiety occurs for the first time with a certain situation, most people believe that, should they confront that same situation again, they would be more than likely to become anxious. Likewise, certain activities or problems may also have become associated over time with discomfort or anxiety. The occurrence of anxiety is unpleasant and so, as any sensible person would, sufferers soon learn to try to anticipate the situations or events likely to trigger their anxiety.

Of course, it is quite helpful to behave in a way to minimize objective danger, such as getting your doctor to check an unusual mole on your arm or avoiding deserted parts of the city late at night. On these occasions the anxiety that causes us to act in these ways will serve a useful purpose. The problem is that when they are anxious, individuals with generalized anxiety will often avoid situations that are not dangerous, such as upsetting TV or newspaper stories, meeting certain people, or anything that might remind them of their fears or worries. Others will put off doing things that they know should be done, or avoid solving their problems. Yet others will unnecessarily seek reassurance from those around them to decrease their fears or doubts.

The problem with these behaviors is that the relief is only temporary.

In practice, the things we avoid become harder and harder to do, and gradually we avoid more and more things.

The need to seek reassurance becomes greater, and more and more reassurance is required to relieve the anxiety.

When anxiety is relieved by something we do, the fear can be made even worse, because the feeling of relief and drop in anxiety following the behavior tell us that the behavior was sensible. Thus, the behavior is reinforced or strengthened; after all, if you can avoid anxiety by acting in a particular way, why not do so? Unfortunately, you just identify more and more situations as difficult and avoid them also.

Then what is the cure? If avoiding the things you fear makes them harder and harder to face, what would happen if you started to confront your fears? If the fear is reinforced by seeking reassurance, what would happen if you prevented yourself from checking? Actually, if you confronted your fears or doubts for long enough, it would eventually go, and the fear the next time you encountered that situation would be less. However, most people don't like to put this to the test, so they keep avoiding those situations or seeking reassurance.

One good way to break behaviors is to start with easy situations and slowly build up enough confidence to face the harder things. The other important strategy is to control the level of the anxiety using the breathing exercise and controlling worrying thoughts, and then stay with the situation until you have become more calm.

But how do you organize such experiences? First, you need to identify all behaviors that might be maintaining anxiety.

You have already made a list of:

- Situations or circumstance that trigger worry or anxiety.
- The situations that you avoid because of anxiety or worry.
- Behaviors you engage in response to your worry.

Make sure that you include things that might not be obvious at first, such as certain topics of conversation or news items, missed opportunities, uncertainty, thoughts of illness or accidents, not accepting invitations, putting things off, or cutting activities short.

Then you plan ways of changing the behavior so that it no longer prevents you from facing what you fear. Some examples are listed below:

Avoiding newspaper items about life-threatening illness.
Being unable to leave work until all correspondence is checked.
Putting off your tax until a few days before the deadline.

Next, rank those situations or circumstances in terms of the anxiety that they cause, or would potentially cause. If the anxiety is too high to allow you to directly change that behavior then:
1. You can break down the behavior into smaller, more manageable steps.
2. You might need to address unrealistic worries about the outcome of this change in behavior.

Example: Avoiding newspaper items about life-threatening illness

Planned task	Predicted anxiety
Read newspaper story about cancer cure	50%
Read newspaper story about cancer – how common it is and its consequences	70%
Read magazine article about personal experience of cancer	75%
Watch ER and other TV programmes with medical themes	90%

Example: Being unable to leave work until all correspondence is checked

Planned task	Predicted anxiety
Don't check e-mail before leaving work	50%
Don't check e-mail after lunch	60%
E-mail unchecked for one day	85%
Leave all new letters unopened and e-mail unchecked for one day	100%

Carefully monitor and record your progress on the sheets provided. This will help you to both structure your progress and give you feedback as to how you are doing. *Make sure a task is attempted every day until you feel comfortable with the situation.*

Planned tasks	Predicted anxiety

Record of homework tasks	Date	Maximum anxiety

SECTION 8

8 Keeping your practice going

Some people have difficulty keeping up practice of their anxiety-management skills. This difficulty may be because they don't think that they are making any progress, even though other people may see a change. Progress is often slow, and sometimes difficult to notice over a number of days. Take care not to underrate your achievements. Learn to praise yourself for your efforts in attempting new ways to deal with difficult situations, as well as your successes. Remember that praising yourself is an important factor in maintaining motivation, particularly in the early stages following treatment.

8.1 Dealing with setbacks

Setbacks can occur occasionally, even in persons who are making excellent progress. When this happens, people often become alarmed and despondent, fearing they have gone back to their very worst. Remember, no matter how badly you feel during a setback, it is very rare for you to go all the way back to your worst level of incapacitation. Also, day-to-day fluctuations in anxiety levels are bound to occur in the period after your treatment, just as in general day-to-day life. It is also important to remember that at these times it may be more difficult to think realistically about situations, and you may find some of your old worries (or some new ones) creeping back into your thinking.

For most people the apparent setback is only a passing phase, due to external factors such as extra work demands, the flu, or school holidays. In such cases, the setback is often viewed as devastating because it has a great deal of emotional meaning for the person who has put considerable effort into gaining control over anxiety. But this effort is not wasted and, after the stressful time passes, you can learn from this experience and again will find you are able to deal with anxiety. We often see this pattern. It is common, however, for people to worry that they will relapse as a result of encountering setbacks.

8.2 Expect to lapse occasionally

A lapse might mean that you start to engage in old unhelpful worries again. This is very different from experiencing a full relapse of your disorder. A relapse would involve a return to levels of symptoms you experienced before treatment and not use any of the techniques you have learned.

So the trick is to not turn a lapse into a relapse and exaggerate the lapse into being bigger than it really is. Most people will have some sort of lapse when they are trying to change their behavior. If you have noticed that you have slipped in your use of the anxiety-management skills, don't say things to yourself such as:

> "I'm really hopeless. I'm right back where I started from. I'll never be able to change."

Instead, you can view your lapse in the following light:

> "I'm disappointed that I have let things slip, but I can deal with that and I'm not going to turn it into an excuse for giving up altogether. Now, I'll get out my Manual and start my practice again."

Therefore, if you have a setback don't add to the problem with all the old catastrophic and unhelpful ideas. Keep practicing all the techniques you have been taught and you will still be making progress.

Of course, many people do stop things like relaxation when they have been feeling okay for some time. This is fine, so long as you keep aware of any stress or anxiety that may be creeping back into your life, and restart the exercises as soon as you become aware of any increase. It will also be important to reinstate such techniques if you have recently experienced any stress or life event.

It may also be helpful to revisit some of the thinking strategies you found useful over treatment. For example, rather than trying to deal with unhelpful worries in your mind, write them down! You will remember that this helps you to distance yourself from your fears and to be more realistic in your thinking.

8.3 Long-lasting change

People with longstanding anxiety have usually suffered for a long time. Most often, anxiety problems will begin in adolescence, but most individuals do not reach treatment until their late 20s or 30s.

In this program, our aim is that you will not only change your reactions and your ability to cope with adversity, but also change the way in which you have learned to think. Such ways of thinking may have become an intrinsic feature of your personality, perhaps even that part of yourself that you consider makes up what is "you". However, this feature turns you into your own worst enemy. In effect, you will eventually need to change the unhelpful aspects of the way you think and behave. You will need to do this in order to make your life more rewarding, to make you more effective and efficient in your work, and to help you to become closer to the people around you.

These changes will not be easy, because changing a fundamental part of the way you think and behave is not easy. But with continued and solid practice of the new skills you have learned, you will continue to make positive changes over future months and even years. Before you realize what has happened, you will find yourself saying:

> "I used to get upset about that, but now I don't!"

SECTION 9

9 Further reading

There is no evidence-based self-help book specifically for GAD available right now. However, this may be useful as a general reference:

Barlow DH, Rapee RM. (1991) *Mastering Stress: A Lifestyle Approach.* Dallas, TX: American Health Publishing Co.

24

Posttraumatic stress disorder

Syndrome

Historical context

Recent years have seen an extraordinary growth in awareness of traumatic stress, not only among health workers but also among the general public. This increased awareness might suggest that mental health professionals have only just discovered the fact that human beings experience a psychological reaction following exposure to trauma or, worse, that the disorder has just been "invented". It is important, therefore, to understand the historical context of PTSD.

The notion that an individual may experience psychological problems following a traumatic experience is not new, with references dating back nearly three thousand years to Homer's *Iliad*. Shakespeare provided several descriptions of traumatic stress reactions, as have other writers throughout history. It was not until early this century, however, that the condition became the focus of interest from a scientific perspective. Several leading figures in the burgeoning field of psychiatry at that time, such as Freud, Kraepelin, and Janet, commented on the existence and nature of traumatic stress reactions following accidents, fires, and other traumatic events. Wartime experiences, notably in the American Civil War and the First World War, prompted physicians to speculate on the cause of posttrauma reactions. The condition was thought initially to be a result of organic damage to the brain caused by explosions on the battlefield and thus the term "shell shock" was coined during the First World War. It was not until later that the psychological basis of the disorder was widely accepted and clinicians began to recognize that terms such as "shell shock", "war neurosis", and "combat fatigue" all referred to the same phenomenon. Gradually, it was acknowledged also that these disorders were essentially no different from traumatic stress reactions seen in civilians following nonmilitary traumas such as transport accidents, fires, natural disasters, and violent assault.

Despite interest in the area over many decades, the disorder was not formally recognized until 1980, with the publication of DSM-III. The term "posttraumatic stress disorder" was proposed and the diagnostic criteria were delineated. With that formal recognition, the area became accepted as a legitimate focus of empirical research and theoretical debate. In 1987, the diagnostic criteria were modified significantly in DSM-III-R and further minor changes were made in the latest edition, DSM-IV. The most recent version of the *International Classification of Diseases*, ICD-10, has included the category of PTSD for the first time.

Diagnostic criteria and clinical presentation

Intense psychological distress is part of a normal human response to overwhelming experiences but, in the majority of people, symptoms progressively ameliorate over the first few months. PTSD is a serious psychiatric disorder that, in its more chronic forms, develops in only a minority of trauma survivors. It represents a failure to integrate the traumatic experience with existing views of the self and the world. Individuals with PTSD remain so captured by the memory of past horror that they have difficulty paying attention to the present. The disorder is characterized by the repeated intrusion into consciousness of painful memories, accompanied by high arousal, as well as by constant attempts to prevent return of the memories by both active and passive avoidance strategies. This pattern of intrusion and avoidance results in a progressive recruitment of symptoms and disability in the period following traumatic exposure.

The first criterion to be met for a diagnosis of PTSD is experience of a traumatic event. Considerable debate has focused on this criterion in an attempt to define how serious a trauma must be before a diagnosis is warranted. Interestingly, the DSM-IV field trials found that, contrary to expectations, the prevalence of PTSD did not increase to any significant degree when less rigorous definitions of the trauma were adopted (Kilpatrick et al., 1997). Nevertheless, DSM-IV places heavy emphasis on the presence of physical threat to the self or others in criterion A1. The individual's response to the event is relevant also, with criterion A2 requiring the presence of "fear, helplessness, or horror". The failure of DSM-IV to specify the timing of such responses has led to considerable confusion, since it is relatively common for distress not to appear until some time after the event has terminated. Examples would include emergency workers who are required to function at a high level during their exposure, as well as those trauma survivors who dissociate during the incident. In practice, the timing of distress is interpreted fairly liberally, with A2 being considered to be met even if the fear, helplessness, or horror does not become apparent until some time after the trauma. While the issue of whether criterion A is met according to the DSM wording is of importance in psycho-legal settings, it is generally not a matter of great significance in clinical practice. If the individual clearly meets the remaining criteria, it may be best to conceptualize the case as PTSD for treatment purposes, even if the traumatic event does not, strictly speaking, comply with the DSM wording.

The second group of criteria is perhaps the most important in understanding traumatic stress, since unpleasant memories of the event dominate the clinical picture (particularly in more acute forms). The B criteria cover re-experiencing of the event in some form; one symptom from this group is required for a diagnosis. Criterion B1 refers to intrusive memories, including images and other perceptions (such as smells or sounds). It is important to note that these memories invade consciousness – it is not simply a matter of ruminating about the experience in a voluntary manner. Dreams and nightmares (criterion B2) are an important diagnostic feature, since they tend to be qualitatively different in PTSD. Traumatic nightmares are usually accompanied by thrashing movements, vocalizations, sweating, and, occasionally, acting out aspects of the dream, often making it impossible for the partner to sleep in the same bed. Although research in the area is sadly lacking, clinical experience suggests also that traumatic nightmares are often accurate replications of the event rather than symbolic representations. Such features are rarely seen in nontraumatic nightmares. Criterion B3 refers to experiences in which the sufferer actually believes that the event is recurring. These dissociative-like phenomena are referred to as "flashbacks". They are actually relatively rare, but are commonly confused with the vivid intrusive images referred to above. Psychological distress (B4) and physical symptoms of arousal when reminded of the trauma (B5) comprise the final two re-experiencing criteria. Such reminders comprise not only the obvious traumatic elements of the event, but may include also a range of idiosyncratic stimuli such as sounds, smells, or even internal states present at the time of the trauma.

The re-experiencing symptoms are highly distressing and result in aversive states of high arousal. In an attempt to reduce the occurrence of these intrusive phenomena, the person is likely to avoid any reminders of the trauma and, in more severe cases, show a pervasive numbing of general responsiveness. These symptoms are categorized together under the C group of criteria and at least three are required for a diagnosis. The first two symptoms in this cluster have something of a phobic quality, describing active attempts at avoidance of activities, places, and people (C1), or thoughts, feelings, and conversations (C2). The lifestyle of someone with PTSD can become progressively more restricted in an attempt to avoid any reminders of the trauma and prevent a recurrence of the painful memories. The remaining symptoms in this cluster may be described as a more passive form of avoidance and are often referred to as emotional numbing. Psychogenic amnesia (C3) may occur for all or part of the traumatic event. Loss of interest in normal activities is common (C4), much as seen in depressive disorders. The trauma survivor may appear detached or become estranged from significant others (C5), a feature often commented upon by the spouse. Criterion C6 refers to a restricted range of affective responses, giving as an example "unable to have loving feelings". Clinical experience suggests that, while this symptom is not unusual in more chronic forms of the disorder, the problem in more acute forms is often the opposite. That is to say, trauma survivors tend to report overwhelming emotions, with highly labile affect (although loving feelings may still elude them). The final symptom in this cluster refers to a sense of fore-shortened future (C7); the person's sense of mortality has been brought home to them to such an extent that it is impossible for them to imagine a long and happy life in the future.

While the DSM-IV includes active avoidance and numbing of responsiveness within the same symptom cluster, there is increasing evidence that the two may represent separate constructs (Foa et al., 1995b). Those authors speculate also that the numbing symptoms are central to the diagnosis of PTSD, differentiating it from more common, but less pathological, psychological responses to trauma. Certainly, clinical experience suggests that, if a trauma survivor does not meet criteria for a formal diagnosis of PTSD, it is often because the person does not have sufficient numbing symptoms.

The final cluster of symptoms are those of persistently increased arousal. Sleep disturbance (criterion D1) appears to be almost universal in the early days posttrauma. Some trauma survivors report that they are frightened to go to sleep because of the intrusive images and nightmares while, for others, fears for their safety are enough to keep them awake. These disturbed patterns often develop into chronic problems with the establishment of habitual poor sleep hygiene. Anger and irritability (D2) are also common. These symptoms can be very destructive to support networks, with the survivor alienating the very people who are trying to help (such as family, friends, and helping professionals). In more chronic PTSD, especially among veteran populations, explosive and consuming anger is often a central component of the initial presentation. Concentration is likely to be disturbed (D3), often as a result of the frequent intrusions. Individuals with PTSD tend to be hypervigilant (D4) – always on the look-out for signs of potential danger – a feature that is often quite noticeable in the clinical interview. The final arousal symptom is that of exaggerated startle response (D5). This is characterized not only by an excessive physiological arousal when startled but also by a failure to habituate to repeated presentations of the startle stimulus. Two of these hy-perarousal symptoms are required for a diagnosis of PTSD.

DSM-IV requires that symptoms in B, C and D have been present for at least 1 month (criterion E). In line with other DSM-IV diagnoses is the requirement that the disturbance must cause significant distress or functional impairment (cri-terion F). The disorder is specified as acute if duration of symptoms is less than 3 months and chronic if 3 months or more. It could be argued that 3 months is a little premature to be referring to the disorder as "chronic". Nevertheless, the distinction is an important one and may prompt appropriate research into phenomenological differences and treatment implications for acute versus chronic presentations of the disorder. Finally, DSM-IV allows for a delayed category if the onset of symptoms was at least 6 months after the trauma.

CASE EXAMPLE

Mr. D., a 38-year-old male, presented for treatment 18 months posttrauma following intense pressure from his wife and work supervisor. He finally agreed to treatment after bursting into tears at a school concert in which his youngest child was appearing.

History of presenting complaint

Mr. D. was working as a night security guard when an armed robbery occurred. Three men wearing balaclavas broke into the building carrying sawn-off shotguns. He was struck on the head (but did not lose consciousness) and was then tied to a chair, gagged, blindfolded, and repeatedly threatened with being killed. At one point, the blindfold and gag were removed to ask him for the safe combination. When he said he did not know it, they again threatened to shoot him. The men stayed for approximately 1 hour, ransacking drawers and cupboards. Throughout this time, Mr. D. feared for his life. He stated that he believed he was going to die and was convinced he would never again see his wife and children. There was little to suggest that he dissociated during the incident, but reported symptoms of high arousal throughout (heart racing, sweating, stomach churning). He was found by a cleaner at 6.00 a.m., taken to hospital, and discharged shortly afterwards.

Following the incident, he stayed at home for several days, too frightened to leave the house. During this time, he was required to repeat the story for police statements. Each retelling was accompanied by high physiological arousal and intense feelings of fear. Since then, he has not discussed the incident with anyone. He returned to work after 1 week, but has remained on special duties. He feels unable to work at nights and has been allocated only "low risk" jobs. Although he is coping adequately with his current work regime, he feels under pressure to return to normal duties and believes he will lose his job if he does not do so soon.

On questioning, it was clear that he had suffered many symptoms typical of posttraumatic stress over the previous 18 months. He was troubled by vivid intrusive images, notably of the gunman's face and the shotgun, although these had reduced in frequency. He was experiencing nightmares several times a week, accompanied by excessive sweating and movement, and had taken to sleeping in a room separate from that of his wife. He was easily distressed by reminders in the media, as well as idiosyncratic stimuli (such as seeing people wearing sunglasses, which reminded him of the double barrels of the shotgun thrust into his face). He avoided talking about the incident, tried to block thoughts from his mind, and had made several changes to his lifestyle in order to avoid potential reminders. Previously a keen sportsman, he had given up all competitive sports (although continued to jog on a regular basis). He noted that his wife complained of him being withdrawn and irritable, no longer showing affection towards her or the children. His consumption of alcohol had increased markedly from occasional social drinking to regular consumption of five or six standard drinks each evening. His sleep had become very disturbed, dropping from an average of 8 hours per night before the incident to 4–5 hours. He reported problems with concentration, being unable to read books or focus on television programs, and complained of problems with memory and decision making. He talked of being hypervigilant when away from home, particularly when out at night (which he tried to avoid if at all possible). The course of symptoms over the previous 18 months had been relatively stable, with a slight reduction in intrusive symptoms accompanied by an increase in avoidance and emotional numbing.

A brief interview with Mr. D.'s wife confirmed the above story. In particular, she emphasized the social withdrawal and emotional numbing aspects of his current presentation, saying that he had become "a different man to the one I've known for the last 18 years".

History

There was no significant prior psychiatric or medical history. The oldest of three children, his childhood was relatively stable, although he reported that he was shy at school and a "bit of a loner" as a child. He described his mother as a nervous woman who tended to shun social contact. His father drank fairly heavily, although Mr. D. did not remember any episodes of associated violence. He described his family as being "no nonsense – when things went wrong you didn't complain or talk about it, just got on with life". He completed school and went on to teacher training. Although he worked for 10 years as a teacher, he never enjoyed it and was pleased to be offered voluntary early retirement. Over the past 7 years he has had several jobs and has been with the security firm for the last 2 years. He married his wife, also a teacher, when they were both at college and has two children aged 7 and 10 years. The relationship is strong, although it has been put under considerable pressure since the trauma. He has many acquaintances, but few (if any) close friends.

Permorbid personality

Mr. D. described himself as being a happy and outgoing person prior to the trauma, although on closer questioning his social contact seemed to revolve almost entirely around sport. Not particularly psychologically minded, his habitual style of coping with stress appeared to be one of avoidance and denial.

Mental state

Mr. D. presented as a casually dressed man of above-average intelligence who appeared haggard and tired. Although initially quite defensive and tense (he insisted on taking a chair facing the door), he loosened up and eventually spoke freely and openly about his history and current problems. His affect varied from flat to dysthymic, often on the edge of tears. He showed little insight and was unable to understand why he had not recovered from the event, seeing it as a sign of weakness. He was pessimistic about the future and reported feeling guilty about his behavior towards his family. There was no evidence of thought disorder, hallucinations, or delusions. Having made the decision to seek treatment, he seemed highly motivated to work on his problems.

Formulation

Mr. D. clearly meets criteria for a diagnosis of chronic PTSD, with evidence of a traumatic experience, several re-experiencing symptoms, widespread avoidance and numbing, and persistent hyperarousal. Although there is evidence also of depression, this seems secondary to the PTSD and would not warrant a separate diagnosis. Despite an absence of prior trauma history or psychiatric problems, there is some evidence of vulnerability in terms of a prior tendency towards anxiety (in both him and his parents) and a pattern of coping with stress characterized by avoidance and denial. Although these strategies have worked well in the past, they have prevented him from integrating his experience and moving on. The traumatic memories remain unchanged and continue to invade consciousness causing frequent distress. His attempts to deal with the memories by increased avoidance, denial, and emotional numbing, while not always successful, have resulted in social and occupational problems.

Other diagnoses of traumatic stress

A new category, acute stress disorder (ASD), was included for the first time in DSM-IV to describe a posttrauma reaction that has been present for less than the 4 weeks required for PTSD. As such, the stressor criterion is identical, and one symptom from each of the re-experiencing, avoidance, and hyperarousal clusters is required. Also required is some evidence of dissociation at the time of, or immediately following, the event (such as feeling numb or in a daze, derealization, depersonalization). The disorder must have been present for between 2 days and 4 weeks, and must not be due to organic factors. Several aspects of the ASD criteria are controversial and an excellent critical review of this new diagnostic category was provided by Bryant and Harvey (1997). Such a diagnosis is important, however, for several reasons. First, it may facilitate access to early treatment that would perhaps be denied to persons without a formal diagnosis. Second, the introduction of ASD will hopefully prompt research into differential treatments (e.g., brief and focused interventions for ASD as compared to intensive treatment for PTSD). Third, it may prompt identification of those factors that determine which survivors will progress from ASD to PTSD and why.

There has been considerable discussion regarding the possible introduction of a new category of traumatic stress disorder to cover the long-term effects of prolonged and repeated abuse. Termed complex PTSD or complicated PTSD, this clinical syndrome was the subject of extensive field trials in preparation for the DSM-IV (Pelcovitz et al., 1997). For a variety of reasons, this category was not included in the final version. This is disappointing, since its inclusion (perhaps as a research criteria set) may have prompted study into both phenomenology and treatment. Interestingly, the ICD-10 has attempted to address this issue with the inclusion of a new category, "Enduring personality change after catastrophic experience". This diagnosis refers to the development of persistent, inflexible, and maladaptive personality features following severe trauma, such as hostility, social withdrawal, feelings of emptiness, hypervigilance, and emotional numbing. Empirical research has yet to investigate the validity or utility of this new diagnostic category.

Comorbidity

It is important to recognize that comorbidity is the norm, rather than the exception, in chronic PTSD. For example, Kulka and his colleagues (1990) reported that 98% of Vietnam veterans with PTSD had, at some stage, qualified for another DSM-III-R diagnosis. The National Comorbidity Survey (Kessler et al., 1995) reported that 88% of men and 79% of women with chronic PTSD meet criteria for at least one other psychiatric diagnosis.

Although not a formal diagnosis, feelings of guilt are reported frequently by survivors of trauma. This symptom was included in DSM-III but was dropped from the revised version in 1987. These feelings of guilt may be about behavior required for survival, about the fact that the individual survived while others did not, or about reactions and behavior since the event. Symptoms of depression are common also following trauma. Indeed, it is clear from the PTSD criteria outlined above that many symptoms overlap between the two diagnostic categories, sometimes presenting a problem for differential diagnosis. Indeed, an additional formal diagnosis is often warranted: major depression is the most common comorbid condition occurring with chronic PTSD (in around 46% of cases; Kessler et al., 1995). Other anxiety disorders, particularly in the form of panic disorder and social phobia, may occur in 20% to 30% of individuals with chronic PTSD. Substance abuse and dependence is a frequent complication, occurring in around 52% of men and 28% of women with chronic PTSD. This use of both licit and illicit drugs is often conceptualized as part of the avoidance and numbing component of PTSD, as the sufferer attempts to block out the painful memories and feelings. Somatic symptoms, including gastrointestinal problems, aches and pains, cardiovascular symptoms, and psychosexual difficulties may be present, particularly in more chronic forms, as well as poor health behavior (such as smoking, poor diet, lack of exercise).

Although this discussion has focused on the comorbid conditions that may occur along with PTSD, it is important to remember also that many of these disorders may develop as sequelae of trauma in the absence of PTSD. It is important to resist the temptation to diagnose PTSD simply because the person has experienced a significant trauma when an alternative diagnosis may be more appropriate.

Prevalence and course

It is clear from recent epidemiological studies that experience of trauma is relatively common, with estimates in the general population ranging from 51% for women and 61% for men (Kessler et al., 1995) to as high as 84% for mixed-gender samples (Vrana and Lauterbach, 1994). Thankfully, by no means all of those people who experience trauma will go on to develop PTSD and, of those who do, many will recover over the first few months following the event.

Estimates of lifetime PTSD prevalence in the general community vary from a low of 1% (Helzer et al., 1987) to around 10% for women and 5% for men (Kessler et al., 1995). Not surprisingly, the nature of the traumatic event is critical in the subsequent development of PTSD, with rape generally resulting in the highest prevalence. Kessler et al. (1995), for example, report that 65% of male and 46% of female rape victims developed PTSD. The lifetime prevalence of PTSD following other traumas varies considerably across studies.

Lifetime prevalence may provide a somewhat misleading picture, since, in many cases, PTSD will remit even in the absence of formal treatment. The National Comorbidity Survey (Kessler et al., 1995) found that around 60% of cases eventually recovered (regardless of whether the person received treatment), with most improvement in the first 12 months. A study of PTSD in victims of nonsexual assault (Riggs et al., 1995) found that 71% of women and 50% of men met PTSD criteria shortly after the assault. By 3 months, only 21% of the women and none of the men remained with PTSD. The same authors report a similar decline for female rape victims over the same period, although the percentages were considerably higher (94% immediately postrape, dropping to 47% by 11 weeks; Rothbaum et al., 1992a). Thus, as a broad guideline, around half of those individuals who develop PTSD in the aftermath of trauma will recover over the first few months without the benefit of formal treatment. After that point, however, the picture becomes less optimistic. Data from several sources (e.g., Solomon, 1989; Kessler et al., 1995) suggest that individuals who still meet criteria for PTSD at about 6 months posttrauma are unlikely to recover without additional assistance. The disorder is likely to assume a chronic course, with symptoms lasting for many decades unless effective interventions are implemented.

It is important to emphasize that PTSD is not a "normal" response to trauma. Rather, it is a serious psychiatric disorder that, at least in its chronic forms, develops in only a minority of trauma survivors. While virtually everybody will develop a psychological reaction in response to a traumatic event, with the help of existing coping strategies and support networks the majority are able to recover without developing serious psychopathology.

Etiology and vulnerability factors

Theoretical models from psychological, social, and biological perspectives have been proposed to explain the development of PTSD. Indeed, the complexity of the disorder, and the high prevalence of comorbidity, is such that a single approach is unlikely to provide an acceptable explanation. Rather, there is a need to develop integrated biopsychosocial models in order to provide a full understanding of the condition. An explanation of all three approaches is beyond the scope of this review and the reader is referred to alternative sources for a summary of the key biological approaches (see Bremner et al., 1999), psychological models (see Foa and Rothbaum, 1998), and sociocultural issues (see Kleber et al., 1995). A review of risk and vulnerability factors in PTSD was provided by Yehuda (1999).

For the purposes of this discussion, vulnerability factors are apparent in three broad domains: pretrauma, peritrauma, and posttrauma. In terms of pretrauma vulnerability factors, research examining demographic factors has been conflicting, with few clear trends emerging. However, there is some evidence to suggest that poor education and low income may be associated with a slightly increased risk of PTSD, and that married men may be at higher risk than unmarried men (Kessler et al., 1999b). There is now clear evidence that females may be more vulnerable than males to the development of PTSD following exposure to trauma (Breslau et al., 1997). There are many potential explanations for this finding from biological, psychological, and sociocultural perspectives. While it may be explained in part by a reluctance on the part of males to report symptoms, it may also be a function of trauma type. Anecdotal evidence would suggest that females are more likely than males to be victims of violence perpetrated by someone they know, resulting in greater disruption of long held beliefs relating to trust, safety, and intimacy.

Several studies have suggested that prior psychiatric history, or a pre-existing tendency towards anxiety and depression, may be a vulnerability factor in the development of PTSD (e.g., Rothbaum et al., 1992b; Blanchard et al., 1996b). The question of prior trauma experience is complex. It is possible that, at certain levels, prior life stress may help to inoculate the individual to subsequent stress, providing an opportunity to learn and practice coping skills and to develop more flexible internal models of the self and the world that can incorporate future trauma more readily. Some support for this suggestion was provided by Ruch and Leon (1983), who found a curvilinear relationship between prior life stress and adjustment to rape. Those survivors with both very high and very low levels of prior life stress fared worst, with those who had experienced moderate levels doing best. However, the bulk of research suggests that a prior history of trauma, particularly childhood physical and sexual abuse, constitutes an important vulnerability factor in the development of PTSD following subsequent trauma (Breslau et al., 1999).

With regard to the characteristics of the event itself (peritrauma variables), research has consistently shown severity of the trauma to be a critical factor in subsequent adjustment (e.g., Kulka et al., 1990; Kessler et al., 1995). More severe events are characterized by factors such as a high degree of life threat, longer duration, complexity, and exposure to the suffering of others. It has been suggested also that predictability and controllability may be important, with people being likely to adjust better to high level events if they are, at least to a degree, expected. For example, people in the military or emergency services are better prepared to routinely cope with events that would be highly traumatic for the general population. An important caveat on the above, however, is that several studies have suggested that perceived life threat during the trauma may be a stronger predictor of subsequent adjustment than the actual level of threat (Creamer et al., 1993; Blanchard et al., 1995).

Finally, posttrauma factors may moderate development of the disorder and facilitate the recovery process. The available research suggests that good social support (Creamer et al., 1993; Green, 1996) and stress-management skills (Foa et al., 1991b) may assist recovery from trauma. It is probable that both of these posttrauma factors assist the victim in managing the distress associated with confronting the traumatic memories, reducing the likelihood of prolonged cognitive and behavioral avoidance. Anecdotal evidence suggests that cultural attitudes towards the event, and the extent to which the experience is validated by the person's social networks, may be important also in facilitating the recovery process.

The assessment of posttraumatic stress disorder

The purpose of this section is to summarize the key areas to be covered in the clinical evaluation of a trauma survivor. More detailed reviews of PTSD assessment are well covered in other work (e.g., Carlson, 1996; Wilson and Keane, 1997). The complexity of the assessment process will depend to a large extent on the context in which it is taking place. In primary health care settings, for example, a relatively quick screening may be all that is required before referring the client on for specialized assessment and treatment. On the other hand, assessing for intensive treatment or for psycho-legal purposes would naturally require a more detailed approach. In either case, the clinician must remain sensitive to the mental state of the client, constantly drawing a delicate balance between providing support to a distressed victim and obtaining reliable and objective information. While an empathic and caring manner is clearly required, an overemphasis on that approach at the expense of a more rigorous assessment may not be in the client's best interest over the longer term.

A comprehensive assessment should include not only mental state, current functioning, and life circumstances, but also details of the traumatic experience, prior history of trauma, and pretrauma functioning. The clinician needs to cover the presence and course of core PTSD symptoms, as well as likely comorbid conditions such as depression, anxiety, and substance abuse. In order to understand the client's reaction to the experience, information must be collected also regarding the broader social context.

In most clinical settings, an unstructured interview will comprise the primary, if not the only, assessment strategy. In suspected cases of PTSD, however, there is often a need for more objective assessment that will stand up to the rigorous scrutiny expected in a psycho-legal context. With our current state of knowledge, there is no "gold standard" for diagnosing PTSD. Rather, a multifaceted approach incorporating information from a variety of sources is recommended. In clinical settings, the combination of a structured clinical interview and self-report inventories comprise the optimum strategy. In research settings, the addition of a third category of data in the form of psychophysiological measures provides an extra degree of objectivity, although this approach is rarely practical in clinical contexts.

Structured clinical interviews

Structured clinical interviews provide the best strategy for making a categorical diagnosis of PTSD and, in many cases, also provide a good indication of severity. Administered by experienced clinicians, they have the potential to provide the ideal combination of a standardized and objective instrument with some degree of clinical judgment. The questions directly address the symptoms of PTSD and an objective scale for each question assists in determining whether that symptom is sufficiently severe to meet criteria. Although some clinicians are concerned that this approach of reading questions to the client from a prepared script is too mechanistic, and interferes with rapport and empathy, this is rarely a problem in clinical practice. On the contrary, experience suggests that survivors of trauma are often reassured by this clear validation of their psychological reactions.

Several well-validated structured interviews for PTSD are available (for a review, see Weiss, 1997). The PTSD Symptom Scale Interview (PSS-I; Foa et al., 1993), the Structured Interview for PTSD (SI-PTSD; Davidson, Smith and Kudler, 1989) and the PTSD Interview (PTSD-I; Watson et al., 1991) are all relatively brief and simple to administer. All provide both categorical and dimensional measures of PTSD symptomatology, and all have demonstrated good psychometric properties. As such, all are recommended for use in routine clinical practice. The Clinician Administered PTSD Scale (CAPS; Blake et al., 1995) is a more detailed and complex instrument designed to overcome many of the limitations of other structured PTSD interviews. Each symptom is assessed for both intensity and frequency and, where possible, each symptom is behaviorally defined. The CAPS has demonstrated strong psychometric properties (Blake et al., 1995) and is an excellent choice for use in research. On the other hand, it is a complex instrument requiring considerable practice and takes anything from 45 to 90 minutes to administer. As such, its use in routine clinical settings is limited.

Self-report measures

A multitude of inventories exist for the assessment of PTSD symptoms and several excellent reviews exist (e.g., Solomon et al., 1996; Norris and Riad, 1997). The best self-report measures are psychometrically robust, relatively nonintrusive, and often (although not always) reasonably inexpensive. They have the advantage of assessing how the clients view their symptoms without being influenced by the presence of an interviewer. Equally, they are easy to fake and may be susceptible to symptom exaggeration or minimization. As such, self-report measures should never be used as the only, or even the primary, diagnostic tool. On the other hand, they can function as excellent screening instruments: those clients who score highly can be targeted for more intensive interview procedures. Finally, they are useful for repeated assessments in assessing change as a function of treatment. The following provides a brief overview of some of the more commonly used self-report instruments that may be useful in the psychological assessment of traumatic stress.

Many of the more comprehensive self-report measures of psychopathology have been used in the assessment of traumatic stress reactions and PTSD. For example, Keane and his colleagues have developed a 49-item PTSD scale from the MMPI (PK subscale; Keane et al., 1984). Similarly, several attempts have been made to derive a PTSD scale from the Symptom Checklist 90-R (SCL-90-R; Derogatis, 1977). The best known of these is the Crime-Related PTSD Scale (CR-PTSD; Saunders et al., 1990). While these global measures of psychopathology have useful research applications, scales developed specifically for traumatic stress are more appropriate in most clinical settings.

The Mississippi Scale (Keane et al., 1988), available in both combat and civilian versions, functions as a good indicator of PTSD severity and has excellent psychometric properties. The recommended cutoff for a probable PTSD diagnosis varies, although 107 was suggested by the original authors. The Penn Inventory (Hammarberg, 1992) is a 26-item scale designed to apply to all types of traumatic event. It requires respondents to select the most appropriate of four possible statements for each question. A cutoff score of 35 provided reasonable sensitivity and specificity in PTSD diagnosis across a range of populations (Hammarberg,

1992). The oldest and most widely used self-report measure for the assessment of traumatic stress is the Impact of Event Scale (Horowitz et al., 1979). This 15-item scale takes about 5 minutes to complete and comparative data are available for a wide range of traumatized populations. Developed prior to the recognition of PTSD in 1980, the scale is limited by its exclusive emphasis on intrusion and avoidance symptoms. In order to address this deficiency, the IES-R has recently been published (Weiss and Marmar, 1997). This revised scale includes additional items that reflect the arousal symptom cluster in PTSD. At this stage, insufficient data are available to comment on the reliability and validity of this new scale.

None of the above scales are tied specifically to the DSM symptoms of PTSD. Rather, they provide a more general evaluation of the severity of traumatic stress reactions. A few currently available scales, on the other hand, are designed to reflect the DSM content exactly. The Posttraumatic Stress Disorder Checklist (PCL; Weathers et al., 1993) covers the 17 PTSD symptoms, with each rated on a five-point scale from "not at all" to "extremely". The scale is brief, taking only 5 minutes to complete, and possesses excellent psychometric qualities (Blanchard et al., 1996a). A score of 50 is recommended as the diagnostic cutoff. Another DSM-specific scale is the self-report version of the PSS-I structured interview discussed above. The PSS-S (Foa et al., 1993) consists of the 17 items rated on a four-point scale from "not at all" to "very much". Finally, the Davidson Trauma Scale (DTS; Zlotnick et al., 1996) is a similar self-report measure allowing for both frequency and intensity ratings. Although the authors report good psychometric properties, additional research is required to provide further validation of this measure.

Malingering and symptom exaggeration

PTSD is a diagnosis that is likely to be associated with various psycho-legal processes. In that context, there has been considerable debate in recent years regarding the extent to which symptoms of PTSD may be fabricated or exaggerated, especially when issues of compensation are involved (Resnick, 1993; Frueh et al., 1997). As with any other psychiatric disorder, it is not possible to completely eliminate the possibility of malingering or symptom exaggeration. Nevertheless, a competent and thorough assessment, utilizing standardized instruments where possible, will minimize inaccuracies.

A detailed discussion of the detection of malingering in PTSD is beyond the scope of this chapter. Briefly, however, a full hand of all 17 PTSD symptoms should always raise suspicions. When inquiring about the presence of specific features, the clinician should ask for examples (e.g., "tell me about the last time you experienced that" or "tell me more – what was that like?"). It is hard for patients to present a credible description of most PTSD symptoms unless they have actually experienced them first-hand. Resnick (1993) suggested that a history of unstable employment or previous incapacitating illnesses, emphasis on re-experiencing (rather than avoidance and numbing) symptoms, and lack of sexual dysfunction or nightmares are all potential indicators of malingering in PTSD. Contradictions in the clinical presentation (such as being unable to work but retaining an active social life, or complaining of emotional detachment and high irritability in the absence of any marital discord) should be a cause for concern. Similarly, several features of PTSD may be directly observable to the clinician during the interview (e.g., hypervigilance, flattened affect) and those observations can be compared with the patient's report. Informant interviews, particularly with a spouse or partner, can shed a great deal of light on the validity of the patient's report. If good diagnostic practices are adopted, it is not an easy task to deceive an experienced clinician with a thorough knowledge of the disorder. Equally, unless we are to adopt an attitude of constant disbelief, assuming that everyone with PTSD is malingering until proved otherwise, occasionally even the best clinicians will be deceived.

Summary

PTSD is a severe psychiatric disorder that develops in a minority of trauma survivors. It is important to distinguish this more severe reaction from normal, albeit highly distressing, reactions that will occur in most people following a traumatic event. The disorder is characterized by intrusive memories of the trauma, attempts to block those memories out, and persistent hyperarousal. The likelihood of developing PTSD is dependent upon a complex interaction of pretrauma vulnerability, severity of the trauma, and the posttrauma recovery environment.

25

Posttraumatic stress disorder

Treatment

Survivors of trauma who do not recover independently, and who go on to develop longer-term problems as a result of their experiences, may require formal treatment. There is also a mounting body of research suggesting that early interventions with high risk survivors may facilitate the recovery process and reduce the prevalence of subsequent PTSD. The purpose of this chapter is to provide a brief overview of common interventions used in the treatment of acute stress disorder (ASD) and PTSD, and to discuss their application as a preventive strategy.

Aims of treatment

It is reasonable to assume that virtually all human beings will experience a psychological reaction to very frightening or upsetting events. This raises questions about what constitutes an adaptive psychological response to trauma and, as a corollary, what are reasonable treatment goals. Severe traumatic events profoundly affect survivors' views of themselves and the world. In most cases, it is reasonable to suggest that the survivor will never be the same person again. Equally, those changes need not all be bad. Recovery from trauma can result in personal growth, with the development of improved coping strategies and more adaptive models of the self and the world.

Ideally, treatment would serve to eliminate all the symptoms of PTSD and return the survivor to pretrauma levels of functioning. In reality, that will not always be possible. As with other disorders, factors such as the severity of the condition, chronicity, and comorbidity (particularly in the form of axis II disorders) are likely to affect treatment efficacy. In acute cases of PTSD with few complications, it is reasonable to expect a high degree of success with relatively few sessions (6 to 10). In such cases, elimination of PTSD symptoms, a return to prior functioning, and low risk of relapse would be achievable goals. (Importantly, this is not to imply that the person will never again experience distressing memories of the event but, rather, that such intrusive phenomena will be infrequent and manageable). On the other hand, treatment goals for a Vietnam veteran with, for example, a 30-year history of PTSD, high levels of comorbid alcohol abuse, and poor social and occupational functioning, would be more conservative. It may be a question of helping that person to manage the symptoms more effectively, reducing their impact on quality of life, relationships, and general functioning.

Psychological treatments: description

Several psychological approaches have been proposed for the treatment of PTSD and excellent reviews of the area can be found elsewhere (e.g., Shalev et al., 1996; Foa and Meadows, 1997). Regrettably, few of those approaches have been the subject of adequately controlled treatment outcome research. The following discussion focuses primarily upon cognitive behavioral approaches, since those have been the most comprehensively studied. However, it should not be assumed that the interventions are the exclusive domain of cognitive behavioral therapy. On the contrary, several of the following strategies (notably exposure to the traumatic memories) are used in some form in a variety of alternative intervention models, including brief psychodynamic approaches and hypnotherapy.

Cognitive behavioral approaches to the treatment of PTSD and related disorders routinely comprise a combination of several components. This discussion is limited to those core components of treatment that have been the subject of empirical evaluation. A more comprehensive guide for clinicians appears in Chapter 26. This section provides an overview of the interventions, while the following section reviews the empirical data.

Anxiety management

PTSD is an anxiety disorder characterized by persistent arousal, with high levels of fear relating to trauma-related memories and external cues. This, in combination with a poor understanding of their own psychological reactions, leaves many survivors feeling vulnerable and out of control. Thus a vital step in the early part of treatment is that of teaching a repertoire of simple strategies to manage the arousal and distress. These interventions do not address the underlying causes and are not usually seen as a treatment for PTSD per se. Rather, they provide ways to manage anxiety and distress when it occurs. As such, they are an important precursor to the painful process of exposure.

Anxiety management may be conceptualized under the three broad headings of physical, cognitive, and behavioral components, with interventions delivered in all three domains. The more physically oriented strategies, which directly address the hyperarousal aspects of traumatic stress reactions, are an excellent starting point. Clinical experience suggests that they often produce rapid effects that not only assist the survivor in feeling better but, perhaps more importantly, improve feelings of self-efficacy and contribute to expectations of recovery. The rationale is straightforward (in terms of a fight–flight response) and it requires little in the way of psychological mindedness. A simple controlled breathing strategy is a good first step, often introduced in the initial treatment session (Foa and Rothbaum, 1998). Progressive muscle relaxation, aerobic exercise, and advice to reduce the intake of stimulants such as caffeine and nicotine are all potentially useful interventions. They assist the person to gain some initial control over the powerful physical symptoms of hyperarousal.

The intrusive nature of traumatic memories, and the tendency of many trauma survivors to ruminate about their experience, suggests the need for some direct cognitive interventions. Some of these, such as thought stopping and distraction techniques, are designed specifically to gain control over the frequency and duration of distressing cognitive events. Others, such as the use of coping self-statements and guided self-dialogue, are intended to modify the content. More intensive cognitive interventions are likely to occur later in treatment and are discussed below.

Behavioral interventions are often appropriate also, targeted to the specific needs of the client. Since traumatic stress reactions often involve social withdrawal and isolation, interventions may include activity scheduling and social reintegration (much as is commonly used in the treatment of depression). This would normally include encouragement to resume normal routines as quickly as reasonably possible after the trauma. While care should be taken to ensure that excessive commitment to work is not used as an avoidance strategy, resumption of a normal routine helps the survivor to regain a sense of structure and control. Other behavioral interventions are useful to address specific areas such as sleep, communication skills, and assertiveness.

Exposure treatments

It is reasonable to assume that all successful treatments of PTSD involve some kind of opportunity to confront the traumatic memories. Exposure-based treatments, widely used in the management of anxiety disorders for many years, constitute a central component of treatments for PTSD. Initially, these approaches were based on the assumption that fear is acquired and maintained by the processes of classical and operant conditioning of stimuli related to the traumatic incident. The concept of extinction, or habituation, has been used to explain fear reduction following prolonged exposure to the traumatic stimuli. More recently, Foa and Kozak (1986) have proposed the notion of emotional processing to explain anxiety reduction during exposure. They suggested that the processing of corrective information results in changes to the traumatic memory network, modifying both the stimulus–response connections and the meaning attached to the experience. Excellent descriptions of exposure treatment in PTSD are provided elsewhere (see Lyons and Keane, 1989; Foa and Rothbaum, 1998) and only a brief overview of the technique will be provided here.

In the treatment of most anxiety disorders, it is generally accepted that live exposure work (known as in vivo) is more efficacious than imaginal exposure. In PTSD, in vivo exposure is used for external cues – activities, places, objects, or people – that have become anxiety provoking as a result of the trauma. In the case of PTSD, however, since the traumatic memories constitute the primary feared stimulus, much of the exposure work will be imaginal, with the client being asked to recount the traumatic experience in detail. In order to optimize the efficacy of imaginal exposure, it is important to maximize both stimulus cues (e.g., sights, sounds, smells) and response cues (e.g., cognitions, affect, somatic sensations). Clients are asked to report on their level of anxiety and distress at regular intervals. In conjunction with the clinician's observations, these indices assist the clinician in pacing the exposure and indicate when anxiety reduction is taking place.

Cognitive restructuring

Cognitive restructuring, based on the work of Beck and his colleagues (1979), is sometimes included under the heading of anxiety management. However, the techniques of cognitive therapy have been used to directly treat the core symptoms of PTSD. Cognitive processing therapy (CPT; Resick and Schnicke, 1992) comprises cognitive restructuring with specific reference to five primary themes: safety, trust, power, self-esteem, and intimacy. Clients in CPT are taught to identify maladaptive cognitions (or "stuck points") and to vigorously challenge them using a list of dispute questions. A detailed description of the procedure has been provided by Resick and Schnicke (1993). Various adaptations of cognitive therapy and CPT have now been trialled in the treatment of PTSD.

Psychological treatments: empirical review

The field of PTSD treatment is progressing rapidly and new outcome studies are beginning to appear in the literature on a regular basis. The following provides an overview of the major studies published at the time of writing. A more detailed review of the various treatment options for PTSD has been published recently by the International Society for Traumatic Stress Studies (Foa et al., 2000).

Anxiety management

Regrettably, few of the anxiety-management strategies described above have been empirically evaluated in isolation for the treatment of traumatic stress reactions. It is difficult, therefore, to comment on the efficacy of any individual component.

Most research has investigated a combination of strategies under the heading of stress inoculation training (SIT). This approach, developed by Meichenbaum (1985), incorporates many of the anxiety-management techniques discussed above and has been used widely in the treatment of female assault victims. While several uncontrolled trials have supported the use of SIT with trauma survivors, only three controlled trials have been published to date.

Resick and her colleagues (1988) compared SIT to assertion training, supportive counseling, and a wait-list control. All active conditions resulted in some symptom reduction, with SIT producing a 27% improvement as compared with 14% deterioration in the wait-list controls. Another study of female assault victims (Foa et al., 1991b) compared SIT with prolonged exposure (PE), supportive counseling, and a wait-list control. Although SIT produced the largest improvement at posttreatment, PE showed a superior outcome at follow-up. Measures of PTSD severity at follow-up showed a 60% reduction for PE, as compared with 49% for SIT and 36% for supportive counseling. Finally, Foa and her colleagues (1999) compared PE, SIT, and their combination in the treatment of female assault victims. SIT demonstrated a 57% improvement on PTSD severity from pretreatment to 12-month follow-up, only marginally worse than PE and comparable to the combination treatment. Importantly, however, the dropout rate was higher for both SIT and the combination treatment than for PE.

Thus, while the available data support the use of anxiety management in the treatment of traumatic stress, conclusions must remain tentative and further research is required. The approach has been evaluated only with female assault victims and only three controlled trials have been published, two of these from the same research group. Nevertheless, clinical experience suggests that anxiety management is a vital step in preparing clients for subsequent exposure treatment.

Exposure treatments

A large body of empirical support now exists for the efficacy of exposure treatment in PTSD, with the first controlled trials published in 1989. In a study of 24 combat veterans, Keane and his colleagues (1989) found significant improvements in anxiety (40% reduction in symptoms) and depression (39% reduction), as well as in the re-experiencing symptoms of PTSD (35% reduction), using imaginal exposure compared with a wait-list control. Similar results have been achieved in other studies of combat veterans with PTSD (e.g., Cooper and Clum, 1989; Boudewyns and Hyer, 1990). While all of those studies suffered some methodological flaws, they provided important preliminary evidence for the benefits of exposure in PTSD, particularly with regard to the re-experiencing symptoms.

As noted above, Foa et al. (1991b) found PE to be marginally superior to SIT, and considerably superior to both supportive counseling and a wait-list control, in

45 female assault survivors with PTSD. As noted above, SIT was superior at posttreatment, but subjects in this group tended to show some relapse at follow-up. Those in the PE group, on the other hand, showed a slower but continued improvement. This finding is interesting, perhaps suggesting that the SIT was effective for symptom management but did little to modify the traumatic memories in the longer term. Thus, while PE is a more difficult and painful process, it does seem to produce more meaningful and lasting curative effects. Also noted above is the second study by the same group (Foa et al., 1999), which confirmed the superiority of PE over both SIT and a combination of the two. The fact that the combination treatment was less effective than PE alone is intriguing. The most likely explanation is that session lengths in all groups were identical. Thus the combination group received less time on exposure and anxiety management than the single modality equivalents. It may be that an extended treatment protocol, allowing adequate time for both components, would prove superior.

Two other studies are worthy of note, since they investigated PTSD patients with a variety of traumatic stressors rather than focusing solely on veterans or female assault victims. Thompson et al. (1995) conducted an open trial with 23 PTSD patients, providing eight weekly exposure sessions. While the results must be interpreted cautiously given the absence of a control condition, significant improvements in PTSD symptoms were obtained across several objective measures. In an interesting variation, Richards et al. (1994) compared imaginal with in vivo exposure in the treatment of PTSD, using a cross-over design. They found surprisingly high symptom reduction of 65% to 80% following treatment, with no patients continuing to meet criteria for PTSD at posttreatment or 1 year follow-up. The only difference between exposure types was found on phobic avoidance, with in vivo being superior regardless of the order of presentation.

In summary, controlled treatment outcome research has consistently provided support for the use of exposure techniques in the treatment of PTSD.

Cognitive restructuring

Resick and Schnicke (1992) evaluated a group version of CPT with 19 rape victims and compared it with a wait-list control group. They reported a 40% reduction in PTSD symptoms in the CPT group, as compared with 1.5% for the wait-list controls. These results are encouraging, although interpretation is hampered by the absence of a credible control treatment. Two recent studies with mixed PTSD samples have addressed this issue by investigating both cognitive therapy and exposure. Marks et al. (1998) compared four treatment approaches: (1) imaginal and in vivo exposure, (2) cognitive restructuring, (3) a combination of exposure and cognitive restructuring, and (4) relaxation. Exposure, cognitive restructuring, and the combination group all produced global improvements, but no significant difference in efficacy was apparent between the groups. Importantly, however, observation of the means reveals that a larger percentage improvement was obtained for the exposure conditions (74% to 81%) than for the cognitive restructuring condition (53%). All three were more effective than relaxation. Similar results were obtained in a comparison of cognitive therapy (adapted from Resick and Schnicke's (1992) model) with imaginal exposure (Tarrier et al., 1999). They found that both treatments were superior to a baseline monitoring period, with improvements of between 27% and 35%, but, again, they found no differences between groups.

Other treatment approaches

Several other nondrug treatments have been proposed for the treatment of PTSD. Regrettably, few of those have an adequate theoretical basis and even fewer have been the subject of controlled clinical research. An exception to the former may be brief psychodynamic approaches and an exception to the latter may be eye movement desensitization and reprocessing (EMDR). Both of those approaches will be discussed briefly. A vast array of other techniques has been proposed, many as "one-session" cures for PTSD. In the absence of either a strong theoretical basis or objective empirical support, most of these do not justify attention in this review. Nevertheless, it remains a possibility that some will prove to be useful interventions and controlled clinical trials are clearly required.

Several clinicians have advocated the use of brief psychodynamic approaches in the treatment of PTSD, although, to date, only one controlled study has appeared in the literature (Brom et al., 1989). That study compared brief psychodynamic therapy with hypnosis, desensitization, and a wait-list control. All active treatments yielded some improvement. Although the authors reported no significant differences across treatment type, Foa and Meadows (1997) noted that inspection of the mean data suggest that psychodynamic approaches were inferior to desensitization (29% as compared with 41% reduction from pre- to posttreatment). While psychodynamic treatment will, no doubt, continue to be widely used in clinical practice, there are insufficient empirical data available at present to evaluate the efficacy of this approach in the treatment of PTSD.

EMDR (Shapiro, 1995) has been the focus of considerable controversy for several reasons, not least of which are the remarkable claims for its efficacy and the fact that it lacks a strong theoretical basis. At first glance, the technique appears to incorporate components of several other approaches, including exposure and cognitive restructuring (albeit presented very briefly). Those components are accompanied by rapid eye movements, which are thought to facilitate processing of the traumatic memories. Although only case studies appeared in the literature over the first few years following the original publication of EMDR, there have since been several controlled studies. A comprehensive review of that research is beyond the scope of this chapter and has been adequately covered elsewhere (McNally, 1999). In summary, the findings are mixed. Several studies have failed to find any objective evidence of improvement in PTSD symptoms following EMDR. Although a number of studies have reported improvement, many of these suffer from methodological flaws rendering the results hard to interpret. However, the only study to compare EMDR with CBT found that the latter (incorporating anxiety management, exposure, and cognitive restructuring) was more effective than EMDR in reducing PTSD pathology at posttreatment, and that this superiority became more evident by 3 month follow-up (Devilly and Spence, 1999). Interestingly, three controlled studies (Renfrey and Spates, 1994; Pitman et al., 1996; Devilly et al., 1998) have suggested that the eye movements themselves may be irrelevant to the efficacy of the procedure. In summary, while the technique shows some promise, further research is required. In the meantime, the continued use of EMDR as one part of a broad clinical approach is probably justifiable. Its use in isolation for the treatment of PTSD cannot be justified on the available data.

Drug treatments

Since several useful reviews of pharmacological interventions in PTSD exist (e.g., Friedman, 1997; Yehuda et al., 1998), this section will attempt to provide only a broad overview of the area. Drug treatments may serve several functions in the treatment of PTSD. First, since confronting the trauma as part of treatment is inevitably distressing, medication may serve as an adjunct to psychological interventions. Drugs may serve to moderate the arousal and distress, allowing the patient to tolerate the difficult process of modifying, and coming to terms with, the traumatic memories. Second, drugs may be used to treat comorbid conditions, such as depression, that may interfere with treatment of the core PTSD symptoms. Finally, pharmacotherapy may be viewed as directly relieving the primary PTSD symptoms, a position that has strengthened with the increasing recognition of biological alterations in PTSD. This, however, remains a goal for the future. To date, no drug has been developed specifically for PTSD and, instead, drugs developed for depression and anxiety have been tested with varying degrees of success.

The new generation of antidepressants, selective serotonin reuptake inhibitors (SSRIs), have emerged recently as the first choice of drug treatments for PTSD. This is despite the fact that few randomized clinical trials have been published to date (van der Kolk et al., 1994; Connor et al., 1999). Those studies reported improvement in civilian samples, but van der Kolk et al. (1994) found that fluoxetine was no better than placebo in treating veterans with combat-related

PTSD. Several open trials have suggested that SSRIs produce marked reductions in overall PTSD symptomatology. In particular, the apparent capacity of SSRIs to reduce the emotionally numbing symptoms of PTSD has provoked much interest, since other drugs have failed to moderate this aspect of the disorder. The SSRIs remain promising medications in the treatment of PTSD, partly because of their purported ability to target the whole syndrome and partly because of the relatively low side-effects profile. Drugs such as trazadone and nefazadone, which are serotonergic antidepressants with both SSRI and 5-hydroxytryptamine type 2 receptor blockade properties, also have potential. Although these are yet to be tested in adequately controlled trials, multisite trials of nefazadone are currently in progress.

Of the older antidepressants, the monoamine oxidase inhibitors (MAOIs) have produced improvements in two out of three randomized trials, particularly with reference to the re-experiencing symptoms. In practice, however, clinicians are reluctant to prescribe these agents because of concerns about the dietary restrictions. The newer breed of MAOIs such as moclobemide, known as reversible inhibitors of monoamine oxidase type A (RIMAs), do not have these problems but have yet to be tested in PTSD. Three randomized trials have investigated tricyclic antidepressants in PTSD, along with numerous open trials and case reports. The results have been mixed and generally moderate in magnitude. With the advent of SSRIs, the tricyclics are no longer a first-line drug in PTSD treatment.

Anxiolytic drugs, particularly the benzodiazepines, have been prescribed widely for PTSD in some clinical settings. While they may produce modest reductions in generalized anxiety, evidence from both randomized and open trials suggests that they are no better than placebo in reducing core PTSD symptoms. Indeed, there is some evidence that they may impede recovery when used in the first few weeks following the trauma (Gelpin et al., 1996). On the other hand, antiadrenergic agents such as clonidine and propranolol may be helpful. Although no randomized trials exist as yet, several open trials suggest improvement in hyperarousal and intrusion symptoms (Yehuda et al., 1998). Further, clonidine has been proposed as a useful intervention in the very acute stages of traumatic stress such as combat stress reaction (Friedman et al., 1993).

Several other classes of medication have been used in the treatment of PTSD, although none has been adequately evaluated at this stage. Open trials of anticonvulsant agents, such as carbamazepine and valproate, have suggested some role for this class of medication in PTSD, particularly with reference to the arousal symptom cluster. Although antipsychotic drugs were used in the past, the advent of more appropriate medications has rendered this class of medication less useful in PTSD, except in cases presenting with frank psychotic symptoms. While suggestions that the endogenous opioid system is dysregulated in PTSD have led to an interest in the use of opioid antagonists, there is little evidence of their efficacy (Yehuda et al., 1998).

In summary, surprisingly few randomized controlled trials have been conducted in the area of drug treatments for PTSD. None have adequately addressed the issue of cessation of medication, although it is reasonable to assume that, if nothing else has changed, relapse would be likely. At this stage, there is little to support pharmacological interventions as an effective "cure" for PTSD. Given the nature and etiology of the disorder, that is, perhaps, hardly surprising. Even the most ardent proponents of pharmacology would recognize the importance of combining drug treatments with psychological interventions. Equally, there is no doubt that considerable efforts will be devoted in the coming years to the search for a PTSD-specific drug.

Prevention and early intervention

PTSD, it would seem, is potentially an ideal candidate for early intervention and prevention, since it is possible to accurately identify the precipitating event. In recent years, there has been considerable debate regarding the extent to which it may be possible to modify the course of traumatic stress reactions, and to facilitate recovery, by means of an early intervention. A whole culture and industry has built up around the assumption that early interventions following trauma are effective.

Primary prevention

Primary prevention aims to reduce the incidence of new cases through intervention before the disorder occurs. These interventions are provided to the whole of the affected population, with no attempt to identify high-risk survivors (although that may be an important outcome of the process). Much debate has revolved around the area of psychological debriefing as described by Mitchell and Bray (1990). As noted by several authors (Kenardy et al., 1996; Rose and Bisson, 1998), there is a paucity of adequate empirical evidence to support the use of brief early interventions, such as debriefing, following trauma. That is not to say that debriefing is not helpful – the methodological problems inherent in the available research simply do not permit firm conclusions to be drawn either way. There is an urgent need for rigorous evaluation of debriefing strategies to answer not only the obvious questions regarding the efficacy of debriefing, but also a range of other very basic questions about which, at present, there is little consensus. What exactly is debriefing? What are the goals? To whom is it suited – which populations and following which types of incident? When should it be provided? Who should provide it? And, perhaps most importantly, can debriefing be harmful? A comprehensive discussion of this debate is beyond the scope of this chapter. Suffice to say that it places mental health professionals in a difficult position in the immediate aftermath of trauma. It is not reasonable to abrogate all responsibility simply because solid empirical data are not yet available; rather, it is incumbent upon health professionals to provide some kind of psychological first aid to survivors of recent trauma. In doing so, it may be necessary to develop general principles by drawing upon our knowledge of preventive strategies in other mental health areas, as well as on our knowledge of effective treatments for PTSD. A discussion of some of those principles appears in Chapter 26.

As a general guide, however, it is important to distinguish between those events that occur within an organizational context and within the expected range of experience (e.g., in the emergency services) from those unpredictable events that are clearly beyond normal expectations (e.g., random acts of extreme violence in the community). The predictable nature of the former, combined with the ongoing structure and support provided by the organization, may render standard interventions such as Critical Incident Stress Management and debriefing as appropriate. However, when working with those populations for whom the only (or main) thing they have in common is their experience of the trauma, it may be preferable not to adopt a CISM or debriefing model. Rather, the focus may be limited to the provision of information and support, with clear guidelines of when and how to obtain professional assistance. This may help to promote expectations of recovery and the use of existing coping strategies and support mechanisms. In the final analysis, however, the field of primary prevention following trauma is characterized, at this stage, by educated guesswork rather than solid empirical data.

Secondary prevention and the treatment of acute stress disorder

Secondary prevention aims to reduce the prevalence of disorders through early identification of problems, with intervention before the disorder becomes severe. Thus the next question is whether it is possible to intervene early, and prevent long-term problems such as PTSD in survivors identified as high risk as a result of their acute response. In this area of prevention, the data are a little more positive. Foa and her colleagues (1995a) investigated the efficacy of a brief prevention program aimed at arresting the development of chronic pathology in assault victims with acute PTSD. (That is to say, participants met all criteria for PTSD except for the duration requirement.) Participants in the active condition received four sessions of cognitive behavioral treatment within a few weeks of the assault and were compared with a wait-list control group. The intervention included education about common reactions to assault, anxiety management, in vivo and imaginal exposure, and cognitive restructuring. Two months postassault, participants who received the active condition had significantly less severe PTSD symptoms than participants in the control condition; 10% of the former group met criteria for PTSD versus 70% of the latter group. Five and a half months postassault, victims in the active condition were significantly less depressed, and had significantly less severe re-experiencing symptoms, than victims in the control condition. Interestingly, the rate of PTSD in the wait-list condition had dropped to 20% by follow-up, providing further evidence of the trend towards recovery over the first 6 months posttrauma, even in the absence of formal treatment.

The advent of ASD as a diagnostic category has provided the opportunity to determine whether specific interventions may prevent the progression from ASD to PTSD. Although only one controlled trial is available at this time, many more are likely to appear in the literature over the coming months. Bryant and colleagues (1998) investigated survivors of civilian trauma with a diagnosis of ASD, comparing a cognitive behavioral therapy (CBT) intervention (similar to that of Foa et al.'s study) with supportive counseling (SC). Only 8% of patients in the CBT group met criteria for PTSD at posttreatment, as compared with 83% in the SC condition. At 6-month follow-up, the figures were 17% and 67%, respectively, with the CBT group showing significantly greater reductions in intrusive, avoidance, and depressive symptomatology. In a subsequent extension of that study, Bryant and colleagues (1999) found that prolonged exposure, as well as a combination of prolonged exposure and anxiety management, were both superior to supportive counseling. Interestingly, the combination treatment was not superior, suggesting that exposure may be the most critical component.

In summary, there is now sufficient evidence to suggest that it is worth targeting symptomatic survivors in the immediate aftermath of trauma with the provision of specific interventions. Such treatment can be expected to significantly reduce the subsequent prevalence of more serious and chronic pathology such as PTSD.

Conclusions

The controlled outcome studies quoted above, at first sight, provide impressive support for various approaches to the treatment of chronic PTSD. However, it is important to be cautious in our optimism. The treatment of chronic PTSD (i.e., of more than 3 months duration) has yet to achieve the levels of efficacy obtainable in the treatment of most other anxiety disorders. As a rule of thumb, around one-third of patients with chronic PTSD do very well following treatment. Another third do reasonably well – although they will probably not meet criteria for a formal diagnosis of PTSD at posttreatment, many problems remain and impairment of psychosocial functioning continues. The final one-third of patients fail to respond in any significant way to treatment. The elucidation of those factors that will predict response to treatment, as well as which treatment modality is suited to which patients, is a major challenge for the field.

26

Posttraumatic stress disorder

Clinician Guide

PTSD is a complex disorder requiring a multistaged intervention. The core components of treatment – psychoeducation, anxiety management, exposure, and cognitive restructuring – overlap with interventions used in the treatment of many other anxiety disorders. The purpose of this chapter is to discuss the application of those strategies to the specific challenges of PTSD, as well as to highlight some contextual treatment issues. Although the field of acute stress disorder (ASD) is in its infancy, preliminary research indicates that the same treatment protocols are applicable to both disorders. Under most circumstances, however, it would be expected that the treatment of ASD would be simpler, and would proceed at a faster rate, than treatment of more chronic PTSD presentations.

The bulk of this chapter addresses the treatment of PTSD as a disorder in itself. In acute presentations, and in people with good pretrauma functioning and intact support networks, such approaches may be all that is required. In most cases, however, by the time the person seeks treatment, the PTSD has become embedded in a range of comorbid conditions and psychosocial dysfunction. This chapter will begin by addressing some of the issues associated with more complex cases before discussing the primary treatment components in detail.

Assessment issues

A detailed discussion of assessment strategies for PTSD was provided in Chapter 24. The purpose of this section is to elucidate some additional factors to be considered when assessing for treatment purposes. A thorough assessment of the patient's history, current psychosocial functioning, and diagnosis is required before an adequate formulation of the case can be made and a management plan developed. A detailed discussion of psychiatric interviewing is beyond the scope of this chapter and only those issues particularly relevant to survivors of trauma will be discussed in this section. Key issues to look for in the history include previous episodes of psychiatric disorder (or simply "bad nerves"), as well as prior treatment experience and pretrauma coping strategies. Identification of these factors will assist in the formulation of realistic treatment goals and selection of intervention strategies with an improved chance of success. It is important also to take a history of prior traumatic experiences. Clearly, this latter area may be highly sensitive and relevant information may not necessarily emerge in the first session. While the utmost care must be taken not to assume the existence of prior trauma on the basis of symptom profile or treatment response, the clinician is nevertheless advised to keep the possibility in mind. Clinical experience suggests that it is not unusual for current presentations to be exacerbated by activation of prior traumatic memory networks, even if the patient does not necessarily make the connection.

The patient's current social context – their "recovery environment" – may impact upon the efficacy of treatment. Thus assessment should include evaluation of support networks and close interpersonal relationships, and should attempt to gauge the attitude of significant others to the person's traumatic experience and psychological response. Social support and validation of the experience by significant others appear to facilitate effective recovery. Active involvement of spouses and partners (with the patient's approval) in both assessment and treatment phases is strongly encouraged. Where social support is obviously lacking, it may be worth attempting to address this issue by means of a skills-development, problem-solving approach in the initial stages of treatment. Evaluation of occupational functioning is important also. Clinical experience suggests that the structure provided by daily routines is important in restoring a sense of control. Equally, an overcommitment to work is often used by PTSD sufferers as an avoidance strategy – keeping busy every minute of the day helps to prevent the memories from returning. Although this, like many avoidance behaviors, may be an effective strategy for some people some of the time, it precludes the possibility of confronting and modifying the traumatic memories and will interfere with longer-term recovery.

Since PTSD is routinely associated with comorbidity, a thorough assessment of other conditions, particularly substance abuse, depression, and other anxiety disorders, is essential in planning an effective intervention strategy. The next section discusses the implications of chronicity and comorbidity for treatment.

Chronicity and comorbidity

Common sense and clinical experience suggest that chronic forms of the disorder will be more difficult to treat than acute presentations. The former are more likely to be associated with secondary comorbidity and other psychosocial sequelae of living with the condition over a long period. There is a world of difference between treating an assault victim with a "clean" PTSD diagnosis a few weeks posttrauma and treating a Vietnam veteran with a 30-year history of the disorder, several failed marriages, an unstable employment history, substance abuse, anger problems, and a pension claim currently pending. It is beyond the scope of this chapter to discuss all the issues associated with the latter example. Suffice to say that issues of good clinical management become of paramount importance. Change will be slow and effective case management is essential. Psychosocial issues other than core PTSD symptoms will need to be addressed, including relationships, occupational functioning, and social reintegration.

The appropriate management of comorbid conditions is, more often than not, an important factor in the treatment of PTSD. The two most common Axis I conditions associated with chronic PTSD are substance abuse and depression. Each of these will be dealt with briefly, although it must be stated at the outset that empirical data on the treatment of comorbid conditions in PTSD are lacking and decisions often need to be based on informed clinical judgment.

Substance abuse

Substance abuse, particularly in the form of alcohol, is a common complication in survivors of trauma. Regular alcohol use, notwithstanding its obvious drawbacks, can be an effective way for PTSD patients to manage the intrusion and arousal symptoms. As such, it is best conceptualized as part of the avoidance and emotional numbing component of the disorder. Care must be taken when asking people to give up this crutch without providing alternative coping strategies. This raises one of the more difficult clinical decisions in the treatment of PTSD: should the substance abuse be treated first, aiming for a period of sobriety prior to addressing the PTSD, or should the two disorders be treated concurrently? There is no easy answer. One argument proposes that the primary reason the person is abusing alcohol is to manage the PTSD symptoms and, thus, amelioration of those symptoms must occur before (or concomitant with) attempting to reduce the substance abuse. The alternative argument proposes that effective processing and modification of the traumatic memories is not possible while the person continues to abuse alcohol or other drugs. Some clinicians believe that the decision can be made on the basis of history: if the person was abusing substances prior to the trauma (even if the abuse has significantly worsened since), then the behavior is not fundamentally trauma related and should be treated separately and prior to the PTSD. If the abuse only commenced following the trauma, it should be treated in conjunction with the traumatic stress.

In the final analysis, it will be a clinical decision based on a range of factors. There is no doubt that sobriety is preferable and that, at the very least, the substance abuse must be under control prior to PTSD treatment. The severity of the abuse is an important consideration and the person must be able to attend treatment without being under the influence of drugs. As a guide, we suggest that the early stages of treatment (as discussed below) can, and should, proceed in conjunction with treatment for the substance abuse, since they are likely to facilitate change in that area. It is doubtful that the more intensive stages of exposure and cognitive restructuring will be effective in the context of ongoing substance abuse.

Depression

The second common comorbid condition in PTSD is depression, again raising the difficult question of which disorder to treat first. As with substance abuse, an evaluation of whether the depression is secondary to the PTSD or a primary disorder in itself may facilitate decision making, although, of course, this is not a clear dichotomy. The severity of the depression will be an important factor also. Milder forms of the disorder are more likely to resolve with improvements in other areas and are less likely to interfere with PTSD treatment. As in the treatment of other anxiety disorders, however, more severe depression is likely to impact negatively on the treatment process and outcome.

Thus, when moderate to severe depression is diagnosed, it is recommended that attention be paid to that disorder prior to addressing the PTSD symptoms. Psychological or pharmacological interventions may be useful. Both of these may have additional advantages in providing some amelioration of core PTSD symptoms, which may, in turn, facilitate subsequent psychological interventions directed at the traumatic memories.

Impediments in treatment

There are many potential impediments to the treatment of PTSD, several of which (such as comorbid conditions and poor rapport or client motivation) are common to any psychological intervention. A few, however, are particularly relevant to PTSD and are worthy of consideration if treatment does not seem to be progressing as expected.

The issue of secondary gain, particularly in the form of monetary compensation, can be a complicating factor in recovery from trauma. There is no clear or automatic relationship – many people who fail to show a good recovery are not seeking compensation, and many who are awaiting the outcome of a claim are still able to benefit considerably from treatment. Nevertheless, in an ideal world, it would be wise to ensure that all compensation claims are resolved prior to commencing treatment. In the real world that is not possible and often the best that can be done is to raise the issue openly and to discuss the implications with the patient. Through this process of open discussion, the clinician may be able to gauge the extent to which the patient feels a need to retain a symptom profile for the purposes of compensation. This, in turn, may influence the goals and type of treatment provided. It may be possible also to convince the patient that a good psychological recovery will, in the long term, contribute more to their happiness and well-being than any compensation payout. Finally, it is advisable for the treating clinician not to provide assessment reports for compensation or other psycho-legal purposes. This is obviously a difficult issue, with the clinician in this situation often arguing that he or she knows the patient best and is therefore in the optimum position to provide such a report. However, the conflict in roles is unavoidable and the blurring of boundaries has the potential to impact negatively on both the treatment and assessment roles. It may be better to explain the situation openly to the patient at the outset, offering instead to refer on to a trusted colleague for the assessment reports.

Reference has already been made to the issue of prior trauma. It is important to reiterate that assumptions by clinicians about the existence of prior trauma, and subsequent attempts to "unearth" previously inaccessible memories, are both unethical and dangerous. Guidelines regarding such procedures are available from most professional organisations. Equally, to ignore the possibility of prior trauma as an influence on current functioning is almost negligent. Thus the clinician must walk a fine line between, on the one hand, encouraging the client to (perhaps unconsciously) generate false memories and, on the other, providing a safe environment in which genuine traumatic experiences can be revealed. Nondirective questions, such as "have you had other experiences in your past that were very frightening or distressing?" or "Have there been times in your life when you've felt like this before?" can be useful in accessing important information. If therapy targeted at the most recent trauma is progressing well, this is unlikely to be an issue. However, if the patient is not progressing as expected, one hypothesis may be the existence of prior traumatic experiences. Revelations of prior trauma provide the clinician with an opportunity to make links between those experiences and the more recent events, with the possibility of treating the earlier traumatic memories more directly if appropriate. It is not unusual, particularly in patients who habitually deal with stress by avoidance and denial (e.g., not uncommon in emergency workers) for the opportunity to make those links to be a turning point in treatment.

Although the issue of guilt will be discussed further below, it warrants separate attention at this stage, since clinical experience suggests that it often interferes with treatment. By definition, those things about which survivors feel most guilty are those that they are most reluctant to acknowledge and admit to another person. This is particularly a problem with veteran populations, since many acts committed in the context of war are unacceptable when viewed later from a civilian

Table 26.1 Stages in the psychological treatment of PTSD

1. Stabilization and engagement
2. Psychoeducation
3. Anxiety management
4. Exposure to the traumatic memories
5. Cognitive restructuring
6. Relapse prevention and maintenance

perspective. As with prior trauma, issues of guilt will often emerge quite naturally during treatment and can be dealt with by normal therapeutic processes. In some cases, however, guilt feelings may be particularly strong and may not be acknowledged even in response to direct questioning. A failure to progress in treatment may prompt the clinician to hypothesize about the existence of unresolved guilt and to gently probe the patient with appropriate questions. Again, clinical experience suggests that an opportunity to acknowledge the guilt, often for the first time, and to re-evaluate those self-appraisals in the context of therapy may be a turning point in treatment.

Treatment process

The major stages of treatment are shown in Table 26.1. As a general guideline, the interventions are presented in the order in which they appear in the table, although we recommend that attempts be made to integrate the exposure and cognitive restructuring components. It is recommended that all treatment sessions be taped so that clients have an opportunity to review and consolidate the information. As noted below, exposure components will be taped separately and therefore we recommend the use of two tapes for each client, one being reserved exclusively for the exposure.

Stabilization and engagement

Individuals with PTSD and related conditions often present for treatment in crisis, particularly in the acute aftermath of trauma. Keane (1995) has noted the importance of some kind of stabilization phase prior to the commencement of a formal intervention directed specifically at the PTSD. If the person is, for example, actively suicidal, in the midst of a major psychosocial crisis, or requires practical assistance with concerns such as personal safety, those issues should be addressed as a matter of priority before embarking on treatment. Survivors will not be in a position to devote resources to their own recovery if there has been a failure to adequately recognize and address those more practical concerns.

Engagement in treatment is often a significant problem in PTSD, particularly in its more chronic forms. First, individuals with PTSD may be unwilling to acknowledge that they have a problem as a result of their traumatic experiences, seeing it as a sign of weakness. They may continue to blame other factors or people (including loved ones) for their difficulties and may continue to use a variety of maladaptive strategies to deal with the unpleasant symptoms. Second, even if they acknowledge the problem, they may be reluctant to seek treatment. This may be through fear of ridicule or a belief that no-one could understand or help. It may also, of course, be a function of the symptom picture of PTSD, characterized as it is by avoidance and a fear of confronting the traumatic experience. Third, even if PTSD sufferers make it into treatment, they may have difficulty forming a therapeutic relationship based on trust and mutual respect that will allow them to reveal their vulnerabilities and to discuss the highly emotive issues associated with the trauma. Spending adequate time in the development of rapport and a strong relationship is therefore usually essential in the treatment of PTSD. The advantage of the following treatment model is that the early stages, such as psychoeducation and symptom management, are relatively unthreatening and provide opportunities for the clinician to demonstrate their knowledge, credibility, and nonjudgmental approach to the client. Thus the therapeutic relationship is able to develop while still covering important ground.

Psychoeducation

Psychoeducation in traumatic stress is an important first step in treatment. It can do much to reduce the secondary distress (about the symptoms) and to enhance the credibility of the therapist and the collaborative nature of the relationship. The sudden onset of symptoms following trauma can be extremely frightening, especially for someone with no prior psychiatric history. The person may believe that they are going crazy and will never recover. A poor understanding of personal reactions may prompt denial, avoidance, and withdrawal, often with associated substance abuse, which may serve to impede recovery. On the other hand, a good understanding of traumatic stress reactions is the first step in cementing the therapeutic relationship, managing symptoms effectively, and working on the recovery process.

The content of this phase would normally include common responses to trauma, much as outlined in the accompanying Patient Treatment Manual. Care should be taken not to minimize these reactions and the commonly used phrase "normal reactions in a normal person to an abnormal event" is not always appropriate. If patients have developed PTSD, their reaction is not (statistically) normal. Even if they do not have the full disorder, their reaction is far from normal in terms of their own experience and the phrase may sound dismissive of the level of distress being experienced. The concept, however, is important and other phrases may be useful (such as "although the problems you've told me about are very unpleasant for you, they are part of a common human response to life threatening events and they will diminish"). Written handouts are very useful to accompany the therapist's words, providing concrete validation for the survivors' personal experiences and reinforcing that their response is not unique. A good rationale for the proposed treatment is vital also: treatment will be difficult and the client needs to know what is going to happen and why.

Symptom management

Most clients presenting with PTSD or other traumatic stress disorders are feeling frightened, vulnerable, and out of control. While the psychoeducation will have helped them to understand what is happening to them, they now need strategies to manage the symptoms in order to regain a feeling of control. A detailed description of the range of possible strategies is beyond the scope of this section and clinicians are referred to other chapters in this book (e.g., Chapters 7, 15 and 23) for excellent descriptions of some key anxiety management interventions. Nevertheless, the following provides a summary under the broad headings of physiological, cognitive, and behavioral strategies as they apply to the treatment of traumatic stress.

It is important not to overwhelm the patient with too many strategies, but rather to think about which will work best for each particular case. Then, if it is worth teaching, it is worth teaching properly. Provide a rationale for, and a description of, the strategy, before modeling and practicing it in the session. Discuss any problems or misunderstandings as they arise and adjust as necessary. It is then vital to emphasize the importance of practicing the skill (often several times a day) in nonstressful environments before attempting to use it to control anxiety in a difficult (particularly trauma-related) situation. It is better to teach and consolidate a few skills well than to provide a plethora of strategies that are poorly understood and unlikely to be effective.

A first step is often to introduce the concept of SUDs – subjective units of distress. (A copy of this scale appears in the Patient Treatment Manual.) This is a "fear thermometer" that clients use to rate their current level of anxiety or distress on a scale of 0 ("perfectly relaxed and calm") to 100 ("the worst imaginable anxiety or distress"). This is important in helping the person to self-monitor the effects of the anxiety-management interventions, providing a more objective measure of their efficacy. It will also be a vital component of the subsequent exposure treatment. Introducing it at this stage has the added benefit of providing the patient with plenty of opportunities to practice rating his or her own anxiety before being asked to do so in the more difficult phase of exposure.

Physiological arousal is a key feature of traumatic stress and any strategy that assists in reducing arousal is likely to be beneficial. This may be particularly important in the acute stages posttrauma – clinical experience suggests that effective arousal management in the first few hours or days may facilitate subsequent recovery. Physically orientated strategies are appealing not only for their efficacy in producing rapid results, but also because they are easy, nonthreatening (and nonpsychological) interventions to use while the patient is still feeling very vulnerable. A first option adopted by many therapists is that of breathing control, an area well covered in several other chapters in this book, as well as in the Patient Treatment Manual (Chapter 27). Progressive muscle and isometric relaxation strategies, also covered well elsewhere in this book, are often useful. Other suggestions involve dietary advice, including the reduction of stimulants such as caffeine and nicotine, as well as aerobic exercise.

Cognitive strategies are usually designed to give the patient some control over the intrusive cognitions, but care must be taken not to give contradictory messages. It should be emphasized that thinking about the trauma is not a bad thing to do – on the contrary, it will be a central component of treatment further down the track. However, it is important to do this in a controlled manner for limited times during the day. If the thoughts are intruding constantly, they simply result in high distress and the person may feel unable to focus on anything else. Thus these strategies will help to limit the time spent thinking about the trauma in order to reduce distress and facilitate a return to more normal functioning. Distraction techniques are commonly used – anything from counting backwards from 100 in 7s to asking patients to describe their current surroundings in great detail. Again, see the Patient Treatment Manual for more information on such strategies. Many people with PTSD are good at imaging. However, if imaginal techniques are to be used for arousal reduction in PTSD, it is essential that the patient, not the therapist, describes the scene, since there is too much danger of unwittingly introducing potentially traumatic elements into the scenario. Some people find imagining a safe place, and describing it in great detail, to be a useful technique that provides not only a distraction from the painful memories but also a sense of security.

Behaviorally orientated techniques usually revolve around scheduling activities and providing structure to the person's day. It is often a good idea to encourage people to resume a normal routine as quickly as reasonably possible following a trauma, although they should be reminded to take it easy and not throw themselves into work as a way of avoiding the unpleasant memories. Scheduling pleasant activities is often important, since the core symptoms of PTSD are likely to produce anhedonia and loss of interest. It is particularly important to recommend that the person makes an effort to undertake activities with other family members. This helps to reduce the social withdrawal and isolation that can place an enormous strain on relationships.

Although the bulk of this section has referred to anxiety management, since that is a fundamental part of treatment for all traumatic stress reactions, more chronic presentations may require symptom management for other problems. Anger is often a primary presenting problem in chronic PTSD (especially in veterans). The consuming and explosive nature of anger, and its impact on social networks, often necessitates direct intervention prior to addressing core PTSD symptoms. Similarly, depression that does not ameliorate over the first few sessions will impact negatively on subsequent treatment and should be addressed. Empirically validated behavioral strategies may be used to address other areas of difficulty such as sleep disturbance, substance abuse, and assertion (see e.g., the Social phobia: Patient Treatment Manual, Chapter 11).

The purpose of the symptom-management component of treatment for PTSD is to help the person to develop some control over the distressing symptoms in the early stages of treatment. The strategies are generally simple and relatively quick to teach and to learn. It is recommended, therefore, that one or two interventions from each of the physical, cognitive, and behavioral domains be provided to the patient over the first few weeks. It is important that some progress is made in symptom management before moving on to the most important aspect of treatment, exposure to the traumatic memories.

Exposure: background issues

While the strategies described above will provide some symptomatic relief, the painful process of exposure to the traumatic memories is thought to be essential for modification of the traumatic memory network and longer-term recovery from trauma. Before discussing the process of exposure treatment in PTSD, it is worth remembering some of the key guidelines for successful exposure treatment and considering their application to PTSD. In particular, exposure should ideally be in vivo, graded, prolonged, repeated, and functional.

First, in vivo exposure is generally considered to be more effective than imaginal exposure. When treating a spider phobic, for example, it is more therapeutic to confront real spiders than to simply imagine them. In PTSD, however, it is neither possible nor desirable to relive the traumatic event. This does not preclude the possibility of in vivo exposure tasks. On the contrary, it is routine practice to generate, with the patient, a hierarchy of feared situations and activities to be confronted one at a time. The feared stimulus in PTSD, however, is actually the traumatic memory and most of the exposure work will be imaginal. The bulk of the following discussion refers to imaginal exposure.

Second, exposure should be conducted in a graded manner by developing a hierarchy of progressively more feared situations and gradually confronting each one in turn. Thus the person is not asked to face the most feared stimulus until he or she is ready to do so. When conducting in vivo exposure, this is often relatively straightforward – a list of feared situations or activities is generated and they are rank ordered in the hierarchy. It is also possible when conducting imaginal exposure with multiply traumatized individuals, such as emergency services workers. Each event can be rated for severity and the imaginal exposure can proceed accordingly. While grading imaginal exposure in the case of single traumas (or each individual incident in the case of multiple traumas) is more problematic, there are several strategies that may be adopted to titrate the exposure. These techniques should be used only if necessary – if the patient can tolerate the anxiety, it is best to move to the most vivid images and the worst details of the trauma as quickly as possible. However, if appropriate, clients may be allowed to skip over the most difficult aspects of the event on initial presentations, but not in later sessions. They may be encouraged to keep their eyes open during initial sessions, but to close them during later exposures, since closing the eyes significantly increases the vividness of the imagery. They may be asked to use the past tense when recounting the event in early sessions (e.g., "I saw him coming towards me"), but to use the present tense in later sessions ("I can see him coming towards me"). Some therapists use techniques such as watching the event from afar, or viewing it on a television screen, in the early sessions. Manipulation of these strategies assists the clinician in grading the level of exposure, even when working imaginally with a single event, and helps to maintain distress and anxiety at levels that are sufficiently high to be optimally therapeutic, yet sufficiently low to be manageable. Equally, it needs to be remembered that this is not always possible in PTSD – activation of one part of the traumatic network is often enough to access the whole memory – and the therapist needs to be prepared for extreme levels of arousal despite the best planning. Either way, before treatment eventually terminates, the person must have been exposed repeatedly to the full details of the memory, in the present tense, with eyes shut, for a sufficiently prolonged period to allow the anxiety to reduce.

The third rule of effective exposure treatment is often handled poorly by novice therapists: each session should be prolonged, continuing until the anxiety has reduced by at least half. It should be remembered that anxiety levels often rise during exposure before they start to drop. Premature termination of exposure while the anxiety is still high runs the risk of incubating, or worsening, the anxiety response. (Indeed, this is what happens in chronic, untreated PTSD. The memories return frequently, but are blocked out again as quickly as possible before the therapeutic effect takes place.) In clinical practice, it is not always possible in PTSD to prolong the session long enough for the anxiety to reduce by half. At the very least, however, a significant reduction must take place before the session is terminated, even if this means prolonging the session longer than usual.

Fourth, each item on the hierarchy needs to be repeated as often as is necessary for it to evoke only minimal anxiety. This repetition may occur within a single session, within multiple sessions, or between sessions as discussed below. Finally, exposure needs to be functional, which means that the affective components of the memory must be accessed along with the stimulus material. Individuals with PTSD become adept at telling their story in a detached, unemotional manner, accessing only part of the traumatic memory network. This process is not likely to be therapeutic. However, a few probing questions are usually sufficient to access the accompanying affect, allowing habituation to occur.

Exposure: the process

An excellent description of the process of exposure in PTSD was provided by Foa and Rothbaum (1998) and readers are referred to that text for a more detailed discussion. Briefly, however, the process is conducted in the following steps. First, a rationale for exposure is provided to the client, including an explanation of habituation. Several examples of possible rationales appear in the Patient Treatment Manual. Second, the patient is reminded of the concept of SUDs as discussed above. Third, a hierarchy of feared situations and activities is constructed – this can comprise anything that the person has tended to avoid since the trauma. In the case of multiple or complex traumas it is often useful to generate two separate lists, one comprising potential targets for in vivo exposure and the other comprising a list of traumatic events for imaginal exposure. Each item on the hierarchy is rated using the SUD Scale to estimate the predicted fear associated with confronting that situation, activity, or memory. Fourth, the therapist works with the client to generate specific in vivo homework assignments from the in vivo hierarchy. Specificity is important here: client and therapist should agree on exactly what will be done, where, how often, and so on. It is important to start with a relatively easy item, ensuring success on the first trial. Thus the patient is asked to begin with an item that is expected to invoke moderate levels of anxiety, with a SUDs of around 50, and to stay in that situation for 30 to 40 minutes or until the anxiety has reduced by half. On subsequent items, an expected SUDs of around 70 is probably optimal. The patient keeps detailed records of the beginning and end SUDs, as well as the timing and duration of each exposure exercise. The item is repeated until it evokes only minimal anxiety before the client moves on to the next item on the list. Each treatment session begins with a review of the in vivo exposure homework and the setting of targets for the next few days.

Imaginal exposure is conducted initially within the treatment session, beginning with a review of the rationale for the process. The prospect of reliving the trauma is likely to cause high anxiety and the patient may require considerable reassurance prior to commencing the imaginal exposure. Then the patient is asked to describe the experience in detail and to continue the description until the event is over and a point of safety is reached. Although Foa and Rothbaum (1998) suggested that the client be told to recount the trauma in the present tense with eyes closed on the first presentation, in routine clinical practice the therapist may decide to titrate the distress by allowing a past-tense narrative with eyes open. This provides an opportunity for an initial sense of mastery and gives the therapist important information about likely difficult points on subsequent exposures. Assuming the SUDs are manageable, however, a move to present tense with eyes closed is recommended as soon as possible. Similarly, the client may be allowed to skip over the worst aspects on earlier sessions. On later presentations, however, the therapist should use prompts with stimulus cues (e.g., "What does he smell like?" or "Describe her face") and response cues (e.g., "What are you feeling now?" or "What are you thinking now?") as appropriate. It is also useful to provide supportive comments throughout the process (e.g., "You're doing really well" or "I know it's difficult, but stay with that image for a while"). As the SUDs gradually reduce over repeated sessions, more attention is paid to the specific elements of the memory that are most distressing. Later sessions may focus primarily on repeated exposure to those most upsetting parts. It is important in these later sessions to maximize the cues in all sensory modalities (sights, sounds, smells, tastes, sensations). Elements of cognitive restructuring are also routinely incorporated into the imaginal exposure, as discussed below.

The client should be asked for a SUDs rating every 5 minutes throughout the exposure, which is recorded by the therapist and discussed at the end of the session. The therapist should not rely exclusively on SUDs reports but, rather, should observe the client closely for signs of distress or avoidance. If the anxiety has reduced appreciably, that should be reinforced. If not, it is important to reassure the client that it will reduce with persistent confrontation of the memory. Adequate time should be allocated at the end of the session to discuss the experience and to unwind. Some therapists provide a separate room for patients to recover in their own time before going home and may use a relaxation procedure at this point.

Repeated exposure to the traumatic memory is best achieved by taping the session and instructing the client to listen to the tape daily at home. Obviously, this component requires some clinical judgment and there may be occasions when the therapist decides that this may not be the best course of action. At the very least, it is important to provide clear structure and guidelines for this homework and to ensure that support is available should the experience prove too distressing. An example of appropriate guidelines for taped exposure homework is provided in the Patient Treatment Manual.

A final point to consider during the exposure process concerns the client's knowledge about the experience. Indeed, it has been suggested that a key to effective recovery from trauma is the ability to answer fundamental questions about what happened and why it happened (Figley, 1985). Therapists often assume that the survivor is clear about all the details – after all, they were there, surely they know what happened? In reality, many survivors of trauma have very confused and fragmented memories of the experience, with a poor understanding of exactly what happened, how it happened, and why it happened. Misunderstandings, and gaps in the memory, may make successful exposure treatment more difficult. Obviously, some of these questions will remain unanswerable and others will resolve as part of the exposure process. However, therapists should be constantly aware of opportunities to fill in gaps in the trauma memory in order to assist the client to "put the pieces of the jigsaw together" and make sense of the experience. Are there other people they can talk to, such as emergency services personnel or others present at the scene? Is there written information from media reports that they can read about the incident, or video footage to view, that would help make sense of what happened? Occasionally, the therapist is able to support and empower the client in accessing such information. The opportunity to find out more about what happened (and possibly why) can do a great deal to assist survivors in understanding, and coming to terms with, their experiences.

Exposure: potential problems

If the above procedure is adhered to in the context of a good therapeutic relationship, there are likely to be few problems encountered. Nevertheless, it can be a powerful experience for both therapist and client, with high levels of emotion associated with attention to the most distressing details of the experience. It is vital that therapists communicate confidence in their ability to cope, and to help the client cope, with whatever emerges during the session. As far as possible, it is best not to encourage the use of anxiety-management strategies during the process of exposure but, rather, to allow the anxiety to habituate of its own accord. However, clinicians should not be afraid to use arousal reduction techniques in sessions where insufficient habituation has taken place over a reasonable period (e.g., 60 minutes) or where it is clear that the level of distress has become intolerable for the client.

If problems occur, they are likely to be associated with some kind of avoidance behavior on the part of the client. Sometimes, this will constitute a form of dissociation characterized by detachment and a failure to engage. There is no doubt that avoidance, or a failure to access the memory network in its entirety (including stimulus, response, and interpretive components) will mitigate against successful exposure treatment. Reassurances of safety, and making the distinction between experiencing the trauma itself and reliving the memory, will often help to minimize avoidance. Foa and Rothbaum (1998) suggested that asking clients to recount the most difficult aspects using a "slow motion" strategy, with thoughts, feelings, and physical sensations slowed down, may help to maintain full engagement and minimize avoidance. An alternative form of dissociation is often mentioned in the context of exposure. This is opposite to the detached, disengaged form described above, characterized instead by an overinvolvement in the memory and a vivid flashback experience as if the event were recurring again. It is not possible to modify the traumatic memory network effectively, incorporating new information, while experiencing a flashback. The therapist should therefore make every effort to bring the client back into the "here and now" before proceeding with the exposure. Instructions to open their eyes, look around, feel the chair, describe the room, check date, time and place, and so on, are all useful in dealing with such dissociative episodes during exposure. Having said that, if the exposure is conducted carefully according to the guidelines described above, such dissociative flashback experiences should be a rare occurrence.

Contraindications for exposure are basically common sense. Timing is important: does the client feel sufficiently in control (having mastered some key symptom management strategies) and is rapport adequate? Acute life crises, current substance abuse, severe psychiatric comorbidity, and a history of noncompliance with treatment should all suggest caution in the use of exposure. While the possibility of iatrogenic effects with exposure, as with any other potent intervention, should not be ignored, the likelihood of adverse reactions can be minimized by sensible clinical practice.

Cognitive restructuring

Cognitive restructuring in PTSD is designed to assist the client in identifying dysfunctional thoughts and beliefs about the world, other people, or themselves that have developed from, or been strengthened by, the traumatic experience. There are many ways to go about the process of cognitive restructuring and good descriptions of its application in PTSD are provided elsewhere (Resick and Schnicke, 1993; Foa & Rothbaum, 1998).

Foa and Rothbaum (1998) identified five common themes of dysfunctional belief (and associated negative thoughts) that frequently occur following trauma. The first two of these relate to pretrauma beliefs about the self and the world, with extreme views in either direction rendering the person vulnerable to poor posttrauma adjustment. On the one hand, a prior negative view of the self may be reinforced by the traumatic experience (e.g., "this proves that I'm really no good"). On the other hand, prior unrealistic beliefs of invulnerability and personal competence may be shattered by the experience, leaving the person confused and insecure. Similarly, pretrauma beliefs about the safety of the world may be affected in the same way. Prior perceptions of the world, and other people, as being dangerous will be reinforced by the trauma, while unrealistic views of the world as always safe will be shattered by the trauma. More flexible and realistic prior views of the self and the world are likely to be associated with improved posttrauma adjustment. The third category relates to beliefs about reactions during the trauma, leading to negative self-perceptions (e.g., "I should have fought back", or "I can't trust myself"). The fourth relates to beliefs about the PTSD symptoms themselves (such as "I'm going crazy" or "I'll never recover"), while the final theme relates to beliefs about the reactions of others (such as "Everyone thinks it was my fault" or "They think I'm overreacting").

The client is helped to identify the negative automatic thoughts and dysfunctional beliefs present following the trauma, and to treat them as hypotheses rather than facts. Therapist and client can then work together in a collaborative fashion to challenge and dispute the negative cognitions, eventually replacing them with more balanced and rational alternatives. While there are several ways to go about this process, it is common to work through a series of questions, as shown in the Patient Treatment Manual. The important point common to all effective cognitive therapy is that the process of challenging and disputing the automatic thoughts and dysfunctional beliefs is an active and rigorous intellectual task. It is not sufficient to simply replace the maladaptive cognitions with an adaptive alternative; the individual must make an effort to really understand why the thought is based upon faulty logic.

Many survivors of trauma seek unrealistic assurances, wishing to replace the distress-producing thoughts with beliefs that are patently untrue. A common example of this is to seek an assurance that they will never experience such an event again. ("If you could promise me that this will never happen again, I'd be alright"). Clearly, it is not possible to provide such an assurance. Rather, the therapist needs to work with the client to realistically evaluate the risks and the potential effects. A common theme in all anxiety disorders is the tendency to overestimate the probability of a bad event occurring, as well as to overestimate the negative consequences should it occur. The latter, of course, are difficult cognitions to challenge in PTSD. However, therapists need to assist clients in focusing on what few positives there are: the fact that they did survive, that they are recovering, and that they have learnt skills that will help them in the extremely unlikely event that it should happen again.

The timing of cognitive restructuring in PTSD is important if its efficacy is to be optimized. Although exposure work is routinely commenced prior to the cognitive interventions, in practice the two are inextricably entwined. Exposure often helps to integrate the fragmented traumatic memory, bringing to light information that casts a new perspective on the event. These new perspectives are often best dealt with by cognitive restructuring. Indeed, it may be postulated that the real therapeutic ingredient of any exposure treatment is actually the processing of new information. Appraisals, interpretations, and beliefs are central to our understanding of traumatic stress, which is characterized by shattered assumptions about fundamental issues such as safety, trust, and personal worth. While some of these may be resolved by a pure exposure paradigm alone, in most cases cognitive restructuring needs to be woven into the later stages of exposure. This is particularly relevant from the perspective of cognitive processing models of PTSD which postulate that the traumatic memory network must be activated before it can be modified. The interpretations and beliefs associated with the experience need to be restructured in the context of the entire memory network. Therapists should therefore be prepared to do at least some of the cognitive challenging work during the later exposure sessions when target thoughts and beliefs are activated.

Working with guilt

Guilt and self-blame deserve a special mention at this point. Guilt is commonly reported and may be part of the process of "working through the trauma" and developing a modified view of the self and the world that is acceptable to the client. Indeed, some research has suggested that guilt in the first few months may actually be associated with improved subsequent recovery (Creamer et al., 1993). Therapists are advised to resist the temptation to dispute guilt-related cognitions too quickly, despite the fact that they may often appear irrational. It may be speculated that guilt, unlike fear or sadness, is something that the survivor is unlikely to be able to discuss with support networks (who are likely to respond immediately with reassurances such as "It wasn't your fault; you did all you could"). Thus, some opportunity to simply ventilate the guilt in a caring and supportive environment may be beneficial.

If the guilt feelings do not resolve, however, cognitive restructuring is indicated. Often this is a case of pointing out the discrepancies between making a value judgment based on the context and information available at the time of the trauma, and making a judgment with the benefit of hindsight and with the adoption of the current context and rules for acceptable behavior. It is inappropriate, for example, to judge an act of violence committed during combat on the basis of peacetime rules and expectations. Kubany (1994) referred to this as an "I should have known better" typology of guilt. He refers also to "Catch 22" guilt: in many situations (particularly war) there is no "right" thing to do – all options are unacceptable. An obvious example is the "kill or be killed" dilemma.

A useful distinction is often made between behavioral guilt and characterological guilt. The former may actually be adaptive, since behavioral changes may restore feelings of security (e.g. "It was my fault I was attacked because I went to a dangerous part of town, on my own, in the early hours of the morning. I won't do that again"). Characterological self-blame, however, is potentially much more problematic ("It was my fault it happened because I'm such a worthless person"). In such cases, the therapist needs to highlight the logical errors inherent in global self-rating, drawing the distinction between a bad, or unwise, behavior and a bad person. This is particularly important when working with someone who did, undeniably, "do something bad" during the traumatic event: e.g., by mistake or design, the person did something that resulted in the death or suffering of innocent others. It is counter-therapeutic to pretend that it did not happen or that it was an acceptable way to behave. Rather, the client needs to be assisted in understanding that it is illogical and unhelpful to generalize from a single mistake or negative act to rate their whole selves. The field of rational emotive therapy (RET) is notably strong on this issue and interested readers are referred to standard RET texts (e.g., Walen et al., 1992) for a more detailed elucidation of this concept.

Relapse prevention and maintenance

In acute PTSD presentations, with little in the way of premorbid psychopathology or comorbidity, a return to normal functioning with low chance of relapse may be possible. Even in such cases, however, and certainly in more chronic and complex cases, it is likely that some vulnerability will remain. Times of high stress, and exposure to (or hearing about) other traumatic events, are potential triggers for some kind of relapse. It is important that clients are prepared for this possibility and that they have strategies to deal with such situations should they arise. In more severe cases, ongoing support from a mental health professional or counseling agency may be required for a considerable period.

In all cases, however, attention should be paid to relapse prevention. This would normally involve several steps. First, the client should be made aware that distress will occur from time to time when he or she is confronted with reminders and that this is a normal part of traumatic stress reactions. Provided that they are not too severe and do not last too long, an ability to accept such lapses philosophically will indicate effective recovery. Second, consideration should be given to identifying likely high-risk times such as reminders of the trauma or news of similar events, experience of another traumatic event, and high-stress times at work or at home. Third, therapist and client should collaboratively develop a written plan to deal with such lapses. Who can the client call (and what are the phone numbers)? What physical, cognitive, and behavioral coping strategies have they found useful and could use at such times? The written plan should include also expectations of recovery, perhaps in the form of self-statements (e.g., "I expect to be upset when reminded of what happened, but that's OK. It's a perfectly normal reaction and I can cope with it. It will pass. Now, what strategies can I use to take control and help myself to feel better?").

The duration and timing of treatment

The question of how many sessions it takes to treat PTSD is impossible to answer, with a multitude of factors determining the duration of treatment. In the best case scenario – e.g., treatment initiated within a few weeks of a single incident trauma, with good pretrauma functioning and strong support networks – it should be possible to cover the above treatment plan in around six sessions. Two studies of early intervention using such approaches (Foa et al., 1995a; Bryant et al., 1998) have used four or five sessions, although these sessions were of one and a half hours duration. Indeed, it is advisable to schedule 90-minute sessions when conducting the exposure components of treatment in PTSD in order to ensure sufficient time for the anxiety to habituate.

A sample five-session treatment plan for an acute presentation is provided below. The more complex the presentation, the more time will be required for each component of treatment, although the general format and structure of the intervention will remain largely the same. In cases with high levels of comorbidity and psychosocial dysfunction, those issues may be addressed before, after, or even in the midst of the suggested treatment plan.

Acute traumatic stress reactions: a five-session ($\times$ $1\frac{1}{2}$ hours) intervention

Note 1: Timing and content are guidelines only.
Note 2: Use two tapes to record sessions, reserving one for exposure components only.

- Session 1
  - Assessment (45 minutes)
  - Psychoeducation (20 minutes)
  - One arousal reduction strategy (e.g., controlled breathing) (15 minutes)
  - Discuss social support (10 minutes)
- Session 2
  - Check homework and coping (15 minutes)
  - Anxiety management (30 minutes)
  - Begin exposure (initial run-through) (45 minutes)
- Session 3
  - Check homework and coping (15 minutes)
  - Continue anxiety management (10 minutes)
  - Exposure (45 minutes)
  - Introduce cognitive restructuring (20 minutes)

- Session 4
  - Check homework and coping (15 minutes)
  - Exposure (45 minutes)
  - Continue cognitive restructuring (30 minutes)
- Session 5
  - Check homework (15 minutes)
  - Cognitive restructuring (15 minutes)
  - Relapse prevention (45 minutes)
  - Closure & termination (15 minutes)

Conclusions

While the treatment of PTSD (and ASD) has come a long way in the past 10 years, there is still much to learn about these complex disorders. Expectations of treatment outcome must remain modest. As a rule of thumb, it can be expected that around one-third of patients will respond very well to treatment, making close to a full recovery. Another one-third will show clear benefits, probably not meeting criteria for a formal diagnosis at posttreatment but continuing to experience milder adjustment problems and interference in social and occupational functioning. Research data are not yet available regarding continued recovery in this subpopulation, although anecdotal evidence would suggest that significant changes from pretrauma functioning may remain in the long term. Often these changes are described by partners in terms of their loved ones being somewhat more withdrawn and less spontaneous than they used to be, with perhaps a slight flattening of affect. The final one-third of patients with PTSD seem to gain little from existing treatment approaches. A major challenge for the field is that of identifying potential nonresponders prior to treatment and designing alternative strategies (perhaps with a more symptom-management, social problem-solving focus) for that group.

27

Posttraumatic stress disorder

Patient Treatment Manual*

This Manual is both a guide to treatment and a workbook for persons who suffer from posttraumatic stress disorder. During treatment, it is a workbook in which individuals can record their own experience of their disorder, together with the additional advice for their particular case given by their clinician. After treatment has concluded, this Manual will serve as a self-help resource enabling those who have recovered, but who encounter further stressors or difficulties, to read the appropriate section and, by putting the content into action, stay well.

Contents

*Parts of this Manual were adapted from *What Is PTSD: Information for Veterans and Their Families*, written by Mark Creamer, David Forbes, and Grant Devilly, and produced by the Australian Centre for Posttraumatic Mental Health, Melbourne, Australia.

SECTION 1

Experience of a traumatic event can shatter a person's life, leaving him or her feeling vulnerable and frightened. It is very important to remember that recovery is possible and that you can lead a normal, happy life again. This does not mean that you will forget what happened to you or that you will never again be distressed by memories and reminders of the event. A certain amount of distress when you think about what happened is part of being a normal, caring human being and we certainly do not want you to have no feelings. However, the distress will become less frequent and more manageable – it will no longer control your life as it may do now. Recovery also does not mean that you will be exactly the same person that you were before the trauma. Such powerful experiences may change people in many ways, not all of them negative. As people recover from trauma, they may find themselves stronger than before, perhaps more caring and with a more balanced and sensible view about what is important in their lives.

By seeking some help, you have taken the first steps to recovery. The purpose of this Manual is to help you through the treatment process in a step-by-step fashion. There is a great deal of information here – take it slowly and read each section as often as necessary until you understand it before moving on. You will be asked to write things down from time to time, so we suggest that you find an exercise book to use for those tasks that you will keep adding to throughout your recovery. Try not to worry if it all seems too difficult at the moment – recovery from trauma is often a long process and you need to take things one day at a time, recognizing small improvements as they occur. It can be a long journey, but it will be worth it.

1 The nature of traumatic stress and posttraumatic stress disorder

At some point in our lives, nearly all of us will experience a very frightening or distressing event that will challenge our view of the world or ourselves. Virtually everyone develops some kind of psychological reaction following such experiences – this is part of a normal human response to extreme stress. Most people will recover over the weeks and months following the incident, with the help of caring family members and friends. For some, however, recovery does not come so easily and more serious problems develop. In those cases, professional help is often required.

Some individuals who experience a traumatic event will go on to develop a chronic condition known as posttraumatic stress disorder (PTSD). The exact numbers are difficult to specify, but anywhere between 5% and 40% of trauma survivors may develop PTSD. The question of why some people are affected more than others has no simple answer – many factors are involved. It seems to be a complex mix of what the person was like before the trauma, his or her experience of other frightening events in the past, the severity of the current trauma, and what else is happening as he or she tries to recover. Regardless of the causes, effective treatment does a great deal to improve the chances of recovery.

1.1 What is a traumatic event?

Trauma is a very personal thing. What traumatizes one person can be of less significance to others. This variation in people's reactions occurs because of their individual personality, beliefs, personal values, and previous experiences (especially of other traumatic events in their life). It occurs also because each person's experience of the incident is unique. However, in all cases the individual has experienced a threatening event that has caused them to respond with intense fear, helplessness, or horror. The threat or injury may be to themselves or to others close to them. Typical traumatic events may be of human origin (such as war experiences, physical assault, sexual assault, accidents, and witnessing the death or injury of others) or of natural origin (such as bushfires, earthquakes, floods, and hurricanes). Overall, there are no hard and fast rules to define trauma.

1.2 What is posttraumatic stress disorder?

PTSD is a psychological response to the experience of intense traumatic events, particularly those that threaten life. It can affect people of any age, culture or gender. Although we have started to hear much more about it in recent years, the condition has been known to exist at least since the times of ancient Greece (more than 2000 years ago) and has been called by many different names. In the American Civil War it was referred to as "soldier's heart", in the First World War it was called "shell shock", while by the Second World War it was known as "war neurosis". In civilian life, terms such as "shock neurosis", "railway spine", and "rape trauma syndrome" were used in the past.

Traumatic stress can be seen as part of a normal human response to intense experiences. While most people recover over the first few months, for many the symptoms do not seem to resolve quickly and, in some cases, may continue to cause problems for the rest of the person's life. It is also common for symptoms to vary in intensity over time. Some people go for long periods without any significant problems, only to relapse when they have to deal with other major life stress. In rare cases, the symptoms may not appear for months, or even years, after the trauma.

1.3 Common symptoms of posttraumatic stress disorder

PTSD is characterized by three main groups of problems. They can be classified under the headings intrusive, avoidant and arousal symptoms.

1.3.1 Intrusive symptoms

Memories, images, smells, sounds, and feelings of the traumatic event can "intrude" into the lives of individuals with PTSD. Sufferers may remain so captured by the memory of past horror that they have difficulty paying attention to the present. People with PTSD report frequent, distressing memories of the event that they wish they did not have. They may have nightmares of the event or other frightening themes. Movement, excessive sweating, and sometimes even acting out the dream while still asleep may accompany these nightmares. They sometimes feel as though the events were happening again; this is referred to as "flashbacks", or "reliving" the event. They may become distressed, or experience physical signs such as sweating, heart racing, and muscle tension, when things happen which remind them of the incident. Overall, these "intrusive" symptoms cause intense distress and can result in other emotions such as grief, guilt, fear, or anger.

Intrusive symptoms of PTSD
- Distressing memories or images of the incident
- Nightmares of the event or other frightening themes
- Flashbacks (reliving the event)
- Becoming upset when reminded of the incident
- Physical symptoms, such as sweating, heart racing, or muscle tension when reminded of the event

---

1.3.2 Avoidance symptoms

Memories and reminders of traumatic events are very unpleasant, causing considerable distress. Therefore, people with PTSD often avoid situations, people, or events that may remind them of the trauma. They try not to think about, or talk about, what happened, and attempt to cut themselves off from the painful feelings associated with the memories. In their attempts to do this, they often withdraw from family, friends, and society in general. They begin to do less and less, no longer taking part in activities they used to enjoy. This may help them to shut out the painful memories, but it can also lead to feelings of isolation and of not belonging to the rest of society. In this way the person can become "numb" to their surroundings and not experience normal everyday emotions such as love and joy, even towards those close to them. Such reactions can lead to depression and problems within the family. They can also lead to severe problems with motivation – people with PTSD often find it hard to make decisions and to "get themselves going". They may have difficulty making the effort to help themselves or even to do things that they would previously have found enjoyable or easy. This can be very hard for family and friends, who often think that the sufferer is just being lazy or difficult.

Avoidance and numbing symptoms of PTSD

- Trying to avoid any reminders of the trauma, such as thoughts, feelings, conversations, activities, places and people
- Gaps in memory – forgetting parts of the experience
- Losing interest in normal activities
- Feeling cut off or detached from loved ones
- Feeling flat or numb
- Difficulty imagining a future

1.3.3 Arousal symptoms

People who have experienced a trauma have been confronted with their own mortality. Their assumptions and beliefs that the world is safe and fair, that other people are basically good, and that "it won't happen to me", have been shattered by the experience. After the event, they see danger everywhere and become "tuned in" to threat. As a consequence, they may become jumpy, on edge, and feel constantly on guard. This can lead to being overly alert or watchful and to having problems concentrating (e.g., not able to read a book for long, getting only a small amount of work completed in a few hours, easily distracted). It is common for sleep to be very disturbed – difficulty getting off, restlessness through the night, or waking early. Sometimes people find that they are frightened to go to sleep because of the nightmares or because they feel unsafe.

Anger is often a central feature in PTSD, with sufferers feeling irritable and prone to angry outbursts with themselves, others around them, and the world in general. In part, the anger is one way of expressing the feelings of being tense and on edge that are associated with PTSD – for some people it is easier to acknowledge anger than fear. In addition, however, this anger results from the feelings of injustice caused by the trauma – a reaction to the gross unfairness of it all. Anger and irritability frequently cause major problems at work, as well as with family and friends.

Arousal symptoms of PTSD

- Sleep disturbance
- Anger and irritability
- Concentration problems
- Constantly on the look out for signs of danger
- Jumpy, easily startled

1.4 Associated problems

PTSD is not the only psychological response to trauma. People may develop a range of other problems that can affect their quality of life, their ability to relate to other people, and their capacity for work. These problems may occur on their own, or as part of the PTSD. Many of these problems are thought to be the result of people trying to control either themselves and their symptoms (such as alcohol and drug abuse) or their environment (such as avoidance behavior and angry outbursts). Also, many of the signs are directly related to stress (such as skin complaints and general aches and pains). Overall, the most commonly associated problems in PTSD are those relating to anxiety, depression, and alcohol or drug use – we will discuss each of these briefly. They can be very disabling to the sufferer, and may affect family members and work colleagues. Many of the following problems develop over time as the person struggles to cope with the PTSD. If you are in the early stages following a trauma, some of the following may not apply to you.

Anxiety

Anxiety is a state of apprehension and worry that something unpleasant is about to happen. It is often accompanied by a range of physical symptoms (such as sweating, racing heart, and breathing difficulties) that are, in themselves, very frightening. Sometimes people experiencing these symptoms believe that they are going to die from a heart attack or go crazy. Anxiety can be specific to certain situations (such as social events, crowded places, or public transport), or it can be a general state of worry about many things in our lives. If you are having significant problems in these areas, be sure to tell your therapist. Treatment (as outlined in other chapters in this book) can be very effective.

Depression

Depression is a general state of low mood and a loss of interest or pleasure in activities that were once enjoyed. Life becomes flat and gray, and nothing seems fun, exciting, or enjoyable anymore. These depressed states can be very intense, leading to a total withdrawal from others and a state of numbness, or they can be lower in intensity – just feeling "down in the dumps". They may last for as little as a few hours or as long as months or even years. In more severe cases, the person may believe that life is no longer worth living. Many people who suffer from PTSD over a long period develop significant problems with depression. Again, it is important to tell your therapist if these problems apply to you. It can be treated effectively with psychological treatments and/or prescription drugs.

Guilt

People with PTSD often report strong feelings of guilt, shame, and remorse. This may be about the fact that they survived while others did not; it may be about what they had to do to survive; it may be related to how they have coped or acted since the trauma. Guilt is often the most difficult thing to talk about, especially if you feel that you did something wrong or acted in a bad way. However, it is very important that you work on those feelings as part of your PTSD treatment, so be sure to tell your therapist about those feelings.

Alcohol and drugs

In an attempt to cope with the unpleasant symptoms, many people turn to alcohol or other drugs. Although they may seem to help in the short term, they prevent the person from recovering effectively and lead to long-term problems. Drug and alcohol abuse impairs the person's ability to function effectively and to relate to other people. It can cause great difficulties in areas such as relationships, work, finances, and violent behavior.

Impact on relationships and work

Traumatized people can become "consumed" by their feelings, which may lead others to believe that they are selfish, thinking only of themselves. Difficulty feeling and expressing emotions (e.g., love and enthusiasm), loss of interest in sex, and reduced participation in activities and hobbies that they used to enjoy before the trauma are common. Traumatized people are often tired and can become cranky and irritable. They may say hurtful things without really considering the implications of what they are saying. All of these symptoms may cause partners to feel rejected and unloved, and the absence of shared enjoyable activities makes it difficult to have a normal family life. It is very important to keep communicating about what is happening – try to be reasonably honest with each other about how you are feeling.

People with PTSD may have difficulty coping with pressure at work. Irritability, jumpiness, mood swings, poor concentration, and memory problems may lead to disputes in the workplace and frequent job changes. Some people with PTSD adopt a workaholic pattern, shutting themselves away in their work and putting in very long hours. This seems to be part of the avoidance component of PTSD – keeping very busy helps to prevent the memories and unpleasant thoughts coming back – but it does not help in the long term. Others find that their problems prohibit them from working effectively at all.

1.5 Why do traumatic stress reactions develop?

It is important to understand where the signs and symptoms of PTSD come from. One of the leading clinicians in the area, Mardi Horowitz, described trauma as an experience that is, by its very nature, overwhelming. It contains lots of new information that is hard to accept or understand. It does not fit with our view of the world or ourselves – the way we think things are or should be. Human beings have a natural tendency to try to make sense of things that happen around them. When people experience a trauma, the event keeps coming back into their mind in an attempt to make sense of what happened. This is the body's natural way of trying to deal with, or come to terms with, difficult experiences and seems to work well for many stressful life events. However, due to the high level of distress associated with memories of more severe trauma, the thoughts and feelings tend to be pushed away to protect the person from this distress. The result is that, whilst the memory may go away for a while, the need for it to be dealt with has not been addressed and it keeps coming back. The movement backward and forward from intrusive thoughts and feelings about the trauma to avoidance and numbing can then continue almost indefinitely unless the cycle is addressed in some way.

Throughout this alternating between short bursts of painful memories and periods of avoidance and numbing, the sense of feeling keyed-up persists. The traumatized person has been through an event that threatened their life, or the life of someone else, so the mind and body stay on alert to make sure that no future potential dangers will be missed. It is safer to get it wrong by overestimating potential threat than to risk the possibility of missing any future threat. The persistent activation of this threat detection system, however, leaves the traumatized person feeling keyed-up or on edge much of the time. In addition, the threat detection system is so sensitive that it is constantly going off when there is no danger in such a way that interferes with the person's capacity to live a normal and happy life.

Traumatic stress reactions, therefore, are sensible and adaptive both as part of survival during the trauma and in attempts to come to terms with the trauma afterward. Once we recognize where these symptoms come from, it is easier to understand the typical traumatic stress reactions. The difficult part is letting go of these reactions now that they have ceased to provide benefit and are interfering with the traumatized person's quality of life.

1.6 The process of treatment and recovery

You have already started the first stage of recovery by acknowledging your reactions to the traumatic event. Presumably, you have also taken the next step of seeking appropriate treatment from a mental health professional. Getting help is often frightening – for many it is a leap into the unknown – but trying to recover from PTSD on your own is much more difficult. Treatment usually involves several stages; we will go through each of these in turn.

PTSD: stages of treatment

1. Crisis stabilization and engagement
2. Education about PTSD and related conditions
3. Strategies to manage the symptoms
4. Trauma focused therapy (confronting the painful memories and feared situations)
5. Cognitive restructuring (learning to think more realistically about what happened)
6. Relapse prevention and ongoing support

It is important to remember that treatment can be painful and hard work. Unfortunately, there is no easy way to get rid of the memories or make them less distressing. There is no magic wand that your therapist can wave or tablet that you can take to make it all go away. But the long-term gains can be enormous: effective treatment can dramatically assist your recovery, helping you to live a normal life once again.

SECTION 2

2 Stabilization of a crisis and engagement in treatment

People who have been through a trauma often have other difficult situations to deal with in the aftermath. These may be legal issues, family disruptions, financial problems, or a multitude of other crises. It is important that any current life crises are resolved, or at least put "on hold", before the real treatment of PTSD can begin. It is not possible to devote the necessary concentration, time, and energy to your recovery if you are constantly worried about your job, your relationship, your children, or other important life areas. That is not to say that you have to be able to solve all those problems before you can work on your PTSD, but you will need to be able to put them to one side for a while to concentrate on your treatment. Therapy is hard work – there is no easy way to do it – and you will need to devote all your personal resources to the task. If other life issues are worrying you, it is important that you discuss these with your therapist as they arise so that they do not interfere too much with your treatment.

The first part of treatment will often be devoted to developing a relationship with the therapist (or the treatment team if you are taking part in a group program). You will need to spend some time getting to know each other, and building trust, if you are to work on the difficult issues. We call this process "engagement". For many people with PTSD, this is a very difficult process – experience of a traumatic event often makes it very hard to trust another person, particularly someone whom you have never met before. In many cases, you will need to tell your therapist about experiences and feelings that you have never discussed with anyone. We need to recognize that this is a difficult process that will take a lot of courage, but it will be worth it and it is the only way to recovery.

SECTION 3

3 Education and information

PTSD can sometimes feel like an incomprehensible cloud that hangs over all areas of the person's life. The first step in treatment is to understand exactly what trauma is, why we have the symptoms we do and, therefore, why it is treated the way it is. In this regard, you have come a long way already by reading the sections above. You need to know what the common signs and symptoms are, and you need to recognize that you are not alone – many people who have experienced traumatic events have responded in exactly the same way you have. You need to understand why the symptoms have appeared – the fact that they were very useful for survival while the traumatic events were happening but that they are no longer useful. They have become "maladaptive" and now serve only to create problems and distress for you. You need to understand what treatment will involve and how it may affect you. It is very important that you feel able to ask your therapist questions about the nature of your problems and the process of treatment. He or she will not have all the answers, but together you will reach a better understanding of what has happened and how you will recover.

Sometimes people who have been through a traumatic event have trouble understanding what happened and why it happened. You may find yourself constantly asking questions such as "How did this happen" or "Why me?". This is partly because, when we are under threat, our attention is very focused on the source of the danger and we do not take in all the other things that are happening around us. We may end up with a distorted and confused memory of the experience, so that it becomes difficult to understand and make sense of the event. This confusion often stops us from being able to put the experience behind us. For this reason, your therapist may help you to find out more about what happened during the event. This process is important in being able to "put the pieces of the jigsaw puzzle together" and make sense of your experience. A good understanding of exactly what happened, and why it happened, often facilitates recovery.

Although we have put this under the heading "Education and information", it is actually something that may happen at several stages throughout treatment and you need to make sure that you are ready before you pursue these options. When you are feeling reasonably confident, however, ask yourself what other information you need to help you to understand what happened and why it happened.

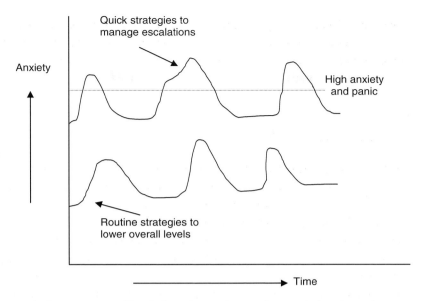

Reducing your general level of tension and managing escalations in anxiety

- Is there anyone else you can talk to who may be able to clarify things for you and help you to reach a better understanding of your experience (such as others who were there, police officers, or ambulance officers)?
- Is there anything you can read that will help to fill in the missing pieces (such as media reports, police statements, or reports from a trial or coroner's inquest)? Sometimes, reading accounts written by other survivors of trauma can be useful in understanding your reactions.
- Occasionally there may even be video footage available from news reports or other sources: is there anything you can watch that will help you to fill in the gaps?

Unfortunately, of course, it is not always possible to fill in all the gaps in your understanding of the event. Sometimes we may never find out exactly what happened (or, more commonly, why it happened) and treatment needs to focus on helping us learn to live with that uncertainty.

SECTION 4

4 Managing anxiety and distress

The next step is to help you to feel more in control of your reactions. We will do this in several parts. First, there are many simple things you can do in your day-to-day life that will make you feel more in control and less distressed. There is nothing magical about these "Hints for coping" – most are simply common sense – but they can make a real difference. The second part involves more specific strategies that your therapist will teach you to control your anxiety and distress. Some of these are useful in lowering your overall level of tension and stress – the more relaxed you are in general, the better you will cope when the memories return or you are confronted with other unexpected difficulties. Everyone experiences increases in anxiety and distress at those times. If your overall level of stress is high, these escalations will take you up into the level of high anxiety and panic (the top graph in the figure above). If your overall level is lower, the shape will be the same – you will still react to negative events, but your anxiety and distress will not reach the same heights (the lower graph in the figure). We will call these "routine strategies", since we want them to become part of your everyday routine. Examples would be regular exercise, rest, sensible diet, and relaxation (see below). Other strategies are designed to help you to deal more specifically with difficult situations when you can feel your anxiety escalating and you are beginning to feel overwhelmed. These require a lot of practice, but are very useful to use when the feelings of distress and anxiety are particularly strong.

4.1 Hints for coping

The following is a list of tips that many people find useful. Do not try to do everything at once. When you have read the following sections, you may wish to stop for a while and work out a "plan of action". Which strategies sound particularly useful for you? Which ones are you prepared to try? We suggest that you select only one or two to begin with. Work out a plan to achieve them, one at a time, and set yourself some realistic goals for the next week. At the end of the week, review your progress: modify your goals if necessary and/or try some additional strategies for the following week. Over time, you will gradually develop a range of coping strategies and changes to your lifestyle that will help you to feel more in control of your symptoms and get more out of life.

- Eat healthy meals. This sounds so simple, but how many of us actually do it? A poor diet (especially junk food with lots of sugar) will increase your stress levels – if in doubt, talk to your general practitioner or a dietician.
- Get regular aerobic exercise such as walking, jogging, swimming, or cycling. Exercise is very effective in managing stress. If you have PTSD, your body is constantly geared up for "fight or flight". Exercise helps to burn up those chemicals (like adrenaline (epinephrine)) that are hyping you up and it will help you to become more relaxed.
- Get enough rest, even if you can't sleep. Rest will help to increase your reserves of strength and energy. (See also "Hints for "sleeping better", below).
- Establish, and try to stick to, daily routines (e.g., go to bed and get up at a set

time, plan your activities for the day). Routine is very important in helping us to feel in control and to function effectively. If you feel able, return to work, study, or other routines as soon as possible but take it easy – don't expect too much of yourself and don't use work as a way of avoiding painful feelings.

- Ask for support and help from your family, friends, church, or other community resources when you need it. This is not a sign of weakness. In general, other people are very keen to help as long as you let them know what you want. If they do not offer, it may simply be because they are unsure of what to do.

- Spend time with other people, but don't feel that you have to talk about the trauma. Talk about football, books, or the weather; go to a movie or a concert; try to do some enjoyable things with others. This is part of resuming a normal life.

- Focus on your strengths and coping skills. It may not feel like it at times, but you have many strengths and strategies to deal with difficult times. Remember that you are not alone. Many other survivors over the centuries have experienced these kinds of problems and the vast majority have recovered well.

Hints for family and friends

Partners and close friends are often at a loss as to how to help someone with PTSD. There are several things that loved ones can do to help the traumatized person. You may find the following suggestions useful.

- If possible, listen and empathize when the traumatized person wants to talk. Remember that it may be very hard for them to express what they are going through. A sympathetic listener is important in minimizing the tendency of people with PTSD to withdraw and "shut down".

- It is best not to say "I understand what you're feeling" (you probably don't, since you haven't been through the same experiences). Instead, show your empathy by comments such as "it must be really difficult for you; I can see that it upsets you; is there anything I can do to help?".

- Spend time with the traumatized person. There is no substitute for personal presence. Just keep doing the usual things that people do together. Do not feel that you have to talk about the trauma or be their counselor. Just being with people who care about them is very important for traumatized individuals. Equally, try to respect the person's need for privacy and private grief at times.

- Don't tell survivors that they are "lucky it wasn't worse" or to "pull themselves together and get over it". They are not consoled by such statements. Tell them, instead, that you're sorry they were involved in such an event, and that you want to understand and assist them.

- Re-assure them that they are now safe.

- Care about each other. Give hugs. Tell each other how much they are appreciated. Offer praise. Make a point of saying something nice to each other every day. Good relationships are characterized by lots of positive interactions, but they require hard work.

Hints for sleeping better

Sleep disturbance is very common in both PTSD and depression. Medication sometimes helps, but it should be used with caution and only as directed by your medical practitioner. There are several simple "nondrug" strategies that you can try that can be very helpful in improving sleep.

- Get into a regular routine. In particular, get up at the same time each morning even if you haven't slept well.
- If you are not asleep within 30 minutes, get up for a while before returning to bed. If you don't drop off within 30 minutes, get up again and so on.
- Try to avoid caffeine (coffee, tea, cola, chocolate) from 6 p.m. onwards. Avoid alcohol and, if possible, cigarettes from dinnertime onwards. Try not to eat a meal within a couple of hours of going to bed.
- Starting a gentle exercise routine and losing some weight often helps with sleep.
- Don't do anything in bed except sleep (and, perhaps, sex): don't watch TV, read, do crosswords, or think about worrying things. Reserve bed for sleeping.
- Get into the habit of doing something relaxing before bed: listen to a relaxation tape or some relaxing music, have a warm bath, slow down!
- Try not to worry about not sleeping: the more you worry about it, the less likely you are to drop off to sleep. You can survive without much sleep, even though you will be tired.
- Sleep, like any habit, takes a while to change. Try to stick to the above guidelines for at least 2 weeks before deciding whether or not they help.

4.2 Overview of anxiety management

When we experience a very frightening or unpleasant event, our body gears itself up to fight the threat or to run away (the "fight or flight" response). If the threat is small and passes, our body quickly returns to normal. If the threat has been major, however, or if there is ongoing danger (or stress), our body remains in a state of alertness ready to react immediately if the threat reappears. This chronic state of alertness affects us in many ways. First, we tend to stay physically hyped up and aroused all the time. Our heart rate and breathing are increased, and our muscles remain tensed up, leading to all sorts of unpleasant physical sensations, aches, and pains. Second, our thinking is affected. We may find it hard to concentrate, remember things, and make decisions. Memories of the trauma, or thoughts of future danger, seem to constantly come to mind even when we do not want them to. Third, our behavior is affected. Experience of the trauma, as well as the unpleasant signs and symptoms that may follow, causes people to feel scared and vulnerable. In an attempt to cope, they may try to withdraw from other people and the outside world, shutting down as a means of self-protection. If we are to effectively manage the anxiety and distress that follows a traumatic experience, we will need to address all three aspects: the physical components, the thoughts, and the behavior.

It is important to remember that the goal is not to make the unpleasant feelings go away altogether – that is neither possible nor desirable. Rather, the goal is to keep them manageable – to keep them under control and to stop them escalating into extreme anxiety and panic. Practice is essential to master most of the following techniques. Try to set aside some time each day (preferably twice a day) to practice. If you wait until you are tense and frightened before you try the technique, it will not work. Once you have practiced them regularly, however, they will become more automatic and effective. They will become important tools in helping you to manage anxiety and distress. Keep a diary of your practice sessions, noting down the SUDs level (see below) before and after. This will give both you and your therapist a good idea of how you are progressing.

The following sections discuss strategies in each of the three domains. Other chapters in this book contain very good descriptions of several anxiety-management strategies. You may wish to talk to your therapist about getting copies of some of the relevant sections.

4.3 Subjective units of distress (SUDs)

As you start to conquer your fears, it becomes very important to have a means of measuring your level of anxiety and distress. We suggest that you use a SUDs scale ranging from 0 to 100 – a kind of fear thermometer – where 0 is feeling perfectly relaxed and 100 is the worst anxiety and distress you can imagine. It is useful to get into the habit of rating your anxiety. That way you become more in touch with your feelings and have a better chance of controlling them. Without some kind of measure, people tend to think in black-and-white terms – you are either anxious or relaxed – when, in reality, there are many shades of gray. Using the SUDs scale will help you to keep your distress level in perspective, e.g., you may be feeling anxious, but it's only 40 – you can handle that. In the exercises that follow, try to rate your distress (using the SUDs scale) before you try the anxiety-management strategy and again afterwards. We hope it will have come down (if only a little).

4.4 Managing the physical symptoms

Several strategies will assist in managing the unpleasant physical symptoms associated with traumatic stress and PTSD. Some of these have been discussed above under the heading "Hints for coping". If you can get some regular gentle exercise,

SUDs: The Fear Thermometer

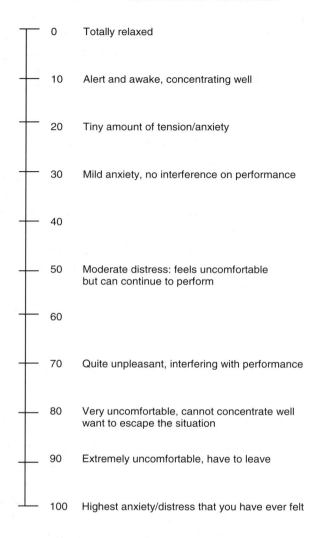

0	Totally relaxed
10	Alert and awake, concentrating well
20	Tiny amount of tension/anxiety
30	Mild anxiety, no interference on performance
40	
50	Moderate distress: feels uncomfortable but can continue to perform
60	
70	Quite unpleasant, interfering with performance
80	Very uncomfortable, cannot concentrate well want to escape the situation
90	Extremely uncomfortable, have to leave
100	Highest anxiety/distress that you have ever felt

eat properly, get enough rest, and try to cut down on stimulants (such as coffee, tea, cola, chocolate, and cigarettes), you will go a long way towards reducing the chronic arousal that is part of PTSD. In this section, we will look at two specific strategies to reduce arousal. The first is a simple breathing control strategy designed to reduce your rate and depth of breathing and help you to feel more relaxed and in control.

Often when people are frightened or upset, they start to breathe faster. An increase in breathing is part of the fight or flight response – we need more oxygen if we are to fight or run away. However, breathing too deeply and too fast when we are not using up a lot of energy tends to make us more anxious and often causes unpleasant physical symptoms such as dizziness, tightness in the chest, and a feeling of being short of breath. When we are upset, we may be told to "take a few deep breaths". However, this is not quite right. When we are feeling anxious or frightened, we don't need to take a deep breath; we need to take a normal breath in and exhale slowly. Breathing out is associated with relaxation, not breathing in. While concentrating on a long, slow exhalation, it's a good idea to say a word like "relax" or "calm" to yourself. Any word that is associated with feeling peaceful and at ease will do fine. Try to drag out the word to match the long, slow exhalation, as in "r-e-e-e-l-a-a-a-x" or "c-a-a-a-a-l-m".

The next thing to remember is to slow your breathing down. Remember that taking in too much air causes an increase in anxiety and unpleasant physical symptoms. So, what we need to do is to slow our breathing down and take in less air. We do this by taking smaller breaths and by pausing between breaths to space them out. It is also important to try to breathe in through your nose, not through your mouth. When you have taken a normal breath in through your nose, hold your breath for a count of 4 before exhaling slowly.

Now, try putting it all together:
- Take in a normal breath through your nose with your mouth closed.
- Pause briefly while you count to 4.
- Exhale very slowly (mouth open or closed, whichever feels most comfortable).
- Say "calm" or "relax" to yourself as you exhale.
- Repeat the whole sequence 6 to 10 times.

Practice this type of breathing at least twice a day. That way, when you become frightened or anxious, you will be ready to use the technique to help you to calm down.

The second physical intervention we will discuss is relaxation training, or progressive muscle relaxation (PMR). The breathing control described above, once you have mastered it, is an excellent strategy for dealing with rapid increases in anxiety that may occur when you experience memories of the trauma or find yourself in a frightening situation. PMR is designed to deal with the more pervasive, chronic tension and stress associated with PTSD. If you can lower your general level of arousal or "uptightness", you will be much less likely to overreact in response to minor perceived threats. This is just like a coiled spring – the more wound up it is, the more likely it is to explode under pressure. The world will seem like a safer place.

PMR is usually done by listening to a tape, which will take you through a series of exercises in which you will be asked to tense up and relax various muscle groups. By gradually working through your whole body, from head to toe, you will achieve a state of physical relaxation that, with practice, you will be able to maintain through much of the day. Your therapist will make a tape for you to use at home. Alternatively, many libraries or community health centers will be able to provide one for you. Excellent descriptions of relaxation training appear in other Patient Treatment Manuals contained in this book and will not be repeated here. If you decide to try this approach (and we strongly recommend that you do), ask your therapist to copy one of the relevant sections for you. Making relaxation a regular part of your daily routine will go a long way to help you in managing the physical symptoms of PTSD.

4.5 Managing problems with thoughts

People with PTSD are often troubled with memories or other unwanted thoughts about the trauma. It is important that you do not try to get rid of these thoughts and memories completely – thinking about what happened is an important part of coming to terms with it and putting it behind you. Equally, it is not helpful to be thinking about it all the time – that simply causes unnecessary distress and prevents you from getting on with your life. So it is a good idea to learn a few strategies to control these unwanted thoughts so that you can limit them to times that do not interfere too much with other activities.

4.5.1 Distraction

One simple way that, with practice, can be very effective is distraction. An obvious example would be getting on with an activity that is absorbing (and we hope enjoyable) to occupy your mind. Can you think of something that you could do to distract yourself? Passive activities (like reading, or watching TV) do not usually work, as your concentration may not be good enough. Rather, you will need to do something more active that involves both physical and mental aspects. Games, crafts, and other creative activities are often good.

It is also good to practice a purely mental distraction technique that you can use anywhere, anytime. There are many things that you could try and the following list provides some examples. They are particularly good because no-one else can see you doing them. Do not try to do them all – pick one or two that feel as though they may work for you and practice regularly. Even with practice, you must expect the thoughts to intrude again from time to time. That's OK – just go back to the distracting thoughts as often as necessary.

Strategies for mental distraction

- *Count and relax:* Breathe normally, as you might when you're just about to drop off to sleep. As you breathe in, count to yourself. As you breathe out, say "relax" to yourself. That is to say, when you breathe in, think "one"; as you breathe out, think "relax"; as you breathe in, think "two", as you breathe out, think "relax"; as you breathe in, think "three", and so on for 10 slow breaths several times a day. Don't worry if other thoughts intrude, just go back to the count and relax.
- *Focus* on a small area (e.g., a square meter (3 foot × 3 foot) on the wall opposite), or on an object, and describe it in minute detail – every line, shadow, and shape.
- *Focus* on your surroundings with all senses: describe in detail to yourself what you can see around you, what you can hear, what you can smell, what you can feel (sensory perceptions of touch, not emotions or anxiety symptoms). Try to describe five things you can see, five you can hear, five you can feel, and so on. This is particularly good as it keeps you in touch with reality "here and now".
- *Mental exercises:* e.g., counting backwards to yourself from 100 in 7s or naming an animal beginning with each letter of the alphabet.
- *Describe* to yourself in great detail a happy experience from the past (e.g., a holiday, a family occasion, a favorite walk). Try to go through every aspect from start to finish.
- *Describe* in detail a place (perhaps from your past) where you feel safe, secure, relaxed, and happy. Where is it, what does it look like and smell like, who is there with you, what time of day is it, how does it feel, and so on.

4.5.2 Thought stopping

Another strategy to deal with unwanted thoughts and memories is known as "thought stopping". This is a simple technique, but surprisingly effective if you are troubled by constant thoughts or "ruminations" about the trauma – if you find yourself thinking about what happened (or might have happened) over and over again. (Note: It should not be used for the brief and very vivid memories that jump into your mind for shorter periods of time.) If you wish to try thought stopping, practice it several times in the following manner. Place an elastic band round your wrist. Now, deliberately bring the unwanted thoughts into your mind and let them run for a minute or so. Then shout the word "STOP!" loudly (it's best to practice this one on your own!) and snap the rubber band against your wrist. This will interrupt your train of thought. Repeat this process over and over again, gradually saying "stop" more and more quietly until eventually (after a dozen or so times) you are whispering it and then saying it just to yourself in your head. Keep snapping the band each time. If you practice that whole process a couple of times a day for several days, you will gain much more control over your thoughts. You will be able to stop the thoughts when you are in public without saying anything out loud (although you may wish to keep the rubber band there for a while as a reminder).

4.5.3 Self-statements

One final area we would like to discuss under the heading of managing thought problems is that of "self-statements". At present, it is likely that many of your thoughts are negative: worrying about the safety of yourself or others, concerned that you will never recover, and so on. These negative thoughts feed into your anxiety and distress, making it much worse. We will address this issue again later. For the time being, we are going to suggest that you simply work out some simple things that you can say to yourself to help you calm down and relax when you are in a difficult situation or when you are feeling overwhelmed by painful memories. A famous psychologist, Donald Meichenbaum, has suggested that we should break up each event into several stages.

Examples of self-statements for coping with stress

1. Preparing for a stressor
   - What is it I have to do?
   - What is the real likelihood of anything bad happening?
   - Don't focus on how bad I feel; think about what I can do about it.
   - I have the support of people who are experienced in dealing with these problems.
   - I have already come a long way towards recovery; I can go the rest of the way.

2. Confronting and handling a stressor
   - One step at a time; I can handle this.
   - Don't think about being afraid or anxious, think about what I am doing.
   - The feelings I'm having are a signal for me to use my coping exercises.
   - There's no need to doubt myself. I have the skills I need to get through.
   - Focus on the plan. Relax ... breath easily; I'm ready to go.

3. Coping with feelings of being overwhelmed
   - Take a gentle breath and exhale slowly.
   - Focus on what is happening now, not what might happen; what is it I have to do?
   - I expect my fear to rise, but I can keep it manageable.
   - This will be over soon. I can do it.
   - This fear may slow me down, but I will not be incapacitated by it.
   - I may feel nauseated and want to avoid the situation, but I can deal with it.
   4. Reinforcing self-statements
   - It was much easier than I thought.
   - I did it – I got through it; each time it will be easier.
   - When I manage the thoughts in my head, I can manage my whole body.
   - I'm avoiding things less and less. I'm making progress.
   - One step at a time – easy does it. Nothing succeeds like success.

First, what can we say to ourselves when we are preparing for something difficult? This helps you to re-evaluate the actual probability of the feared negative event happening – following trauma, most people overestimate the likelihood of danger. Second, what can we say as we approach and enter the difficult situation? This will help to reduce the desire to avoid and run away (which will only make it more difficult next time). The third stage is dealing with the feelings of anxiety and distress as they arise (to prevent them from becoming overwhelming), and the final stage is when looking back on the episode. Several examples of things you could try saying to yourself are provided in the box above.

Read the examples carefully and work out a few self-statements that you feel comfortable with. Then write them on a card that you can carry with you so that it's handy when you need it. When you know you are about to do something difficult, it's a good idea to set aside some time to prepare specific cards for the occasion. For example, if you are going into the city, you may write something like this on a small card that you can carry with you:

> It's natural to be nervous about going into the city given my traumatic experiences, but the likelihood of anything bad happening is very remote. Just relax and slow down my breathing. I may not feel great, but I can cope. Now, what is it that I need to do?

Like everything else, the more you practice using these self-statements, the more effective they will be in helping you to manage your anxiety at difficult times. This will become especially important as we move on to the next stage of treatment.

4.6 Changing behaviors

As we noted above, one feature of PTSD is that people lose interest in normal activities and withdraw into themselves, cutting off from friends and things they used to enjoy. This is a particular difficulty if you are not working. It is important to address this problem directly, even if you do not feel like it. Doing nothing provides lots of opportunities for the memories to come back and is a sure way of making you feel depressed and anxious.

When you get up in the morning (or the night before), make a plan of what you will do that day. Take a sheet of paper and write down the hours (say, from 9.00 a.m. to 9.00 p.m.) on the left-hand side. Then fill in each hour with what you intend to do. If you are working, that will take up much of the day. If not, you will need to try to find worthwhile activities to take up your time. Having some structure and routine to your day will do a great deal to help you feel more in control. Try to put in a broad range of activities but do not expect too much of yourself.

Possible activities for your daily timetable
- Some exercise: walk, swim, cycle ride, gym
- Some work: jobs around the house, study, chores, voluntary work
- Something for fun: a movie, museum, art gallery, zoo, window shopping
- Some social activities: visit friends, meet someone for coffee, a club or society
- Some anxiety-management practice: relaxation, breathing, self-statements
- Some time for other therapy homework

4.7 Arousal and anger

The strategies above are important in helping you deal with anger as well as anxiety. Anger often acts as a stumbling block to recovery, preventing you from moving on to the next stage of treatment. The physical aspects of tension and high arousal are similar in both anxiety and anger, but the triggers that set off the feelings will often be different. Try to identify the kinds of situation that lead you to become angry – the first step in managing your anger is being prepared for it. Take a sheet of paper and jot down a list of things that are likely to set you off. A major difficulty with anger is that it escalates so quickly that it becomes very hard to control. If you can recognize the warning signs and intervene early, you will have a much better chance of doing something about it. Think back to the last time that you were angry and jot down a list of the first signs that appeared. (What happened to you physically? What happened to your thoughts? What happened to your behavior?). Once you are more aware of the triggers and the early warning signs, you will be in a much better position to use the strategies described above to control your anger.

We will briefly look at three extra strategies that people find useful for dealing with anger in PTSD. They are all common sense, but can be very effective:

- *Delay:* As we said, anger escalates very quickly so you need to find a way to stop yourself making that first angry response. Take a few slow, easy breaths and count to 10 before you react.
- *Time Out:* If you feel the anger beginning to escalate, try to remove yourself from the situation. This does not mean storming out in a rage. It means explaining to the person you are with that you are not thinking too clearly and that you need a 5-minute break. Go outside or into another room and use some of the strategies described above to calm down. Then go back and try again.
- *Planning:* Once you have identified the triggers, it is important to use that information to prepare yourself for high-risk situations. If you are going to do something that you know is likely to make you angry, choose a good moment (e.g., no other distractions, not too tired or hungry, plenty of time). Practice what you will do or say in your head beforehand.

SECTION 5

5 Exposure therapy: confronting feared situations

The next part of treatment is the most difficult and painful – confronting the feared situations and traumatic memories. It is also the most important. Your therapist will not start this process until you are ready and will take you through at a pace that you can manage. Most people find that it is not nearly as difficult as they expect it to be and there is often a tremendous sense of relief and achievement as the feared situations and painful memories are confronted and dealt with.

Not surprisingly, anxiety frequently causes people to stay away from frightening situations. It is quite normal for people to want to escape or avoid situations, thoughts, memories, or feelings that are painful or distressing. However, this is one of the major impediments to recovery. Avoidance and escape provide temporary relief – the anxiety reduces – but the next time the person encounters that situation again, he or she is likely to become anxious long before it is planned to occur. We call this "anticipatory anxiety". The more the situation is avoided, the more the person continues to believe that it is dangerous. Further, even if the person does not avoid, the anxiety may continue to build once they are in the situation. Very often people believe that if they do not leave the situation they will "lose control", "go crazy", "have a heart attack", or have some other dire consequences. At the very least, they are likely to believe that the unpleasant feelings will be intolerable. Exposure therapy aims to show that this is not the case by helping the person to confront the feared situation. The important thing to remember when you are confronting something that you are frightened of (whether it is a situation or a memory) is that the *anxiety will come down* if you stay there long enough. There is no answer to the question of how long is enough. In some cases, the anxiety may drop considerably in 15 to 20 minutes. In other cases, it may take as long as an hour or more but it will reduce eventually. It is vital that you try to stay in the feared situation long enough for the anxiety to reduce. It is important to note also that anxiety often increases before it starts to drop. This temporary increase is often enough to make people avoid or escape – it is vital that you stay with the feared situation through this phase until the anxiety reduces. This pattern is shown in the figure overleaf. You will notice that the drop in anxiety is not smooth – you may notice occasional small increases – but the general trend is downwards. Exposure is done in a controlled and gradual fashion so that discomfort is kept manageable. By building upon repeated successes in facing these feared situations, you will eventually be able to confront them without anxiety and no longer avoid them.

In many ways, this approach is common sense. Let's take an example of a little boy who is standing on the beach when a big wave knocks him over. He becomes

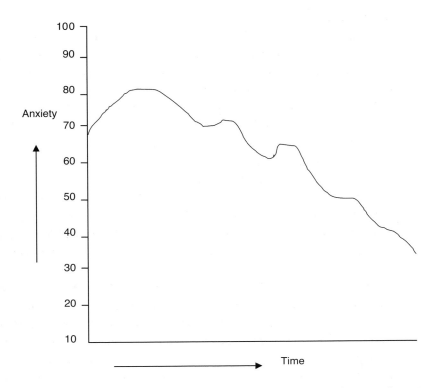

very frightened of the sea and refuses to go to the beach the next day. How would his mother or father help? In order to overcome the fear, his parents may take him for a walk along the beach, staying away from the sea, holding his hand and reassuring him. Gradually, they walk closer and closer to the water's edge. Eventually, the boy is able to go into the sea again unaided. This is a simple example, but exactly the same process applies to treating more severe and complex fears in adults.

This section discusses confronting activities, places, people, or objects that you have become frightened of since the trauma. We call this type of exposure "in vivo". In vivo simply means "in real life". When we are confronting memories, we have to do it in imagination, so we call it imaginal exposure – which is discussed in the next section. In conducting exposure treatment, your therapist will work with you in constructing a hierarchy – a list of feared situations in order of difficulty. Treatment involves tackling each item, one at a time, and moving on to the next only when you are confident to do so. More difficult items may be broken up into several steps. Exposure treatment can be difficult and painful, but it is the most effective way of treating many anxieties.

5.1 Planning your program

1. Draw up a list of goals that you would like to achieve. These are likely to comprise places and activities that you have avoided since the trauma. The goals should be very specific and should vary from relatively easy to extremely difficult. Don't worry if the worst ones seem unachievable at the moment – they will become easier as you progress through the others. List them in order of difficulty, starting with the easiest. For example:
   - To be able to go shopping at the local shopping center
   - To be able to catch public transport into the city
   - To go back to where the trauma occurred

   As a general rule, as you work through the list you should be aiming to confront situations that produce a SUDs level of around 70. For the first one or two, however, we suggest that you start with ones that are a little easier than that (say, around 50) – it is important that you experience some success early on in the process.

2. If something is too hard to try in one go, break it down into smaller steps. For example, if you were assaulted in a particular park, the first step may be to go to the end of the street and look at the park from a distance. The second may be to go to the edge of the park, the third to walk into the park a short distance, and the final one to go back to the spot where the assault occurred.

3. You may want to work on more than one item at any one time, but do not overwhelm yourself. When you have mastered one (i.e., you are able to do it with minimal anxiety), move on to the next more difficult one.

5.2 Implementing your program

1. Try to do at least one of your selected goals every day. Avoiding something one day will set you back, as you will have built up the fear you are trying to reduce. Sometimes you will have bad days and feel that you are not progressing. It is important to still do something, although you may choose just to go over steps that you have already mastered.

2. You will need to do each step several times until you master it. Once you can do it without too much anxiety, it is still important to do it once in a while to make sure you don't slip back. The general rule is: *the more you fear it, the more frequently you need to confront it.*

3. Keep a careful record of your progress. Take a sheet of paper and divide it into columns. In the first, write down your goal. In the second, note the date. In the third and fourth, write the time you started and (when you get back) the time you finished. In the fifth, write down the maximum SUDs you reached and in the sixth the SUDs level when you left the situation. The final column should be

used for making any comments about the exercise. This will help both you and your therapist keep track of your exposure progress.

5.3 Practicing the steps

1. Try to relax using the techniques described above before you start. Get yourself as calm as possible.
2. Mentally rehearse the activity. Go through it in your mind and work out strategies to deal with difficult aspects. Practice the coping self-statements that you will say to yourself when you become distressed. Good preparation will make success more likely.
3. Go about the exercise in a slow and relaxed manner – give yourself plenty of time.
4. Keep an eye on your SUDs throughout the exercise. If they become very high (80 or more) before you've reached your goal, stop and wait for a while until the anxiety comes down a bit. When you feel ready, move on again slowly.
5. Try to stay in the situation until you feel yourself calming down. Ideally, the SUDs should reduce by half (e.g., from 70 to 35). The longer you remain in the situation, the calmer you will become and the faster you will overcome your fears.
6. Never leave the situation while your anxiety is still high. Try to face the fear, accept it, let it fade away, and then either move on or return. If you leave while the anxiety is still high it will be more difficult next time. Remind yourself that you have done really well to get this far; just hang in there until the anxiety comes down.
7. Congratulate yourself for your achievements. This is very hard work and you deserve a pat on the back. Don't put yourself down by saying that you could do this kind of thing easily before the trauma or that anyone should be able to do it without getting upset. It's a vital part of your recovery.

SECTION 6

6 Exposure therapy: confronting the memories

A form of exposure therapy is also used to treat distressing memories of the trauma. We call it "imaginal exposure". In Section 5, we talked about confronting feared situations such as places, people, and activities. In cases of PTSD, however, the most "feared situation" is actually the painful memories of your experience. These memories are so frightening, and cause so much distress, that the person tries to avoid or escape from them by blocking them out. Imaginal exposure treatments are used to assist in confronting the memories. Exposure is only one term used to describe this process. Some people talk about "trauma focus work", "working through the trauma", "coming to terms with the experience" or simply "confronting the memories".

6.1 What is imaginal exposure?

There are many analogies used to explain this process to PTSD sufferers before treatment commences. The following examples from our clinical practice may help you to understand what will happen and why it is important.

After a trauma, we often try to file away our memory of what happened, putting it to the back of our mind. It's as if we are trying to pack the event away into a box. We then use a little strength to keep the lid tightly closed and try to leave it undisturbed. However, over time, two things happen. Firstly, our strength begins to wane and it becomes more of an effort to keep it sealed (that is, to stop the memories from coming back). Secondly, due to the pressure, the box begins to lose its shape and small cracks begin to appear. What we experience as symptoms (such as memories of the trauma, and having nightmares and disturbed sleep) is like the content of the box spilling out through these cracks. This is usually very frightening, so we try to avoid anything that reminds us of the trauma. We try to stop thinking and talking about what happened and how we felt. In this way, the content of the box becomes a "ghost" which we have learned to fear and which we are terrified of confronting. As part of therapy, we are going to open the box and inspect the content for what it really is. We will talk through what happened and how you felt. We will be inspecting the "ghosts" that have been created and throwing away any maladaptive and distressing beliefs you may have about the event. We find that once the trauma has been dealt with in this manner the symptoms become much less severe and less frequent.

Another analogy talks about the dentist:

When dentists work on a decayed tooth, they don't just slap the filling on top of the decay. If they did, it might be fine for a few weeks or months, but the problems would keep coming back as the tooth continued to deteriorate. Instead, they spend some time drilling and scraping, cleaning out all the decay before putting the tooth back together. This is a very unpleasant and painful process, but we know it is worth going through this short-term pain for the long-term gain. Traumatic memories are a bit like tooth decay. We need to make sure that we have confronted all aspects of the trauma before we try to put the event behind us. We need to give ourselves time to face up to even the worst parts of the experience so that there are no skeletons in the closet to come and haunt us in the future. Like the dentist's drilling, it is a painful process but an important part of recovery.

A final analogy comes from the work of Edna Foa, one of the leading experts in the treatment of PTSD:

Suppose you have eaten a very large and heavy meal that you are unable to digest. This is an uncomfortable feeling. But when you have digested the food, you feel a great sense of relief.

Flashbacks, nightmares, and troublesome thoughts continue to occur because the traumatic event has not been adequately digested. Treatment will help you to start digesting your heavy memories so that they will stop interfering with your daily life. (E. B. Foa and B. O. Rothbaum (1998) *Treating the Trauma of Rape*, p. 160)

Exposure-based treatments are not for everybody. In some cases, if the trauma occurred many years ago and the memories are not causing too much of a problem, it may be best not to drag everything up again. Talk to your therapist about whether this approach would be beneficial for you.

6.2 Therapist-assisted imaginal exposure

Confronting the traumatic memories is a very difficult and painful process, and is best done with the help of an experienced therapist. There are several steps that your therapist will take you through. First, the therapist will provide an explanation of the process, including what you will be doing, why you are doing it, and a reminder on the SUD scale, as well as answering any questions you may have. Next, the therapist will work with you to develop a hierarchy of painful memories in much the same way as you developed a list of goals for your in vivo exposure above. If you have experienced several traumatic events, this may be simple enough. You will need to think about each event and rank them in order of how distressing they are for you to remember. If you have only experienced one event that is causing you problems, you will not need to generate a hierarchy.

The therapist will then ask you to go through the selected event or experience in great detail, starting at the beginning and continuing through to the end, to a point where you felt relatively safe. In order to keep the distress manageable, you may initially be allowed to keep your eyes open, to talk in the past tense (e.g., "I was walking along the path when I saw him coming towards me"), and to skip some of the worst details. For the procedure to be fully effective, however, you will need to build up (perhaps over several sessions) to making your account as vivid and detailed as possible. You will need to talk through the whole event with your eyes closed and in the present tense (e.g., "I am walking along the path and I can see him coming towards me"), since this makes it much more real for you. You will need to be careful that you do not miss any of the details, even (or perhaps especially) the worst ones. Remember that we do not want to leave any skeletons in the closet to come out and worry you in the future. Your therapist will repeat this process many times in the same session and/or in subsequent sessions. However, the more often you go through it the quicker you will recover, so your therapist may tape the session and ask you to listen to the tape every day at home. Again, this is not an easy process, but sticking to the following steps will help you through it and help to ensure that it provides the maximum benefit.

- Step 1: Preparation.
  - Plan an activity to do immediately afterwards (e.g., go for a walk, visit or ring a friend; do an enjoyable absorbing activity, *not* an addictive activity like watching TV or drinking, or an emotional shutdown like hiding away on your own).
  - Choose a private place with no interruptions (take the phone off the hook, let others know you are not to be disturbed).
  - Identify two people you can contact immediately if you need help: keep their phone numbers handy.
  - Briefly relax yourself and try to clear your mind of other thoughts and worries: note down your SUDs level on a piece of paper.
- Step 2: Confront the memory safely.
  - Listen to the tape and try to focus on what is being said: try not to imagine other, more frightening parts – just concentrate on the tape.
  - Equally, try to imagine it happening as if you were experiencing it again. What can you see, hear, smell, touch, taste? What are you feeling and thinking?
  - When reminded to do so on the tape, note your SUDs level. If it is above 90, take a moment to remind yourself where you are; you are safe here and now; you can feel as upset as you need to in the memory.
  - Don't stop the tape in the middle: stick with the memory through to the end.
- Step 3: At the end of the tape, pause and open your eyes.
  - Look around, feel the chair, remind yourself where you are and that you are safe.
  - Note your SUDs level and use an arousal management strategy if necessary (such as breathing control or relaxation).
- Step 4: Process the memory by writing down some or all of:
  - What new (or old) pieces of the memory did you discover or became clearer?
  - Are you now thinking differently about any aspects?
  - What feelings or thoughts are going through your mind right now?
  - What parts of the memory are still too upsetting to remember or accept?
  - What do you still want to change about the event or its aftermath? How can you achieve that?
  - What did you do that you should be able to feel good about?
- Step 5: Relax and do your planned activity.

6.3 Self-directed imaginal exposure

Many people find it difficult to do imaginal exposure to traumatic memories on their own. The process is too painful and they need the support and structure provided by a therapist. However, it is not impossible. Indeed, many people who recover from trauma without professional help are doing just that. They are thinking about the trauma often enough, for long enough, and in enough detail for the memory to lose the worst of its associated distress and for it to become modified and "sorted out" in their own mind. If you are going to attempt the process without a therapist, writing down the memory is often a useful way of doing it. (Indeed, it may be helpful to do this even if you are working with a therapist, although we suggest that you discuss it with him or her first.)

The assignment described below (and the one appearing in the Section 7.1) is adapted from the work of two American psychologists, Patricia Resick and Monica Schnicke. Follow the steps outlined in Section 6.2 when doing the task (substituting the writing for listening to the tape). Make sure you read through those steps carefully and prepare yourself properly before attempting the assignment. Select a suitable time and place so that you have enough privacy and sufficient time to do the task properly.

This task is important in helping you to sort out exactly what happened. The process of "putting the pieces of the jigsaw puzzle together" seems to be very important in getting over the incident. It also works in a similar way to the imaginal exposure described above – the more you confront the painful memories and the bad feelings associated with them, the less powerful and distressing they will become.

The task is to take a sheet of paper – an exercise book would be ideal – and write out a detailed account of exactly what happened. (Interestingly, research suggests that it is much more effective if you write it out by hand rather than using a word processor.) Include as many sensory details as possible (sights, sounds, smells, and so on). Also try to include all the thoughts and feelings that you had during the event. Do not stop yourself from feeling the emotions – although it is painful, that is part of the recovery process. If you become too distressed, you can stop writing for a while but try to continue again as soon as possible. It is important to keep writing until you reach the end (and a point of relative safety), even if that takes a long while. Make a note of your SUDs level in the margin every few minutes – this is important to compare your levels when you reread or rewrite the account. You can rewrite the account as often as you like, putting in more details or different perspectives as they come to you. On days when you do not rewrite the account, read it to yourself at least once. Again, stick to the steps outlined above when you do this. If you have kept a note of the SUDs levels in the margin, you will notice them dropping over time as you repeat the process. You will need to repeat the task until your SUDs are reasonably low throughout (say, a maximum of about 30).

6.4 Exposure: can I cope with it?

Exposure is a very difficult and painful process, but it is the only way to recovery. As we noted above, it is usually not as difficult as you fear it will be and most people get an enormous sense of achievement when they have confronted the memory or other feared situation. If you have read (and practiced) the sections above, you now have several strategies that will help you to manage your anxiety and distress. These are very useful to use both before and after the exposure exercises. If necessary, you can use them during the exposure exercises also, although we recommend that you do this only if you really need to. It is better to confront the full anxiety and allow it to reduce of its own accord than it is to use other strategies to bring it down. However, it is important that you do not feel overwhelmed at any time. Despite the best of intentions (in terms of preparing your hierarchies and confronting only situations or memories that you feel ready for) the anxiety will, sometimes, be greater than you expect. On those occasions, by all means use your coping strategies if necessary.

SECTION 7

7 Cognitive restructuring

One effect that exposure may have is to bring to the surface unhelpful thoughts and beliefs that have arisen as a result of your experiences. In order to recover effectively from the trauma, it may be necessary to challenge those thoughts and beliefs (we call them "cognitions"), and try to replace them with something more rational and realistic. In PTSD, this process is best carried out in conjunction with the process of exposure, modifying the unhelpful cognitions as they arise.

Following a traumatic experience, people may be left with a range of negative thoughts about what happened, as well as about themselves and the world. For example, many people are left feeling vulnerable and insecure. They may think that the world has become a dangerous place and that other people are nasty, cruel, and out to take advantage. Similarly, many people experience feelings of guilt and shame following trauma. They may think that they are bad or evil for acting in the way they did during or after the incident; they may think that what happened was their fault; they may see themselves as weak or inadequate for not coping better. Sometimes, there may be elements of truth in these thoughts. Usually, however, they are completely untrue or, at least, grossly exaggerated. This kind of thinking leads to all sorts of unpleasant emotions such as depression and guilt, anxiety and fear, and anger. An important part of recovery involves identifying those maladaptive thoughts, challenging them, and replacing them with a more realistic view of yourself and the world.

Cognitive restructuring is a procedure whereby people's thoughts, beliefs and interpretations about past experiences are identified and mistakes in thinking are highlighted. For example, it may be that the person is thinking in "black-and-white terms" – seeing things (or other people) as all good or all bad – when in reality the world holds much that is "gray". It may not be perfect, but it's not all bad either. The person may be overgeneralizing (e.g., "no-one can be trusted") or overfocusing on the negatives and minimizing the positives about their situation. They may see one negative thing as confirmation that they are not coping, while ignoring other evidence that they are, in fact, coping quite well. A common problem in PTSD is that people base their interpretations about what happened, themselves, or the world upon only a fragment of the memory (the part that repeatedly comes back) rather than on information that places that aspect in a broader context. Once these faulty thought patterns are discovered, it is the goal of cognitive therapy to replace them with more adaptive, realistic and flexible beliefs. This, of course, includes re-evaluating our experiences and, in particular, the traumatic event. It is a difficult process that can take a lot of hard work, but it can be very effective in minimizing and managing unpleasant emotions.

7.1 The process of cognitive restructuring

As with several other components of treatment, the other Patient Treatment Manuals in this book contain some excellent descriptions of the process of cognitive restructuring. If you are working with a therapist, you may wish to ask him or her to copy some of the relevant sections for you. In this section, we will talk briefly about how to go about identifying and challenging your unhelpful thoughts with specific reference to trauma. A good starting point is to do another assignment – this one follows on well from the exercise discussed in Section 6.3.

The task this time is to write at least one page on what your experience of the event *means* to you. In particular, how has it changed your beliefs, views, and ideas about yourself, other people, and the world? What views or beliefs have been strengthened? Which ones have changed? Try to write something under each of the following headings:

- My beliefs about myself have changed since the trauma in the following ways.
- My beliefs about other people have changed since the trauma in the following ways.
- My beliefs about the world have changed since the trauma in the following ways.

In answering those questions, you may want to think about issues such as how you feel about yourself (self-esteem), your personal safety, trusting others, thoughts about control and power, intimacy with others, what kind of society we live in, etc. Any ways in which you think the event has changed your ideas, thoughts and beliefs.

The next stage is to pick one of the key themes that is leading you to feel an unpleasant emotion. Which one makes you feel angry? Or frightened? Or guilty? Or sad? Try to express it as a single statement of opinion, such as "all men are bad" or "it was all my fault". In particular, look for statements beginning with "I", such as "I'm weak and hopeless" or "I'm not safe anywhere". Write this thought or belief at the top of a clean sheet in your exercise book. Then go through and try to answer the following questions. Some of them may not apply to every thought, but most will – they will help you to re-evaluate whether your thoughts and beliefs are really true.

What is the evidence? Here we want you to become a scientist and really think about the objective evidence for and against the thought. Is it really true? Are you 100% sure? Do the facts of the situation back up what you think or contradict it? Write out all the evidence you can think of for and against the thought. In most cases, you will find that it is not completely true. (Indeed, it may turn out to be completely false.)

What alternative views are there? How do other people think about this? Would other people agree with you? Is there another way of looking at it? Are there other explanations? Try to generate as many alternative explanations as you can and review the evidence for and against them. When you look at it objectively, which explanation is most likely to be correct?

Am I thinking in all-or-nothing, black-and-white terms? Am I using terms like all, always, never? Nothing is all bad or all good, no person is either perfect or worthless. Try to look for a more balanced view, with a more realistic assessment of the situation.

Am I overestimating my responsibility? Things happen for all sorts of complex reasons, many of which we may never understand. Be very careful not to take too much responsibility for things over which you do not have control.

Are my judgments based on how I feel, rather than what is actually happening? If you feel guilty, you are likely to assume things must have been your fault. If you feel frightened, you may assume that you are not safe. If you feel depressed, you may assume that things will never get better. Feelings are not a good basis on which to make rational judgments. Put the feelings to one side for a moment and look for objective evidence.

Am I over-focusing on one aspect and forgetting other aspects? Am I looking only at the negative side and ignoring the neutral or positive things? If we focus only on small parts of the whole picture, we will end up with a very distorted view of reality.

How likely is it? Am I confusing a low probability with a high probability? How likely is it that what you fear will actually happen? Understandably, many trauma survivors fear a recurrence of the event but, realistically, how likely is it?

Am I underestimating what I can do about it? Am I putting myself in the role of helpless victim? What can I do to make things better or safer for myself? Taking some control – doing something about it – is an important part of recovery.

What will happen if I continue to think like this? Is this kind of thinking helping me to recover? Will it help me to live a happy and relaxed life? Are there any benefits to thinking this way? If not, it is worth working hard to try to let go of the irrational negative thoughts.

When you have written an answer to all (or most) of the above questions, go back and reconsider the original thought. Do you still believe it? Is it still a rational statement of reality? If yes, try to go through the above process again – talking to others who can be more objective may help. Do not expect all the negative thoughts to disappear at once – it is hard work and you will need to go through the process many times to shift those ideas. If the thought does not seem entirely rational now, can you come up with a more realistic version of the original thought? Remember that we are not talking here about positive thinking – that is just as unrealistic and very fragile. We do not want to pretend that everything is rosy when it is not. We do not want to minimize what you went through. Equally, we do not want to overemphasize the negatives. Recovery is difficult, but you can make progress; life will not always be safe, but do not exaggerate the dangers. For example, if the original thought was "all men are bad", a more rational alternative may be "some men are bad, but by no means all – most men are actually caring, safe, friendly people". If the original thought was "I'm not safe anywhere" the rational alternative may be "I am safe in most places most of the time – I will be careful not to put myself in dangerous situations, but I do not need to worry constantly about getting hurt again".

SECTION 8

8 Relapse prevention

The final stage of treatment will look at relapse prevention. Recovery is not just about getting better; it is about staying better. Some simple strategies will help you to get through difficult times in the future. There are a few simple points to remember in relapse prevention:

- *Lapses are to be expected from time to time:* When you are reminded of your traumatic experience (such as hearing of a similar event, or experiencing something else frightening) it is natural for you to become a little distressed. This is part of a normal human reaction and, as long as it is not too severe or lasts too long, you should not consider it to be a problem. You can cope with being upset for a while. It becomes a problem if you are not expecting it and you tell yourself that you have "fallen in a heap" or that you are "back to square one". Simply use it as a reminder to practice your coping strategies a bit more for a few days.

- *Be aware of the early warning signs:* Keep an eye on yourself and try to notice when you are not coping so well. The earlier that you can recognize that things are not right, the easier it will be to do something about it. The longer you leave it, the worse it will get, and the more difficult it will become to pull yourself out again. It will be easier to recognize the early warning signs if you are aware of the kinds of things that may precipitate a lapse.

- *Identify high risk situations:* Spend some time thinking about what kinds of things may cause you to become upset – the more prepared you are, the better you will cope. The kinds of things that upset most trauma survivors are powerful reminders or news of similar incidents, an experience similar to the original trauma, and other life stresses such as financial or family problems. What kinds of things may cause you to become upset and think about the trauma again?

- *Generate a plan to cope:* Write down on a card what you will do if and when you are upset again about the trauma. The kinds of things to include are:
  - *Who will you call?* Write down the names and phone numbers.
  - *Physical coping strategies:* Which arousal management strategies worked best for you? Write down one or two (such as breathing control, go for a walk, listen to the relaxation tape) as a reminder to do them.
  - *Cognitive coping strategies:* Write out a coping self-statement that you can use such as "I expect to feel upset when I'm reminded of what happened, but that's okay – I may not like it but I can cope with it. I don't have to make it worse by exaggerating it. Now, what can I do to make myself feel better?" You may wish also to jot down any other strategies that worked well for you such as your favorite distraction technique or thought stopping.
  - *Behavioral coping strategies:* Write down one or two things you can do to get you back on track – visit a friend, go to a movie, get involved in an engrossing hobby or task.

- *Be positive:* Remind yourself that you expected this from time to time and that you will get over it quickly. Try to view it as an opportunity to practice your skills and become a stronger person.

- *Get professional help if necessary:* No matter how well you have recovered from the original trauma, sometimes a relapse may be just too much for you to cope with alone. Don't hesitate to get some professional help if necessary. It does not mean that you are weak or that you are back to square one, simply that you need some extra support to get over a difficult time. It may require only one or two sessions.

SECTION 9

9 Concluding comments

If you have worked your way through this Manual, with or without a therapist, you will have come a long way to recovering from an experience that changed your life. As we noted at the beginning, you will never be quite the same person again. But over the course of your recovery you have learnt many new skills that will stand you in good stead in the future. Importantly, you have faced one of the worst things that life can throw at you and you have come through it. You have survived. Give yourself a pat on the back and remember that, if you can deal with this, you can deal with almost anything.

SECTION 10

10 Recommended resources

The following books are available from most large bookstores, many smaller ones, and some news-stands. If in doubt, ask whether the book can be ordered. We also suggest that you use your local library to gain access to some of these books. When you read these or any similar books on the management of anxiety, remember that they are best regarded as guidelines only. Be critical in both a positive and negative sense when reading these books, so that you get what is best for you out of them. Most of these books are inexpensive.

10.1 Books

Allen JG. (1999) *Coping With Trauma: A Guide To Self Understanding.* Washington, DC: American Psychiatric Press.

Herbert C and Wetmore A. (1999) *Overcoming Traumatic Stress: A Self Help Guide Using Cognitive Behavioral Techniques.* London: Robinson Publishing Ltd.

Matsakis A. (1996) *I Can't Get Over It: A Handbook For Trauma Survivors,* 2nd Edition. Oakland CA: New Harbinger Publications.

Matsakis A. (1998) *Trust After Trauma: A Guide To Relationships For Survivors And Those Who Love Them.* Oakland CA: New Harbinger Publications.

Rosenbloom D, Williams MB and Watkins B. (1999) *Life After Trauma: A Workbook For Healing.* New York: Guilford.

Schiraldi GR. (2000) *The Posttraumatic Stress Disorder Sourcebook.* Lincolnwood, IL: Lowell House Publications.

10.2 Internet resources

There is also considerable information available on the internet. As a starting point, the following websites contain a great deal of useful information for both therapists and survivors of trauma:

US National Center for PTSD: www.ncptsd.org

David Balwyn's trauma information pages: www.trauma-pages.com

International Society for Traumatic Stress Studies: www.istss.org

Australian Centre for Posttraumatic Mental Health: www.acpmh.unimelb.edu.au

28

Conclusions

Part of this book has been quite conventional. The reviews of the syndromes and treatments in relation to panic and agoraphobia, social phobia, specific phobias, obsessive–compulsive disorder, generalized anxiety disorder and posttraumatic stress disorder are brief, succinct overviews designed for busy clinicians. The discussion of general issues in the etiology and treatment of the anxiety disorders is also essential information for the practicing clinician. The Clinician Guides and the Patient Treatment Manuals are, however, quite unusual. These Guides and Manuals need to be placed in context.

There is an art and a science to good medical practice. Because the science tends to predominate, the art of treatment is seldom discussed, either at a general or a specific level. Elsewhere, we have called attention to the need for the elements of good clinical care to be made explicit. Good clinical care needs to be taught to trainee psychiatrists and clinical psychologists for use with patients for whom there is no specific remedy immediately applicable to their disorder (Andrews, 1993a). This book is different. It is about treating persons with chronic anxiety disorders who, if expertly treated with specific remedies, can be expected to recover. This recovery has been made possible by the scientific advances that have occurred in our understanding of the treatment of the anxiety disorders. Much of this book is focused on the cognitive behavioral treatments simply because the instructions for prescribing medications are relatively simple and, courtesy of advertising by the pharmaceutical industry, do not need repeating in a book on the treatment of anxiety disorders. The cognitive behavioral treatments are less well known and, being both nonproprietary and not for profit, are neither as widely promoted nor as readily available as are the drug therapies.

There is a greater problem. The amount of evidence for the efficacy of psycho-therapy is less plentiful than the evidence that is routinely provided by the pharmaceutical industry to the national regulatory authorities in each country. This evidence is provided as part of the process of having products cleared for marketing and, in many countries, for subsidy. In the first edition of this book, much of the evidence about the efficacy of cognitive behavioral therapy came from trials in which the progress of treated groups were compared to their own pretreated status, or else were compared to the progress of wait-list or no treatment control groups.

While aggregating evidence of effectiveness from such trials can be satisfactory, in the final analysis evidence from randomized placebo controlled trials is necessary. This type of trial is necessary to control for the three factors that can produce improvement even when the treatment being studied has no specific value. The first of these factors is spontaneous remission of the disorder over the duration of treatment and assessment. Spontaneous remission is likely to be more important when this duration extends over months or years. The next factor is regression to the mean. Persons with chronic and fluctuating disorders seek treatment when their symptoms are most disabling and, with the passage of time and even in the absence of treatment, these symptoms will improve to their average level, thus imitating treatment-related benefit. The last of these confounds is the placebo effect, which identifies the improvement that occurs due to the morale-raising effect of seeing an interested clinician and expecting to benefit from a notionally effective treatment. In a randomized controlled design, a placebo control group controls for all these factors whereas wait-list or no-treatment control groups satisfy only the first two.

Randomized placebo controlled trials are the standard method by which the efficacy of a new treatment is assessed. The most informative design is a placebo controlled comparison trial in which the new treatment is compared with a placebo and with a proven and accepted treatment. Even so, the results of a single trial should be taken cautiously, because – even given the control – chance factors might have contributed to the improvement observed in the treated group. Once replicated by independent scientists, acceptance of the finding depends on two other factors. The first factor is the power of the treatment as measured by the superiority over the placebo treatment, for this power indicates the likely robustness of the finding. The second factor is the number of subjects in the trials, for this will indicate the probability that the results will be applicable to other subjects. These issues are not completely independent and stronger treatments are usually accepted on evidence from fewer subjects, given that the proviso of independent replication is met.

The number of replication studies in the literature varies with the length of time a treatment has been available, the funds for such research, and the ease of mounting a placebo controlled trial. For example, when alprazolam was introduced for panic disorder, the manufacturer funded a series of multicenter and multinational placebo and comparison trials of the drug. The placebo, an inert replica tablet, was simple to manufacture, measurement was standardized, and the results at the end of treatment were clear. In contrast, there are relatively few multicenter placebo controlled trials of cognitive behavioral therapies in the anxiety disorders, in part because there is no economic imperative that necessitates funding of such trials, and in part because of the greater difficulty of designing an ethical placebo. The ideal placebo treatment for a nondrug treatment is continued good clinical care of persons in the control group over the duration of the trial – good clinical care in which the clinician provides support and advice about how the patient should deal with their problems, but advice that stops short of recommending any of the components of the nondrug treatment being investigated. Trials in which a nondrug therapy are compared to an established drug therapy that is in turn compared to a placebo tablet coupled with continuing clinical management are also satisfactory (e.g., Elkin et al., 1989; Marks et al., 1993). These trials free the investigators from the more difficult task of having to mount a nondrug placebo condition.

Drug therapies are regulated in most countries and approved for use only after being assessed for efficacy and safety. There have been calls to regulate the nondrug therapies (Sartorius et al., 1993) and, once regulation occurs, the demands for acceptable evidence about efficacy and safety will follow. We identified the English language randomized placebo controlled trials of nondrug therapies for anxiety disorders (Andrews et al., 1992) to determine whether they would be likely to satisfy an interested regulatory agency. Bearing in mind that acceptance depends not only on independent replication but also on strength of benefit and number of subjects, we used the data from a traditional power analysis (80% chance of a significant result at $p < 0.5$) to set an arbitrary threshold to identify registerable treatments at the equivalent of four minimum-sized significant trials or better. This arbitrary threshold meant that if the average superiority over placebo for a particular treatment was 0.5 effect size or standard deviation (SD) units, then the number of subjects in the treated groups in the individual trials should total more than 200. Whereas, if the average effect size was 1.0, then 52 subjects would be required; and, if the average effect size was 2.0, then the total number of subjects required need only exceed 16. At the time of the first edition of this book it was important to show that the cognitive behavioral therapies (CBTs) would, if treated like drug therapies, be suitable for registration and subsidy.

CBT for three anxiety disorders met such stringent criteria (Andrews, 1996b):
Panic disorder/agoraphobia: We located five randomized controlled studies from five independent research groups (Chambless et al., 1982; Telch et al., 1985; Klosko et al., 1990; Beck et al., 1992; Marks et al., 1993) that showed the CBTs in panic disorder and agoraphobia to be an average of 1.26 SD units superior to placebo treatment. The content of the therapies varied, covering aspects of behavioral control of anxiety, cognitive therapy of panic, exposure to feared situations, and to the experience of panic symptoms. The total number of

patients in the active treatment groups was 73, double the number required to meet the threshold requirements at this level of effectiveness.

Generalized anxiety disorder: We located four randomized controlled trials in generalized anxiety disorder that compared CBT with an appropriate placebo condition (Borkovec et al., 1987; Lindsay et al., 1987; Power et al., 1989, 1990). The treatments were well defined and the cognitive therapies were based on the procedures described by Beck and Emery (1979) but also included relaxation training and graded exposure where appropriate. The average effect size from the 57 subjects in the four trials was 2.07, considerably above the threshold required.

Obsessive–compulsive disorder: Four randomized placebo-controlled trials were identified (Roper et al., 1975; Marks et al., 1980, 1988, Lindsay et al., 1997) in which graded exposure, coupled with response prevention, was utilized as the specific treatment. The mean effect size was 1.81, and the number of patients in the treatment groups was 33, very few indeed but above the threshold required.

There is supporting evidence that, unlike the drug remedies, the benefits of these treatments are stable and continue for months or years after treatment has concluded. The number of studies and the number of subjects in the studies is small compared with the amount of evidence for effectiveness of drugs in these disorders. While this difference in the number of studies is the result of both the money available and the ease of doing the drug trials, it remains important that the proponents of the nondrug therapies see that more studies are done. It will be clear from the chapters of this second edition that more research has been done and that now there is sufficient evidence for the efficacy of CBT in social phobia and posttraumatic stress disorder as well as in panic, generalized anxiety disorder and obsessive–compulsive disorder.

That CBT works is established (Nathan and Gorman, 1998). The larger question is whether it is more cost effective than the alternative therapies. Hofmann and Barlow (1999) considered such data to be lacking but offered a model that compared CBT in anxiety disorders to the costs of three different drug therapies. In the initial months the costs of CBT were greater but, as no further treatment was required, the costs of the repeated visits to the doctor and the costs of continuing the medications meant that within the year the costs of drug treatments exceeded the costs of CBT. When a treatment is both more effective and cheaper it is said to dominate the alternative treatments. Our modeling for the clinical practice guidelines for the Royal Australian and New Zealand College of Psychiatrists is showing, exactly as we showed in depression (Andrews et al., 2000), that CBT for panic disorder/agoraphobia dominates the drug therapies in that it is both cheaper and more effective.

There is both an art and a science to good clinical practice. The scientific information from the randomized placebo controlled trials has been summarized in the chapters on treatment and operationalized in the Patient Treatment Manuals. Although the content of these Manuals is based on research, the form of the Manuals – how the techniques are sequenced, how each technique is presented and reinforced with patient exercises – is the result of our clinical experience over 20 years of treating patients with these disorders. Thus the manuals contain both art and science.

The Clinician Guides are again different. As new staff members joined the Clinical Research Unit for Anxiety Disorders and took responsibility for conducting these treatment programs, we discovered an increase in their effectiveness as therapists that reached an asymptote after they had treated their third or fourth group. Discussing these findings, we concluded that it was not their technical competence at guiding patients through the Manuals that had changed but rather their ability to recognize and manage difficulties that individual patients experienced with aspects of the program. For this reason we began to write a series of Clinician Guides.

Like the Patient Treatment Manuals, these Clinician Guides were initially written to a set design. However, we soon realized that, while all difficulties were at times evident with patients regardless of diagnosis, there were domains of difficulty particularly associated with certain disorders. Furthermore, it became evident that the way of presenting the solutions differed depending on the patient's principal diagnosis. The Clinician Guides in this book are therefore both specific and general; each is written from the viewpoint of a clinician treating only patients with that particular diagnosis but each contains information of general importance in the treatment of patients with any of the anxiety disorders. Thus the Clinician Guides are our view of the art of clinical practice.

References

Abramowitz JS, Foa EB. (1998) Worries and obsessions in individuals with obsessive–compulsive disorder with and without comorbid generalized anxiety disorder. *Behaviour Research and Therapy*, **36**, 695–700.

Adler CM, Craske MG, Kirschenbaum S, Barlow DH. (1989) "Fear of panic": an investigation of its role in panic occurrence, phobic avoidance, and treatment outcome. *Behaviour Research and Therapy*, **27**, 391–6.

Agras SW, Sylvester D, Oliveau D. (1969) The epidemiology of common fears and phobias. *Comprehensive Psychiatry*, **10**, 439–47.

Akiskal HS. (1998) Toward a definition of generalized anxiety disorder as an anxious temperament type. *Acta Psychiatrica Scandinavica*, **98** (Suppl. 393), 66–73.

Alnaes R, Torgersen S. (1988a) DSM-III symptom disorders (axis I) and personality disorders (axis II) in an outpatient population. *Acta Psychiatrica Scandinavica*, **78**, 348–55.

Alnaes R, Torgersen S. (1988b) The relationship between DSMIII symptom disorders (axis I) and personality disorders (axis II) in an outpatient population. *Acta Psychiatrica Scandinavica*, **78**, 485–92.

Amies PL, Gelder MG, Shaw PM. (1983) Social phobia: a comparative clinical study. *British Journal of Psychiatry*, **142**, 174–9.

Amir N, Foa EB, Coles ME. (1998) Automatic activation and strategic avoidance of threat-relevant information in social phobia. *Journal of Abnormal Psychology*, **107**, 285–90.

Anderson DJ, Noyes R, Crowe RR. (1984) A comparison of panic disorder and generalized anxiety disorder. *American Journal of Psychiatry*, **141**, 572–5.

Andrews G. (1981) A prospective study of life events and psychological symptoms. *Psychological Medicine*, **77**, 795–801.

Andrews G. (1988) Stressful life events and anxiety. In Burrows G, Noyes R, Roth M (Eds), *Handbook of Anxiety*, Vol. 2: *Classification, Etiological Factors and Associated Disorders*. Amsterdam: Elsevier.

Andrews G. (1990a) Neurosis, personality and cognitive behaviour therapy. In McNaughton N, Andrews G (Eds), *Anxiety*. Dunedin: Otago University Press.

Andrews G. (1990b) Classification of neurotic disorders. *Journal of the Royal Society of Medicine*, **83**, 606–7.

Andrews G. (1990c) England: an innovative community psychiatric service. *Lancet*, **335**, 1087–8.

Andrews G. (1991) Anxiety, personality and anxiety disorders. *International Review of Psychiatry*, **3**, 293–302.

Andrews G. (1993a) The essential psychotherapies. *British Journal of Psychiatry*, **162**, 447–51.

Andrews G. (1993b) Panic and generalized anxiety disorders. *Current Opinion in Psychiatry*, **6**, 191–4.

Andrews G. (1996a) Comorbidity and the general neurotic syndrome. *British Journal of Psychiatry*, **168** (Suppl. 30), 76–84.

Andrews G. (1996b) Talk that works: the rise of cognitive behaviour therapy. *British Medical Journal*, **313**, 1501–2.

Andrews G. (2000) The anxiety disorder inclusion and exclusion criteria in DSM-IV and ICD-10. *Current Opinion in Psychiatry*, **13**, 139–41.

Andrews G, Craig A. (1988) Prediction of outcome after treatment for stuttering. *British Journal of Psychiatry*, **153**, 236–40.

Andrews G, Moran C. (1988) Exposure treatment of agoraphobia with panic attacks: are drugs essential? In Hand I, Wittchen H-U (Eds), *Panic and Phobias II. Treatments and Variables Affecting Course and Outcome.* Heidelberg: Springer-Verlag.

Andrews G, Peters L. (1998) Psychometric properties of the CIDI. *Social Psychiatry and Psychiatric Epidemiology*, **33**, 80–8.

Andrews G, Tennant CC, Hewson D, Vaillant G. (1978) Life event stress, social support, coping style and risk of psychological impairment. *Journal of Nervous and Mental Disease*, **16**, 307–16.

Andrews G, Pollock C, Stewart G. (1989) The determination of defense style by questionnaire. *Archives of General Psychiatry*, **46**, 455–60.

Andrews G, Neilson MD, Hunt C, Stewart GW, Kiloh LG. (1990a) Diagnosis, personality and the long-term outcome of depression. *British Journal of Psychiatry*, **157**, 13–18.

Andrews G, Stewart G, Allen R, Henderson, AS. (1990b) The genetics of six neurotic disorders: a twin study. *Journal of Affective Disorders*, **19**, 23–9.

Andrews G, Stewart G, Morris-Yates A, Holt P, Henderson S. (1990c) Evidence for a general neurotic syndrome. *British Journal of Psychiatry*, **157**, 6–12.

Andrews G, Crino RD, Hunt C, Lampe L, Page A. (1992) *A List of Essential Psychotherapies.* Proceedings of the Annual Conference of the Royal Australian and New Zealand College of Psychiatrists. Canberra: Royal Australian and New Zealand College of Psychiatrists.

Andrews G, Page AC, Neilson MD. (1993a) Sending your teenagers away: controlled stress decreases neurotic vulnerability. *Archives of General Psychiatry*, **50**, 585–9.

Andrews G, Singh M, Bond, M. (1993b) The Defense Style Questionnaire. *Journal of Nervous and Mental Disease*, **181**, 246–56.

Andrews G, Hall W, Teesson M, Henderson S. (1999a) *The Mental Health of Australians.* Canberra: Commonwealth Department of Health and Aged Care.

Andrews G, Slade T, Peters L. (1999b) Classification in psychiatry: ICD-10 versus DSM-IV. *British Journal of Psychiatry*, **174**, 3–5.

Andrews G, Henderson S, Hall W. (2001a) Prevalence, comorbidity, disability and service utilisation: an overview of the Australian national mental health survey. *British Journal of Psychiatry*, **178**, 145–53.

Andrews G, Issakidis C, Carter G. (2001b) The shortfall in mental health service utilization. *British Journal of Psychiatry*, **179**, 417–25.

Andrews G, Sanderson K, Corry J, Lapsley HM. (2000) Using epidemiological data to model efficiency in reducing the burden of depression. *Journal of Mental Health Policy and Economics*.

APA (American Psychiatric Association). (1980) *Diagnostic and Statistical Manual of Mental Disorders*, 3rd Edition (DSM-III). Washington, DC: American Psychiatric Association.

APA (American Psychiatric Association). (1987) *Diagnostic and Statistical Manual of Mental Disorders*, 3rd Edition, Revised (DSM-III-R). Washington, DC: American Psychiatric Association.

APA (American Psychiatric Association). (1994) *Diagnostic and Statistical Manual of Mental Disorders*, 4th Edition (DSM-IV). Washington, DC: American Psychiatric Association.

Arntz A, van den Hout M. (1996) Psychological treatments of panic disorder without agoraphobia: cognitive therapy versus applied relaxation. *Behaviour Research and Therapy*, **34**, 113–21.

Aronson TA, Logue CM. (1987) On the longitudinal course of panic disorder: development history and predictors of phobic complications. *Comprehensive Psychiatry*, **28**, 344–55.

Arts W, Hoogduin K, Schaap C, De Haan E. (1993) Do patients suffering from obsessions alone differ from other obsessive compulsives? *Behaviour Research and Therapy*, **31**, 119–32.

Baillie AJ, Lampe LA. (1998) Avoidant personality disorder: empirical support for DSM-IV revisions. *Journal of Personality Disorders*, **12**, 23–30.

Bakker A, van Balkom AJLM, Spinhoven P, Blaauw BMJW, van Dyck R. (1998) Follow-up on the treatment of panic disorder with or without agoraphobia: a quantitative review. *Journal of Nervous and Mental Disease*, **186**, 414–19.

Baldwin D, Bobes J, Stein DJ, Scharwachter I, Faure M. (1999) Paroxetine in social phobia/social anxiety disorder. *British Journal of Psychiatry*, **175**, 120–6.

Ballenger JC, Davidson JRT, Lecrubier Y, Nutt DJ, Bobes J, Beidel DC, Ono Y, Westenberg HGM. (1998) Consensus statement on social anxiety disorder from the International Consensus Group on Anxiety and Depression. *Journal of Clinical Psychiatry*, **59** (Suppl. 17), 54–60.

Bandelow B. (1995) Assessing the efficacy of treatments for panic disorder and agoraphobia: II. The Panic and Agoraphobia Scale. *International Clinical Psychopharmacology*, **10**, 73–81.

Bandelow B, Sievert K, Roethemeyer M, Hajak G, Ruther E. (1995). What treatments do patients with panic disorder and agoraphobia get? *European Archives of Psychiatry & Clinical Neuroscience*, **245**, 165–71.

Bandura A. (1977) Self-efficacy: toward a unifying theory of behavioural change. *Psychological Review*, **84**, 191–215.

Barlow DH. (1988) *Anxiety and Its Disorders: The Nature and Treatment of Anxiety and Panic*. New York: Guilford.

Barlow DH. (1997). Cognitive-behavioral therapy for panic disorder: current status. *Journal of Clinical Psychiatry*, **58** (Suppl. 2), 32–7.

Barlow DH. (2000) Unraveling the mysteries of anxiety and its disorders from the perspective of emotion theory. *American Psychologist*, **51**, 1247–63.

Barlow DH, Craske MG. (1988) The phenomenology of panic. In Rachman S, Maser JD (Eds),

Panic: Psychological Perspectives. Hillsdale, NJ: Lawrence Erlbaum.

Barlow DH, Wincze J. (1998) DSM-IV and beyond: what is generalized anxiety disorder. *Acta Psychiatrica Scandinavica*, **98** (Suppl. 393), 23–9.

Barlow DH, O'Brien GT, Last CG. (1984) Couples treatment of agoraphobia. *Behavior Therapy*, **15**, 41–58.

Barlow DH, Blanchard EB, Vermilyea JA, Vermilyea BB, Di Nardo PA. (1986a) Generalized anxiety and generalized anxiety disorder: description and reconceptualization. *American Journal of Psychiatry*, **143**, 40–4.

Barlow DH, Di Nardo PA, Vermilyea BB, Vermilyea JA, Blanchard EB. (1986b) Comorbidity and depression among the anxiety disorders: issues in classification and diagnosis. *Journal of Nervous and Mental Disease*, **174**, 63–72.

Barlow DH, Craske MG, Cerny JA, Klosko JS. (1989) Behavioral treatment of panic disorder. *Behavior Therapy*, **20**, 261–82.

Barlow DH, Rapee RM, Brown TA (1992) Behavioral treatment of generalized anxiety disorder. *Behavior Therapy*, **23**, 551–70.

Barlow DH, Esler JL, Vitali AE. (1998) Psychosocial treatments for panic disorders, phobias, and generalized anxiety disorder. In Nathan PE, Gorman JM (Eds), *A Guide to Treatments that Work.* New York: Oxford University Press.

Basoglu M, Lax T, Kasvikis Y, Marks IM. (1988) Predictors of improvement in obsessive–compulsive disorder. *Journal of Anxiety Disorders*, **2**, 299–317.

Baumgarten HG, Grozdanovic Z. (1998) The role of serotonin in obsessive–compulsive disorder. *British Journal of Psychiatry*, **173** (Suppl. 35), 13–20.

Beck AT. (1976) *Cognitive Therapy and the Emotional Disorders.* New York: International Universities Press.

Beck AT. (1988) Cognitive approaches to panic disorder. In Rachman S, Maser JD (Eds), *Panic: Psychological Perspectives.* Hillsdale, NJ: Lawrence Erlbaum.

Beck AT, Emery G. (1979) *Cognitive Therapy of Anxiety and Phobic Disorders.* Philadelphia, PA: Center for Cognitive Therapy.

Beck AT, Ward CH, Mendelson M, Mock J, Erbaugh J. (1961) An inventory for measuring depression. *Archives of General Psychiatry*, **4**, 53–63.

Beck AT, Rush AJ, Shaw BF, Emery G. (1979) *Cognitive Therapy of Depression.* New York: Guilford Press.

Beck AT, Emery G, Greenberg R. (1985) *Anxiety Disorders and Phobias: A Cognitive Perspective.* New York: Basic Books.

Beck AT, Epstein N, Brown G, Steer RA. (1988) An inventory for measuring clinical anxiety: Psychometric properties. *Journal of Consulting and Clinical Psychology*, **56**, 893–7.

Beck AT, Sokol L, Clark DM, Berchick R, Wright F. (1992) A crossover of focused cognitive therapy for panic disorder. *American Journal of Psychiatry*, **149**, 778–83.

Beidel DC. (1998) Social anxiety disorder: etiology and early clinical presentation. *Journal of Clinical Psychiatry*, **59**, 27–31.

Bekker MHJ. (1996) Agoraphobia and gender: a review. *Clinical Psychology Review*, **16**, 129–46.

Bellodi L, Scuito G, Diafera G, Ronchi P, Smereldi E. (1992) Psychiatric disorders in the families of patients with obsessive compulsive disorder. *Psychiatry Research*, **42**, 111–20.

Benson H. (1976) *The Relaxation Response.* London: Collins & Sons.

Bernadt MW, Silverstone P, Singleton W. (1980) Behavioral and subjective effects of beta-adrenergic blockade in phobic subjects. *British Journal of Psychiatry,* **137,** 452–7.

Bernstein DA, Allen GJ. (1969) Fear Survey Schedule (II): normative data and factor analysis. *Behaviour Research and Therapy,* **7,** 403–7.

Berrios GE. (1985) Obsessional disorders during the nineteenth century: terminology and classificatory issues. In Bynum WF, Porter R, Shepherd M. (Eds), *The Anatomy of Madness,* Vol. 1, *People and Ideas.* London, New York: Tavistock Publications.

Bienvenu OJ, Eaton WW. (1998) The epidemiology of blood–injection–injury phobia. *Psychological Medicine,* **28,** 1129–36.

Bienvenu OJ, Nestadt G, Eaton WW. (1998) Characterizing generalized anxiety: temporal and symptomatic thresholds. *Journal of Nervous and Mental Disease,* **186,** 51–6.

Biran M, Wilson GT. (1981) Treatment of phobic disorders using cognitive and exposure methods: a self-efficacy analysis. *Journal of Consulting and Clinical Psychology,* **49,** 886–99.

Biran M, Augusto F, Wilson GT. (1981) In vivo exposure vs cognitive restructuring in the treatment of scriptophobia. *Behaviour Research and Therapy,* **19,** 525–32.

Black A. (1974) The natural history of obsessional neurosis. In Beech HR (Ed), *Obsessional States.* London: Methuen.

Black DW, Noyes R. (1990). Co-morbidity and obsessive compulsive disorder. In Masser JD, Cloninger CR (Eds), *Comorbidity of Mood and Anxiety Disorders.* Washington DC: American Psychiatric Press.

Black DW, Noyes R, Goldstein RB, Blum N. (1992) A family study of obsessive compulsive disorder. *Archives of General Psychiatry,* **49,** 362–8.

Black DW, Noyes R, Pfohl B, Goldstein RB, Blum N. (1993) Personality disorder in obsessive-compulsive volunteers, well comparison subjects and their first degree relatives. *Archives of General Psychiatry,* **150,** 1226–32.

Blake DD, Weathers F, Nagy LM, Kaloupek DG, Klauminzer G, Charney DS, Keane TM. (1995) The development of a clinician administered PTSD scale. *Journal of Traumatic Stress,* **8,** 75–90.

Blanchard EB, Hickling EJ, Mitnick N, Taylor AE, Loos WR, Buckley TC. (1995) The impact of severity of physical injury and perception of life threat in the development of posttraumatic stress disorder in motor vehicle accident victims. *Behaviour Research and Therapy,* **33,** 529–34.

Blanchard EB, Hickling EJ, Taylor AE, Loos WR, Forneris CA, Jaccard J. (1996a) Who develops PTSD from motor vehicle accidents? *Behaviour Research and Therapy,* **34,** 1–10.

Blanchard EB, Jones-Alexander J, Buckley TC, Forneris CA. (1996b) Psychometric properties of the PTSD Checklist (PCL). *Behaviour Research and Therapy,* **34,** 669–73.

Blazer D, Hughes D, George LK. (1987) Stressful life events and the onset of a generalized anxiety syndrome. *American Journal of Psychiatry,* **144,** 1178–83.

Blazer DG, Hughes D., George LK, Swartz M, Boyer R. (1991).Generalized anxiety disorder. In Robins LN, Regier DA (Eds), *Psychiatric Disorders in America.* New York: The Free Press.

Bobes J. (1998) How is recovery from social anxiety disorder defined? *Journal of Clinical Psychiatry,* **59** (Suppl. 17), 12–16.

Boerner RJ, Moeller H-J. (1997) The value of selective serotonin re-uptake inhibitors (SSRIs) in the treatment of panic disorder with and without agoraphobia. *International Journal of Psychiatry in Clinical Practice*, 1, 59–67.

Bonn JA, Readhead CPA, Timmons BH. (1984) Enhanced behavioral response in agoraphobic patients pretreated with breathing retraining. *Lancet*, ii, 665–9.

Boone ML, McNeil DW, Masia CL, Turk CL, Carter LE, Ries BJ, Lewin MR. (1999) Multimodal comparisons of social phobia subtypes and avoidant personality disorder. *Journal of Anxiety Disorders*, 13, 271–92.

Borkovec TD, Costello E (1993) Efficacy of applied relaxation and cognitive-behavioral therapy and the treatment of generalized anxiety disorder. *Journal of Consulting and Clinical Psychology*, 61, 611–19.

Borkovec TD, Whisman MA. (1996) Psychosocial treatment for generalized anxiety disorder. In Mavissakalian MR, Prien RF (Eds), *Long-term Treatments of Anxiety Disorders*. Washington, DC: American Psychiatric Press, pp. 171–99.

Borkovec TD, Robinson E, Pruzinsky T, Depree JA. (1983) Preliminary exploration of worry: some characteristics and processes. *Behaviour Research and Therapy*, 21, 9–16.

Borkovec TD, Mathews AM, Chambers A, Ebrahimi S, Lytle R, Nelson R. (1987) The effects of relaxation training with cognitive or nondirective therapy and the role of relaxation-induced anxiety in the treatment of generalized anxiety. *Journal of Consulting and Clinical Psychology*, 55, 883–8.

Borkovec TD, Ray WJ, Stoeber J. (1998) Worry: a cognitive phenomenon intimately linked to affective, physiological, and interpersonal behavioral processes. *Cognitive Therapy and Research*, 22, 561–76.

Bouchard S, Pelletier MH, Gauthier JG, Côté Laberge B. (1997) The assessment of panic using self-report: a comprehensive survey of validated instruments. *Journal of Anxiety Disorders*, 11, 89–111.

Boudewyns PA, Hyer L. (1990) Physiological response to combat memories and preliminary outcome in Vietnam veteran PTSD patients treated with direct therapeutic exposure. *Behavior Therapy*, 21, 63–87.

Bourdon KH, Boyd JH, Rae DS, Burns BJ, Thompson JW, Locke BZ. (1988) Gender differences in phobias: results of the ECA community survey. *Journal of Anxiety Disorders*, 2, 227–41.

Bourque P, Ladouceur R. (1980) An investigation of various performance-based treatments with agoraphobics. *Behaviour Research and Therapy*, 18, 161–70.

Bouton ME, Kenney FA, Rosengard C. (1990) State-dependent fear extinction with two benzodiazepine tranquilizers. *Behavioral Neuroscience*, 104, 44–55.

Bouwer C, Stein DJ. (1998) Use of the selective serotonin reuptake inhibitor citalopram in the treatment of generalized social phobia. *Journal of Affective Disorders*, 49, 79–82.

Bowman D, Scogin F, Floyd M, Patton E, Gist L. (1997). Efficacy of self-examination therapy in the treatment of generalized anxiety disorder. *Journal of Counseling Psychology*, 44, 267–73.

Boyd J. (1986) Use of mental health services for the treatment of panic disorder. *American Journal of Psychiatry*, 143, 1569–74.

Brantley PJ, Mehan DJ, Ames SC, Jones GN. (1999) Minor stressors and generalized anxiety disorder among low-income patients attending primary care clinics. *Journal of Nervous and*

Mental Disease, **187**, 435–40.

Brawman-Mintzer O, Lydiard B, Emmanual N, Payeur R, Johnson M, Roberts J, Jarrell MP, Ballenger JC. (1993). Psychiatric comorbidity in patients with generalized anxiety disorder. *American Journal of Psychiatry*, **150**, 1216–18.

Breier A, Charney DS, Heninger GR. (1985) The diagnostic validity of anxiety disorders and their relationship to depressive illness. *American Journal of Psychiatry*, **142**, 787–97.

Breitholtz E, Johansson B, Öst LG. (1999) Cognitions in generalized anxiety disorder and panic disorder patients. A prospective approach. *Behaviour Research and Therapy*, **37**, 533–44.

Bremner JD, Southwick SM, Charney DS. (1999) The neurobiology of posttraumatic stress disorder: an integration of animal and human research. In Saigh PA, Bremner JD (Eds), *Posttraumatic Stress Disorder: A Comprehensive Text*. Needham Heights, MA: Allyn & Bacon, pp. 103–43.

Breslau N, Davis GC. (1985) Further evidence on the doubtful validity of generalized anxiety disorder (letter). *Psychiatry Research*, **16**, 177–9.

Breslau N, Davis GC, Andreski P, Peterson EL, Schultz LR. (1997) Sex differences in posttraumatic stress disorder. *Archives in General Psychiatry*, **54**, 1044–8.

Breslau N, Chilcoat S, Kessler R, Davis G. (1999) Previous exposure to trauma and PTSD effects of subsequent trauma. *American Journal of Psychiatry*, **156**, 902–7.

Brom D, Kleber RJ, Defares PB. (1989) Brief psychotherapy for post traumatic stress disorders. *Journal of Consulting and Clinical Psychology*, **57**, 607–12.

Brown GW, Harris TO. (1978) *Social Origins of Depression: A Study of Psychiatric Disorder in Women*. London: Tavistock.

Brown TA, Barlow DH. (1992). Comorbidity among anxiety disorders: implications for treatment and DSM-IV. *Journal of Consulting and Clinical Psychology*, **60**, 835–44.

Brown TA, Moras K, Zinbarg RE, Barlow DH. (1993) Diagnostic and symptom distinguishability of generalized anxiety disorder and obsessive-compulsive disorder. *Behavior Therapy*, **24**, 227–40.

Brown TA, DiNardo PA, Barlow DH. (1994) *Anxiety Disorders Interview Schedule for DSM-IV (ADIS-IV)*. Albany, NY: Graywind.

Brown TA, Marten PA, Barlow DH. (1995) Discriminant validity of the symptoms constituting the DSM-III-R and DSM-IV associated symptom criterion of generalized anxiety disorder. *Journal of Anxiety Disorders*, **9**, 317–28.

Brown TA, Chorpita BF, Korotitsch W, Barlow DH. (1997) Psychometric properties of the Depression Anxiety Stress Scales (DASS) in clinical samples. *Behaviour Research and Therapy*, **35**, 79–89.

Brown TA, Chorpita BF, Barlow DH. (1998) Structural relationships among dimensions of the DSM-IV anxiety and mood disorders and dimensions of negative affect, positive affect, and autonomic arousal. *Journal of Abnormal Psychology*, **107**, 179–92.

Bruch MA, Heimberg RA, Hope DA. (1991) States of mind model and cognitive change in treated social phobics. *Cognitive Therapy and Research*, **15**, 429–41.

Bryant RA, Harvey AG. (1997) Acute stress disorder: a critical review of diagnostic issues. *Clinical Psychology Review*, **17**, 757–73.

Bryant RA, Harvey AG, Dang ST, Sackville T, Basten C. (1998) Treatment of acute stress disorder: a comparison of cognitive behavior therapy and supportive counseling. *Journal of Consulting and Clinical Psychology*, **66**, 862–6.

Bryant RA, Sackville T, Dang ST, Moulds M, Guthrie R. (1999). Treating acute stress disorder: an evaluation of cognitive behavior therapy and supporting counseling techniques. *American Journal of Psychiatry*, **156**, 1780–6.

Burgess IS, Jones LN, Robertson SA, Radcliffe WN, Emerson E, Lawler P, Crow TJ. (1981) The degree of control exerted by phobic and non-phobic verbal stimuli over the recognition behaviour of phobic and non-phobic subjects. *Behaviour Research and Therapy*, **19**, 223–34.

Burke M, Drummond LM, Johnston DW. (1997). Treatment of choice for agoraphobic women: exposure or cognitive-behaviour therapy? *British Journal of Clinical Psychology*, **36**, 409–20.

Burns LE. (1980) The epidemiology of fears and phobias in general practice. *Journal of International Medical Research*, **8**, 1–7.

Burns GL, Keortge SG, Formea GM, Sternberger LG. (1996) Revision of the Padua Inventory of obsessive compulsive disorder symptoms: distinctions between worry, obsessions and compulsions. *Behaviour Research and Therapy*, **34**, 163–73.

Burvill PW. (1990) The epidemiology of psychological disorders in general medical settings. In Sartorius N, Goldberg D, De Girolamo G, Costa E, Silva J, Lecrubier Y, Wittchen H-U (Eds), *Psychological Disorders in General Medical Settings*. Toronto: Hogrefe and Huber.

Butler G. (1989a) Issues in the application of cognitive and behavioral strategies in the treatment of social phobia. *Clinical Psychology Review*, **9**, 91–106.

Butler G. (1989b) Phobic disorders. In Hawton K, Salkovskis PM, Kirk J, Clarke DM (Eds), *Cognitive-Behaviour Therapies for Psychiatric Problems: A Practical Guide*. Oxford: Oxford University Press.

Butler G. (1993) Predicting outcome after treatment for generalised anxiety disorder. *Behaviour Research and Therapy*, **31**, 211–13.

Butler G, Booth RG. (1991) Developing psychological treatments for generalized anxiety disorder. In Rapee RM, Barlow DH (Eds), *Chronic Anxiety, Generalized Anxiety Disorder and Mixed Anxiety–Depression*. New York: Guilford.

Butler G, Mathews A. (1983) Cognitive processes in anxiety. *Advances in Behaviour Research and Therapy*, **5**, 51–62.

Butler G, Cullington A, Munby M, Amies P, Gelder M. (1984) Exposure and anxiety management in the treatment of social phobia. *Journal of Consulting and Clinical Psychology*, **52**, 642–50.

Butler G, Fennell M, Robson P, Gelder M. (1991) Comparison of behaviour therapy and cognitive behaviour therapy in the treatment of generalized anxiety disorder. *Journal of Consulting and Clinical Psychology*, **59**, 167–75.

Cahill SP, Carrigan MH, Frueh BC. (1999) Does EMDR work? And if so, why? A critical review of controlled outcome and dismantling research. *Journal of Anxiety Disorders*, **13**, 5–33.

Cameron OG, Thyer BA, Nesse RM, Curtis GC. (1986) Symptom profiles of patients with DSM-III anxiety disorders. *American Journal of Psychiatry*, **143**, 1132–7.

Campos PE, Solyom L, Koelink A. (1984) The effects of timolol maleate on subjective and physiological components of air travel phobia. *Canadian Journal of Psychiatry*, **29**, 570–4.

Cannon WB. (1927) *Bodily Changes in Pain, Hunger, Fear, and Rage*. New York: Appelton-

Century-Crofts.

Carlson EB. (1996) *Trauma Research Methodology.* Lutherville, MD: Sidran Press.

Casacalenda N, Boulenger J-P. (1998) Pharmacologic treatments effective in both generalized anxiety disorder and major depressive disorder: clinical and theoretical implications. *Canadian Journal of Psychiatry*, **43**, 722–30.

Castle DJ, Deale A, Marks IM, Cutts F, Chadhoury Y, Stewart A. (1994) Obsessive–compulsive disorder: prediction of outcome from behavioural psychotherapy. *Acta Psychiatrica Scandinavica*, **89**, 393–8.

Cath DC, van der Wetering BJM, van Woerkom TCAM, Hoogduin CAL, Roos, RAC, Rooijmans HGM. (1992) Mental play in Gilles de la Tourette's syndrome and obsessive compulsive disorder. *British Journal of Psychiatry*, **161**, 542–5.

Chaleby KS, Raslan A. (1990) Delineation of social phobia in Saudi Arabians. *Social Psychiatry and Psychiatric Epidemiology*, **25**, 324–7.

Chambless DL. (1988) Body sensations questionnaire. In Hersen M, Bellack A (Eds), *Dictionary of Behavioral Assessment Techniques.* New York: Pergamon.

Chambless DL. (1990) Spacing of exposure sessions in treatment of agoraphobia and simple phobia. *Behavior Therapy*, **18**, 225–32.

Chambless DL, Gracely EJ. (1989) Fear of fear and the anxiety disorders. *Cognitive Therapy and Research*, **13**, 9–20.

Chambless DL, Mason J. (1986) Sex, sex-role stereotyping and agoraphobia. *Behaviour Research and Therapy*, **24**, 231–5.

Chambless DL, Foa EB, Groves GA, Goldstein AJ. (1982) Exposure and communications training in the treatment of agoraphobia. *Behaviour Research and Therapy*, **20**, 219–31.

Chambless DL, Caputo GC, Bright P, Gallagher R. (1984) Assessment of fear in agoraphobics: the Body Sensations Questionnaire and the Agoraphobic Cognitions Questionnaire. *Journal of Consulting and Clinical Psychology*, **52**, 1090–7.

Chambless DL, Caputo GC, Jasin SE, Gracely EJ, Williams C. (1985) The Mobility Inventory for Agoraphobia. *Behaviour Research and Therapy*, **23**, 35–44.

Chambless DL, Goldstein AA, Gallagher R, Bright P. (1986) Integrating behavior therapy and psychotherapy in the treatment of agoraphobia. *Psychotherapy: Theory, Research, and Practice*, **23**, 150–9.

Chambless DL, Tran GQ, Glass CR. (1997) Predictors of response to cognitive-behavioral group therapy for social phobia. *Journal of Anxiety Disorders*, **11**, 221–40.

Chorpita BF, Tracey SA, Brown TA, Collica TJ, Barlow DH. (1997) Assessment of worry in children and adolescents: an adaptation of the Penn State Worry Questionnaire. *Behaviour Research and Therapy*, **35**, 569–81.

Chouinard G, Goodman W, Greist J, Jenike M, Rasmusson S, White K, Hackett E, Gaffney M, Bick P. (1990) Results of a double blind placebo controlled trial of a new serotonin uptake inhibitor, sertraline, in the treatment of obsessive compulsive disorder. *Psychopharmacology*, **26**, 279–84.

Clark DB, Agras WS. (1991) The assessment and treatment of performance anxiety in musicians. *American Journal of Psychiatry*, **148**, 598–605.

Clark DM. (1986) A cognitive approach to panic. *Behaviour Research and Therapy*, **24**, 461–70.

Clark DM. (1988) A cognitive model of panic attacks. In Rachman S, Maser JD (Eds), *Panic: Psychological Perspectives.* Hillsdale, NJ: Lawrence Erlbaum.

Clark DM, Hemsley DR. (1982) The effects of hyperventilation: individual variability and its relation to personality. *Journal of Behavior Therapy and Experimental Psychiatry*, **13**, 41–7.

Clark DM, Wells A. (1995) A cognitive model of social phobia. In Heimberg RG, Liebowitz MR, Hope DA, Schneier FR (Eds), *Social Phobia: Diagnosis, Assessment and Treatment.* New York: Guilford Press, pp. 69–93.

Clark DM, Salkovskis PM, Chalkley AJ. (1985) Respiratory control as a treatment for panic attacks. *Journal of Behavior Therapy and Experimental Psychiatry*, **16**, 23–30.

Clark LA, Watson D. (1991) Tripartite model of anxiety and depression: psychometric evidence and taxonomic implications. *Journal of Abnormal Psychology*, **100**, 316–36.

Clarke JC, Jackson JA. (1983) *Hypnosis and Behavior Therapy.* New York: Springer-Verlag.

Clum GA. (1989) Psychological interventions vs. drugs in the treatment of panic. *Behavior Therapy*, **20**, 429–57.

Clum GA, Knowles SL. (1991) Why do some people with panic disorder become avoidant? A review. *Clinical Psychology Review*, **11**, 295–313.

Clum GA, Broyles S, Borden J, Watkins PL. (1990) Validity and reliability of the panic attack symptoms and cognitions questionnaires. Special Issue: DSM-IV and the psychology literature. *Journal of Psychopathology and Behavioral Assessment*, **12**, 233–45.

Clum GA, Clum GA, Searles R. (1993) A meta-analysis of treatments for panic disorder. *Journal of Consulting and Clinical Psychology*, **61**, 317–26.

Cohen J. (1992) A power primer. *Psychological Bulletin*, **112**, 155–9.

Coles ME, Heimberg RG. (2000) Patterns of anxious arousal during exposure to feared situations in individuals with social phobia. *Behaviour Research and Therapy*, **38**, 405–24.

Connolly J, Hallam RS, Marks IM. (1976) Selective association of fainting with blood–injury–illness fear. *Behaviour Research and Therapy*, **7**, 8–13.

Connor KM, Davidson JRT. (1998) Generalized anxiety disorder: neurobiological and pharmacotherapeutic perspectives. *Biological Psychiatry*, **44**, 1286–94.

Connor KM, Sutherland SM, Tupler LA, Malik ML, Davidson JRT. (1999) Fluoxetine in post-traumatic stress disorder – randomised, double-blind study. *British Journal of Psychiatry*, **175**, 17–22.

Constans JI, Penn DL, Ihen GH, Hope DA. (1999) Interpretive biases for ambiguous stimuli in social anxiety. *Behaviour Research and Therapy*, **37**, 643–51.

Cooper NA, Clum GA. (1989) Imaginal flooding as a supplementary treatment for PTSD in combat veterans: a controlled study. *Behavior Therapy*, **20**, 381–91.

Cooper PJ, Eke M. (1999) Childhood shyness and maternal social phobia: a community study. *British Journal of Psychiatry*, **174**, 439–43.

Copp JE, Schwiderski UE, Robinson DS. (1990) Symptom comorbidity in anxiety and depressive disorders. *Journal of Clinical Psychopharmacology*, **10** (3, Suppl.), 52S–60S.

Costa P, Herbst JH, McCrae RR, Siegler IC. (2000) Personality at midlife: stability, intrinsic maturation, and response to life events. *Assessment*, **7**, 365–78.

Costa PT, McCrae RR. (1992) Normal personality assessment in clinical practice: the NEO personality inventory. *Psychological Assessment*, **4**, 5–13.

Cottraux J. (1989) Behavioural psychotherapy for obsessive compulsive disorder. *International Review of Psychiatry*, **1**, 227–34.

Cottraux J, Messy P, Marks IM, Mollard E, Bouvard M. (1993) Predictive factors in the treatment of obsessive–compulsive disorders with fluvoxamine and/or behaviour therapy. *Behavioural Psychotherapy*, **21**, 45–50.

Cox BJ, Direnfeld DM, Swinson RP, Norton GR. (1994) Suicidal ideation and suicide attempts in panic disorder and social phobia. *American Journal of Psychiatry*, **151**, 882–7.

Cox BJ, Ross L, Swinson RP, Direnfeld DM. (1998) A comparison of social phobia outcome measures in cognitive-behavioral group therapy. *Behavior Modification*, **22**, 285–97.

Craig A, Franklin J, Andrews G. (1984) A scale to measure locus of control of behaviour. *British Journal of Medical Psychology*, **7**, 173–80.

Craske MG, Rapee RM, Barlow DH. (1988) The significance of panic – expectancy for individual patterns of avoidance. *Behavior Therapy*, **19**, 577–92.

Craske MG, Rapee RM, Jackel L, Barlow DH. (1989) Qualitative dimensions of worry in DSM-III-R generalized anxiety disorder subjects and nonanxious controls. *Behaviour Research and Therapy*, **27**, 397–402.

Craske MG, Barlow DH, O'Leary TA. (1992). *Mastery of Your Anxiety and Worry*. Albany, NY: Graywind.

Craske MG, Rowe M, Lewin M, Noriega-Dimitri R. (1997) Interoceptive exposure versus breathing retraining within cognitive-behavioural therapy for panic disorder with agoraphobia. *British Journal of Clinical Psychology*, **36**, 85–99.

Creamer M, Burgess P, Buckingham WJ, Pattison P. (1993) Post-trauma reactions following a multiple shooting: a retrospective study and methodological inquiry. In Wilson JP, Raphael B (Eds), *The International Handbook Of Traumatic Stress Syndromes*. New York: Plenum Press.

Crino R, Andrews G. (1996a) Obsessive compulsive disorder and axis I comorbidity. *Journal of Anxiety Disorders*, **10**, 37–46.

Crino R, Andrews G. (1996b) Personality disorder in obsessive–compulsive disorder: a controlled study. *Journal of Psychiatric Research*, **30**, 29–38.

Crowe RR. (1985) The genetics of panic disorder and agoraphobia. *Psychiatric Developments*, **2**, 243–8.

Crowe RR, Noyes R, Pauls DL, Sylmen D. (1983) A family study of panic disorder. *Archives of General Psychiatry*, **40**, 1065–9.

Curtis GC, Nesse RM, Buxton M, Wright J, Lippman D. (1976) Flooding in vivo as a research tool and treatment method for phobias: a preliminary report. *Comprehensive Psychiatry*, **17**, 153–60.

Da Roza Davis J, Gelder M. (1991) Long-term management of anxiety states. *International Review of Psychiatry*, **3**, 5–17.

Dager SR, Cowley DS, Dunner DL. (1987) Biological markers in panic states: lactate-induced panic and mitral valve prolapse. *Biological Psychiatry*, **22**, 339–59.

Daiuto AD, Baucom DH, Epstein N, Dutton SS. (1998). The application of behavioral couples therapy to the assessment and treatment of agoraphobia: implications of empirical research. *Clinical Psychology Review*, **18**, 663–87.

Davey GCL, Levy S. (1998) Catastrophic worrying: personal inadequacy and a perseverative iterative style as features of the catastrophizing process. *Journal of Abnormal Psychology*, **107**, 576–86.

Davidson J, Smith R, Kudler H. (1989) Validity and reliability of the DSM-III criteria for posttraumatic stress disorder. Experience with a structured interview. *Journal of Nervous and Mental Disease*, **177**, 336–41.

Davidson JRT, Potts NLS, Richichi EA, Krishnan R, Ford SM, Smith R, Wilson WH. (1993) Treatment of social phobia with clonazepam and placebo. *Journal of Clinical Psychopharmacology*, **13**, 423–8.

Davidson JRT, Hughes DC, George LK, Blazer DG. (1994) The boundary of social phobia: exploring the threshold. *Archives of General Psychiatry*, **51**, 975–83.

de Haan E, Hoogduin K, Buitelaar J, Keijsers G. (1998) Behaviour therapy versus clomipramine for the treatment of obsessive compulsive disorder in children and adolescents. *Journal of the American Academy of Child and Adolescent Psychiatry*, **37**, 1022–9.

De Loof C, Zandbergen H, Lousberg T, Pols H, Griez E. (1989) The role of life events in the onset of panic disorder. *Behaviour Research and Therapy*, **27**, 461–3.

De Ruiter C, Garssen B, Rijken H, Kraaimaat F. (1989a) The hyperventilation syndrome in panic disorder, agoraphobia, and generalized anxiety disorder. *Behaviour Research and Therapy*, **27**, 447–52.

De Ruiter C, Rijken H, Garssen B, Kraaimaat F. (1989b) Breathing retraining, exposure, and a combination of both, in the treatment of panic disorder with agoraphobia. *Behaviour Research and Therapy*, **27**, 647–55.

De Silva P, Rachman SJ. (1984) Does escape behaviour strengthen agoraphobic avoidance? A preliminary study. *Behaviour Research and Therapy*, **22**, 87–91.

De Veaugh-Geiss J, Katz RJ, Landau P. (1989) Preliminary results from a multicentre trial of clomipramine in obsessive compulsive disorder. *Psychopharmacology Bulletin*, **25**, 36–40.

DeFries JC, Gervais MC, Thomas EA. (1978) Response for 30 generations of selection for open field activity in laboratory mice. *Behavior Genetics*, **8**, 3–13.

den Boer JA. (1998) Pharmacotherapy of panic disorder: Differential efficacy from a clinical viewpoint. *Journal of Clinical Psychiatry*, **59**, 30–6.

Denney DR, Sullivan DJ, Thiry MR. (1977) Participant modelling and self-verbalization training in the reduction of spider fears. *Journal of Behavior Therapy and Experimental Psychiatry*, **8**, 247–53.

Derogatis LR. (1977) *SCL-90 Revised Version Manual-1*. Baltimore, MD: Johns Hopkins School of Medicine.

Devilly G, Spence S. (1999) The relative efficacy and treatment distress of EMDR and a cognitive-behavior trauma treatment protocol in the amelioration of posttraumatic stress disorder. *Journal of Anxiety Disorders*, **13**, 131–57.

Devilly G, Spence S, Rapee R. (1998) Statistical and reliable change with eye movement desensitization and reprocessing: treating trauma within a veteran population. *Behavior Therapy*, **29**, 435–55.

DeWit DJ, Ogborne A, Offord DR, MacDonald K. (1999) Antecedents of the risk of recovery from DSM-III-R social phobia. *Psychological Medicine*, **29**, 569–82.

Di Nardo PA, Barlow DH. (1988) *Instructions for the Anxiety Disorders Interview Schedule –*

Revised. Albany, NY: Center for Anxiety Disorders.

Di Nardo PA, O'Brien GT, Barlow DH, Waddell MT, Blanchard EB. (1983) Reliability of DSM-III anxiety disorder categories using a new structured interview. *Archives of General Psychiatry*, **40**, 1070–4.

Di Nardo PA, Guzy LT, Bak RM. (1988) Anxiety response patterns and etiological factors in dog-fearful and non-fearful subjects. *Behaviour Research and Therapy*, **26**, 245–52.

Dibartolo PM, Brown TA, Barlow DH. (1997) Effects of anxiety on attentional allocation and task performance: an information processing analysis. *Behaviour Research and Therapy*, **35**, 1101–11.

Dickinson A. (1980) *Contemporary Animal Learning Theory.* London: Cambridge University Press.

Dryden W. (1985) Challenging but not overwhelming: a compromise in negotiating homework assignments. *British Journal of Cognitive Psychotherapy*, **3**, 77–9.

Dubovsky SL. (1990) Generalized anxiety disorder: new concepts and psychopharmacologic therapies. *Journal of Clinical Psychiatry*, **51** (Suppl.), 3–10.

Dugas MJ, Freeston MH, Ladouceur R, Rheaume J, Provencher M., Boisvert JM. (1998a). Worry themes in primary GAD, secondary GAD, and other anxiety disorders. *Journal of Anxiety Disorders*, **12**, 253–61.

Dugas MJ, Gagnon F, Ladouceur R, Freeston MH. (1998b) Generalized anxiety disorder: a preliminary test of a conceptual model. *Behaviour Research and Therapy*, **36**, 215–26.

Duncan-Jones P. (1987) Modelling the aetiology of neurosis: long-term and short-term factors. In Cooper B (Ed), *Psychiatric Epidemiology: Progress and Prospects.* London: Croom Helm.

Dunner DL, Ishiki D, Avery DH, Wilson LG, Hyde TS. (1986) Effect of alprazolam and diazepam on anxiety and panic attacks in panic disorder. *Journal of Clinical Psychiatry*, **47**, 458–60.

Durham RC, Allan T. (1993) Psychological treatment of generalised anxiety disorder. A review of the clinical significance of results in outcome studies since 1980. *British Journal of Psychiatry*, **163**, 19–26.

Durham RC, Murphy T, Allan T, Richard K, Treliving LR, Fenton GW. (1994) Cognitive therapy, analytic psychotherapy and anxiety management training for generalised anxiety disorder. *British Journal of Psychiatry*, **165**, 315–23.

Durham RC, Allan T, Hackett CA. (1997) On predicting improvement and relapse in generalized anxiety disorder following psychotherapy. *British Journal of Clinical Psychology*, **36**, 101–19.

Durham RC, Fisher PL, Treliving LR, Hau CM, Richard K, Stewart JB. (1999) One year follow-up of cognitive therapy, analytic psychotherapy and anxiety management training for generalized anxiety disorder: symptom change, medication usage and attitudes to treatment. *Behavioural and Cognitive Psychotherapy*, **27**, 19–35.

D'Zurilla TJ. (1986) *Problem Solving Therapy: A Social Competence Approach to Clinical Intervention.* New York: Springer-Verlag.

D'Zurilla TJ, Goldfried MR (1971) Problem solving and behaviour modification. *Journal of Abnormal Psychology*, **8**, 107–26.

Eaton WW, Dryman A, Weissman MM. (1991) Panic and phobia. In Robins LN, Regier DA

(Eds), *Psychiatric Disorders in America: The Epidemiological Catchment Area Study*. New York: Free Press.

Eaton WW, Anthony JC, Romanoski A, Tien A, Gallo J, Cai G, Neufeld K, Schlaepfer T, Laugharne J, Chen LS. (1998) Onset and recovery from panic disorder in the Baltimore Epidemiologic Catchment Area follow-up. *British Journal of Psychiatry*, **173**, 501–7.

Ehlers A, Margraf J, Davies S, Roth WT. (1988) Selective processing of threat cues in subjects with panic attacks. *Cognition and Emotion*, **2**, 201–20.

Ehlers A, Margraf J, Roth WT. (1986a) The authors' reply. *Psychiatry Research*, **19**, 165–7.

Ehlers A, Margraf J, Roth WT, Taylor CB, Maddock RJ, Sheikh J, Kopell ML, McClenahan KL, Gossard D, Blowers GH, Agras WS, Kopell BS. (1986b) Lactate infusions and panic attacks: do patient and controls respond differently? *Psychiatry Research*, **17**, 295–308.

Eley TC, Plomin R. (1997) Genetic analyses of emotionality. *Current Opinion in Neurobiology*, **7**, 279–84.

Elkin I, Shea T, Watkins JT, Imber SD, Sotsky SM, Collins JF, Glass DR, Pilkonis PA, Leber WR, Docherty JP, Fiester SJ, Parloff MB. (1989) National Institute of Mental Health treatment of depression collaborative research program. *Archives of General Psychiatry*, **46**, 971–82.

Ellis A. (1957) Outcome of employing three techniques of psychotherapy. *Journal of Clinical Psychology*, **13**, 344–50.

Ellis A. (1962) *Reason and Emotion in Psychotherapy*. New York: Lyle Stuart.

Ellis A, Harper RA. (1975) *A New Guide to Rational Living*. North Hollywood, CA: Wilshire.

Emmelkamp PMG. (1979) The behavioral study of clinical phobias. In Hersen M, Eisler RM, Miller PM (Eds), *Progress in Behavior Modification*, Vol. 8. New York: Academic Press.

Emmelkamp PMG. (1982) *Phobic and Obsessive–Compulsive Disorders: Theory, Research, and Practice*. New York: Plenum Press.

Emmelkamp PMG, Beens H. (1991) Cognitive therapy with obsessive–compulsive disorder: a comparative evaluation. *Behaviour Research and Therapy*, **29**, 293–300.

Emmelkamp PMG, Felten M. (1985) Cognitive and physiological changes during prolonged exposure in vivo: a comparison with agoraphobics as subjects. *Behaviour Research and Therapy*, **23**, 219–23.

Emmelkamp PMG, Wessels H. (1975) Flooding in imagination vs. flooding in vivo: a comparison with agoraphobics. *Behaviour Research and Therapy*, **13**, 7–15.

Emmelkamp PMG, van der Helm M, van Zantin BL, Plochg I. (1980) Treatment of obsessive compulsive patients: the contribution of self-instructional training to the effectiveness of exposure. *Behaviour Research and Therapy*, **18**, 61–6.

Emmelkamp PMG, Mersch P-P, Vissia E. (1985a) The external validity of analogue outcome research: evaluation of cognitive and behavioural interventions. *Behavior Research and Therapy*, **23**, 83–6.

Emmelkamp PMG, Mersch P-P, Vissia E, van der Helm M. (1985b) Social phobia: a comparative evaluation of cognitive and behavioral interventions. *Behavior Research and Therapy*, **23**, 365–9.

Emmelkamp PMG, Visser S, Hoekstra RJ. (1988) Cognitive therapy versus exposure in vivo in the treatment of obsessive–compulsives. *Cognitive Therapy and Research*, **12**, 103–14.

Endicott J, Spitzer RL. (1978) A diagnostic interview: the schedule for affective disorders and schizophrenia. *Archives of General Psychiatry*, **35**, 837–44.

Eng W, Heimberg RG, Coles ME, Schneier FR, Liebowitz MR. (2000) An empirical approach to subtype identification in individuals with social phobia. *Psychological Medicine*, **30**, 1345–57.

Eysenck HJ. (1990) *Rebel With a Cause: The Autobiography of Hans Eysenck*. London: W.H. Allen.

Eysenck HJ, Eysenck SGB. (1975) *Manual of the Eysenck Personality Questionnaire (Junior and Adult)*. Kent, England: Hodder and Stoughton.

Falloon I, Mueser K, Gingerich S, Rappaport S, McGill C, Hole V. (1988) *Behavioural Family Therapy*. Buckingham: Buckingham Mental Health Service.

Faravelli C. (1985) Life events preceding the onset of panic disorder. *Journal of Affective Disorders*, **9**, 108–12.

Faravelli C, Pallanti S. (1989) Recent life events and panic disorder. *American Journal of Psychiatry*, **146**, 622–6.

Faravelli C, Webb T, Ambonetti A, Fonnesu F, Sessarego A. (1985) Prevalence of traumatic early life events in 31 agoraphobic patients with panic attacks. *American Journal of Psychiatry*, **142**, 1493–4.

Fava GA, Savron G, Zielezny M, Grandi S, Rafanelli C, Conti S. (1997) Overcoming resistance to exposure in panic disorder with agoraphobia. *Acta Psychiatrica Scandinavica*, **95**, 306–12.

Feske U, Perry KJ, Chambless DL, Renneberg B, Goldstein AJ. (1996) Avoidant personality disorder as a predictor for treatment outcome among generalized social phobics. *Journal of Personality Disorders*, **10**, 174–84.

Figley CR. (1985) *Trauma And Its Wake*. New York: Brunner/Mazel.

First MB, Spitzer RL, Gibbon M, Williams JBN. (1997) *Structured Clinical Interview for DSM-IV Axis I Disorders – Clinician Version*. Washington, DC: American Psychology Press.

Fisher PL, Durham RC. (1999) Recovery rates in generalized anxiety disorder following psychological therapy: an analysis of clinically significant change in the STAI-T across outcome studies since 1990. *Psychological Medicine*, **29**, 1425–34.

Flament MF, Whitaker A, Rapoport JL, Davies M, Berg CZ, Kalikow K, Sleery W, Shaffer D. (1988) Obsessive compulsive disorder in adolescence: an epidemiological study. *Journal of the American Academy of Child and Adolescent Psychiatry*, **27**, 764–71.

Fleming B, Falk A. (1989) Discriminating factors in panic disorder with and without agoraphobia. *Journal of Anxiety Disorders*, **3**, 209–19.

Foa EB. (1979) Failure in treating obsessive compulsives. *Behaviour Research and Therapy*, **17**, 169–79.

Foa EB, Kozak MJ. (1985) Treatment of anxiety disorders: implications for psychotherapy. In Tuma AH, Maser JD (Eds), *Anxiety and the Anxiety Disorders*. Hillsdale, NJ: Lawrence Erlbaum.

Foa EB, Kozak MJ. (1986) Emotional processing of fear: exposure to corrective information. *Psychological Bulletin*, **99**, 20–35.

Foa EB, Meadows EA. (1997) Psychosocial treatments for posttraumatic stress disorder: a critical review. *Annual Review of Psychology*, **48**, 449–80.

Foa EB, Rothbaum BO. (1998) *Treating the Trauma of Rape: Cognitive-Behavioral Therapy for PTSD*. New York: Guilford Press.

Foa EB, Tillmans A. (1980) The treatment of obsessive compulsive neurosis. In Goldstein A, Foa EB (Eds), *Handbook of Behavioural Interventions: A Clinical Guide*. New York: Wiley.

Foa EB, Jameson JS, Turner RM, Payne LL. (1980) Massed vs. spaced exposure sessions in the treatment of agoraphobia. *Behaviour Research and Therapy*, **18**, 333–8.

Foa EB, Steketee GS, Grayson JB. (1981) Success and failure in treating obsessive–compulsives. *Biological Psychiatry*, **5**, 1099–1102.

Foa EB, Grayson JB, Steketee G, Doppelt HG, Turner RM, Latimer PR. (1983a) Success and failure in behavioral treatment of obsessive compulsives. *Journal of Consulting and Clinical Psychology*, **51**, 287–97.

Foa EB, Steketee GS, Grayson JB, Doppelt HG. (1983b) Treatment of obsessive–compulsives: when do we fail? In Foa EB, Emmelkamp PMG (Eds), *Failures in Behavior Therapy*. New York: Wiley.

Foa EB, Steketee GS, Ozarow BJ. (1985) Behaviour therapy with obsessive compulsives: from therapy to treatment. In Mavissakalian M, Turner SM, Michelsen L (Eds), *Obsessive Compulsive Disorder: Psychological and Pharmacological Treatments*. New York: Plenum Press.

Foa EB, Feske U, Murdock TB, Kozak MJ, McCarthy PR. (1991a) Processing of threat-related information in rape victims. *Journal of Abnormal Psychology*, **100**, 156–62.

Foa EB, Rothbaum BO, Riggs DS, Murdock TB. (1991b) Treatment of posttraumatic stress disorder in rape victims: a comparison between cognitive-behavioral procedures and counseling. *Journal of Consulting and Clinical Psychology*, **59**, 715–23.

Foa EB, Riggs DS, Dancu CV, Rothbaum BO. (1993) Reliability and validity of a brief instrument for assessing post-traumatic stress disorder. *Journal of Traumatic Stress*, **6**, 459–73.

Foa EB, Hearst-Ikeda ID, Perry KJ. (1995a) Evaluation of a brief cognitive-behavioral program for the prevention of chronic PTSD in recent assault victims. *Journal of Consulting and Clinical Psychology*, **63**, 948–55.

Foa EB, Riggs DS, Gershuny BS. (1995b) Arousal, numbing, and intrusion: symptom structure of PTSD following assault. *American Journal of Psychiatry*, **152**, 116–20.

Foa EB, Dancu CV, Hembree EA, Jaycox LH, Meadows EA, Street GP. (1999) A comparison of exposure therapy, stress inoculation training, and their combination for reducing posttraumatic stress disorder in female assault victims. *Journal of Consulting and Clinical Psychology*, **67**, 194–200.

Foa EB, Keane TM, Friedman MJ. (2000) *Effective Treatments for PTSD*. New York: Guilford Press.

Fones CSL, Manfro GG, Pollack MH. (1998) Social phobia: an update. *Harvard Review of Psychiatry*, **5**, 247–59.

Forsyth JP, Chorpita BF. (1997) Unearthing the non-associative origins of fears and phobias: a rejoinder. *Journal of Behavior Therapy and Experimental Psychiatry*, **28**, 297–305.

Foulds J, Wiedmann K, Patterson J, Brooks N. (1990) The effects of muscle tension on cerebral circulation in blood-phobic and non-phobic subjects. *Behaviour Research and Therapy*, **28**, 481–6.

Franklin JA. (1987) The changing nature of agoraphobic fears. *British Journal of Clinical Psychology*, **26**, 127–33.

Franklin JA. (1990a) Behavioural therapy for panic disorder. In McNaughton N, Andrews G (Eds), *Anxiety*. Dunedin: Otago University Press.

Franklin JA. (1990b) Agoraphobia: its nature, development and treatment. Unpublished doctoral dissertation. Sydney: University of New South Wales.

Franklin JA. (1991) Agoraphobia. *International Review of Psychiatry*, **3**, 151–62.

Franklin JA, Andrews G. (1989) Stress and the onset of agoraphobia. *Australian Psychologist*, **24**, 203–19.

Freeston MH, Rheaume J, Letarte H, Dugas MJ, Ladouceur R. (1994) Why do people worry? *Personality and Individual Differences*, **17**, 791–802.

Freeston MH, Dugas MJ, Ladouceur R. (1996a) Thoughts, images, worry and anxiety. *Cognitive Therapy and Research*, **20**, 265–73.

Freeston MH, Rheaume J, Ladouceur R. (1996b) Correcting faulty appraisals of obsessional thoughts. *Behavior Research and Therapy*, **34**, 433–46.

Freeston M, Ladoucer R, Gagnon F, Thibodeau N, Rheaume J, Letarte H, Bujold A. (1997) Cognitive-behavioral treatment of obsessive thoughts: a controlled study. *Journal of Consulting and Clinical Psychology*, **65**, 405–13.

Friedman MJ. (1997) Drug treatment for PTSD: answers and questions. *Annals of the New York Academy of Science*, **821**, 359–71.

Friedman, MJ, Charney, DS, Southwick SM. (1993) Pharmacotherapy for recently evacuated military casualties. *Military Medicine*, **158**, 493–7.

Friend P, Andrews G. (1990) Agoraphobia without panic attacks. In McNaughton N, Andrews G (Eds), *Anxiety*. Dunedin: Otago University Press.

Frueh BC, Gold PB, de Arellano MA. (1997) Symptom overreporting in combat veterans evaluated for PTSD: differentiation on the basis of compensation seeking status. *Journal of Personality Assessment*, **68**, 369–84.

Furmark T, Tillfors M, Everz P-O, Marteinsdottir I, Gefvert O, Fredrickson M. (1999) Social phobia in the general population: prevalence and sociodemographic profile. *Social Psychiatry and Psychiatric Epidemiology*, **34**, 416–24.

Furmark T, Tillfors M, Stattin H, Ekselius L, Fredrikson M. (2000) Social phobia subtypes in the general population revealed by cluster analysis. *Psychological Medicine*, **30**, 1335–44.

Fyer AJ. (1987) Simple phobia. *Modern Problems in Pharmacopsychiatry*, **22**, 174–92.

Fyer AJ, Mannuzza S, Gallops MS, Martin LY, Aaronson C, Gorman JM, Liebowitz MR, Klein DF. (1990) Familial transmission of simple phobias and fears: a preliminary report. *Archives of General Psychiatry*, **47**, 252–6.

Gale C, Oakley-Browne M. (2000) Extracts from "Clinical Evidence": anxiety disorder. *British Medical Journal*, **321**, 1204–7.

Garssen B, van Veenendaal W, Bloemink R. (1983) Agoraphobia and the hyperventilation syndrome. *Behaviour Research and Therapy*, **21**, 643–9.

Garssen B, de Ruiter C, van Dyck R. (1992) Breathing retraining: a rational placebo? *Clinical Psychology Review*, **12**, 141–53.

Garvey MJ, Noyes R, Cook B. (1987) Does situational panic disorder represent a specific panic disorder subtype? *Comprehensive Psychiatry*, **28**, 329–33.

Garvey MJ, Cook B, Noyes R. (1988) The occurrence of a prodrome of generalized anxiety in panic disorder. *Comprehensive Psychiatry*, **29**, 445–9.

Gelder M. (1979) Behavior therapy for neurotic disorders. *Behavior Modification*, **3**, 469–95.

Gelenberg AJ, Lydiard RB, Rudolph RL, Aguiar L, Haskins JT, Salinas E. (2000). Efficacy of venlafaxine extended-release capsules in nondepressed outpatients with generalized anxiety disorder: a 6-month randomized controlled trial. *Journal of the American Medical Association*, **283**, 3082–8.

Gelernter CS, Uhde TW, Cimbolic P, Arnkoff DB, Vittone BJ, Tancer ME, Bartko JJ. (1991) Cognitive behavioural and pharmacological treatments of social phobia: a controlled study. *Archives of General Psychiatry*, **48**, 938–45.

Gelpin E, Bonne O, Peri T, Brandes D, Shalev AY. (1996) Treatment of recent trauma survivors with benzodiazepines: a prospective Study. *Journal of Clinical Psychiatry*, **57**, 390–4.

George MS, Trimble MR, Ring HA, Sallee FR, Robertson MM. (1993) Obsessions in obsessive–compulsive disorder with and without Gilles de la Tourette's syndrome. *American Journal of Psychiatry*, **150**, 93–7.

Gittleson NL. (1966) Depressive psychosis in the obsessional neurotic. *British Journal of Psychiatry*, **112**, 883–7.

Goldberg DP, Lecrubier Y. (1995) Form and frequency of mental disorders across centres. In Ustun TB, Sartorius N (Eds), *Mental Illness in General Health Care: An International Study. US:* New York: Wiley.

Goldfried MR, Davison GC. (1976) *Clinical Behavior Therapy*. New York: Holt, Rinehart and Winston.

Goldstein AJ, Chambless DL. (1978) A reanalysis of agoraphobia. *Journal of Behavior Therapy and Experimental Psychiatry*, **1**, 305–13.

Goodman WK, Price LH, Rasmussen SA, Mazure C, Fleischman RL, Hill C, Heninger G, Charney D. (1989) The Yale–Brown Obsessive Compulsive Scale 1. Development, use and reliability. *Archives of General Psychiatry*, **46**, 1006–11.

Goodman WK, Price LH, Delgado PL, Palumbo J, Krystal JH, Nagy LM, Rasmussen SA, Heninger GR, Charney DS. (1990) Specificity of serotonin re-uptake inhibitors in the treatment of obsessive–compulsive disorder: comparison of fluvoxamine and desipramine. *Archives of General Psychiatry*, **47**, 577–85.

Goodman WK, McDougle CJ, Price LH. (1992) Pharmacotherapy of obsessive–compulsive disorder. *Journal of Clinical Psychiatry*, **53** (4, Suppl.), 29–37.

Goodwin D, Guze S, Robins E. (1969) Follow up studies in obsessional neurosis. *Archives of General Psychiatry*, **20**, 182–7.

Gorman JM, Papp LA. (1990) Chronic anxiety: deciding the length of treatment. *Journal of Clinical Psychiatry*, **51** (Suppl.), 11–15.

Gorman JM, Askanazi J, Liebowitz MR, Fyer AJ, Stein J, Kinney JM, Klein DF. (1984) Response to hyperventilation in a group of patients with panic disorder. *American Journal of Psychiatry*, **141**, 857–61.

Gorman JM, Liebowitz MR, Fyer AJ, Stein MB. (1989) A neuroanatomical hypothesis for panic disorder. *Journal of Clinical Psychopharmacology*, **5**, 298–301.

Gosling SD, John OP. (1999) Personality dimensions in nonhuman animals: a cross-species review. *Current Directions in Psychological Science*, **8**, 69–75.

Gould RA, Clum GA. (1995) Self-help plus minimal therapist contact in the treatment of panic disorder: a replication and extension. *Behavior Therapy*, **26**, 533–46.

Gould RA, Clum GA, Shapiro D. (1993) The use of bibliotherapy in the treatment of panic: a preliminary investigation. *Behavior Therapy*, **24**, 241–52.

Gould RA, Buckminster S, Pollack MH, Otto MW, Yap L. (1997a) Cognitive-behavioral and pharmacological treatment for social phobia: a meta-analysis. *Clinical Psychology: Science and Practice*, **4**, 291–306.

Gould RA, Otto MW, Pollack MH, Yap L. (1997b) Cognitive behavioural and pharmacological treatment of generalized anxiety disorder: a preliminary meta-analysis. *Behavior Therapy*, **28**, 285–305.

Gournay KJM. (1991) The failure of exposure treatment in agoraphobia: implications for the practice of nurse therapists and community psychiatric nurses. *Journal of Advanced Nursing*, **16**, 1099–109.

Gray JA. (1988) A neuropsychological basis of anxiety. In Last CA, Hersen M (Eds), *Handbook of Anxiety Disorders*. Elmsford, NY: Pergamon Press.

Gray JA, McNaughton N. (2000) *The Neuropsychology of Anxiety*, 2nd Edition. New York: Oxford University Press.

Green BL. (1996) Traumatic stress and disaster: mental health effects and factors influencing adaptation. In Mak FL, Nadelson CC (Eds), *International Review of Psychiatry*, Vol. 2. Washington, DC: American Psychiatric Press.

Greist J, Chouinard G, DuBoff E, Halaris A, Kim SW, Koran L, Liebowitz M, Lydiard RB, Rasmussen S, White K, Sikes C. (1995) Double blind parallel comparison of three doses of sertraline and placebo in outpatients with obsessive compulsive disorder. *Archives of General Psychiatry*, **52**, 289–95.

Greist JH. (1990a) Medication management of obsessive compulsive disorder. *Today's Therapeutic Trends*, **7**, 13–27.

Greist JH. (1990b) Treatment of obsessive–compulsive disorder: psychotherapies, drugs and other somatic treatments. *Journal of Clinical Psychiatry*, **51** (8, Suppl.), 44–50.

Greist JH. (1998) The comparative effectiveness of treatments for obsessive–compulsive disorder. *Bulletin of the Meninger Clinic*, **62** (Suppl. A), A65–A81.

Greist JH, Marks IM, Berlin F, Gourney K, Noshirvani, H. (1980) Avoidance versus confrontation of fear. *Behavior Therapy*, **11**, 1–14.

Griez E, van den Hout MA. (1982) Effects of carbon dioxide–oxygen inhalations on subjective anxiety and some neurovegetative parameters. *Journal of Behavior Therapy and Experimental Psychiatry*, **13**, 27–32.

Griez E, Zandbergen J, Lousberg H, van den Hout M. (1988) Effects of low pulmonary CO_2 on panic anxiety. *Comprehensive Psychiatry*, **29**, 49–58.

Grossberg JM. (1965) Successful behavior therapy in a case of speech phobia ("stage fright"). *Journal of Speech and Hearing Disorders*, **30**, 285–8.

Hafner RJ, Marks IM. (1976) Exposure in vivo of agoraphobics: contributions of diazepam, group exposure, and anxiety evocation. *Psychological Medicine*, **6**, 71–88.

Hamilton M. (1959) The assessment of anxiety states by rating. *British Journal of Medical Psychology*, **2**, 50–9.

Hammarberg M. (1992) Penn Inventory for Posttraumatic Stress Disorder: psychometric properties. *Psychological Assessment*, **4**, 67–76.

Hansen AMD, Hoogduin CAL, Scaap C, de Haan E. (1992) Do drop-outs differ from successfully treated obsessive compulsives. *Behaviour Research and Therapy*, **30**, 547–50.

Heide FJ, Borkovec TD. (1984) Relaxation-induced anxiety: mechanisms and theoretical implications. *Behaviour Research and Therapy*, **22**, 1–12.

Heimberg R. (1989) Cognitive and behavioral treatments for social phobia: a critical analysis. *Clinical Psychology Review*, **9**, 107–28.

Heimberg RG, Becker RE, Goldfinger K, Vermilyea BA. (1985) Treatment of social phobia by exposure, cognitive restructuring, and homework assignments. *Journal of Nervous and Mental Disease*, **173**, 236–45.

Heimberg RG, Hope DA, Rapee RM, Bruch MA. (1987) The validity of the Social Avoidance and Distress Scale and the Fear of Negative Evaluation Scale with social phobic patients. *Behaviour Research and Therapy*, **26**, 407–10.

Heimberg RG, Dodge CS, Hope DA, Kennedy CR, Zollo LJ. (1990a) Cognitive behavioral group treatment for social phobia: comparison with a credible placebo control. *Cognitive Therapy and Research*, **14**, 1–23.

Heimberg RG, Hope DA, Dodge CS, Becker RE. (1990b) DSMIIIR subtypes of social phobia: comparison of generalized social phobics and public speaking phobics. *Journal of Nervous and Mental Disease*, **178**, 172–9.

Heimberg RG, Salzman DG, Holt CS, Blendell KA. (1993) Cognitive behavioral group treatment for social phobia: effectiveness at five-year follow-up. *Cognitive Therapy and Research*, **17**, 1–15.

Heimberg RG, Juster HR, Hope DA, Mattia JI. (1995) Cognitive-behavioral group treatment: description, case presentation and empirical support. In Stein MB (Ed), *Social Phobia: Clinical and Research Perspectives*. Washington, DC: American Psychiatric Press.

Heimberg RG, Liebowitz MR, Hope DA, Schneier FR, Holt CS, Welkowitz LA, Juster HR, Campeas R, Bruch MA, Cloitre M, Fallon B, Klein DF. (1998) Cognitive behavioral group therapy vs. phenelzine therapy for social phobia: 12 week outcome. *Archives of General Psychiatry*, **55**, 1133–41.

Helzer JE, Robins LN, McEvoy L. (1987) Posttraumatic stress disorder in the general population: findings from the Epidemiological Catchment Area Survey. *New England Journal of Medicine*, **317**, 1630–4.

Herzberg A. (1941) Short treatment of neuroses by graduated tacks. *British Journal of Medical Psychology*, **19**, 36–51.

Hibbert GA, Chan M. (1989) Respiratory control: its contribution to the treatment of panic attacks. *British Journal of Psychiatry*, **154**, 232–6.

Hibbert GA, Pilsbury D. (1989) Hyperventilation in panic attacks: ambulant monitoring of transcutaneous carbon dioxide. *British Journal of Psychiatry*, **155**, 805–9.

Hoaken P, Schnurr R. (1980) Genetic factors in obsessive–compulsive disorder: a rare case of discordant monozygotic twins. *Canadian Journal of Psychiatry*, **25**, 167–72.

Hodgson RJ, Rachman S. (1977) Obsessional–compulsive complaints. *Behaviour Research and Therapy*, **15**, 389–95.

Hoehn-Saric R. (1998) Psychic and somatic anxiety: worries, somatic symptoms and physiological changes. *Acta Psychiatrica Scandinavica*, **98** (Suppl. 393), 32–8.

Hoehn-Saric R, McLeod DR, Zimmerli WD. (1988) Differential effects of alprazolam and imipramine in generalized anxiety disorder: somatic versus psychic symptoms. *Journal of Clinical Psychiatry*, **49**, 293–301.

Hoffart A. (1995) Cognitive mediators of situation fear in agoraphobia. *Journal of Behavior Therapy and Experimental Psychiatry*, **26**, 313–20.

Hoffart A. (1998) Cognitive and guided mastery therapy of agoraphobia: long-term outcome and mechanisms of change. *Cognitive Therapy and Research*, **22**, 195–207.

Hoffart A, Hedley LM. (1997) Personality traits among panic disorder with agoraphobia patients before and after symptom-focused treatment. *Journal of Anxiety Disorders*, **11**, 77–87.

Hofmann SG. (2000) Self-focused attention before and after treatment of social phobia. *Behaviour Research and Therapy*, **38**, 717–25.

Hofmann SG, Barlow DH. (1999) The costs of anxiety disorders: implications for psychosocial interventions. In Miller NE, Magruder KM (Eds), *Cost Effectiveness of Psychotherapy*. New York: Oxford University Press.

Hofmann SG, Lehman CL, Barlow DH. (1997) How specific are specific phobias? *Journal of Behavior Therapy and Experimental Psychiatry*, **28**, 233–40.

Hohagen F, Winkelmann G, Rasche-Raeuchle H, Hand I, Koenig, A, Muenchau N, Hiss H, Geiger-Kabisch C, Kaeppler C, Schramm P, Rey E, Aldenhoff J, Berger M. (1998) Combination of behaviour therapy with fluvoxamine in comparison with behaviour therapy and placebo: results of a multicentre study. *British Journal of Psychiatry*, **173** (Suppl. 35), 71–78.

Holland RL, Musch BC, Hindmarch I. (1999) Specific effects of benzodiazepines and tricyclic antidepressants in panic disorder: comparisons of clomipramine with alprazolam SR and adinazolam SR. *Human Psychopharmacology*, **14**, 119–24.

Hollander E, Kaplan A, Allen A, Cartwright C. (2000) Pharmacotherapy for obsessive–compulsive disorder. *Psychiatric Clinics of North America*, **23**, 643–56.

Holt CS, Heimberg RG, Hope DA. (1992) Avoidant personality disorder and the generalized subtype of social phobia. *Journal of Abnormal Psychology*, **101**, 318–25.

Holt PE, Andrews G. (1989a) Provocation of panic: three elements of the panic reaction in four anxiety disorders. *Behaviour Research and Therapy*, **27**, 253–61.

Holt PE, Andrews G. (1989b) Hyperventilation and anxiety in panic disorder, social phobia, GAD, and normal controls. *Behaviour Research and Therapy*, **27**, 453–60.

Holzer JC, Goodman WK, McDougle, CJ, Baer L, Boyarsky BK, Leckman JF, Price LH. (1994) Obsessive–compulsive disorder with and without a chronic tic disorder: a comparison of symptoms in 70 patients. *British Journal of Psychiatry*, **164**, 469–73.

Hoogduin CAL, Diuvenvoorden HJ. (1988) A decision model in the treatment of obsessive–compulsive neurosis. *British Journal of Psychiatry*, **152**, 516–21.

Hope DA, Gansler DA, Heimberg RG. (1989) Attentional focus and causal attributions in social phobia: implications from social psychology. *Clinical Psychology Review*, **9**, 49–60.

Hope DA, Rapee RM, Heimberg RG, Dombeck MJ. (1990) Representations of self in social phobia: vulnerability to social threat. *Cognitive Therapy and Research*, **14**, 177–89.

Hope DA, Heimberg RG, Bruch MA. (1995) Dismantling cognitive-behavioral group therapy for social phobia. *Behaviour Research and Therapy*, **33**, 637–50.

Hornsveld H, Garssen B, Dop MF, van Spiegel P. (1990) Symptom reporting during voluntary hyperventilation and mental load: implications for diagnosing hyperventilation syndrome. *Journal of Psychosomatic Research*, **34**, 687–97.

Horowitz M, Wilner N, Alvarez W. (1979) Impact of Event Scale: a measure of subjective stress. *Psychosomatic Medicine*, **41**, 209–18.

Hudson JI, Pope HG (1990) Affective spectrum disorder: does antidepressant response identify a family of disorders with a common pathophysiology? *American Journal of Psychiatry*, **147**, 552–64.

Hunt C, Andrews G. (1992) Measuring personality disorder: the use of self-report questionnaires. *Journal of Personality Disorder*, **6**, 125–33.

Hunt C, Andrews G. (1998) The long-term outcome of panic disorder and social phobia. *Journal of Anxiety Disorders*, **12**, 395–406.

Hunt C, Singh M. (1991) Generalized anxiety disorder. *International Review of Psychiatry*, **3**, 215–29.

Hunt C, Issakidis C, Andrews G. (2002) DSM-IV Generalized Anxiety Disorder in the Australian National Survey of Mental Health and Well-Being. *Psychological Medicine*, in press.

Ingram IM. (1961). The obsessional personality and obsessional illness. *American Journal of Psychiatry*, **117**, 1016–19.

Insel TR. (1988) Obsessive–compulsive disorder: new models. *Psychopharmacology*, **24**, 365–9.

Insel TR, Hoover C, Murphy DL. (1983) Parents of patients with obsessive–compulsive disorder. *Psychological Medicine*, **13**, 807–11.

International Multicenter Clinical Trial Group on Moclobemide in Social Phobia. (1997) Moclobemide in social phobia: a double-blind, placebo controlled clinical study. *European Archives of Psychiatry and Clinical Neuroscience*, **24**, 71–80.

Issakidis C, Andrews G. (2002). Service utilisation for anxiety in an Australian community sample. *Social Psychiatry and Psychiatric Epidemiology*, in press.

Ito LM, de Araujo LA, Hemsley DR, Marks IM. (1995) Beliefs and resistance in obsessive compulsive disorder: observations from a controlled study. *Journal of Anxiety Disorders*, **9**, 269–81.

Ito LM, Noshirvani H, Basoglu M, Marks IM. (1996) Does exposure to internal cues enhance exposure to external cues in agoraphobia with panic? *Psychotherapy and Psychosomatics*, **65**, 24–8.

Jacobson E. (1962) *You Must Relax*. New York: McGraw-Hill.

Jenike MA. (1990) The pharmacological treatment of obsessive compulsive disorders. *International Review of Psychiatry*, **2**, 411–25.

Jenike MA, Baer L, Mininchiello WE, Schwartz CE, Carey RJ. (1986) Concomitant obsessive compulsive disorder and schizotypal personality disorder. *American Journal of Psychiatry*, **143**, 530–2.

Jenike MA, Baer L, Summergrad P, Mininchiello WE, Holland A, Seymour R. (1990a) Sertraline in obsessive–compulsive disorder: a double blind comparison with placebo. *American Journal of Psychiatry*, **147**, 923–8.

Jenike MA, Hyman S, Baer L, Holland A, Mininchiello WE, Buttolph L, Summergrad P,

Seymour R, Ricciardi J. (1990b) A controlled trial of fluvoxamine in obsessive–compulsive disorder: implications for a serotonergic theory. *American Journal of Psychiatry*, **140**, 1209–15.

Jerremalm A, Jansson L, Öst L-G. (1986) Cognitive and physiological reactivity and the effects of different behavioral methods in the treatment of social phobia. *Behavior Research and Therapy*, **24**, 171–80.

Joffe RT, Regan JP. (1988). Personality and depression. *Journal of Psychiatric Research*, **22**, 279–86.

Jones M, Menzies R. (1997a) Danger ideation reduction therapy (DIRT): preliminary findings with three obsessive compulsive washers. *Behavior Research and Therapy*, **35**, 955–60.

Jones M, Menzies R. (1997b) The cognitive mediation of obsessive–compulsive handwashing. *Behavior Research and Therapy*, **35**, 843–50.

Joorman J, Stober J. (1999) Somatic symptoms of generalized anxiety disorder from the DSM-IV: associations with pathological worry and depression symptoms in a nonclinical sample. *Journal of Anxiety Disorders*, **13**, 491–503.

Judd LL, Kessler RC, Paulus MP, Zeller PV, Wittchen H-U, Kunovac JL. (1998) Comorbidity as a fundamental feature of generalized anxiety disorders: results from the National Comorbidity Study (NCS). *Acta Psychiatrica Scandinavica*, **98** (Suppl. 393), 6–11.

Kagan J, Reznick JS, Snidman N. (1988) Biological basis of childhood shyness. *Science*, **240**, 167–71.

Kahn RJ, McNair DM, Lipman RS, Covi L, Rickels K, Downing R, Fisher S, Frankenthaler LM. (1986) Imipramine and chlordiazepoxide in depressive and anxiety disorders. *Archives of General Psychiatry*, **43**, 79–85.

Kamin LJ. (1968) Attention-like processes in classical conditioning. In Jones MR (Ed), *Miami Symposium on the Prediction of Behavior: Aversive Stimuli.* Coral Gables, FL: University of Miami Press.

Karno M, Golding JM, Sorenson SB, Burnam MA. (1988) The epidemiology of obsessive–compulsive disorder in five U.S. communities. *Archives of General Psychiatry*, **45**, 1094–9.

Kasper S. (1998) Social phobia: the nature of the disorder. *Journal of Affective Disorders*, **50** (Suppl.), S3–S9.

Katon W, Vitaliano PP, Russo J, Jones M, Anderson K. (1987) Panic disorder: spectrum of severity and somatization. *Journal of Nervous and Mental Disease*, **175**, 12–19.

Keane T. (1995) The role of exposure therapy in the psychological treatment of PTSD. *Clinical Quarterly of the National Center for PTSD*, **5**, 2–6.

Keane TM, Malloy PF, Fairbank JA. (1984) Empirical development of an MMPI subscale for the assessment of combat-related posttraumatic stress disorder. *Journal of Consulting and Clinical Psychology*, **52**, 888–91.

Keane TM, Caddell JM, Taylor KL. (1988) Mississippi Scale for combat-related posttraumatic stress disorder: three studies in reliability and validity. *Journal of Consulting and Clinical Psychology*, **56**, 85–90.

Keane TM, Fairbank JA, Caddell JM, Zimering RT. (1989) Implosive (flooding) therapy reduces symptoms of PTSD in Vietnam combat veterans. *Behavior Therapy*, **20**, 245–60.

Keijsers GPJ, Hoogduin CAL, Schaap CPDR. (1994) Predictors of treatment outcome in the behavioural treatment of obsessive–compulsive disorder. *British Journal of Psychiatry*, **165**, 781–6.

Kenardy JA, Webster RA, Lewin TJ, Carr VJ, Hazell PL, Carter GL. (1996) Stress debriefing and patterns of recovery following a natural disaster. *Journal of Traumatic Stress*, **9**, 37–50.

Kendall PC, Lipman AJ. (1991) Psychological and pharmacological therapy: methods and modes for comparative outcome research. *Journal of Consulting and Clinical Psychology*, **59**, 78–87.

Kendell RE, Discipio WJ. (1970) Obsessional symptoms and obsessional personality traits in depressive illness. *Psychological Medicine*, **1**, 65–72.

Kendler KS, Neale MC, Kessler RC, Heath AC, Eaves LJ. (1992a) The genetic epidemiology of phobias in women: the interrelationship of agoraphobia, social phobia, situational phobia, and simple phobia. *Archives of General Psychiatry*, **49**, 273–81.

Kendler KS, Neale MC, Kessler RC, Heath AC, Eaves LJ. (1992b) Major depression and generalized anxiety disorder. Same genes, (partly) different environments? *Archives of General Psychiatry*, **49**, 716–22.

Kendler KS, Neale MC, Kessler RC, Heath AC, Eaves LJ. (1993) Panic disorder in women: a population-based twin study. *Psychological Medicine*, **23**, 397–406.

Kendler KS, Karkowski LM, Prescott CA. (1999) Fears and phobias: reliability and heritability. *Psychological Medicine*, **29**, 539–53.

Kerr WJ, Dalton JW, Gliebe PA. (1937) Some physical phenomena associated with the anxiety state and their relation to hyperventilation. *Annals of Internal Medicine*, **11**, 961–75.

Kessler RC, McGonagle KA, Zhao S, Nelson CB, Hughes M, Eshleman S, Wittchen H-U, and Kendler KS. (1994) Lifetime and 12 month prevalence of DSM-III-R psychiatric disorders in the United States. Results from the National Comorbidity Survey. *Archives of General Psychiatry*, **51**, 8–19.

Kessler RC, Sonnega A, Bromet E, Hughes M, Nelson CB. (1995) Posttraumatic stress disorder in the National Comorbidity Survey. *Archives of General Psychiatry*, **52**, 1048–60.

Kessler RC, Stein MB, Berglund P. (1998) Social phobia subtypes in the National Comorbidity Survey. *American Journal of Psychiatry*, **155**, 613–19.

Kessler R, Sonnega A, Bromet E, Hughes M, Nelson C, Breslau N. (1999a) Epidemiological risk factors for trauma and PTSD. In Yehuda R (Ed), *Risk Factors For Posttraumatic Stress Disorder*. Washington, DC: American Psychiatric Press.

Kessler RC, Stang P, Wittchen H-U, Stein M, Walters EE. (1999b) Lifetime co-morbidities between social phobia and mood disorders in the US National Comorbidity Survey. *Psychological Medicine*, **29**, 555–67.

Kilic C, Curran HV, Noshirvani H, Marks, IM, Basoglu M. (1999) Long-term effects of alprazolam on memory: a 3.5 year follow-up of agoraphobia/panic patients. *Psychological Medicine*, **29**, 225–31.

Kilpatrick DG, Resnick HS, Freedy JR, Pelcovitz D, Resick P, Roth S, van der Kolk B. (1997) The posttraumatic stress disorder field trial: evaluation of the PTSD construct: criteria A through E. In Widiger TA, Frances AJ, Pincus HA, First MB, Ross R, Davis W (Eds), *DSM-IV Sourcebook*, Vol. IV. Washington DC: American Psychiatric Press.

Kirk J. (1989) Cognitive-behavioural assessment. In Hawton K, Salkovskis PM, Kirk J, Clarke

DM (Eds), *Cognitive-Behaviour Therapies for Psychiatric Problems: A Practical Guide.* Oxford: Oxford University Press.

Klass ET, DiNardo PA, Barlow DH. (1989) DSM-III-R personality diagnoses in anxiety disorder patients. *Comprehensive Psychiatry*, **30**, 251–8.

Kleber RJ, Figley CR, Gersons BP. (1995) *Beyond Trauma: Cultural and Societal Dynamics.* New York: Plenum Press.

Klein DF. (1964) Delineation of two drug-responsive anxiety syndromes. *Psychopharmacologia*, **5**, 397–408.

Klein DF. (1981) Anxiety reconceptualized. In Klein DF, Rabkin JG (Eds), *Anxiety: New Research and Changing Concepts.* New York: Raven Press.

Klein DF, Ross DC. (1986) Response of panic patients and normal controls to lactate infusions. *Psychiatry Research*, **19**, 163–4.

Kleinknecht RA. (1987) Vasovagal syncope and blood/injury fear. *Behaviour Research and Therapy*, **25**, 175–8.

Kleinknecht RA, Lenz J. (1989) Blood/injury fear, fainting and avoidance of medically-related situations: a family correspondence study. *Behaviour Research and Therapy*, **27**, 537–47.

Klosko JS, Barlow DH, Tassinari R, Cerny JA. (1990) A comparison of alprazolam and behavior therapy in treatment of panic disorder. *Journal of Consulting and Clinical Psychology*, **58**, 77–84.

Knowles JA, Mannuzza S, Fyer AJ. (1995) Heritability of social anxiety. In Stein MB (Ed), *Social Phobia: Clinical and Research Perspectives.* Washington, DC: American Psychiatric Press, pp. 147–62.

Kobak KA, Greist J, Jeffersen JW, Katzelnick DJ, Henk HJ. (1998) Behavioral versus pharmacological treatments of obsessive–compulsive disorder: a meta-analysis. *Psychopharmacology*, **136**, 205–16.

Kopenon H, Lepola U, Leinonen E, Jokinen R, Penntinen J, Turtonen J. (1997) Citalopram in the treatment of obsessive–compulsive disorder: an open trial. *Acta Psychiatrica Scandinavica*, **96**, 121–9.

Kringlen E. (1965). Obsessional neurotics: a long term follow-up. *British Journal of Psychiatry*, **111**, 709–22.

Kronig M, Apter J, Asnis G, Bystritsky A, Curtis G, Ferguson J, Landbloom R, Munjak D, Reisenberg R, Robinson D, Roy-Byrne P, Phillips K, Du Pont I. (1999) Placebo controlled multicentre study of sertraline treatment for obsessive–compulsive disorder. *Journal of Clinical Psychopharmacology*, **19**, 172–6.

Krueger RF. (1999) The structure of common mental disorders. *Archives of General Psychiatry*, **56**, 921–6.

Krueger RF, Caspi A, Moffitt TE. (2000) Epidemiological personology: the unifying role of personality in population based research on problem behaviors. *Journal of Personality*, **68**, 967–98.

Kubany ES. (1994) A cognitive model of guilt typology in combat-related PTSD. *Journal of Traumatic Stress*, **7**, 3–19.

Kulka RA, Schlenger WE, Fairbank JA, Hough RL, Jordan BK, Marmar CR, Weiss DS. (1990) *Trauma and the Vietnam Generation: Report of Findings from the National Vietnam Veterans*

Readjustment Study. New York: Brunner/Mazel.

Kushner MG, Sher KJ, Beitman BD. (1990) The relation between alcohol problems and the anxiety disorders. *American Journal of Psychiatry*, **147**, 685–95.

Lader M, Scotto J. (1998) A multicentre double-blind comparison on hydroxyzine, buspirone and placebo in patients with generalized anxiety disorder. *Psychopharmacology*, **139**, 402–6.

Ladouceur R. (1983) Participant modelling with or without cognitive treatment for phobias. *Journal of Consulting and Clinical Psychology*, **51**, 942–4.

Ladouceur R, Blais F, Freeston MH, Dugas MJ. (1998) Problem solving and problem orientation in generalized anxiety disorder. *Journal of Anxiety Disorders*, **12**, 139–152.

Ladouceur R, Dugas MJ, Freeston MH, Leger E, Gagnon F, Thibodeau N. (2000a). Efficacy of a cognitive-behavioural treatment for generalized anxiety disorder: evaluation in a controlled clinical trial. *Journal of Clinical and Consulting Psychology*, **68**, 957–64.

Ladouceur R, Gosselin P, Dugas MJ. (2000b). Experimental manipulation of intolerance of uncertainty: a study of a theoretical model of worry. *Behaviour Research and Therapy*, **38**, 933–41.

Lampe LA. (2000) Social phobia: a review of recent research trends. *Current Opinion in Psychiatry*, **13**, 149–55.

Lang PJ. (1979) A bioinformational theory of emotional imagery. *Psychophysiology*, **6**, 495–511.

Langlois F, Freeston MH, Ladouceur R. (2000a) Differences and similarities between obsessive intrusive thoughts and worry in a non-clinical population: study 1. *Behavior Research and Therapy*, **38**, 157–73.

Langlois F, Freeston MH, Ladouceur R. (2000b). Differences and similarities between obsessive intrusive thoughts and worry in a non-clinical population: study 2. *Behavior Research and Therapy*, **38**, 175–89.

Last CG. (1987) Simple phobias. In Michaelson L, Ascher LM (Eds), *Anxiety and Stress Disorders*. New York: Guilford.

Last CG, Barlow DH, O'Brien GT. (1984) Precipitants of agoraphobia: role of stressful life events. *Psychological Reports*, **54**, 567–70.

Last CG, Strauss CC. (1989) Obsessive–compulsive disorder in childhood. *Journal of Anxiety Disorders*, **3**, 295–302.

Leary MR, Kowalsky RM. (1995) The self-presentation model of social phobia. In Heimberg RG, Liebowitz MR, Hope DA, Schneider FR. (Eds), *Social Phobia: Diagnosis, Assessment and Treatment*. New York: Guilford.

Lecrubier Y. (1998) Comorbidity in social anxiety disorder: impact on disease burden and management. *Journal of Clinical Psychiatry*, **59**, 33–7.

Lecrubier Y, Weiller E. (1997) Comorbidities in social phobia. *International Journal of Clinical Psychopharmacology*, **12** (Suppl. 6), 17–21.

Lelliot PT, Noshirvani HF, Basoglu M, Marks IM, Montiero WO. (1988) Obsessive–compulsive beliefs and treatment outcome. *Psychological Medicine*, **18**, 697–702.

Lenane MC, Swedo SE, Leonardo H, Pauls DL, Sceery W, Rapoport JL. (1990) Psychiatric disorders in first degree relatives of children and adolescents with obsessive compulsive disorder. *Journal of the American Academy of Child and Adolescent Psychiatry*, **29**, 407–12.

Lepine J-P, Pelissolo A. (1998) Social phobia and alcoholism: a complex relationship. *Journal of*

Affective Disorders, **50** (Suppl.), S23–S28.

Levis DJ, Hare NA. (1977) A review of the theoretical, rational, and empirical support for the extinction process in implosive (flooding) therapy. In Hersen M, Eisler RM, Miller PM (Eds), *Progress in Behavior Modification*, Vol. 4. New York: Academic Press.

Ley R. (1988) Hyperventilation and lactate infusion in the production of panic attacks. *Clinical Psychology Review*, **8**, 1–18.

Liebowitz MR. (1987) Social phobia. *Modern Problems of Pharmacopsychiatry*, **22**, 141–73.

Liebowitz MR, Gorman JM, Fyer AJ, Klein DF. (1985) Social phobia: review of a neglected anxiety disorder. *Archives of General Psychiatry*, **42**, 729–36.

Liebowitz MR, Gorman JM, Fyer AJ, Campeas R, Levin AP, Sandberg D, Hollander E, Papp L, Goetz D. (1988) Pharmacotherapy of social phobia: an interim report of a placebo-controlled comparison of phenelzine and atenolol. *Journal of Clinical Psychiatry*, **49**, 252–7.

Liebowitz MR, Ballenger J, Barlow DH, Davidson J, Foa EB, Fyer A. (1990) New perspectives on anxiety disorders in DSM-IV and ICD-10. *Drug Therapy*, **20** (Suppl.), 129–36.

Liebowitz MR, Schneier FR, Hollander E, Welkowitz LA, Saoud JB, Feerick J, Campeas R, Fallon BA, Street L, Gitow A. (1991) Treatment of social phobia with drugs other than ben-zodiazepines. *Journal of Clinical Psychiatry*, **52** (11, Suppl.), 10–15.

Liebowitz MR, Schneier F, Campeas R, Hollander E, Hatterer J, Fyer A, Gorman J, Papp L, Davies S, Gully R, Klein DF. (1992) Phenelzine vs. atenolol in social phobia: a placebo-controlled comparison. *Archives of General Psychiatry*, **49**, 290–300.

Lindsay M, Crino R, Andrews G. (1997) Controlled trial of exposure and response prevention in obsessive–compulsive disorder. *British Journal of Psychiatry*, **171**, 135–9.

Lindsay WR, Gamsu CV, McLaughlin E, Hood EM, Espie CA. (1987) A controlled trial of treatments for generalized anxiety. *British Journal of Clinical Psychology*, **26**, 3–15.

Lopatka C, Rachman S. (1995) Perceived responsibility and compulsive checking: an experi-mental analysis. *Behaviour Research and Therapy*, **33**, 673–84.

Loranger AW. (1988) *Personality Disorder Examination (PDE) Manual*. Yonkers, NY: DV Communications.

Loranger AW, Janca A, Sartorius N. (1997) *Assessment and Diagnosis of Personality Disorders: The ICD-10 International Personality Disorder Examination (IPDE)*. Cambridge: Cambridge University Press.

Lorin K, McElroy S, Davidson J, Rasmussen S, Hollander E, Jenike M. (1996) Fluvoxamine versus clomipramine for obsessive–compulsive disorder: a double blind comparison. *Journal of Clinical Psychopharmacology*, **16**, 121–9.

Lovibond PF. (1998) Long-term stability of depression, anxiety and stress syndromes. *Journal of Abnormal Psychology*, **107**, 520–6.

Lovibond PF, Lovibond SH. (1995) The structure of negative emotional states: comparison of the Depression Anxiety Stress Scales (DASS) with the Beck Depression and Anxiety Invento-ries. *Behaviour Research and Therapy*, **33**, 335–43.

Lowry TP. (1967) *Hyperventilation and Hysteria*. Springfield, IL: Charles C. Thomas.

Lucock MP, Salkovskis PM. (1988) Cognitive factors in social anxiety and its treatment. *Behaviour Research and Therapy*, **26**, 297–302.

Lum LC. (1983) Psychological considerations in the treatment of hyperventilation syndromes.

Journal of Drug Research, **8**, 1867–72.

Lydiard RB, Ballenger JC, Rickels K, for the Abecarnil Work Group. (1997). A double-blind evaluation of the safety and efficacy of abecarnil, alprazolam, and placebo in outpatients with generalized anxiety disorder. *Journal of Clinical Psychiatry*, **58** (Suppl. 11), 11–18.

Lyons J, Keane T. (1989) Implosive therapy for the treatment of combat-related PTSD. *Journal of Traumatic Stress*, **2**, 137–52.

Mackintosh NJ. (1983) *Conditioning and Associative Learning*. Oxford: Oxford University Press.

MacLeod C, McLaughlin K. (1995) Implicit and explicit memory bias in anxiety: a conceptual replication. *Behaviour Research and Therapy*, **33**, 1–14.

MacLeod C, Mathews A, Tata P. (1986) Attentional bias in emotional disorders. *Journal of Abnormal Psychology*, **95**, 15–20.

Magarian GJ. (1982) Hyperventilation syndromes: infrequently recognized common expressions of anxiety and stress. *Medicine*, **61**, 219–36.

Magee WJ, Eaton WW, Wittchen HU, McGonagle KA, Kessler RC. (1996) Agoraphobia, simple phobia and social phobia in the National Comorbidity Survey. *Archives of General Psychiatry*, **53**, 159–68.

Mahgoub OM, Abdel-Hafiez HB. (1991) Pattern of obsessive–compulsive disorder in eastern Saudi Arabia. *British Journal of Psychiatry*, **158**, 840–2.

Maier W, Gaensicke M, Freyberger HJ, Linz M, Heun R, Lecrubier Y. (2000) Generalized anxiety disorder (ICD-10) in primary care from a cross-cultural perspective: a valid diagnostic entity? *Acta Psychiatrica Scandinavica*, **101**, 29–36.

Mannuzza S, Fyer AJ, Martin LY, Gallops MS, Endicott J, Gorman J, Liebowitz MR, Klein DF. (1989) Reliability of anxiety assessment: I. Diagnostic agreement. *Archives of General Psychiatry*, **46**, 1093–101.

Mannuzza S, Schneier FR, Chapman TF, Liebowitz MR, Kelin DF, Fyer AJ. (1995) Generalized social phobia: reliability and validity. *Archives of General Psychiatry*, **52**, 230–7.

March JS, Mulle K, Harbel B. (1994) Behavioral psychotherapy for children and adolescents with obsessive–compulsive disorder: an open trial of a new protocol driven treatment package. *Journal of the American Academy of Child Psychiatry*, **33**, 331–41.

Marchand A, Goyer LR, Dupuis G, Mainguy N. (1998) Personality disorders and the outcome of cognitive-behavioural treatment of panic disorder with agoraphobia. *Canadian Journal of Behavioural Science*, **30**, 14–23.

Margraf J, Ehlers A, Roth WT. (1986) Sodium lactate infusions and panic attacks: a review and critique. *Psychosomatic Medicine*, **48**, 23–51.

Margraf J, Taylor CC, Ehlers A, Roth WT, Agras WS. (1987) Panic attacks in the natural environment. *Journal of Nervous and Mental Disease*, **175**, 558–65.

Markowitz JS, Weissman MM, Quellette R, Lish JD, Klerman GL. (1989) Quality of life in panic disorder. *Archives of General Psychiatry*, **46**, 984–92.

Marks IM. (1969) *Fears and Phobias*. Oxford: Heinemann.

Marks IM. (1970) The classification of phobic disorders. *British Journal of Psychiatry*, **116**, 377–86.

Marks IM. (1975) Behavioral treatments of phobic and obsessive–compulsive disorders: a critical appraisal. In Hersen M, Eisler RM, Miller PM (Eds), *Progress in Behavior Modification*,

Vol. 1. New York: Academic Press.

Marks IM. (1978) Behavioral psychotherapy of adult neurosis. In Bergin AE, Garfield S (Eds), *Handbook of Psychotherapy and Behavior Change*. New York: John Wiley and Sons.

Marks IM. (1985) Behavioral treatment of social phobia. *Psychopharmacology*, **21**, 615–18.

Marks IM. (1987) *Fears, Phobias and Rituals: Panic, Anxiety, and Their Disorders*. New York: Oxford University Press.

Marks IM. (1988) Blood–injury phobia: a review. *American Journal of Psychiatry*, **145**, 1207–13.

Marks I, Dar R. (2000) Fear reduction by psychotherapies: recent findings, future directions. *British Journal of Psychiatry*, **176**, 507–11.

Marks IM, Crowe M, Drewe E, Young J, Dewhurst WG. (1969) Obsessive–compulsive neurosis in identical twins. *British Journal of Psychiatry*, **115**, 991–8.

Marks IM, Hodgson R, Rachman S. (1975) Treatment of chronic obsessive–compulsive neurosis by in-vivo exposure. *British Journal of Psychiatry*, **127**, 344–64.

Marks IM, Stern R, Mawson D, Cobb J, McDonald R. (1980) Clomipramine and exposure for obsessive compulsive rituals. *British Journal of Psychiatry*, **136**, 1–25.

Marks IM, Lelliot P, Bosaglu M, Noshirvani H, Montiero W, Cohen D, Kasvikis Y. (1988) Clomipramine, self exposure and therapist aided exposure for obsessive–compulsive rituals. *British Journal of Psychiatry*, **151**, 522–34.

Marks IM, Swinson RP, Basoglu M, Kuch K, Noshirvan H, O'Sullivan G, Lelliott P, Kirby M, McNamee G, Sengun S, Wickwire K. (1993) Alprazolam and exposure alone and combined in panic disorder with agoraphobia. A controlled study in London and Toronto. *British Journal of Psychiatry*, **162**, 776–87.

Marks I, Lovell K, Noshirvani H, Livanou M, Thrasher S. (1998) Treatment of posttraumatic stress disorder by exposure and/or cognitive restructuring. *Archives of General Psychiatry*, **55**, 317–25.

Marks M. (1989) Behavioural psychotherapy for generalized anxiety disorder. *International Review of Psychiatry*, **1**, 235–44.

Marshall JR. (1992) The psychopharmacology of social phobia. *Bulletin of the Meninger Clinic*, **56** (2, Suppl.), A42–A49.

Marshall WL. (1985) The effects of variable exposure in flooding therapy. *Behaviour Research and Therapy*, **16**, 117–35.

Marten PA, Brown TA, Barlow DH, Borkovec TD, Shear MK, Lydiard RB. (1993) Evaluation of the ratings comprising the associated symptom criterion of DSM-III-R generalized anxiety disorder. *Journal of Nervous and Mental Disease*, **181**, 676–82.

Maser JD. (1998) Generalized anxiety disorder and its comorbidities: disputes at the boundaries. *Acta Psychiatrica Scandinavica*, **98** (Suppl. 393), 12–22.

Mathers C, Vos T, Stephenson C. (1999) *The Burden of Disease and Injury in Australia*. Canberra, ACT: Australian Institute of Health and Welfare.

Mathews AM, MacLeod C. (1986) Discrimination of threat cues without awareness in anxiety states. *Journal of Abnormal Psychology*, **5**, 131–8.

Mathews AM, Gelder MG, Johnston DW. (1981) *Agoraphobia: Nature and Treatment*. New York: Guilford.

Mathews A, Mogg K, May J, Eysenck MJ. (1989) Implicit and explicit memory bias in anxiety.

Journal of Abnormal Psychology, **8**, 193–4.

Mattick RP, Clarke JC. (1998) Development and validation of measures of social phobia scrutiny fear and social interaction anxiety. *Behaviour Research and Therapy*, **36**, 455–70.

Mattick RP, Peters L. (1988) Treatment of severe social phobia: effects of guided exposure with and without cognitive restructuring. *Journal of Consulting and Clinical Psychology*, **56**, 251–60.

Mattick RP, Peters L, Clarke JC. (1989) Exposure and cognitive restructuring for social phobia: a controlled study. *Behavior Therapy*, **20**, 3–23.

Mattick RP, Andrews G, Hadzi-Pavlovic D, Christensen H. (1990) Treatment of panic and agoraphobia: an integrative review. *Journal of Nervous and Mental Disease*, **178**, 567–76.

Mattick RP, Page A, Lampe L. (1995) Cognitive and behavioural aspects. In Stein MB (Ed), *Social Phobia: Clinical and Research Perspectives*. Washington, DC: American Psychiatric Press.

Mauri M, Sarno N, Rossi VM, Armani A, Zambotto S, Cassano GB, Akiskal HS. (1992) Personality disorders associated with generalized anxiety, panic, and recurrent depressive disorders. *Journal of Personality Disorders*, **6**, 162–7.

Mavissakalian M. (1988) The relationship between panic, phobia, and anticipatory anxiety in agoraphobia. *Behaviour Research and Therapy*, **26**, 235–40.

Mavissakalian M, Barlow DH. (1981) *Phobia: Psychological and Pharmacological Treatment*. New York: Guilford Press.

Mavissakalian M, Hamann MS, Jones B. (1990). DSM-III personality disorders in obsessive–compulsive disorder: changes with treatment. *Comprehensive Psychiatry*, **5**, 432–7.

McDougle C, Epperson N, Pelton G, Wasylink S, Price L. (2000) A double blind placebo controlled study of risperidone addition in serotonin reuptake inhibitor-refractory obsessive–compulsive disorder. *Archives of General Psychiatry*, **57**, 794–801.

McGuffin P, Mawson D. (1980) Obsessive–compulsive neurosis: two identical twin pairs. *British Journal of Psychiatry*, **137**, 285–7.

McNally RJ. (1981) Phobias and preparedness: instructional reversal of electrodermal conditioning to fear-relevant stimuli. *Psychological Reports*, **48**, 175–80.

McNally RJ. (1990) Psychological approaches to panic disorder: a review. *Psychological Bulletin*, **108**, 403–19.

McNally RJ. (1999) Research on eye movement desensitization and reprocessing (EMDR) as a treatment for PTSD. *PTSD Research Quarterly of the National Center for PTSD*, **10**, 1–7.

McNally RJ, Foa EB. (1987) Cognition and agoraphobia: bias in the interpretation of threat. *Cognitive Therapy and Research*, **11**, 567–82.

McNally RJ, Steketee GS. (1985) The etiology and maintenance of severe animal phobias. *Behaviour Research and Therapy*, **23**, 431–5.

McNally RJ, Foa EB, Donnell CD. (1989) Memory bias for anxiety information in patients with panic disorder. *Cognition and Emotion*, **3**, 27–44.

McNally RJ, Kaspi SP, Riemann BC, Zeitlin SB. (1990a) Selective processing of threat cues in post-traumatic stress disorder. *Journal of Abnormal Psychology*, **9**, 398–402.

McNally RJ, Riemann BC, Kim E. (1990b) Selective processing of threat cues in panic disorder. *Behaviour Research and Therapy*, **28**, 407–12.

McPherson FM, Brougham L, McLaren S. (1980) Maintenance of improvement in agoraphobic patients treated by behavioral methods – four year follow-up. *Behaviour Research and Therapy*, **18**, 150–2.

Meehl PE. (1954) *Clinical Versus Statistical Prediction: A Theoretical Analysis and a Review of the Evidence*. Minneapolis, MN: University of Minnesota Press.

Meichenbaum D. (1977) *Cognitive Behavior Modification*. New York: Plenum Press.

Meichenbaum D. (1985) *Stress Inoculation Training*. New York: Pergamon Press.

Menzies RG, Clarke JC. (1995) The etiology of phobias: a non-associative account. *Clinical Psychology Review*, **15**, 23–48.

Mersch PPA, Emmelkamp PMG, Bogels SM, van der Sleen J. (1989) Social phobia: individual response patterns and the effects of cognitive and behavioral interventions. *Behavior Research and Therapy*, **27**, 421–34.

Mersch PPA, Jansen MA, Arntz A. (1995). Social phobia and personality disorder: severity of complaint and treatment effectiveness. *Journal of Personality Disorders*, **9**, 143–59.

Meyer TJ, Miller ML, Metzger RL, Borkovec TD. (1990) Development and validation of the Penn State Worry Questionnaire. *Behaviour Research and Therapy*, **28**, 487–95.

Michelson LK, Marchione K. (1991) Behavioral, cognitive, and pharmacological treatments of panic disorder with agoraphobia: critique and synthesis. *Journal of Consulting and Clinical Psychology*, **59**, 100–14.

Mick MA, Telch MJ. (1998) Social anxiety and history of behavioral inhibition in young adults. *Journal of Anxiety Disorders*, **12**, 1–20.

Miguel EC, Coffey BJ, Baer L, Savage CR, Rauch SL, Jenike MA. (1995) Phenomenology of intentional repetitive behaviors in obsessive–compulsive disorder and Tourette's disorder. *Journal of Clinical Psychiatry*, **56**, 246–55.

Miller WR, Page AC. (1991) Warm turkey: other paths to abstinence. *Journal of Substance Abuse Treatment*, **8**, 227–32.

Miller WR, Rollnick S. (1991) *Motivational Interviewing: Preparing People to Change Addictive Behaviors*. New York: Guilford Press.

Mineka S. (1988) A primate model of phobic fears. In Eysenck HJ, Martin I (Eds), *Theoretical Foundations of Behaviour Therapy*. New York: Plenum Press.

Mineka S, Zinbarg R. (1996) Conditioning and ethological models of anxiety disorders: stress-in-dynamic-context anxiety models. In Hope DA. (Ed), (1996) *Nebraska Symposium on Motivation, 1995: Perspectives on Anxiety, Panic, and Fear. Current Theory and Research in Motivation*, Vol. 43, Lincoln, NE: University of Nebraska Press.

Missri JC, Alexander S. (1978) Hyperventilation syndrome: a brief review. *Journal of the American Medical Association*, **240**, 2093–6.

Mitchell JT, Bray G. (1990) *Emergency Services Stress*. Engelwood Cliffs, NJ: Prentice Hall.

Molina S, Borkovec TD, Peasley C, Person D. (1998) Content analysis of worrisome streams of consciousness in anxious and dysphoric participants. *Cognitive Therapy and Research*, **22**, 109–23.

Montgomery SA. (1998) Implications of the severity of social phobia. *Journal of Affective Disorders*, **50**, S17–S22.

Moran C. (1986) Depersonalization and agoraphobia associated with marijuana use. *British*

Journal of Medical Psychology, **9**, 187–96.

Morgan H, Raffle C. (1999) Does reducing safety behaviours improve treatment response in patients with social phobia? *Australian and New Zealand Journal of Psychiatry*, **33**, 503–10.

Morgenstern J, Langenbucher J, Labouvie E, Miller KJ. (1997) The comorbidity of alcoholism and personality disorders in a clinical population: prevalence rates and relation to alcohol typology. *Journal of Abnormal Psychology*, **106**, 74–84.

Mowrer O. (1960) *Learning Theory and Behaviour*. New York: John Wiley and Sons.

Mulder RT, Sellman JD, Joyce PR. (1991) The comorbidity of anxiety disorders with personality, depressive, alcohol and drug disorders. *International Review of Psychiatry*, **3**, 253–64.

Mullaney JA, Trippett CJ. (1979) Alcohol dependence and phobias: clinical description and relevance. *British Journal of Psychiatry*, **135**, 565–73.

Munby J, Johnston DW. (1980) Agoraphobia: long-term follow-up of behavioural treatment. *British Journal of Psychiatry*, **135**, 418–27.

Mundo E, Bianchi L, Bellodi L. (1997) Efficacy of fluvoxamine, paroxetine and citalopram in the treatment of obsessive–compulsive disorder: a single blind study. *Journal of Clinical Psychopharmacology*, **17**, 267–71.

Munjack DJ. (1984) The onset of driving phobias. *Journal of Behavior Therapy and Experimental Psychiatry*, **15**, 305–8.

Munjack DJ, Baltazar PL, Bohn PB, Cabe DD, Appleton AA. (1990) Clonazepam in the treatment of social phobia: a pilot study. *Journal of Clinical Psychiatry*, **51** (5, Suppl.), 35–40.

Muris P, Merckelbach H. (1997) Treating spider phobics with eye movement desensitization and reprocessing: a controlled study. *Behavioural and Cognitive Psychotherapy*, **25**, 39–50.

Muris P, Merckelbach H, van Haaften H, Mayer B. (1997) Eye movement desensitisation and reprocessing versus exposure in vivo. A single-session crossover study of spider-phobic children. *British Journal of Psychiatry*, **171**, 82–6.

Muris P, Merckelbach H, Holdrinet I, Sijsenaar M. (1998) Treating phobic children: effects of EMDR versus exposure. *Journal of Consulting and Clinical Psychology*, **66**, 193–8.

Murphy MT, Michelson LK, Marchione K, Marchione N, Testa S. (1998) The role of self-directed in vivo exposure in combination with cognitive therapy, relaxation training, or therapist-assisted exposure in the treatment of panic disorder with agoraphobia. *Journal of Anxiety Disorders*, **12**, 117–38.

Murray CJL, Lopez AD. (1996) *The Global Burden of Disease*. Cambridge, MA: Harvard University Press.

Myers JK, Weissman MM, Tischler GL, Holzer CE, Leaf PJ, Orvaschel H, Anthony JC, Boyd JH, Burke JD, Kramer M, Stoltzman R. (1984) Six-month prevalence of psychiatric disorders in three communities: 1980–1982. *Archives of General Psychiatry*, **41**, 959–67.

Nathan P, Gorman J. (1998) *A Guide to Treatments that Work*. New York: Oxford University Press.

Nestadt G, Samuels J, Riddle M, Bienvenu J, Liang K-Y, LaBuda M, Walkup J, Grados M, Hoehn-Saric R. (2000) A family study of obsessive–compulsive disorder. *Archives of General Psychiatry*, **57**, 358–63.

Neufeld KJ, Swartz KL, Beinvenu OJ, Eaton WW, Cai G. (1999) Incidence of DIS/DSM-IV social phobia in adults. *Acta Psychiatrica Scandinavica*, **100**, 186–92.

Newman MG. (2000) Recommendations for a cost-offset model of psychotherapy allocation using generalized anxiety disorder as an example. *Journal of Consulting and Clinical Psychology*, **68**, 549–55.

Newman MG, Kenardy J, Herman S, Taylor CB. (1997) Comparison of palm-top-assisted brief cognitive-behavioral treatment to cognitive-behavioral treatment for panic disorder. *Journal of Consulting and Clinical Psychology*, **65**, 178–83.

Nezu AM. (1986) Efficacy of a social problem-solving therapy approach for unipolar depression. *Journal of Consulting and Clinical Psychology*, **54**, 196–202.

NHMRC (National Health and Medical Research Council). (1991) *Guidelines for the Prevention and Management of Benzodiazepine Dependence.* Monograph Series No. 3. Canberra, ACT: Australian Government Publishing Service.

Nisita C, Petracca A, Akiskal HS, Galli L, Gepponi I, Cassano GB. (1990) Delimitation of generalized anxiety disorder: clinical comparisons with panic and major depressive disorders. *Comprehensive Psychiatry*, **31**, 409–15.

Norris FH, Riad JK. (1997) Standardized self-report measures of civilian trauma and posttraumatic stress disorder. In Wilson J, Keane T (Eds), *Assessing Psychological Trauma and PTSD.* New York: Guilford Press.

Norton GR, McLeod L, Guertin J, Hewitt PL, Walker JR, Stein MB. (1996) Panic disorder or social phobia: which is worse? *Behaviour Research and Therapy*, **34**, 273–6.

Noshirvani HF, Kasvikis YG, Marks IM, Tsakiris F, Montiero WO. (1991) Gender divergent aetiological factors in obsessive–compulsive disorder. *British Journal of Psychiatry*, **158**, 260–3.

Noyes R, Clancy J, Garvey M, Anderson DJ. (1987a) Is agoraphobia a variant of panic disorder or a separate illness? *Journal of Anxiety Disorders*, **1**, 3–13.

Noyes R, Clarkson C, Crowe RR, Yates WR, McChesney CM. (1987b) A family study of generalized anxiety disorder. *American Journal of Psychiatry*, **144**, 1019–24.

Noyes R, Moroz G, Davidson JRT, Liebowitz MR, Davidson A, Siegel J, Bell J, Cain JW, Curlik S, Kent T, Lydiard R, Mallinger AG, Pollack MH, Rapaport M, Rasmussen SA, Hedges D, Schweizer E, Uhlenhuth EH (1997) Moclobemide in social phobia: a controlled dose–response trial. *Journal of Clinical Psychopharmacology*, **17**, 247–54.

Nunn JD, Stevenson RJ, Whalan G. (1984) Selective memory effects in agoraphobic patients. *British Journal of Clinical Psychology*, **23**, 195–201.

Nutt DJ, Bell CJ, Malizia AL. (1998) Brain mechanisms of social anxiety disorder. *Journal of Clinical Psychiatry*, **59**, 4–9.

Oakley ME, Padesky CA. (1990) Cognitive therapy for anxiety disorders. In Hersen M, Eisler RM, Miller PM (Eds), *Progress in Behavior Modification*, Vol. 26. Newbury Park, CA: Sage.

O'Brien GT. (1981) Clinical treatment of specific phobias. In Mavissakalian M, Barlow DH (Eds), *Phobia: Psychological and Pharmacological Treatment.* New York: Guilford.

Oei TPS, Moylan A, Evans L. (1991) Validity and clinical utility of the Fear Questionnaire for anxiety disorder patients. *Journal of Consulting and Clinical Psychology*, **3**, 391–7.

Oei TPS, Llamas M, Evans, L. (1997) Does concurrent drug intake affect the long-term outcome of group-cognitive behaviour therapy in panic disorder with or without agoraphobia? *Behaviour Research and Therapy*, **35**, 851–7.

Oei TPS, Llamas M, Devilly GJ. (1999) The efficacy and cognitive processes of cognitive behaviour therapy in the treatment of panic disorder with agoraphobia. *Behavioural and Cognitive Psychotherapy*, **27**, 63–88.

Offord DR, Boyle MH, Campbell D, Goering P, Lin E, Wong M, Racine A. (1996) One-year prevalence of psychiatric disorder in Ontarians 15 to 64 years of age. *Canadian Journal of Psychiatry*, **41**, 559–63.

Öhman A. (1986) Face the beast and fear the face: animal and social fears as prototypes for evolutionary analyses of emotion. *Psychophysiology*, **23**, 123–45.

Öhman A, Eriksson A, Olofsson C. (1975a) One-trial learning and superior resistance to extinction of autonomic responses conditioned to potentially phobic stimuli. *Journal of Comparative and Physiological Psychology*, **8**, 619–27.

Öhman A, Erixon G, Lofberg I. (1975b) Phobias and preparedness: phobic versus neutral pictures as conditioned stimuli for human autonomic responses. *Journal of Abnormal Psychology*, **4**, 41–5.

Öhman A, Freidrikson M, Hugdahl K, Rimmo P. (1976) The premise of equipotentiality in human classical conditioning: conditioned electrodermal responses to potentially phobic stimuli. *Journal of Experimental Psychology: General*, **105**, 331–7.

Okasha A, Saad A, Khalil AH, Seif El Dawla A, Yehia N. (1994) Phenomenology of obsessive compulsive disorder; a transcultural study. *Comprehensive Psychiatry*, **35**, 191–7.

Oliver N, Page AC. (2002). Fear reduction during in-vivo exposure to blood–injection stimuli: distraction vs attentional focus. *British Journal of Clinical Psychology*, in press.

Ollendick TH. (1995) Cognitive behavioral treatment of panic disorder with agoraphobia in adolescents: a multiple baseline design analysis. *Behavior Therapy*, **26**, 517–31.

Ontiveros A, Fontaine R. (1990) Social phobia and clonazepam. *Canadian Journal of Psychiatry*, **35**, 439–41.

Öst L-G. (1978) Behavioral treatment of thunder and lightning phobics. *Behaviour Research and Therapy*, **16**, 197–207.

Öst L-G. (1987a) Age at onset in different phobia. *Journal of Abnormal Psychology*, **6**, 223–9.

Öst L-G. (1987b) Applied relaxation: description of a coping technique and review of controlled studies. *Behaviour Research and Therapy*, **25**, 397–409.

Öst L-G. (1989) One session treatment for specific phobias. *Behaviour Research and Therapy*, **27**, 1–7.

Öst L-G, Breitholtz E. (2000). Applied relaxation vs. cognitive therapy in the treatment of generalized anxiety disorder. *Behaviour Research and Therapy*, **38**, 777–90.

Öst L-G, Jerremalm A, Johansson J. (1981) Individual response patterns and the effects of different behavioral methods in the treatment of social phobia. *Behavior Research and Therapy*, **19**, 1–16.

Öst L-G, Lindahl I-L, Sterner U, Jerremalm A. (1984a) Exposure in vivo vs applied relaxation in the treatment of blood phobia. *Behaviour Research and Therapy*, **22**, 205–16.

Öst L-G, Sterner U, Lindahl, I-L. (1984b) Physiological responses in blood phobics. *Behaviour Research and Therapy*, **22**, 109–17.

Öst L-G, Sterner U. (1987) Applied tension: a specific method for treatment of blood phobia. *Behaviour Research and Therapy*, **25**, 25–9.

Öst L-G, Sterner U, Fellenius J. (1989) Applied tension, applied relaxation, and the combination in the treatment of blood phobia. *Behaviour Research and Therapy*, **27**, 109–21.

O'Sullivan G, Noshirvani H, Marks I, Montiero W, Lelliot P. (1991) Six year follow-up after exposure and clomipramine therapy for obsessive compulsive disorder. *Journal of Clinical Psychiatry*, **52**, 150–5.

Otto MW, Pollack MH, Gould RA, Worthington JJ, McArdle ET, Rosenbaum JF. (2000) A comparison of the efficacy of clonazepam and cognitive-behavioral group therapy for the treatment of social phobia. *Journal of Anxiety Disorders*, **14**, 345–58.

Overbeek T, Rikken J, Schruers K, Griez E. (1998) Suicidal ideation in panic disorder patients. *Journal of Nervous and Mental Disease*, **186**, 577–80.

Page AC. (1991a) Simple phobias. *International Review of Psychiatry*, **3**, 175–84.

Page AC. (1991b) An assessment of structured diagnostic interviews for adult anxiety disorders. *International Review of Psychiatry*, **3**, 265–78.

Page AC. (1993) *Don't Panic! Overcoming Anxiety, Phobias and Tension.* Sydney: Gore Osment.

Page AC. (1994a) Panic provocation in the treatment of agoraphobia: a preliminary investigation. *Australian and New Zealand Journal of Psychiatry*, **28**, 82–6.

Page AC. (1994b) Blood–injury phobia. *Clinical Psychology Review*, **14**, 443–61.

Page AC. (1994c) Distinguishing panic disorder and agoraphobia from social phobia. *Journal of Nervous and Mental Disease*, **182**, 611–17.

Page AC. (1996) Blood–injury–injection fears in medical practice. *Medical Journal of Australia*, **164**, 189.

Page AC. (1998a) Assessment of panic disorder. *Current Opinion in Psychiatry*, **11**, 137–41.

Page AC. (1998b) Blood–injury–injection fears: nature, assessment, and management. *Behaviour Change*, **15**, 160–4.

Page AC, Andrews G. (1996) Do specific anxiety disorders show specific drug problems? *Australian and New Zealand Journal of Psychiatry*, **30**, 410–14.

Page AC, Bennett K, Carter O, Smith J, Woodmore K. (1997) The Blood-Injection Symptom Scale (BISS): assessing a structure of phobic symptoms elicited by blood and injections. *Behaviour Research and Therapy*, **35**, 457–64.

Parker G, Wilhelm K, Mitchell P, Austin M-P, Roussos J, Gladstone G. (1999). The influence of anxiety as a risk to early onset major depression. *Journal of Affective Disorders*, **52**, 11–17.

Pato MT, Zohar-Kadouch R, Zohar J, Murphy DL. (1988) Return of symptoms after discontinuation of clomipramine in patients with obsessive compulsive disorder. *American Journal of Psychiatry*, **145**, 1521–5.

Pauls DL, Bucher KD, Crowe RR, Noyes R. (1980) A genetic study of panic disorder pedigrees. *American Journal of Human Genetics*, **32**, 639–44.

Pauls DL, Alsobrook JP, Goodman W, Rasmussen S, Leckman JF. (1995) A family study of obsessive–compulsive disorder. *American Journal of Psychiatry*, **152**, 76–84.

Pavlov IP. (1927) *Conditioned Reflexes.* London: Oxford.

Pelcovitz D, van der Kolk B, Roth S, Mandel F, Kaplan S, Resick P. (1997) Development of a criteria set and a Structured Interview for Disorders of Extreme Stress (SIDES). *Journal of Traumatic Stress*, **10**, 3–16.

Penfold K, Page AC. (1999). Distraction enhances within-session fear reduction during in vivo exposure. *Behavior Therapy*, **30**, 607–21.

Perse TL, Greist JH, Jefferson JW, Rosenfeld R, Dar R. (1987) Fluvoxamine treatment of obsessive–compulsive disorder. *American Journal of Psychiatry*, **144**, 1543–8.

Peters L (2000) Discriminant validity of the social phobia anxiety inventory (SPAI), the Social Phobia Scale (SPS) and the social interaction anxiety scale (SIAS). *Behaviour, Research and Therapy*, **38**, 943–50.

Peters L, Andrews G. (1995) Procedural validity of the computerized version of the Composite International Diagnostic Interview (CIDI-Auto) in the anxiety disorders. *Psychological Medicine*, **25**, 1269–80.

Peters L, Slade T, Andrews G. (1999) A comparison of ICD-10 and DSM-IV criteria for posttraumatic stress disorder. *Journal of Traumatic Stress*, **12**, 335–43.

Phillips K, Fulker DW, Rose RJ. (1987) Path analysis of seven fear factors in adult twin and sibling pairs and their parents. *Genetic Epidemiology*, **4**, 345–55.

Pigott TA, Pato MT, Bernstein SF, Grover GN, Hill JL, Tolliver TJ, Murphy DL. (1990) Controlled comparison of clomipramine and fluoxetine in the treatment of obsessive–compulsive disorder: behavioural and biological results. *Archives of General Psychiatry*, **47**, 926–32.

Pitman RK, Orr SP, Altman B, Longpre RE, Poire RE, Macklin ML. (1996) Emotional processing during eye movement desensitization and reprocessing therapy of Vietnam veterans with chronic posttraumatic stress disorder. *Comprehensive Psychiatry*, **37**, 419–29.

Pollack MH, Worthington JJ, Manfro GG, Otto MW, Zucker BG. (1997). Abecarnil for the treatment of generalized anxiety disorder: a placebo-control comparison of two dosage ranges of abecarnil and buspirone. *Journal of Clinical Psychiatry*, **58** (Suppl. 11), 19–23.

Pollack MH, Otto MW, Worthington JJ, Manfro GG, Wolkow R. (1998) Sertraline in the treatment of panic disorder: a flexible-dose multicenter trial. *Archives of General Psychiatry*, **55**, 1010–16.

Pollard CA, Pollard HJ, Corn KJ. (1989) Panic onset and major events in the lives of agoraphobics: a test of contiguity. *Journal of Abnormal Psychology*, **8**, 318–21.

Poulton R, Andrews G. (1992) Personality as a cause of adverse life events. *Acta Psychiatrica Scandinavica*, **85**, 35–8.

Power KG, Jerrom DWA, Simpson RJ, Mitchell MJ, Swanson S. (1989) A controlled comparison of cognitive-behaviour therapy, diazepam and placebo in the management of generalized anxiety. *Behavioural Psychotherapy*, **17**, 1–14.

Power KG, Simpson RJ, Swanson V, Wallace LA. (1990) A controlled comparison of cognitive-behaviour therapy, diazepam, and placebo, alone and in combination, for the treatment of generalized anxiety disorder. *Journal of Anxiety Disorders*, **4**, 267–92.

Quality Assurance Project. (1985) Treatment outlines for the anxiety states. *Australian and New Zealand Journal of Psychiatry*, **19**, 138–51.

Quality Assurance Project. (1990) Treatment outlines for paranoid, schizotypal and schizoid personality disorders. *Australian and New Zealand Journal of Psychiatry*, **24**, 339–50.

Rabavilas HD, Boulougouris JC, Perissaki C. (1979) Therapist qualities related to outcome with exposure in vivo in neurotic patients. *Journal of Behaviour Therapy and Experimental Psychiatry*, **10**, 293–9.

Rachman SJ. (1974) Primary obsessional slowness. *Behaviour Research and Therapy*, **12**, 9–18.

Rachman SJ. (1981) Part 1. Unwanted intrusive cognitions. *Advances in Behavior Research and Therapy*, **3**, 89–99.

Rachman SJ. (1984) Agoraphobia: a safety-signal perspective. *Behaviour Research and Therapy*, **22**, 59–70.

Rachman SJ. (1990) The determinants and treatment of simple phobias. *Advances in Behaviour Research and Therapy*, **12**, 1–30.

Rachman SJ. (1991) Neo-conditioning and classical theory of fear acquisition. *Clinical Psychology Review*, **11**, 155–73.

Rachman SJ. (1993) Obsessions, responsibility and guilt. *Behaviour Research and Therapy*, **31**, 149–54.

Rachman SJ. (1997) A cognitive theory of obsessions. *Behavior Research and Therapy*, **35**, 379–91.

Rachman S, Bichard S. (1988) The overprediction of fear. *Clinical Psychology Review*, **8**, 303–12.

Rachman SJ, Craske M, Tallman K, Solyom C. (1986) Does escape behavior strengthen agoraphobic avoidance? A replication. *Behavior Therapy*, **17**, 366–84.

Raguram R, Bhide AY. (1985) Patterns of phobic neurosis: a retrospective study. *British Journal of Psychiatry*, **147**, 557–60.

Rapee RM. (1985a) Distinctions between panic disorder and generalized anxiety disorder: clinical presentation. *Australian and New Zealand Journal of Psychiatry*, **19**, 227–32.

Rapee RM. (1985b) A case of panic disorder treated with breathing retraining. *Journal of Behavior Therapy and Experimental Psychiatry*, **16**, 63–5.

Rapee RM. (1991a) The conceptual overlap between cognition and conditioning in clinical psychology. *Clinical Psychology Review*, **11**, 193–204.

Rapee RM. (1991b) Generalized anxiety disorder: a review of clinical features and theoretical concepts. *Clinical Psychology Review*, **11**, 419–40.

Rapee RM. (1995) Descriptive psychopathology of social phobia. In Heimberg RG, Leibowitz MR, Hope DA, Schneier FR (Eds), *Social Phobia: Diagnosis, Assessment, and Treatment*. New York: Guilford Press.

Rapee RM, Barlow DH. (1990) The assessment of panic disorder. In McReynolds P, Rosen JC, Chelune G (Eds), *Advances in Psychological Assessment*, Vol. 7. New York: Plenum Press.

Rapee RM, Heimberg RG. (1997) A cognitive-behavioural model of anxiety in social phobia. *Behaviour Research and Therapy*, **35**, 741–56.

Rapee RM, Lim L. (1992) Discrepancy between self and observer ratings of performance in social phobics. *Journal of Abnormal Psychology*, **101**, 728–31.

Rapee RM, Murrell E. (1988) Predictors of agoraphobic avoidance. *Journal of Anxiety Disorders*, **2**, 203–18.

Rapee RM, Mattick RP, Murrell E. (1986) Cognitive mediation in the affective component of spontaneous panic attacks. *Journal of Behavior Therapy and Experimental Psychiatry*, **17**, 245–53.

Rapee RM, Sanderson WC, Barlow DH. (1988) Social phobia features across the DSM-III-R anxiety disorders. *Journal of Psychopathology and Behavioural Assessment*, **10**, 287–99.

Rapee RM, Litwin EM, Barlow DH. (1990) Impact of life events on subjects with panic disorder and on comparison subjects. *American Journal of Psychiatry*, **147**, 640–4.

Rapoport JL. (1990) The walking nightmare: an overview of obsessive–compulsive disorder. *Journal of Clinical Psychiatry*, **51** (11, Suppl.), 25–8.

Raskin M, Peeke HVS, Dickman W, Pinsker H. (1982) Panic and generalized anxiety disorders: developmental antecedents and precipitants. *Archives of General Psychiatry*, **39**, 687–9.

Rasmussen SA, Eisen JL. (1992) The epidemiology and clinical features of obsessive–compulsive disorder. *Psychiatric Clinics of North America*, **15**, 743–58.

Rasmussen S, Eisen J. (1997) Treatment strategies for chronic and refractory obsessive–compulsive disorder. *Journal of Clinical Psychiatry*, **58** (Suppl. 13), 9–13.

Rasmussen S, Tsuang MT. (1986) Clinical characteristics and family history of DSMIII obsessive–compulsive disorder. *American Journal of Psychiatry*, **143**, 317–22.

Ratnasuriya RH, Marks IM, Forshaw DM, Hymas NFS. (1991) Obsessive slowness revisited. *British Journal of Psychiatry*, **159**, 273–4.

Rayment P, Richards J. (1998) Fear of autonomic arousal and use of coping strategies as predictors of agoraphobic avoidance in panic disorder. *Behaviour Change*, **15**, 228–36.

Regier DA, Narrow WE, Rae DS. (1990) The epidemiology of anxiety disorders: the epidemiologic catchment area (ECA) experience. *Journal of Psychiatric Research*, **24**, 3–14.

Regier DA, Rae DS, Narrow WE, Kaebler CT, Schatzberg AF. (1998) Prevalence of anxiety disorders and their comorbidity with mood and addictive disorders. *British Journal of Psychiatry*, **173** (Suppl. 34), 24–8.

Reich J, Noyes R, Troughton E. (1987) Dependent personality disorder associated with phobic avoidance in patients with panic disorder. *American Journal of Psychiatry*, **144**, 323–89.

Renfrey G, Spates CR. (1994) Eye movement desensitization. A partial dismantling study. *Journal of Behavior Therapy and Experimental Psychiatry*, **25**, 231–9.

Rescorla RA. (1968) Probability of shock in the presence and absence of CS in fear conditioning. *Journal of Comparative and Physiological Psychology*, **6**, 1–5.

Rescorla RA. (1988) Pavlovian conditioning: it's not what you think it is. *American Psychologist*, **43**, 151–60.

Resick PA, Schnicke MK. (1992) Cognitive processing therapy for sexual assault victims. *Journal of Consulting and Clinical Psychology*, **60**, 748–56.

Resick PA, Schnicke MK. (1993) *Cognitive Processing Therapy for Sexual Assault Victims: A Treatment Manual.* Newbury Park, CA: Sage Publications.

Resick PA, Jordan CG, Girelli SA, Hutter CK, Marhoefer-Dvorak S. (1988) A comparative outcome study of behavioral group therapy for sexual assault victims. *Behavior Therapy*, **19**, 385–401.

Resnick PJ. (1993) Defrocking the fraud: the detection of malingering. *Israel Journal of Psychiatry and Related Sciences*, **30**, 93–101.

Richards DA, Lovell K, Marks, IM. (1994) Post-traumatic stress disorder: evaluation of a behavioral treatment program. *Journal of Traumatic Stress*, **7**, 669–80.

Rickels K. (1987) Antianxiety therapy: potential value of long-term treatment. *Journal of Clinical Psychiatry*, **48** (12, Suppl.), 7–11.

Rickels K, Schweizer E. (1990) The clinical course and long-term management of generalized anxiety disorder. *Journal of Clinical Psychopharmacology*, **10** (3, Suppl.), 101S–10S.

Riddle MA, Scahil L, King R, Hardin MT, Towbin KE, Ort SI, Leckman JF, Cohen DJ. (1990) Obsessive–compulsive disorder in children and adolescents: phenomenology and family history. *Journal of the American Academy of Child and Adolescent Psychiatry*, **29**, 766–72.

Rickels K, Downing R, Schweizer E, Hassan, H. (1993a). Antidepressants for the treatment of generalised anxiety disorder: a placebo-controlled comparison of imipramine, trazodone and diazepam. *Archives of General Psychiatry*, **50**, 884–95.

Rickels K, Schweizer E, Weiss S, Zavodnick S. (1993b) Maintenance drug treatment of panic disorder, II: short- and long-term outcome after drug taper. *Archives of General Psychiatry*, **50**, 61–8.

Rickels K, Schweizer E, DeMartinis N, Mandos L, Mercer C. (1997). Gepirone and diazepam in generalized anxiety disorder: a placebo-controlled trial. *Journal of Clinical Psychopharmacology*, **17**, 272–277.

Ries BJ, McNeil DW, Boone ML, Turk CL, Carter LE, Heimberg RG. (1998) Assessment of contemporary social phobia verbal report instruments. *Behaviour Research and Therapy*, **36**, 983–94.

Riggs DS, Hiss H, Foa EB. (1992) Marital distress and the treatment of obsessive–compulsive disorder. *Behavior Therapy*, **23**, 585–97.

Riggs DS, Rothbaum BO, Foa EB. (1995) A prospective examination of symptoms of posttraumatic stress disorder in victims of nonsexual assault. *Journal of Interpersonal Violence*, **10**, 201–14.

Riskind JH, Beck AT, Brown G, Steer RA. (1987) Taking the measure of anxiety and depression: validity of the reconstructed Hamilton scales. *Journal of Nervous and Mental Disease*, **22**, 474–8.

Riskind JH, Moore R, Harman B, Hohmann AA, Beck AT, Stewart B. (1991) The relation of generalized anxiety disorder to depression in general and dysthymic disorder in particular. In Rapee RM, Barlow DH (Eds), *Chronic Anxiety. Generalized Anxiety Disorder and Mixed Anxiety–Depression*. New York: Guilford.

Robins LN, Regier DA. (1991) *Psychiatric Disorders in America*. New York: Macmillan.

Rocca P, Fonzo V, Scotta M, Zanalda E, Ravizza L. (1997). Paroxetine efficacy in the treatment of generalized anxiety disorder. *Acta Psychiatrica Scandinavica*, **95**, 444–50.

Roemer L, Borkovec M, Posa S, Borkovec TD. (1995) A self-report diagnostic measure of generalized anxiety disorder. *Journal of Behaviour Therapy and Experimental Psychiatry*, **26**, 345–50.

Roper G, Rachman S, Marks I. (1975) Passive and participant modelling in exposure treatment of obsessive-compulsive neurotics. *Behaviour Research and Therapy*, **13**, 271–9.

Rose RJ, Ditto WB. (1983) A developmental-genetic analysis of common fears from early adolescence to early adulthood. *Child Development*, **54**, 361–8.

Rose S, Bisson J. (1998) Brief early interventions following trauma: a systematic review of the literature. *Journal of Traumatic Stress*, **11**, 697–710.

Rosenberg CM. (1968) Complications of obsessional neurosis. *British Journal of Psychiatry*, **114**, 477–8.

Roth DL, Holmes DS. (1985) Influence of physical fitness in determining the impact of stressful life events on physical and psychological health. *Psychosomatic Medicine*, **47**, 164–73.

Roth M. (1984) Agoraphobia, panic disorder and generalized anxiety disorder: some implications of recent advances. *Psychiatric Developments*, **2**, 31–52.

Roth M, Argyle N. (1988) Anxiety, panic and phobic disorders: an overview. *Journal of Psychiatric Research*, **22** (1, Suppl.), 33–54.

Rothbaum BO, Foa EB, Riggs DS, Murdock T, Walsh W. (1992) A prospective examination of post-traumatic stress disorder in rape victims. *Journal of Traumatic Stress*, **5**, 455–75.

Roy-Byrne PP, Cowley DS (1998) Pharmacological treatment of panic, generalized anxiety, and phobic disorders. In Nathan PE, Gorman JM (Eds), *A Guide to Treatments That Work*. New York: Oxford University Press.

Roy-Byrne P, Mellman TA, Uhde TW. (1988) Biological findings in panic disorder: neuroendocrine and sleep-related abnormalities. *Journal of Anxiety Disorders*, **2**, 17–29.

Roy-Byrne PP, Wingerson D. (1992) Pharmacotherapy of anxiety disorders. In Tasman A, Riba MB (Eds), *Review of Psychiatry*, Vol. 11. Washington DC: American Psychiatric Press.

Ruch LO, Leon JJ. (1983) Sexual assault trauma and trauma change. *Women and Health*, **8**, 5–21.

Safren SA, Heimberg RG, Horner KJ, Juster HR, Schneier FR, Liebowitz MR. (1999) Factor structure of social fears: the Liebowitz Social Anxiety Scale. *Journal of Anxiety Disorders*, **13**, 253–70.

Salaberria K, Echeburua E. (1998) Long-term outcome of cognitive therapy's contribution to self-exposure *in vivo* to the treatment of generalized social phobia. *Behavior Modification*, **22**, 262–84.

Salkovskis PM. (1989) Obsessions and compulsions. In Scott J, Williams JMG, Beck A (Eds), *Cognitive Therapy in Clinical Practice*. London: Routledge.

Salkovskis PM, Kirk J. (1997) Obsessive–compulsive disorder. In Clark DM, Fairburn CG (Eds), *Cognitive Behaviour Therapy: Science and Practice*. New York: Oxford University Press.

Salkovskis PM, Westbrook D. (1989) Behaviour therapy and obsessional ruminations: can failure be turned into success? *Behaviour Research and Therapy*, **27**, 149–60.

Salkovskis PM, Jones DRO, Clark DM. (1986a) Respiratory control in the treatment of panic attacks: replication and extension with concurrent measurement of behaviour and PCO. *British Journal of Psychiatry*, **148**, 526–32.

Salkovskis PM, Warwick HMC, Clark DM, Wessels DJ. (1986b) A demonstration of acute hyperventilation during naturally occurring panic attacks. *Behaviour Research and Therapy*, **24**, 91–4.

Salkovskis PM, Atha C, Storer D. (1990) Cognitive-behavioural problem solving in the treatment of patients who repeatedly attempt suicide. *British Journal of Psychiatry*, **157**, 871–6.

Salkovskis PM, Clark DM, Hackman A. (1991) Treatment of panic attacks using cognitive therapy without exposure or breathing retraining. *Behaviour Research and Therapy*, **29**, 161–6.

Sanavio E. (1988) Obsessions and compulsions: the Padua Inventory. *Behaviour Research and Therapy*, **26**, 169–77.

Sanderson WC, Barlow DH. (1990) A description of patients diagnosed with DSM-III-R GAD. *Journal of Nervous and Mental Disease*, **178**, 588–91.

Sanderson WC, Wetzler S. (1991) Chronic anxiety and generalized anxiety disorder: issues in comorbidity. In Rapee RM, Barlow DH (Eds), *Chronic Anxiety. Generalized Anxiety Disorder and Mixed Anxiety–Depression*. New York: Guilford, pp. 119–35.

Sanderson WC, Rapee RM, Barlow DH. (1989) The influence of an illusion of control on panic attacks induced via inhalation of 5.5% carbon dioxide-enriched air. *Archives of General Psychiatry*, **46**, 157–62.

Sanderson WC, Di Nardo PA, Rapee RM, Barlow DH. (1990). Syndrome co-morbidity in patients diagnosed with DSM IIIR anxiety disorder. *Journal of Abnormal Psychology*, **99**, 308–12.

Sanderson WC, Raue PJ, Wetzler S. (1998) The generalizability of cognitive behavior therapy for panic disorder. *Journal of Cognitive Psychotherapy*, **12**, 323–30.

Sandler IN, Lakey B. (1982) Locus of control as a stress moderator: the role of control perceptions and social support. *American Journal of Community Psychology*, **10**, 65–72.

Sartorius N, de Girolamo G, Andrews G, German GA, Eisenberg L. (1993) *Treatment of Mental Disorders*. Washington, DC: American Psychiatric Press.

Saunders BE, Arata CM, Kilpatrick DG. (1990) Development of a crime-related posttraumatic stress disorder scale for women within the Symptom Checklist 90 Revised. *Journal of Traumatic Stress*, **3**, 439–48.

Saxena S, Rauch SL. (2000) Functional neuroimaging and the neuroanatomy of obsessive compulsive disorder. *Psychiatric Clinics of North America*, **23**, 563–86.

Saxena S, Brody AL, Schwartz JM, Baxter LR. (1998) Neuroimaging and frontal-subcortical circuitry in obsessive–compulsive disorder. *British Journal of Psychiatry*, **173** (Suppl. 35), 26–37.

Scherrer JF, True WR, Xian H, Lyons MJ, Eisen SA, Goldberg J, Lin N, Tsuang MT. (2000). Evidence for genetic influences common and specific to symptoms of generalized anxiety and panic. *Journal of Affective Disorders*, **57**, 25–35.

Schmidt NB. (1999) Panic disorder: cognitive behavioral and pharmacological treatment strategies. *Journal of Clinical Psychology in Medical Settings*, **6**, 89–111.

Schmidt NB, Woolaway-Bickel K, Trakowski J, Santiago H, Storey J, Koselka M, Cook J. (2000) Dismantling cognitive behavioral treatment for panic disorder: questioning the utility of breathing retraining. *Journal of Consulting and Clinical Psychology*, **68**, 417–24.

Schneier FR, Martin LY, Liebowitz MR, Gorman MD, Fyer AJ. (1989) Alcohol abuse in social phobia. *Journal of Anxiety Disorders*, **3**, 15–23.

Schneier FR, Spitzer RL, Gibbon M, Fyer AJ, Liebowitz, MR. (1991) The relationship of social phobia subtypes and avoidant personality disorder. *Comprehensive Psychiatry*, **32**, 496–502.

Schneier FR, Johnson J, Hornig CD, Liebowitz MR, Weissman MM. (1992) Social phobia: comorbidity and morbidity in an epidemiological sample. *Archives of General Psychiatry*, **49**, 282–8.

Schneier FR, Goetz D, Campeas R, Fallon B, Marshall R, Liebowitz MR. (1998) Placebo-controlled trial of moclobemide in social phobia. *British Journal of Psychiatry*, **172**, 70–7.

Schulte D. (1997) Behavioural analysis: does it matter? *Behavioural and Cognitive Psychotherapy*, **25**, 231–49.

Schwartz (1998) Neuroanatomical aspects of cognitive behavioural therapy response in obsessive–compulsive disorders. An evolving perspective on brain and behaviour. *British Journal of*

Psychiatry, **173**, 38–44.

Schweizer E, Rickels K, Weiss S, Zavodnick S. (1993) Maintenance drug treatment of panic disorder, I: results of a prospective, placebo controlled comparison of alprazolam and imipramine. *Archives of General Psychiatry*, **50**, 51–60.

Scupi BS, Maser JD, Uhde TW. (1992) The National Institute of Mental Health Panic Questionnaire: an instrument for assessing clinical characteristics of panic disorder. *Journal of Nervous and Mental Disease*, **180**, 566–72.

Seligman M. (1971) Phobias and preparedness. *Behavior Therapy*, **2**, 307–20.

Shalev AY, Bonne O, Eth S. (1996) Treatment of posttraumatic stress disorder: a review. *Psychosomatic Medicine*, **58**, 165–82.

Shapiro F. (1995) *Eye Movement Desensitization and Reprocessing: Basic Principles, Protocols and Procedures.* New York: Guilford Press.

Shaw P. (1979) A comparison of three behaviour therapies in the treatment of social phobia. *British Journal of Psychiatry*, **134**, 620–3.

Shear MK, Maser JD. (1994) Standardized assessment for panic disorders research: a conference report. *Archives of General Psychiatry*, **51**, 346–54.

Sheikh JI, Cassidy EL. (2000) Treatment of anxiety disorders in the elderly: issues and strategies. *Journal of Anxiety Disorders*, **14**, 173–90.

Sherry GS, Levine BA. (1980) An examination of procedural variables in flooding therapy. *Behavior Therapy*, **11**, 148–55.

Skoog G, Skoog I. (1999) A 40 year follow-up of patients with obsessive–compulsive disorder. *Archives of General Psychiatry*, **56**, 121–7.

Slade T, Andrews G. (2001) DSM-IV and ICD-10 generalized anxiety disorder: discrepant diagnoses and associated disability. *Social Psychiatry and Psychiatric Epidemiology*, **36**, 45–51.

Smail P, Stockwell T, Canter S, Hodgson R. (1984) Alcohol dependence and phobic anxiety states. *British Journal of Psychiatry*, **144**, 53–7.

Soechting I, Taylor S, Freeman W, De Koning E, Segerstrom S, Thordarson D. (1998) In vivo exposure for panic disorder and agoraphobia: Does a cognitive rationale enhance treatment efficacy? In Sanavio E (Ed), *Behavior and Cognitive Therapy Today: Essays in Honor of Hans J. Eysenck.* Oxford: Elsevier.

Solomon S, Keane T, Newman E, Kaloupek D. (1996) Choosing self-report measures and structured interviews. In Carlson EB (Ed), *Trauma Research Methodology.* Lutherville, MD: Sidran Press.

Solomon Z. (1989) A 3-year prospective study of post-traumatic stress disorder in Israeli combat veterans. *Journal of Traumatic Stress*, **2**, 59–73.

Solyom L, Ledwidge B, Solyom C. (1986) Delineating social phobia. *British Journal of Psychiatry*, **149**, 464–70.

Spiegel DA, Bruce TJ. (1997) Benzodiazepines and exposure-based cognitive behavior therapies for panic disorder: conclusions from combined treatment trials. *American Journal of Psychiatry*, **154**, 773–81.

Spielberger CD, Gorusch RL, Lushene R, Vagg PR, Jacobs GA. (1983) *Manual for the State–Trait Anxiety Inventory.* Palo Alto, CA: Consulting Psychologists Press.

Spitzer RL, Williams JB, Gibbon M, First MB. (1995) *Structured Clinical Interview for DSM-IV –*

Patient Version (SCID-P, Version 2.0). Washington, DC: American Psychiatric Press.

Stanley MA, Novy DM. (2000) Cognitive-behavior therapy for generalized anxiety in late life: an evaluative overview. *Journal of Anxiety Disorders*, **14**, 191–207.

Stanley MA, Beck JG, Glassco JD. (1996). Treatment of generalized anxiety in older adults: A preliminary comparison of cognitive-behavioural and supportive approaches. *Behavior Therapy*, **27**, 565–81.

Starcevic V, Bogojevic G. (1997) Comorbidity of panic disorder with agoraphobia and specific phobia: relationship with the subtypes of specific phobia. *Comprehensive Psychiatry*, **38**, 315–20.

Starcevic V, Bogojevic G. (1999) The concept of generalized anxiety disorder: between the too narrow and too wide diagnostic criteria. *Psychopathology*, **32**, 5–11.

Starkman MN, Zelnik TC, Nesse RM, Cameron OG. (1985) Anxiety in patients with pheochromocytomas. *Archives of Internal Medicine*, **145**, 248–52.

Stein M, Forde D, Anderson G, Walker J. (1997) Obsessive–compulsive disorder in the community: an epidemiologic survey with clinical reappraisal. *American Journal of Psychiatry*, **154**, 1120–6.

Stein MB. (1998) Neurobiological perspectives on social phobia: from affiliation to zoology. *Biological Psychiatry*, **44**, 1277–85.

Stein MB, Chavira, DA. (1998) Subtypes of social phobia and comorbidity with depression and other anxiety disorders. *Journal of Affective Disorders*, **50** (Suppl.), S11–S16.

Stein MB, Chartier MJ, Hazen Al, Kozak MV, Tancer ME, Lander S, Furer P, Chubaty D, Walker JR. (1998a) A direct-interview family study of generalized social phobia. *American Journal of Psychiatry*, **155**, 90–7.

Stein MB, Liebowitz MR, Lydiard RB, Pitts CD, Bushnell W, Gergel I. (1998b) Paroxetine treatment of generalized social phobia (social anxiety disorder): a randomized controlled trial. *Journal of the American Medical Association*, **220**, 708–13.

Stein MB, Fyer AJ, Davidson JRT, Pollack MH, Wiita B. (1999) Fluvoxamine treatment of social phobia (social anxiety disorder): a double-blind, placebo-controlled study. *American Journal of Psychiatry*, **156**, 756–60.

Steptoe A, Wardle J. (1988) Emotional fainting and the psychophysiologic response to blood and injury: autonomic mechanisms and coping strategies. *Psychosomatic Medicine*, **50**, 402–17.

Stern R. (1978) *Behavioural Techniques: A Therapist's Manual*. New York: Academic Press.

Stern RS, Marks IM. (1973) Brief and prolonged flooding: a comparison of agoraphobic patients. *Archives of General Psychiatry*, **28**, 270–6.

Stöber J. (1998) Worry, problem elaboration and suppression of imagery: the role of concreteness. *Behaviour Research and Therapy*, **36**, 751–6.

Stöber J, Borkovec TD. (In press) Reduced concreteness of worry in generalized anxiety disorder: findings from a therapy study. *Cognitive Therapy and Research*.

Stravynski A. (1983) Behavioral treatment of psychogenic vomiting in the context of social phobia. *Journal of Nervous and Mental Disease*, **171**, 448–51.

Stravynski A, Greenberg D. (1989) Behavioural psychotherapy for social phobia and dysfunction. *International Review of Psychiatry*, **1**, 207–18.

Stravynski A, Greenberg D. (1998) The treatment of social phobia: a critical assessment. *Acta Pyschiatrica Scandinavica*, **98**, 171–81.

Stravynski A, Marks I, Yule W. (1982) Social skills problems in neurotic outpatients. *Archives of General Psychiatry*, **39**, 1378–85.

Stravynski A, Lamontagne Y, Lavellee Y-J. (1986) Clinical phobias and avoidant personality disorder among alcoholics admitted to an alcoholism rehabilitation setting. *Canadian Journal of Psychiatry*, **31**, 714–19.

Stravynski A, Arbel N, Bounader J, Gaudette G, Lachance L, Borgeat F, Fabian J, Lamontagne Y, Sidoun P, Todorov C. (2000) Social phobia treated as a problem in social functioning: a controlled comparison of two behavioural group approaches. *Acta Psychiatrica Scandinavica*, **102**, 188–98.

Sturgis ET, Scott R. (1984) Simple phobia. In Turner SH (Ed), *Behavioural Theories and Treatment of Anxiety*. New York: Plenum Press.

Swedo SE, Rapoport JL, Leonard H, Lenane M, Cheslow D. (1989) Obsessive–compulsive disorder in children and adolescents: clinical phenomenology of 70 consecutive cases. *Archives of General Psychiatry*, **46**, 335–41.

Tallis F, Eysenck M, Mathews A. (1992) A questionnaire for the measurement of nonpathological worry. *Personality and Individual Differences*, **13**, 161–8.

Tarrier N, Pilgrim H, Sommerfield C, Faragher B, Reynolds M, Graham E, Barrowclough C. (1999) A randomized trial of cognitive therapy and imaginal exposure in the treatment of chronic posttraumatic stress disorder. *Journal of Consulting and Clinical Psychology*, **67**, 13–18.

Taylor FK. (1966) *Psychopathology: Its Causes and Symptoms*. Oxford: Butterworths.

Taylor S. (1996) Meta-analysis of cognitive-behavioral treatments for social phobia. *Journal of Behavioral and Experimental Psychiatry*, **27**, 1–9.

Taylor S, Woody S, Koch WJ, McLean P, Paterson RJ, Anderson KW. (1997) Cognitive restructuring in the treatment of social phobia. *Behavior Modification*, **21**, 487–511.

Telch MJ, Agras WS, Taylor CB, Roth WT, Gallen C. (1985) Combined pharmacological and behavioural treatment for agoraphobia. *Behaviour Research and Therapy*, **23**, 325–35.

Telch MJ, Brouillard M, Telch CF, Agras WF, Taylor CB. (1989) Role of cognitive appraisal in panic-related avoidance. *Behaviour Research and Therapy*, **27**, 373–83.

Telch MJ, Schmidt NB, Jaimez TL, Jacquin KM, Harrington PJ. (1995) Impact of cognitive-behavioral treatment on quality of life in panic disorder patients. *Journal of Consulting and Clinical Psychology*, **63**, 823–30.

Tellegen A. (1982) *Brief Manual for the Multidimensional Personality Questionnaire*. Minneapolis, MN: University of Minnesota.

Tennant CC, Andrews G. (1976) A scale to measure the stress of life events. *Australian and New Zealand Journal of Psychiatry*, **10**, 27–32.

Teusch L, Boehme H. (1999). Is the exposure principle really crucial in agoraphobia? The influence of client-centered "nonprescriptive" treatment on exposure. *Psychotherapy Research*, **9**, 115–23.

Thayer JF, Friedman BH, Borkovec TD. (1996) Autonomic characteristics of generalized anxiety disorder and worry. *Biological Psychiatry*, **39**, 255–66.

Thomas SE, Thevos AK, Randall CL. (1999) Alcoholics with and without social phobia: a comparison of substance use and psychiatric variables. *Journal of Studies on Alcohol,* **60,** 472–9.

Thompson JA, Charlton PFC, Kerry R, Lee D. (1995) An open trial of exposure therapy based on deconditioning for post-traumatic stress disorder. *British Journal of Clinical Psychology,* **34,** 407–16.

Thyer B, Himle J, Curtis G. (1985a) Blood–injury–illness phobia: a review. *Journal of Clinical Psychology,* **41,** 451–9.

Thyer BA, Parrish RT, Curtis GC, Nesse RM, Cameron OG. (1985b) Ages of onset of DSM-III anxiety disorders. *Comprehensive Psychiatry,* **26,** 113–22.

Tollefson GD, Birkett M, Koran L, Genduso L. (1994) Continuation treatment of OCD: double blind and open label experience with fluoxetine. *Journal of Clinical Psychiatry,* **55** (10, Suppl.), 69–76.

Torgersen S. (1979) The nature and origin of common phobic fears. *British Journal of Psychiatry,* **134,** 343–51.

Torgersen S. (1983) Genetic factors in anxiety disorders. *Archives of General Psychiatry,* **40,** 1085–9.

Torgersen S. (1986) Childhood and family characteristics in panic and generalized anxiety disorders. *American Journal of Psychiatry,* **143,** 630–2.

Tseng W-H. (1973) Psychopathologic study of obsessive–compulsive neurosis in Taiwan. *Comprehensive Psychiatry,* **14,** 139–150.

Tseng W-S, Asai M, Kitanishi K, McLaughlin DG, Kyomen H. (1992) Diagnostic patterns of social phobia: comparison in Tokyo and Hawaii. *Journal of Nervous and Mental Disease,* **180,** 380–5.

Turgeon L, Marchand A, Dupuis G. (1998) Clinical features in panic disorder with agoraphobia: a comparison of men and women. *Journal of Anxiety Disorders,* **12,** 539–53.

Turk CL, Heimberg RG, Orsillo SM, Holt CS, Gitow A, Street LL, Schneier FR, Liebowitz MR. (1998) An investigation of gender differences in social phobia. *Journal of Anxiety Disorders,* **12,** 209–23.

Turner SM, Beidel DC. (1989) Social phobia: clinical syndrome, diagnosis, and comorbidity. *Clinical Psychology Review,* **9,** 3–18.

Turner SM, Beidel DC, Dancu CV, Keys DJ. (1986) Psychopathology of social phobia and comparison of avoidant personality disorder. *Journal of Abnormal Psychology,* **95,** 389–94.

Turner SM, McCanna M, Beidel DC. (1987) Validity of the Social Avoidance and Distress and Fear of Negative Evaluation scales. *Behaviour Research and Therapy,* **25,** 113–15.

Turner SM, Beidel DC, Dancu CV, Stanley MA. (1989) An empirically derived inventory to measure social fears and anxiety: the social phobia and anxiety inventory. *Psychological Assessment: A Journal of Consulting and Clinical Psychology,* **1,** 35–40.

Turner SM, Beidel DC, Borden JW, Stanley MA, Jacob RG. (1991) Social phobia: axis I and II correlates. *Journal of Abnormal Psychology,* **100,** 102–6.

Turner SM, Beidel DC, Stanley MA. (1992a) Are obsessional thoughts and worry different cognitive phenomena? *Clinical Psychology Review,* **12,** 257–70.

Turner SM, Beidel DC, Townsley RM. (1992b) Social phobia: a comparison of specific and generalized subtypes and avoidant personality disorder. *Journal of Abnormal Psychology*, **101**, 326–31.

Turner SM, Beidel DC, Jacob RG. (1994) Social phobia: a comparison of behavior therapy and atenolol. *Journal of Consulting and Clinical Psychology*, **62**, 350–8.

Turner SM, Beidel DC, Wolff PL, Spaulding S, Jacob RG. (1996) Clinical features affecting treatment outcome in social phobia. *Behavior Research and Therapy*, **34**, 795–804.

Tweed JL, Schoenbach VJ, George LK, Blazer DG. (1989) The effects of childhood parental death and divorce on six-month history of anxiety disorders. *British Journal of Psychiatry*, **154**, 823–8.

Uhde TW, Boulenger JP, Roy-Byrne PP, Geraci MP, Vittone BJ, Post RM. (1985) Longitudinal course of panic disorder: clinical and biological considerations. *Progressive Neuro-Psycho-pharmacology and Biological Psychiatry*, **9**, 39–51.

Üstün TB, Von Korff M. (1995) Primary mental health services: access and provision of care. In Ustun TB, Sartorius N. (Eds), *Mental Illness in General Health Care: An International Study.* New York: Wiley.

Vaillant GE. (1971) Theoretical hierarchy of adaptive ego mechanisms. *Archives of General Psychiatry*, **24**, 107–18.

Van Ameringen M, Mancini C, Streiner D. (1994) Sertraline in social phobia. *Journal of Affective Disorders*, **31**, 141–5.

Van Ameringen M, Mancini C, Oakman JM. (1998) The relationship of behavioural inhibition and shyness to anxiety disorder. *Journal of Nervous and Mental Disease*, **186**, 425–31.

van Balkom AJLM, Bakker A, Spinhoven P, Blaauw BMJW, Smeenk S, Ruesink B. (1997) A meta-analysis of the treatment of panic disorder with or without agoraphobia: a comparison of psychopharmacological, cognitive-behavioral, and combination treatments. *Journal of Nervous and Mental Disease*, **185**, 510–16.

van Balkom AJLM, de Haan E, van Oppen P, Spinhoven P, Hoogduin KAL, van Dyck R. (1998) Cognitive and behavioral therapies alone and in combination with fluvoxamine in the treatment of obsessive–compulsive disorder. *Journal of Nervous and Mental Disease*, **186**, 492–9.

van dam-Baggen R, Kraaimaat F. (2000) Group social skills training or cognitive group therapy as the clinical treatment of choice for generalized social phobia? *Journal of Anxiety Disorders*, **14**, 437–51.

van der Kolk BA, Dreyfuss D, Michaels M, Shera D, Berkowitz R, Fisler R, Saxe G. (1994) Fluoxetine in posttraumatic stress disorder. *Journal of Clinical Psychiatry*, **55**, 517–22.

van Oppen P, de Haan E, van Balkom AJL, Spinhoven P, Hoogduin K, van Dyck R. (1995) Cognitive therapy and exposure in vivo in the treatment of obsessive–compulsive disorder. *Behaviour Research and Therapy*, **33**, 379–90.

van Velzen CJM, Emmelkamp PMG, Scholing A. (1997) The impact of personality disorders on behavioral treatment outcome for social phobia. *Behaviour Research and Therapy*, **35**, 889–900.

van Zijderveld GA, Veltman DJ, van Dyck R, van Doornen LJP. (1999) Epinephrine-induced panic attacks and hyperventilation. *Journal of Psychiatric Research*, **33**, 73–8.

Vermilyea BB, Barlow DH, O'Brien GT. (1984) The importance of assessing treatment integrity:

an example in the anxiety disorders. *Journal of Behavioral Assessment*, **6**, 1–11.

Versiani M, Nardi AE, Mundim FD, Alves AB, Liebowitz MR, Amrein R. (1992) Pharmacotherapy of social phobia: a controlled study with moclobemide and phenelzine. *British Journal of Psychiatry*, **161**, 353–60.

Videbech T. (1975) The psychopathology of anancastic endogenous depression. *Acta Psychiatrica Scandinavica*, **52**, 336–73.

Vitaliano PP, Katon W, Russo J, Maiuro RD, Anderson K, Jones M. (1987) Coping as an index of illness behavior in panic disorder. *Journal of Nervous and Mental Disease*, **175**, 78–83.

Vrana S, Lauterbach D. (1994) Prevalence of traumatic events and post-traumatic psychological symptoms in a nonclinical sample of college students. *Journal of Traumatic Stress*, **7**, 289–302.

Wade WA, Treat TA, Stuart GL. (1998). Transporting an empirically supported treatment for panic disorder to a service clinic setting: a benchmarking strategy. *Journal of Consulting and Clinical Psychology*, **66**, 231–9.

Walen S, DiGuiseppe, R, Dryden W. (1992). *A Practitioners Guide to Rational-Emotive Therapy*, 2nd edition. New York: Oxford University Press.

Walk J. (1956) Self-ratings of fear in a fear-invoking situation. *Journal of Abnormal and Social Psychology*, **2**, 171–8.

Walker JR, Stein MB. (1995) Epidemiology. In Stein MB (Ed.) *Social Phobia: Clinical and Research Perspectives*. Washington, DC: American Psychiatric Press.

Warren R, Zgourides GD. (1991) *Anxiety Disorders: A Rational-Emotive Perspective*. New York: Pergamon Press.

Watson CG, Juba MP, Manifold V, Kucala T, Anderson PED. (1991) The PTSD interview: rationale, description, reliability, and concurrent validity of a DSM-III based technique. *Journal of Clinical Psychology*, **47**, 179–88.

Watson D, Friend R. (1969) Measurement of social-evaluative anxiety. *Journal of Consulting and Clinical Psychology*, **33**, 448–57.

Watson J, Rayner R. (1920) Conditioned emotional reactions. *Journal of Experimental Psychology*, **3**, 1–14.

Watson JP, Gaind GE, Marks IM. (1971) Prolonged exposure: a rapid treatment for phobias. *British Medical Journal*, **1**, 13–15.

Weathers FW, Litz BT, Herman DS, Huska JA, Keane TM. (1993) The PTSD Checklist (PCL): reliability, validity, and diagnostic utility. Paper presented at the 9th Annual Conference of the ISTSS, San Antonio.

Weiller E, Bisserbe J-C, Boyer P, Lepine J-P, Lecrubier Y. (1996) Social phobia in general health care: an unrecognised undertreated disabling disorder. *British Journal of Psychiatry*, **168**, 169–74.

Weiss D. (1997) Structured clinical interview techniques. In Wilson J, Keane T. (Eds), *Assessing Psychological Trauma and PTSD*. New York: Guilford Press.

Weiss D, Marmar C. (1997) The Impact of Event Scale – Revised. In Wilson J, Keane T. (Eds), *Assessing Psychological Trauma and PTSD*. New York: Guilford Press.

Weiss JH. (1989) Breathing control. In Lindemann C (Ed), *Handbook of Phobia Therapy: Rapid Symptom Relief in Anxiety Disorders*. Northvale, NJ: Aronson.

Weissman MM, Klerman GL, Markowitz JS, Quellette R. (1989) Suicidal ideation and suicide attempts in panic disorder and attacks. *New England Journal of Medicine,* **321,** 1209–14.

Welkowitz LA, Papp LA, Cloitre M, Liebowitz MR, Martin LY, Gorman JM. (1991) Cognitive-behavior therapy for panic disorder delivered by pharmacologically oriented clinicians. *Journal of Nervous and Mental Disease,* **179,** 473–7.

Wells A. (1994). A multi-dimensional measure of worry: development and preliminary validation of the anxious thoughts inventory. *Anxiety, Stress and Coping,* **6,** 289–99.

Wells A, Carter K. (1999) Preliminary tests of a cognitive model of generalized anxiety disorder. *Behaviour Research and Therapy,* **37,** 585–94.

Wells A, Papageorgiou C. (1998) Social phobia: effects of external attention on anxiety, negative beliefs, and perspective taking. *Behavior Therapy,* **29,** 357–70.

Wells A, Papageorgiou C. (1999) The observer perspective: biased imagery in social phobia, agoraphobia, and blood/injury phobia. *Behaviour Research and Therapy,* **37,** 653–8.

Wells A, Papageorgiou C. (2001) Social phobic interoception: effects of bodily information on anxiety, beliefs and self-processing. *Behaviour Research and Therapy,* **39,** 1–11.

Whisman MA. (1990) The efficacy of booster maintenance sessions in behavior therapy: review and methodological critique. *Clinical Psychology Review,* **10,** 155–70.

White J, Keenan M. (1990) Stress control: a pilot study of large group therapy for generalized anxiety disorder. *Behavioural Psychotherapy,* **18,** 143–6.

Whitehead WE, Robinson A, Blackwell B, Stutz R. (1978) Flooding treatment of phobias: does chronic diazepam increase effectiveness? *Journal of Behavior Therapy and Experimental Psychiatry,* **9,** 219–25.

WHO (World Health Organization). (1990) *International Classification of Diseases, 10th revision (ICD-10).* Geneva: World Health Organization.

WHO (World Health Organization). (1993) *The ICD-10 Classification of Mental and Behavioural Disorders: Diagnostic Criteria for Research.* Geneva: World Health Organization.

Wilhelm S, Otto MW, Zucker BG, Pollack MH. (1997) Prevalence of body dysmorphic disorder in patients with anxiety disorders. *Journal of Anxiety Disorders,* **11,** 499–502.

Williams JMG, Watts FN, MacLeod C, Mathews A. (1997). *Cognitive Psychology and the Emotional Disorders,* 2nd Edition. New York: Wiley.

Williams SL, Falbo J. (1996) Cognitive and performance-based treatments for panic attacks in people with varying degrees of agoraphobic disability. *Behaviour Research and Therapy,* **34,** 253–64.

Williams SL, Turner SM, Peer DF. (1985) Guided mastery and performance desensitization treatments for severe agoraphobia. *Journal of Consulting and Clinical Psychology,* **53,** 237–47.

Wilson GT. (1996). Manual-based treatments: the clinical application of research findings. *Behaviour Research and Therapy,* **34,** 295–314.

Wilson JP, Keane TM. (1997) *Assessing Psychological Trauma and PTSD.* New York: Guilford.

Wilson PH. (1992) Relapse prevention: conceptual and methodological issues. In Wilson PH (Ed), *Principles and Practice of Relapse Prevention.* New York: Guilford, pp. 1–22.

Wittchen H-U, Robins LN, Cottler N, Sartorius N, Burke JD, Regier D. (1991) Cross-cultural feasibility, reliability and sources of variance of the Composite International Diagnostic Interview (CIDI). The Multicentre WHO/ADAMHA Field Trials. *British Journal of Psychiatry,* **159,** 645–53.

Wittchen H-U, Kessler RC, Zhao S, Abelson J. (1995) Reliability and clinical validity of UM-CIDI DSM-III-R generalized anxiety disorder. *Journal of Psychiatric Research*, **29**, 95–110.

Wittchen H-U, Stein MB, Kessler RC. (1999) Social fears and social phobia in a community sample of young adults: prevalence, risk factors and comorbidity. *Psychological Medicine*, **29**, 309–23.

Wittchen H-U, Zhao Z, Kessler RC, Eaton WW. (1994) DSM-III-R generalized anxiety disorder in the National Comorbidity Survey. *Archives of General Psychiatry*, **51**, 355–64.

Wlazlo Z, Schroeder-Hartwig K, Hand I, Kaiser G, Munchau N. (1990) Exposure in vivo vs. social skills training for social phobia: long-term outcome and differential effects. *Behavior Research and Therapy*, **28**, 181–93.

Wolpe J. (1958) *Psychotherapy by Reciprocal Inhibition*. Stanford, CA: Stanford University Press.

Woodman CL, Noyes R, Black DW, Schlosser S, Yagla, SJ. (1999) A 5-year follow-up study of generalized anxiety disorder and panic disorder. *Journal of Nervous and Mental Disease*, **187**, 3–9.

Woodruff R, Pitts F. (1964) Monozygotic twins with obsessional illness. *American Journal of Psychiatry*, **120**, 1075–80.

Woody SR, Chambless DL, Glass CR. (1997) Self-focused attention in the treatment of social phobia. *Behaviour Research and Therapy*, **35**, 117–29.

Yaryura-Tobias JA, Neziroglu FA. (1983) *Obsessive–Compulsive Disorders: Pathogenesis, Diagnosis, Treatment*. Basel: Marcel Dekker.

Yehuda R. (1999) *Risk Factors for Posttraumatic Stress Disorder*. Washington, DC: American Psychiatric Press.

Yehuda R, Marshall R, Giller E. (1998) Psychopharmacological treatment of post-traumatic stress disorder. In Nathan P, Gorman J (Eds), *A Guide to Treatments that Work*. New York: Oxford University Press, pp. 377–97.

Yerkes RM, Dodson JD. (1908) The relation of strength of stimulus to rapidity of habit-formation. *Journal of Comparative Neurology and Psychology*, **18**, 459–82.

Yonkers KA, Warshaw MG, Massion, AO, Keller MB. (1996). Phenomenology and course of generalized anxiety disorder. *British Journal of Psychiatry*, **168**, 308–13.

Yonkers KA, Zlotnick C, Allsworth J, Warshaw M, Shea T, Keller MB. (1998) Is the course of panic disorder the same in women and men? *American Journal of Psychiatry*, **155**, 596–602.

Zak J, Miller JA, Sheehan DV, Fanous BSL. (1988) The potential role of serotonin re-uptake inhibitors in the treatment of obsessive compulsive disorder. *Journal of Clinical Psychiatry*, **49** (Suppl.), 23–9.

Zinbard RE, Barlow DH. (1996) Structure of anxiety and the anxiety disorders: a hierarchical model. *Journal of Abnormal Psychology*, **105**, 181–93.

Zitrin CM, Klein DF, Woerner MG, Ross DC. (1983) Treatment of phobias: I. Comparison of imipramine hydrochloride and placebo. *Archives of General Psychiatry*, **40**, 125–38.

Zlotnick C, Davidson J, Shea MT, Pearlstein T. (1996) Validation of the Davidson Trauma Scale in a sample of survivors of childhood sexual abuse. *Journal of Nervous and Mental Disease*, **184**, 255–7.

Index